T0320913

"Mason's second edition seamlessly weaves stories of human neurological conditions, historical observations and neurobiological facts into a highly readable, informative and insightful story. The author has done a stellar job of relating details of development, anatomy, and cell function to medical problems. This is of great importance as it reinforces the concept that virtually everything you learn about neurobiology has medical significance. Nothing essential is omitted, even a lay person could pick up this book and easily learn about basic neurobiology and the clinical processes caused by its dysfunction. The material is strongly tied to clinical conditions and provides a unique level of understanding of the different neuropathological processes—I recommend it enthusiastically, particularly for medical students and health care professional trainees interested in the nervous system."—**Howard L. Fields, MD, PhD**, Professor of Neurology, University of California San Francisco, San Francisco, CA

"Now it its second edition, *Medical Neurobiology* is an absorbing work, sole authored by Peggy Mason. Living up to the first word in the title, the book focuses exclusively on humans and provides an enriched view of how the brain makes us what we are as individuals. It is written with uncommon clarity. This is a synthesis, not only of systems and cellular functions in the brain, but also of malfunctions accompanying disease. This broad task is organized and presented as a build from the basics to the complexities such as perception and motor function. As such, *Medical Neurobiology* would be attractive to physicians at almost any level or field of training that wish to enrich their understanding of this remarkable organ but also crave a highly accessible read."—**James L. Madara, MD**, CEO, American Medical Association, former Dean and Health System CEO, University of Chicago, Chicago, IL

"My opinion of this book is admittedly biased because I love the brain as much as Dr. Mason does. That being said, as in any discipline, there are some books that are better than others and I can objectively say that this second edition of her book *Medical Neurobiology* is one of the very best books in its class. Dr. Mason has managed yet again to produce an erudite, comprehensive, and superbly explained account of the current state of the field as should be understood by the medical or graduate student. I wish I had used *Medical Neurobiology* 2nd Edition as a neurobiology textbook in graduate school, preferably with Dr. Mason as the professor."—**Oné R. Pagán, PhD**, Department of Biology, West Chester University, West Chester, PA, Author *of The First Brain: the Neuroscience of Planarians*, Oxford University Press.

"Dr. Mason, author of the remarkably clear, concise and accessible second edition of *Medical Neurobiology*, has accomplished the astonishing feat of turning a textbook into a page turner. The topics covered range from normal human neuroanatomy to the functional implications of injury to nervous system components and/or loss of connectivity of specific brain regions. All topics are presented in such a well-defined, straightforward and logical manner that even the most neuro-naïve reader can (and will) master the material. This book is perfect for first year medical neuroscience training and for undergraduate biology students with an interest in how the nervous system works and what happens when neural signaling goes wrong. This book is exemplary in combining clarity and thoroughness in melding two highly complex topics."—**Lorna W. Role, PhD**, Department of Neurobiology and Behavior, Stony Brook University, Stony Brook, NY

"Conveying the essentials of the (dys)function of the most complicated organ in the body, the very organ that makes us who we are, is a daunting task. Peggy Mason has achieved this by presenting the essence of knowledge of brain function, from cells to networks, in a way that it will "stick" in the student's brain well after the course. *Medical Neurobiology* is engaging and enjoyable to read, while including practical information that all physicians should know. The text on this complex topic captures today's readers interest and imagination, rather than being an encyclopedic stockpile of reference information. The book liberally highlights critical concepts throughout, helping the reader organize their thoughts as they read. Figures nicely illustrate complex concepts. *Medical Neurobiology* is a well-organized, highly digestible, text that will surely have a positive impact on neuroscience education in medicine for years to come."—**Larry J. Young, PhD**, Department of Psychiatry, Emory University, Atlanta, GA

MEDICAL NEUROBIOLOGY

SECOND EDITION

Peggy Mason, PhD

DEPARTMENT OF NEUROBIOLOGY

UNIVERSITY OF CHICAGO

CHICAGO, IL

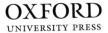

OXFORD

UNIVERSITY PRESS

OXFORD
UNIVERSITY PRESS

Oxford University Press is a department of the University of Oxford. It furthers
the University's objective of excellence in research, scholarship, and education
by publishing worldwide. Oxford is a registered trade mark of Oxford University
Press in the UK and certain other countries.

Published in the United States of America by Oxford University Press
198 Madison Avenue, New York, NY 10016, United States of America.

© Oxford University Press 2017

First Edition published in 2011

Library of Congress Cataloging-in-Publication Data
Names: Mason, Peggy (Neurobiologist), author.
Title: Medical neurobiology / by Peggy Mason.
Description: Second edition. | New York, NY : Oxford University Press, [2017]
| Includes bibliographical references and index.
Identifiers: LCCN 2016028872 | ISBN 9780190237493 (alk. paper)
Subjects: | MESH: Nervous System Physiological Phenomena | Nervous System Diseases
Classification: LCC QP355.2 | NLM WL 102 | DDC 612.8--dc23 LC record available at https://lccn.loc.gov/2016028872

CONTENTS

PREFACE TO SECOND EDITION

Over the past six years, since the publication of the first edition of this book, I have taught more than 400 second-year medical students at the University of Chicago Pritzker School of Medicine. These students inspired me with their insight, curiosity, ideas, and kindness. I was also greatly changed by teaching "Understanding the Brain: The Neurobiology of Everyday Life," a massively open online course (MOOC) that I was able to offer to the lay public through Coursera. Thousands of MOOC students taught me facts, but, more importantly, they reinforced for me how much people care about the workings of the nervous system. People care because the misdeeds of the nervous system affect them, altering their selves and their relationships in ways that diseases of no other organ system can do. It is with these concerns in mind that I revised this book. I rededicated myself to communicating both the basic science and clinical relevance of the nervous system to future physicians. My hope is that physicians will learn from this book how to talk with medical precision about the nervous system. Of equal or greater importance, I hope that readers will develop the skill of speaking plainly and compassionately with patients and their loved ones during what is often a frightening and vulnerable time.

PREFACE TO FIRST EDITION

At the start of the 20th century, medical education in North America was almost universally substandard with few or no requirements for admission, graduation, or competency. In 1905, the American Medical Association boldly recommended broad changes including admission requirements, as well as an initial 2-year curriculum in basic science.[1] Over the ensuing decade, these recommendations were implemented in American and Canadian medical schools and have continued, with some modifications, to the current time. Currently, a full year of basic science by basic scientists is taught at most North American medical schools. A minority of the basic scientists who teach these courses have a medical degree, and an even smaller proportion are practicing clinicians. As a result, a tension has built up between the basic interests and abilities of the scientist teachers and the clinical interests and goals of the students desirous to be physicians. Basic scientists teach what is important to them more than what is clinically relevant, assuming that the medical students will receive clinical training in future courses on pathophysiology taught by clinicians. The medical students feel as though they are being asked to learn material that has varied relevance to their future profession. The fact that the goals of students and teachers differ hinders communication and frustrates both students and teachers. The innocent bystander hurt by this problem is the subject itself, the beautiful world of neurobiology.

I taught in the first-year medical neurobiology course at the University of Chicago for 15 years and directed this course for 7 years, encountering directly the tension between basic science and medicine. Throughout most of my participation in medical neurobiology, I taught what I considered fundamental neurobiological principles, along with the occasional clinical anecdote thrown in to pique the student's interest. A few years ago, however, I had the opportunity and pleasure of talking in depth with four medical students[2]—Markus Boos, Eileen Rhee, Vance Broach, and Jasmine Lew. The conversation occasioned an epiphany from which this book was born. My epiphany centered on (1) the volume of information that medical students must master in 2 years, from gross anatomy and histology to physiology, microbiology, and neurobiology; and (2) the impressive sincerity of medical students' desires to be great physicians and to help people.[3] Understanding medical students' sincere altruism led to my recognition that any resistance that I perceived on the part of the students to learning course material was not attributable to disinterest or lack of motivation. Rather, students were making a realistic assessment of how to go from college-level biology to practicing medicine in 4 short years and were allotting their time and energy accordingly.

With my newfound insight, I looked anew at the material that we taught in medical neurobiology. I realized that a more comfortable union between basic science and clinical interests could and indeed *should* be forged. I now believe that what students deserve from a first-year, basic science neurobiology course is a logical framework that allows them to understand how the nervous system influences the breadth of human biology. An introductory course in neurobiology for medical students should *not* be designed to teach neurology. Rather, the goal should be to communicate the relevance of the nervous system to the practice of *every medical specialty* from cardiology to dermatology, neonatology, pediatrics, geriatrics, pulmonology, ophthalmology, and so on.

A single book in a single voice that teaches fundamental neurobiological concepts important to clinical practice was my objective in writing this textbook. Because this book is aimed more at the future internist than the

---

1. Council on Medical Education of the American Medical Association, JAMA 44:1470–75, 1905.

2. At the time, all were students and now all are physicians.

3. It is my impression that the vast majority of medical students are motivated by some degree of altruism. In contrast, students pursue a Ph.D. degree in science for a number of reasons including the intellectual thrill, curiosity, the fun of laboratory work, and also in some, but certainly not all, cases the desire to improve human health. The often dichotomous motivations of basic scientists and physicians are another source of potential misunderstanding.

future neurologist, no topic is covered in an encyclopedic fashion and thus this book is *not* a reference book. There are many outstanding reference books on topics related to the nervous system. Many of these were invaluable to me as I prepared this book. There are a number of excellent texts on neuroanatomy, neurology, and neuroscience that I encourage those of you whose interest is piqued to explore further.

No author is an island, and I certainly have benefited from the generosity and insight provided by countless individuals. In particular, I thank the hundreds of medical and graduate students whom I have taught over the years.

Questions like "How do we sense wet?" have permitted me to see neurobiology afresh and also pushed me to learn new pieces of neurobiology. I feel particularly grateful to the Pritzker class of 2009 who, as my post-epiphany guinea pigs, worked with me to hone my ideas for how medical neurobiology should be taught. These students worked hard, they engaged the brain, struggled with the material, and most importantly, respected the brain—all that this basic scientist could ever ask for. My hope for this book is that it will catalyze more and more medical students to fully engage and appreciate the wonders of the nervous system.

ACKNOWLEDGMENTS

Numerous people have aided me along the way. I thank past and present members of my laboratory for tolerating my absences and also indulging my off-topic digressions. These include Haozhe Shan, Inbal Ben-Ami Bartal, Kevin Hellman, Madelyn Baez, Maria Sol Bernardez Sarria, Nora Molasky, Thaddeus Brink, Wendy Tong, and Yuri Sugano. Colleagues at the University of Chicago and elsewhere have been generous and patient with me. I want to specifically thank Emily Joy Bembeneck (my etymology guru), Bob Burke, Dominic Catalano, Ruth Anne Eatock, Howard Fields, Aaron Fox, Jay Goldberg, Elizabeth Grove, Javad Hekmat-Penah, Philip Lloyd, Dan Margoliash, Scott Mendelson, Bob Perlman, Peter Pytel, Cliff Ragsdale, Anthony Reder, Peter Redgrave, Callum Ross, Clif Saper, Steve Shevell, Sangram Sisodia, Murray Sherman, Tom Thach, and Steve Waxman for their willingness to discuss and debate the mysteries of neural function and structure over the years. For generously and patiently responding to my questions, I am indebted to Ben Barres, Jack Feldman, Stanford Gregory, Jon Levine, Courtenay Norbury, and Ruediger Thalmann. I am grateful to the University of Chicago and to my chairman, Murray Sherman, for support and encouragement throughout the years of this project.

A few people deserve special mention for help above and beyond either my expectations or my due. Philip Lloyd patiently read and commented on chapters on neural signaling over and over again, as well as on many additional chapters. His comments were always an entertaining blend of scientific rigor and wry humor. Philip saved me from numerous sloppy blunders, and I am more grateful than a forever supply of heirloom tomatoes can express. Bob Perlman has been an invaluable friend and source of encouragement. I have run to Bob repeatedly to understand the influence of evolution on our bodies and brains. Bob never disappoints. Bob possesses a unique blend of thoughtfulness, logical clarity, and compassion that I treasure. My friend and colleague, Kevin Hellman, has generously accompanied me on this journey with humor, knowledge and a positive attitude that buoyed my spirits time after time. Despite all of the help from my wonderful colleagues, mistakes remain. These mistakes are entirely due to my own shortcomings and stubbornness.

Craig Panner, my editor at Oxford University Press, believed in this project long before it was deserving of his faith. I remain both perplexed and deeply appreciative for his nearly immediate confidence in me and the project. Craig's calm served as the perfect antidote to this first-time author's occasional panic, and I am indebted to him for that.

My parents, Jane and Arthur Mason, have been a source of unfailing support and love all of my life. I am lucky to still rely on them in my advanced years. Over the years, my mother, a *Science News* devotee, has sent me hundreds of articles containing the word "brain." Many of those articles have been valuable, and ideas from a few have found their way into this text. Even more valuable has been the faith and belief in me expressed by both of my parents in every possible way and on every possible occasion. My debt to and love for them are infinite.

This book simply would not have been written without the support and love of Gisèle Perreault, my partner in love and life. Gisèle repeatedly agreed to put our life together on hold in order for me to concentrate wholly on this book. She supported me emotionally when my energy flagged. Just as importantly, Gisèle challenged and pushed me in the honest way of a true partner. I would never have completed this project without her. I can never thank her enough.

Peggy Mason
Chicago, IL
2016

MEDICAL NEUROBIOLOGY

SECTION 1

INTRODUCTION TO MEDICAL NEUROBIOLOGY

1.

INTRODUCTION TO THE NERVOUS SYSTEM

THE NERVOUS SYSTEM RUNS LIFE

In the midst of his exciting, glamorous Parisian life as the successful editor of the leading French fashion magazine *Elle*, Jean-Dominique Bauby suffered a massive stroke that rendered him "locked-in." The 43-year-old Bauby could not move his arms or legs nor could he speak, grimace, smile, sit, point, or hold up his head. He could not nod his assent nor signal his dissent. The only way that Bauby could communicate with the outside world was by blinking, the most commonly spared motor function in locked-in patients. Using this last tendril of self-expression, Bauby "wrote" a riveting account of his internal world, an account that was published as *The Diving Bell and the Butterfly* just days before he died of pneumonia. Despite the "diving bell" that confined him, Bauby's mind "takes flight like a butterfly . . . [setting] out for Tierra del Fuego or King Midas' Court." Bauby's personality is untouched; he shows humor when he writes of his relief at finally being able to wear his own clothes: "If I must drool, I may as well drool on cashmere." Bauby's experience while locked-in is remarkable for both the magnitude of what he lost and the profound humanity that he retained.

The most impactful loss in locked-in syndrome is the inability to move with purpose, the loss of voluntary movement. On the other hand, much of the nervous system is operating normally. Locked-in individuals still see, smell, hear, follow normal sleep–wake rhythms, and, most importantly, live rich lives filled with memories, thoughts, and emotion. Improvement from the incapacitation wreaked by locked-in syndrome is rare and usually extremely limited, although a tiny number of locked-in patients show dramatic, even apparently complete, improvement.

Patients with locked-in syndrome exhibit both negative and positive signs of the damage in their nervous system.

Negative signs are clinical symptoms that result from the failure of a system to produce a function. Inabilities to move (paralysis), see (blindness), and hear (deafness) are examples of negative signs. In contrast, *positive signs* are symptoms in which an abnormal symptom occurs in place of or in addition to normal functioning. For example, Bauby sensed parts of his body and face as numb, other parts as assaulted by pins and needles, and still other areas as the source of burning pain. The sensations of pins and needles that follow a part of the body "falling asleep" are positive signs that healthy people may experience. Excess, unwanted movements, such as tics, are examples of positive motor signs.

Individuals with locked-in syndrome are not able to live independently, instead relying on people and machines for basic functions such as nutrition and voiding. Yet locked-in people around the world have achieved awe-inspiring feats: writing books, earning advanced degrees, "running" marathons, building rich social relationships, growing and changing their selves. Invariably, the accomplishments of locked-in patients are achieved in partnership with those who love and care for them. The family and friends who support a locked-in patient travel their own journey as they grapple with the changes wrought by an injured brain. Along with the locked-in individual, they also experience, first-hand and in dramatic fashion, the power of the human nervous system, the subject of this book.

Locked-in syndrome is defined by a loss of voluntary movement and invariably involves impairments in perception and homeostasis while leaving abstract cognitive function untouched. These four functions—perception, voluntary movement, homeostasis, and abstract or higher function—are integral to human well-being. Since disturbances in any of these functions will motivate an individual to seek medical help, they are the focus of this book.

PERCEPTION IS INTERPRETATIVE RATHER THAN AN EXACT REPRESENTATION OF INTERNAL AND EXTERNAL STIMULI

Perception refers to conscious awareness of changes in the internal milieu or external environment. It is part of, but not the entirety of, *sensation*, an umbrella category that includes unconscious processing of sensory information. For example, changes in blood oxygen levels are sensed but not perceived, whereas optical information from this page activates sensory pathways that ultimately result in visual perception. Note that, in psychology, the term "sensation" is typically used to refer to unconscious aspects of sensory processing exclusively.

Perception is achieved by a liberal, context-specific interpretation of the world rather than by a faithful capture of external energy, such as that performed by cameras and audio recorders. This strategy pays off because correctly detected sensory components are far poorer at predicting meaning than are expectation and context (Fig. 1-1). Given the looseness with which sensory information is incorporated into perceptual meaning, it is no surprise that we sense things that are not actually there as well as fail to sense things that are there.

The challenge of perception stems from the interpretation needed for stimulus information to be useful. People with *visual agnosia* ("agnosia" is Greek for "without knowledge, ignorance") fail to understand visual objects and dramatically illustrate the challenge of perceptual interpretation. The title character in Oliver Sacks's "The Man Who

Mistook His Wife for a Hat," Dr. P., describes an object that is handed to him as "about six inches in length, a convoluted red form with a linear green attachment" but cannot name the object. His detailed description clearly indicates a working visual system, but Dr. P. cannot interpret what he sees, something that most of us do without thought or effort. Yet, upon smelling the mysterious object, Dr. P. instantly identifies it as "an early rose," indicating that, unlike Dr. P's visual system, his olfactory system has access to stored knowledge and language production. Visual agnosia exemplifies the distinct challenges of sensing, perceiving, and usefully interpreting sensory information.

MOTOR PATHWAYS ARE THE ONLY AVENUE AVAILABLE FOR SELF-EXPRESSION

The movement of skeletal muscles provides the only way that humans have to express themselves, whether explicitly through speech or writing or more implicitly through posture, facial expression, and eye movements. Thus, the ultimate outcome of the motor system is human nature itself. The only way to access the approximately 750 skeletal muscles of the body is via the roughly 100,000 *motoneurons* in the spinal cord and brainstem that send processes out to terminate on skeletal muscle cells. For this reason, the great neurophysiologist Charles Sherrington called motoneurons the *final common pathway*, an unavoidable bottleneck that must be navigated to achieve willful expression.

Skeletal muscles cannot operate independently but only contract when activated by a very special type of neuron, the *motoneuron*. Located centrally, within the spinal cord and brainstem, motoneurons send a process out of the central nervous system (CNS) to contact skeletal muscle fibers via a *neuromuscular junction*. Any complete lesion of motoneurons or the neuromuscular junction can block all movements of the involved muscle.

Motoneurons are not "smart," and they require instructions that come from several sources. Incoming sensory input allows for adjusting movements to accommodate surprises in the external world, such as unexpected obstacles. Neurons in upper *motor control centers* instruct motoneuron activity to direct a variety of actions from those that are entirely deliberate to more automatized and stereotyped ones such as chewing. Cortical motor control centers are critical to fine movements of the digits, face, and mouth. Brainstem motor control centers are critical for the maintenance of posture and stereotypical movements such as

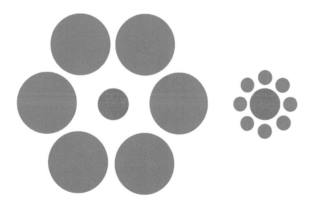

Figure 1-1 In the Ebbinghaus illusion, circles of the same size are perceived as smaller when surrounded by large circles (*left*) and larger when surrounded by small circles (*right*). You can check that the two green circles are the same size by occluding the rings of surrounding lavender circles. Because perception of this illusion persists independently of color, the colors used here serve only an aesthetic purpose.

breathing, swallowing, and locomotion. Communication between upper motor control centers and motoneurons is one-way only in that motoneurons do not "talk back" to motor control centers. Thus, descending pathways from motor control centers to motoneurons form the *motor hierarchy*. Sufficient impairment to the integrity of the motor hierarchy can block subsets of movements while leaving other types intact. In locked-in syndrome, the motor hierarchy pathway is lesioned, resulting in patients losing willful control of voluntary muscles.

Acting alone, the motor hierarchy would not produce recognizable movements. Two modulatory loops, one through the *cerebellum* (diminutive or little brain) and one through the *basal ganglia*, are required. Through the cerebellum's modulation of motor control centers, movements become smooth and well-coordinated. The cerebellum is necessary for coordinating complex movements involving several muscles or ones that require fine control. One can think of the cerebellum as a conductor, not needed by the soloist or even a string quartet, but essential to the coordination of an orchestra. The cerebellum uses sensory feedback from past motor experiences to adjust movements to changing conditions and thereby ensure that the movements we make are those that we intend to make.

We all have only one set of muscles, and each muscle can do only one thing at a time. It is not possible look to the right and look to the left at the same time. Without practice, it is not even possible to move one arm up and down while moving the other side to side. Although many component actions are easy, performing two or more actions simultaneously is difficult and requires practice. The limitation is not in the muscles, motoneurons, motor control centers, or even in the cerebellum. The only obstacle to performing multiple actions simultaneously is the basal ganglia. The basal ganglia choose to do one or a very few related actions while simultaneously suppressing all other movement. The brain's "chooser" is the basal ganglia. Just as the number of actions that an individual can make at one time is limited, so is the number of perceptions, emotions, motivations, or thoughts. The basal ganglia choose perceptions, thoughts, and emotions as well as movements.

HOMEOSTASIS IS THE PROCESS OF ENSURING THAT BODILY VARIABLES STAY WITHIN A PREFERRED RANGE

The human body operates best within certain physiological ranges, and these ranges are maintained by homeostatic functions that regulate internal body temperature, blood pressure, heart rate, electrolyte balance, body weight, sleep–wake cycles, and the like. Neuronal defense of the body's physiology occurs largely unconsciously through use of skeletal muscle, smooth muscle, cardiac muscle, and glands. Different combinations of purposeful and automatic actions contribute to a continuum of homeostatic functions that range from completely unconscious (e.g., hormone release) to those with a large voluntary component, such as keeping warm in the cold.

Homeostasis is often modeled as a feedback system akin to a home's thermostat. However, a thermostat is "dumb" and only reacts to changes after they occur. In contrast, the brain is "smart," and, whenever possible, anticipates challenges to homeostasis. For instance, saliva and insulin, a hormone released by the pancreas that regulates glucose metabolism, are released in anticipation of eating. Anticipatory homeostatic adjustments require the forebrain.

The word "homeostasis" comes from the Greek *homeo-*, meaning "similar" or "same," and *stasis*, meaning "standing." Despite its etymological roots in standing-still, homeostasis is not a system that maintains a uniform internal milieu. The brain does not clamp the internal milieu of the body into one fixed state. Instead, the preferred state of the body changes across the day and night cycle, from one activity to another, and as the external environment changes. For example, the cardiovascular system operates in vastly different ways in a person reading on a couch, taking a school entrance exam, or out for a morning jog. The brain ensures that the body's internal milieu aligns with an individual's activities, even as those activities change drastically.

HUMANS REVEL IN HIGHER ABSTRACT BRAIN FUNCTIONS

Higher brain functions include language, attention, volition, emotion, memory, and the ability to socially interact with others. Our understanding of abstract brain functions relies on findings from psychology, psychiatry, and neurology as well as on basic neuroscience. For example, the lateralization of human language to the left cortex in most individuals was described by Pierre Paul Broca, a French clinician. Even now, most of our understanding of language comes from human studies, although we are starting to benefit from the study of communication in nonhuman animals.

To understand how the brain produces neural function, basic neuroanatomical terminology is needed. A fundamental division, based on embryonic origin and adult anatomy, exists between the central (CNS) and peripheral (PNS) nervous systems (Fig. 1-2). The *brain* is the part of the CNS contained within the *cranium*, and the *spinal cord* is the part of the CNS contained within the spinal canal within the vertebral column. Although the optic nerve and retina are derived from the embryonic brain, they migrate out of the cranium. Yet the retina, present at the back of the eye, is enveloped within the same meninges as the brain and therefore shares its environment with the brain. This arrangement means that the retina is the most accessible part of the CNS; the retina and optic nerve, both part of the CNS, are not within the cranium and therefore not part of the brain, but they provide an important and accessible "window" to the brain.

Three specialized membranes, termed *meninges*, form a fence around the CNS. The PNS is located outside this fence. The integrity of the meninges is essential for the

mechanical and chemical protection of the CNS. The outermost meningeal layer, the *dura mater* or simply *dura*, is a tough membrane that protects the CNS from penetration. The *arachnoid mater*, deep to the dura, forms a fluid-resistant sac around the brain and spinal cord. The innermost meninges, the *pia mater*, is a very thin and delicate membrane separated from the arachnoid by the subarachnoid space, within which the brain's own special fluid, *cerebrospinal fluid* or *CSF*, flows.

The PNS has three components (Fig. 1-2). Primary sensory neurons reside in spinal and cranial *sensory ganglia*. They carry information into the central nervous system that, upon reaching the cerebral cortex, allows us to perceive sound, taste, smell, touch, vibration, warmth, head position, and so on. *Autonomic ganglia*, of either the *sympathetic* or *parasympathetic* variety, are located in the body and head. They contain neurons critical to homeostasis through control of smooth muscle, cardiac muscle, and glands. The overall effects of sympathetic and parasympathetic activity oppose each other, with sympathetic pathways supporting energy expenditure during periods of arousal, fight, or flight, and parasympathetic activation supporting energy accumulation during periods of recuperation, rest, and digestion. Although autonomic pathways are necessary for homeostasis, they are not sufficient, as the example of breathing, which depends on skeletal muscle, clearly illustrates. The final component of the PNS is the *enteric nervous system*, which consists of roughly 1 billion neurons that sit in the lining of the gut. The enteric nervous system is necessary for normal digestion and passage of food through the body. Connections between the gut's little brain and the CNS enable the CNS to influence digestion, as happens when a strong emotion alters gut motility.

CNS anatomy is complex and is best framed in terms of its embryonic development from simpler albeit transient structures. The earliest embryonic divisions of the CNS are regional compartments that develop into the *spinal cord, hindbrain, midbrain,* and *forebrain* of the adult (Fig. 1-3). As development progresses, the embryonic forebrain splits into the *diencephalon* and *telencephalon*. Although, strictly speaking, the words "diencephalon" and "telencephalon" refer to developmental structures, there are no words in common usage to refer to the adult derivatives. Therefore, we will use these terms to refer to adult regions even as we acknowledge the inherent etymological compromise. In the adult, the telencephalon comprises the *cerebral cortex*, core elements of the *basal ganglia* (*striatum* and *pallidum*), and *amygdala*, whereas the diencephalon includes the *thalamus* and *hypothalamus* (Fig. 1-3C). Some basic neuroanatomical

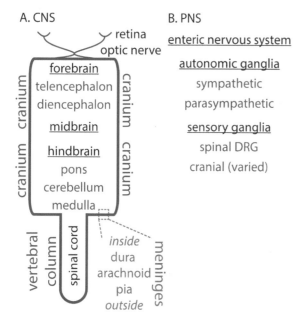

Figure 1-2 The nervous system is divided into the central (A) and peripheral (B) nervous systems by the meninges. The central nervous system (CNS) consists of the brain within the cranium, the spinal cord within the vertebral column, and the retina and optic nerve. The retina and optic nerve, both part of the CNS, are not within the cranium and therefore not part of the brain; yet they provide an important and accessible "window" to the brain. The forebrain, midbrain, and hindbrain make up the brain. The peripheral nervous system (PNS) consists of the enteric nervous system lining the digestive tract, autonomic ganglia of two types, and sensory ganglia associated with spinal and cranial nerves.

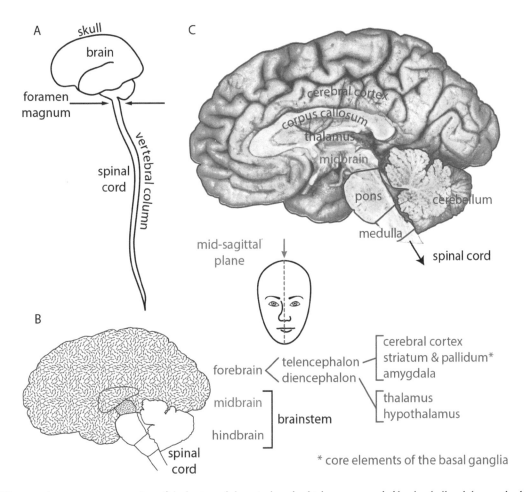

Figure 1-3 A: The central nervous system consists of the brain and the spinal cord, which are surrounded by the skull and the vertebral column, respectively. The foramen magnum is the large hole at the base of the skull where the brain and spinal cord meet. B: A mid-sagittal (see center inset) cartoon of the human brain is shown with the developmental compartments of the hindbrain, midbrain, and forebrain labeled. The forebrain comprises the diencephalon, consisting of the thalamus and hypothalamus, and the telencephalon, which consists of the cerebral cortex, striatum and pallidum, and amygdala. C: A mid-sagittal view of the human brain is shown with major parts of the hindbrain, midbrain, and forebrain labeled. The visible parts of the forebrain are the cerebral cortex, corpus callosum, and thalamus. The midbrain has no subdivisions. The hindbrain consists of the medulla, pons, and cerebellum.   Photograph in C reprinted with permission of deArmond S et al., *Structure of the human brain: A photographic atlas*. New York: Oxford University Press, 1989.

terms are based on anatomical rather than developmental considerations. The *brainstem* is the back part of the brain, consisting of the hindbrain and midbrain. Although they share a common hindbrain origin, the *pons, cerebellum,* and *medulla* appear distinct in the adult (Fig. 1-3C).

MAPPING FUNCTION ONTO STRUCTURE

Using the basic neuroanatomical terminology just introduced, we can now map the functions of the nervous system onto neuroanatomical structures. Perception, voluntary movement, and homeostasis are all distributed through pathways that involve the spinal cord, brainstem, and forebrain. In contrast, higher abstract function depends entirely on the forebrain. In particular, the cerebral cortex, the laminated outer rind of the forebrain, is critical to cognitive function, to processing and understanding events and surroundings, setting and achieving goals, and remembering the past. The forebrain is able to adjust behavior based on previous experiences and provides us with the requisite skills to navigate among family members, friends, and strangers as the social animals that we are.

Perception and voluntary movement comprise our incoming and outgoing interfaces with the world but traverse different routes. Sensory information enters the CNS either at the level of the spinal cord, brainstem, or forebrain. For example, touch information from the body enters the spinal cord, hearing information comes into the hindbrain, and visual information enters the forebrain. Regardless of where sensory information enters the CNS, it must traverse the CNS to reach the cerebral cortex in order for conscious perception to occur.

Motoneurons in the spinal cord control movements of the arms and legs, whereas those in the brainstem control muscles of the neck, face, and oral cavity (Fig. 1-4). The forebrain has no direct connection to muscles but contains motor control centers that initiate deliberate actions—*Simon says* put your hand on your head—or emotional ones—a wince in pain. Motor control centers in the brainstem are critical to postural maintenance, eye movements, chewing, and other subconscious movements. Beyond the motor hierarchy, the cerebellum and basal ganglia play critical roles in voluntary motor control.

To maintain homeostasis, sensory information from the body enters the spinal cord and brainstem, where it triggers automatic or unconscious reactions. For example, in reaction to a mild decrease in ambient levels of oxygen, as occurs routinely in the passenger cabin of an airplane, we breathe more rapidly. Sensory information also engages more conscious adjustments, such as dressing warmly in winter, through ascending connections to the forebrain. Descending messages from the forebrain and brainstem reach neurons in the forebrain, brainstem, and spinal cord

to coordinate hormone release with autonomic adjustments and volitional actions.

Bauby's stroke nearly obliterated the middle portion of the brainstem (the pons), resulting in the loss of functions that depend on that part of the brainstem and, even more vitally, on functions that depend on *connections*, analogous to streets or highways, traveling through this region (Fig. 1-3C). Bauby's grave condition resulted primarily from the latter: the stroke's disruption of connections. Bauby's stroke specifically disconnected the forebrain and rostral brainstem from the caudal brainstem and spinal cord. Disconnecting the forebrain from most of the brainstem and all of the spinal cord has profound effects on perception, voluntary movement, and homeostasis. However, higher brain functions depend entirely on the forebrain and do not involve any connections that travel through the pons. Therefore, higher brain functions are unaffected in locked-in syndrome.

Somatosensory information from the body enters into the spinal cord and then *ascends* (i.e., it travels from caudal to rostral) to the forebrain to give rise to perceptions of touch, pain, temperature, and so on (Fig. 1-4). Visual and olfactory information from the eyes and nose comes directly into the forebrain. A pontine stroke therefore affects somatosensation but not vision or olfaction. The motor message for purposeful movement that originates in the cerebral cortex must reach motoneurons in the brainstem and spinal cord that in turn innervate voluntary muscles. A pontine stroke interrupts connections between the forebrain and virtually all motoneurons, leaving locked-in patients unable to move at will. Finally, locked-in patients have poor control over most homeostatic defense systems. Because the forebrain is disconnected from the brainstem and spinal cord, locked-in patients cannot kiss a loved one, swallow saliva, or willfully release urine.

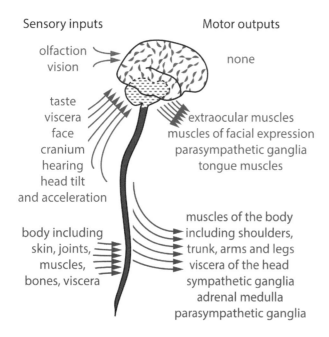

Figure 1-4 A: The sensory inputs to and motor outputs from the central nervous system (CNS) are mapped onto a cartoon of the brain and spinal cord. Sensory inputs reach all parts of the brain, whereas motor outputs only arise from the brainstem and spinal cord. Note that the motor outputs listed include both voluntary movements, using skeletal muscles, and autonomic motor outputs that ultimately influence smooth muscle, cardiac muscle, and glands.

A GUIDE TO OUR JOURNEY THROUGH THE NERVOUS SYSTEM

The two fundamental building blocks of the nervous system are neural communication and neuroanatomy. Foundations in both topics must be mastered. After learning the neurons and glial cells that comprise the nervous system (Chapter 2), we start with the anatomy of the nervous system (Section 2) before moving on to neural communication (Section 3). With these basics of neurophysiology and neuroanatomy in hand, we are ready to tackle how the brain "works" by examining perception (Section 4), voluntary movement (Section 5), and homeostasis (Section 6).

This book is intended as a travel guide for the human brain. It is my hope to communicate to you the profound power and beauty of brain function while providing you with a memorable and enjoyable trip. Bon voyage!

ADDITIONAL READING

Bauby J-D. *The Diving Bell and the Butterfly*. New York: Alfred A. Knopf; 1997.

Sacks O. *The Man Who Mistook His Wife for a Hat*. New York: Touchstone Books; 1985.

2.

CELLS OF THE NERVOUS SYSTEM

NEURONS AND GLIA

NEURONS AND GLIA

Neurons and *glia* populate the nervous system. Neurons are the stars of the show, the cells that receive all the credit, and, beyond a few paragraphs here and there, neurons are nearly the sole focus of this book. Yet there are roughly as many glial cells as there are neurons in the human brain. Just as the extras rather than the actors make a crowd scene, glia are critical to the development and function of the nervous system, providing necessary supportive services to adult neurons. Their demise is at the core of diseases such as multiple sclerosis. Malfunctioning glia are important in the pathophysiology of some primary brain tumors, neurodegenerative diseases, and other neurological conditions. Furthermore, glia-targeting treatments may hold promise in treating a broad range of diseases as well as in facilitating improvement after stroke. Thus, while the developmental, structural, environmental, and repair services of glia hold far less glory than do the lofty functions of neurons, neurons cannot survive and function without glia, just as a theatrical production would grind to a halt without the stage crew and production staff. In this chapter,

we learn the cell biology of neurons, glia, and their progenitor cells and then apply this understanding to a range of clinical issues such as brain tumors and neurodegenerative diseases.

THE NERVOUS SYSTEM DERIVES FROM EMBRYONIC ECTODERM

Embryologically, the nervous system arises from ectoderm, one of three germ layers of the embryo. Ectoderm also gives rise to skin. Three regions of ectoderm are specified that give rise to neurons and glia, as well as to a variety of non-neuronal tissues (Fig. 2-1). The three regions that give rise to neurons and glia are:

- The *neural tube* derives from a sheet of *neuroectoderm* called the *neural plate* and runs most of the length of the embryo (detailed in Chapter 3). Neurons and glia of the central nervous system (CNS) derive from neural tube progenitor cells. A small number of *non-neuronal* tissues, such as the *choroid epithelium* lining the brain's ventricles and the *pineal gland*, also derive from neural tube.

- At the lateral edges of the neural plate, as it closes to form the neural tube, the *neural crest* originates. Neural crest cells are motile, and they migrate to specific locations throughout the body and head of the embryo. Neural crest–derived cells generate the bulk of the peripheral nervous system (PNS), glia and neurons alike, and also give rise to *many* non-neuronal tissues such as dermal bone (e.g., skull), melanocytes, arachnoid, and pia.

- *Placodes*, present in the head region only, flank the anterior neural crest and neural tube. Placodes, thickenings within the ectodermal layer, are the origin of most peripheral sensory ganglia of the head. Placodes also give rise to several non-neuronal structures such as the lens, sclera, anterior pituitary, and hair cells of the inner ear.

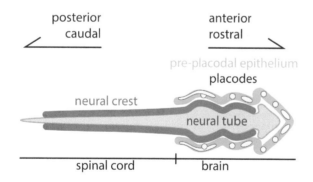

Figure 2-1 This cartoon shows a dorsal view of the early embryo with rostral to the right and caudal to the left. Immediately surrounding the neural tube is neural crest, which gives rise to most of the peripheral nervous system. Within the primordial head region of the developing embryo, neuroepithelium develops into pre-placodal ectoderm (*blue*), which eventually populates seven bilateral pairs of placodes (*yellow*), five of which give rise to sensory neurons associated with cranial nerves.

In sum, *the nervous system derives from three embryonic sources, all of which arise from ectoderm*. The general rule is that the neural tube gives rise to the CNS, whereas the PNS arises from primarily neural crest with a contribution from placodes to sensory ganglia within the head (see Table 2-1). Neural tube, neural crest, and placodes all also give rise to a number of non-neural tissues, some highly important to nervous system function (e.g., arachnoid, hair cells) and others not closely related to the nervous system (e.g., melanocytes).

The embryology of the nervous system provides us with a way to understand genetic disorders that involve varied symptoms that, despite appearing unrelated, are connected by a common developmental lineage. For example, patients with *Waardenburg syndrome* have mutations in genes that regulate neural crest development. These patients present with symptoms that appear unrelated to each other until one realizes that all derive from disruption of normal neural crest development. Predominant symptoms of Waardenburg syndrome include deafness, lack of pigment in areas of the skin and hair, blue eyes, and a facial appearance characterized by wide-set eyes, low hairline, and a uni-brow. The deafness occurs because inner ear development, normally directed by neural crest–derived cells, is disrupted. The lack of pigmentation in skin and eyes can be accounted for by a problem with neural crest–derived melanocytes. Changes in neural crest-directed development of facial bones, muscles, and tendons produce a characteristic facial appearance. Some patients exhibit additional neurological problems such as digestive problems associated with incomplete development of the enteric nervous system.

Waardenburg syndrome exemplifies developmental disorders in having an at-first-glance odd but at-second-glance coherent collection of symptoms that are related to each other solely by a shared developmental history.

NEURONS ARE CHARACTERIZED BY COLLECTIVELY UNIQUE TRAITS

In many organs of the body such as the kidneys, lungs, and even the relatively complex pancreas, there are a few, typically well under a dozen, different types of cells. "If you've seen one lung cell, you've seen them all" is only a slight exaggeration. In contrast, there are *thousands* of different types of neurons. Just as the Milky Way, despite appearing as a continuous spread of light, is an aggregation of hundreds of billions of *individually distinct* stars that differ in location, age, color, and mass, the human brain contains 75–95 billion individual neurons that differ from one another in location, appearance, connections, physiological characteristics, and, ultimately, function.

Despite their heterogeneity, *neurons share the following group of traits that are not collectively shared by any other cell type*:

• Derived embryologically from ectoderm

• Terminally differentiated and not dividing

• Connected to another neuron on the input (motoneurons, preganglionic motor neurons), output (primary sensory afferents), or both (central neurons) ends

Table 2-1 **NEURAL AND NON-NEURAL DERIVATIVES OF NEURAL TUBE, NEURAL CREST, AND PLACODES**

	CNS DERIVATIVES	PNS DERIVATIVES	NON-NEURAL DERIVATIVES
Neural tube	Spinal cord Brain		Pineal gland Choroid epithelium
Neural crest		Enteric nervous system Autonomic ganglia Dorsal root ganglia Peripheral glia Trigeminal ganglia (most neurons)	Arachnoid mater Pia mater Skull, jaw, teeth Cartilage of head Melanocytes Merkel cells Chromaffin cells of adrenal medulla Sclera, cornea Hair cells of inner ear Middle ear ossicles Glandular connective tissue of head and neck . . . . and many more
Placode	GNRH cells of hypothalamus	Sensory neurons associated with cranial nerves I, V (minority), VII, VIII, IX, X	Lens Anterior pituitary

- Transfer information through the mechanism of *synaptic transmission*

- Have an elaborate morphology that typically includes distinct cellular regions

Let's start with the final characteristic. A typical neuron has four anatomical subregions (Fig. 2-2). Each of these different cellular regions plays a primary role in a different neuronal function. The regions and their roles are, in brief:

- *Soma* or *cell body*: Houses DNA-containing nucleus along with extensive protein-making machinery; critical to cell health

- *Dendrites*: Branching processes, or extensions, that collect incoming information

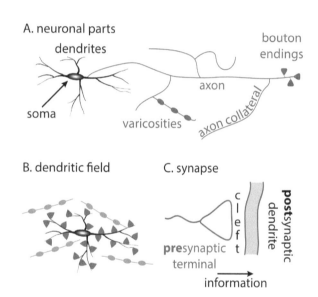

A. neuronal parts

B. dendritic field

C. synapse

Figure 2-2 A: A typical neuron has a soma or cell body, dendrites (*black*), and an axon with synaptic terminals (*red*). The daughter processes from a parent dendrite are called branches, whereas processes coming off a parent axon are called collaterals. Axons and axon collaterals communicate via synaptic terminals in the form of either bouton endings or varicosities. The appearance of varicosities resembles slightly flattened pearls on a necklace, with the axon being the metaphorical necklace. Dendrites receive information, and a neuron's axon carries information to target cells. B: The dendritic field is the information-receiving zone of a neuron. Neurons may receive an enormous number of synaptic inputs from bouton endings, varicosities, or both, throughout this field or arbor. C: At classical chemical synapses, a bouton ending and a dendrite are in close apposition, enabling communication from the presynaptic cell's bouton to the target, or postsynaptic, element (typically a dendrite). The arrow shows the primary direction of information transfer across a synapse. Although the membranes of pre- and postsynaptic cells come very close to each other at classical synapses, they are separated by a narrow divide called the synaptic cleft. Note that these cartoons are not to scale but are drawn for illustrative purposes.

- *Axon*: A process that extends past the immediate locale and serves to send information to cells at many distant locales

- *Synaptic terminals*: Small swellings from where information is sent across a physical divide to another cell

Now, we consider each of these compartments in turn.

As is true for all cells in the body, the neuronal soma (*somata* is the plural) houses the nucleus, endoplasmic reticulum, Golgi apparatus, lysosomes, and other organelles that support cellular life. The rough endoplasmic reticulum in neurons is particularly active, synthesizing large quantities of proteins. Consequently, when stained with basophilic dyes, neuronal rough endoplasmic reticulum stands out prominently as *Nissl substance*. Staining brain sections for Nissl substance reveals the distribution of neuronal cell bodies and provides an easy and useful picture that can be used to readily identify gross changes or abnormalities in pathological specimens.

Dendrites, the primary receiving zone of the neuron, receive the bulk of the input to a neuron. The entirety of the dendritic branches, from large proximal branches to thin distal ones, is called the *dendritic tree* or *dendritic arbor*. The dendritic arbor represents the receiving volume for a neuron; only synaptic terminals within the arbor may provide input to the neuron. Some, but not all, neurons have dendrites with a multitude of small protuberances called *dendritic spines* or simply spines. One common type of spine is knob-like in appearance with a globe-shaped head that is linked to the main dendrite by a very thin process, the neck. Inputs preferentially contact spine heads, which form a subcellular locus for changes associated with many forms of learning. Spines are thought to house anatomical changes central to storing memories.

Input to the entire dendritic arbor is summed up and electrically conducted toward the soma. All input—strong or weak, fast or slow, excitatory or inhibitory—is integrated across both space (different dendritic branches) and time (see Chapter 10). If the summed electrical signal is sufficient, a neuron may then release neurotransmitter at a synaptic terminal. Synaptic terminals take the form of either *bouton endings* or *varicosities*. At a classical synapse, a *presynaptic* cell's bouton ending communicates to a specific target, typically the dendrite of a *postsynaptic* cell (Fig. 2-3). The bouton and dendrite are in close apposition but separated by a narrow divide called the *synaptic cleft* (see Box 2-1). In contrast, varicosities participate in what is a far less specific form of communication that is often termed paracrine or *volume transmission*. Neurotransmitter

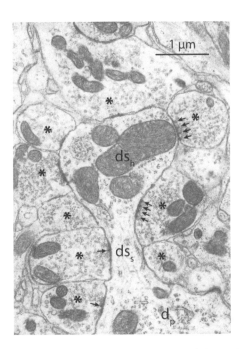

Figure 2-3 An electron micrograph of synaptic terminals (*asterisks*) blanketing the head (*ds_h*) and shaft (*ds_s*) of a dendritic spine in the rat cochlear nucleus. The presynaptic axonal terminals contain synaptic vesicles, filled with neurotransmitter, that are released into the synaptic cleft at synaptic densities (*arrows*) and bind receptors on the postsynaptic dendrite. d_p, parent dendrite. Photomicrograph is reprinted from Peters A. Palay SL, deF Webster H. *The fine structure of the nervous system: Neurons and their supporting cells.* 3rd edition. New York: Oxford University Press, 1991.

Cajal made manifold contributions to neuroscience. Although he was a pure anatomist, looking at Golgi-stained sections day in and day out, Cajal's genius was that he *saw* function from structure, intuiting process from the static picture afforded him by the light microscopes of the late 19th and early 20th centuries. In other words, Cajal's ideas were inspired by, rather than literally adherent to, the microscopic images from which he could not possibly have detected the synaptic cleft that separates neurons. Cajal's genius is further evident in his proposal that *neural information normally flows in one direction, from the dendrites and soma to the axon.* This idea, termed the law of *dynamic polarization,* now accepted as the rule, holds that after traveling down the axon, information crosses over a physical divide to the dendrites and soma of another cell. This point of transfer, the place where two independent neuronal units communicate, is a *synapse,* a term popularized by Sir Charles Sherrington at the end of the 19th century. More important than popularizing the term "synapse," Sherrington, the first great neurophysiologist and winner of the 1932 Nobel Prize in Physiology or Medicine, recognized *the potential of the synapse to integrate excitatory and inhibitory information from multiple sources.*

Box 2-1 THE NEURON DOCTRINE

In the 1830s, two German scientists, Schleiden and Schwann, advanced the idea that plants and animals are made up of small units called *cells.* Cell doctrine was applied to the whole body, except the central nervous system (CNS), where one large continuum or syncytium was postulated. Then, in 1873, Camillo Golgi developed a silver impregnation method, now known as the Golgi stain, which marks cells in their entirety—a great advancement over previously available somatic stains. The Golgi stain does not stain every cell, as "Nissl" staining does. Only a discernible number of neurons are stained (up to about 5%), enabling stained neurons to be followed and studied against a largely unstained background. (Why some cells are stained and others not in any one tissue section appears random and remains mysterious.) Using Golgi's staining technique, Ramon y Cajal, the greatest neuroanatomist of all time, "saw" anatomical gaps between neuronal elements. Instead of a continuous, reticulated network, Cajal championed the neuron doctrine: *Each neuron is an entity unto itself that closely contacts but is not continuous with other neurons.* Cajal and Golgi shared the Nobel Prize in Physiology or Medicine in 1906, although Golgi never subscribed to the neuron doctrine; indeed, Golgi used his Nobel Prize lecture to argue, incorrectly, that the brain is one continuous reticulated tissue.

released from a varicosity may reach any postsynaptic element present within the vicinity. *Regardless of the particular morphology, the essence of synaptic communication is the transfer of information from a presynaptic terminal to target, postsynaptic cells.*

In some neurons, the synaptic terminal is at or very close to the soma. However, most neurons *transfer electrical signals over long distances,* and, for this, an axon is required. The axon, often referred to as a *fiber,* arises from a point on or close to the soma, and it is at this *axon hillock* that graded synaptic inputs are "translated" into the language of *action potentials,* all-or-none electrical potentials that can be propagated over long distances without diminution or failure. Thus, information, in the format of patterned trains of action potentials, travels down an axon to postsynaptic targets. The morphological axon and the physiological action potential are intertwined so that either both are present or both absent. The determining factor in this regard is whether neurons communicate information to distant cells: those that do have axons and action potentials. In contrast, neurons that communicate only within the immediate vicinity of the soma have neither axons nor action potentials. For example, intrinsic retinal neurons send information to nearby cells, and they lack an axon and do not *fire* action potentials.

Axons are unique to neurons; no other cell type has as long processes as do neurons. The longest neuronal processes can be more than a meter long (see Box 2-2). This means that the axonal process of a typical neuron (5–25 microns in diameter) contains more than 99.9% of the total neuronal volume. When all of an axon's branches, or collaterals, are taken into account, the total length of an axon may be more than 4 meters. The fact that small neuronal somata, comprising no more than 0.1% of the neuronal volume, can support long processes and do so for the decades of an individual's life represents a tremendous biological achievement and places the failure of this process in some individuals into context.

Critical to building and maintaining neurons in their vastness is a highway system that provides transport between the soma and the synaptic terminals of even the longest neurons. Neurons transport substances both from the soma to synaptic terminals and from synaptic terminals back to the soma. *Anterograde axonal transport* carries substances made in the soma, such as neuropeptides, neurotransmitter-synthesizing enzymes, and mitochondria, to synaptic terminals where these substances are used. *Retrograde axonal transport* carries substances from the synaptic terminals back to the soma. For example, synaptic terminals may pick up a trophic factor from a target cell and transport this factor back to the soma (see Box 2-3). In addition, protein "waste" is transported from the synaptic terminal to the soma for removal by lysosomes.

Box 2-2 THE DIMENSIONS OF SINGLE NEURONS VARY BY MANY ORDERS OF MAGNITUDE

The longest neuronal processes stretch from the foot to the medulla, a distance of 1.4 meters or more in most adults. To put this into perspective, if we represent an average neuronal soma of 25 microns[1] in diameter by a baseball, then a thin process with a 2-micron diameter would be represented by a cylinder that is about the width of a chopstick. The length of this "chopstick process" would be almost 3 miles (~5km) long in a person of average height and more than 3.5 miles in a tall individual. These staggering anatomical proportions highlight the biological challenges that neurons face in maintaining function throughout the extent of the entire cell.

[1] A micron, symbolized as μm, is 1/1000th of a millimeter; for those not familiar with the metric system, a millimeter corresponds to less than 0.04 inches. Thus, neurons have a diameter of only a few thousandths of an inch.

Box 2-3 RETROGRADE AXONAL TRANSPORT IS USED BY NEURONS TO SIGNAL A HEALTHY CONNECTION TO THE TARGET CELL BUT CAN BE HIJACKED BY VIRUSES

Trophic factors released from target cells can be picked up by synaptic terminals and then transported back to the soma via "backward" movement along the axon. The movement from the synaptic terminal to the soma is considered *retrograde* or backward because it proceeds in the opposite direction from normal information flow. In the event of damage to either the axon or the synaptic terminal, retrograde transport is interrupted and trophic factors do not make it back to the soma. In this way, news of damage can reach the soma, which may be quite a distance away. For example, muscle fibers release factors that the terminals of motoneurons pick up. Interruption of the retrograde signal from muscle to motoneuron soma results in the motoneurons undergoing *chromatolysis*, a form of degeneration that can be detected using a Nissl stain. Chromatolysis is triggered by the absence of muscle-released factors transported back to the motoneuron soma.

The transport of trophic factors from the terminal to the soma provides neurons with continual assurance: "All is well." Unfortunately, this healthy process can be hijacked for nefarious purposes. Several *neurotropic* viruses are picked up at peripheral terminals and retrogradely transported to the parent somata. For example, *poliovirus*, the causative agent of poliomyelitis, is picked up at the muscle by the terminals of motoneurons and ultimately can lead to the death of infected motoneurons, resulting in paralysis of the muscles involved. *Varicella zoster virus*, the causative agent of chickenpox, can be picked up by the terminals of sensory neurons and transported back to the parent somata in a sensory ganglion. Zoster virus can remain in an inactive state in the sensory neuron somata for decades. In some individuals, the virus reactivates, causing an outbreak of *herpes zoster* (see Chapter 17).

The intracellular trafficking of molecules going to and from the soma requires both infrastructure and vehicles for transportation. The neuronal *cytoskeleton* is the highway's infrastructure and is comprised of actin, a neuron-specific *neurofilament*, and *microtubules*. The microtubules form dynamic lanes that are extended or retracted, stabilized or destabilized largely through the action of a microtubule-associated protein called *tau*. Tau's role in axonal transport may be key to its role in neurodegenerative disease (see later discussion in the section "Diverse Neurodegenerative Diseases Share Common Mechanisms of Pathogenesis"). Moving along the microtubules are *dynein* and *kinesin*, two molecular motors that serve as vehicles to shuttle cargo up or down an axon. Transport occurs with an energetic cost as one adenosine triphosphate (ATP) molecule fuels a step of about 8 nm, meaning that a single trip across a distance of 1 meter would require more than 100 million molecules of ATP, which, to place in perspective, is less than a femtomole of ATP.

The raison d'être of an axon is to serve as a conduit or transmission cable for neural signals sent across a distance to reach the actual launching sites for neuronal communication, the synaptic terminals. The speed at which an axon supports action potential conduction, or travel, depends on the width of the axon and on whether the axon is wrapped in *myelin*, the insulation that wraps tightly around axons. Myelin enables the rapid axonal conduction of action potentials at velocities greater than 1 m/s. Myelin surrounds some but not all axons. Axons that have a myelin wrap are *myelinated*, and those that lack myelin are *unmyelinated*. The axons with the fastest conduction times are large in diameter and heavily myelinated. Axons that are unmyelinated conduct action potentials very slowly. In general, myelin is heaviest and most prevalent in axons that serve motor purposes, such as the axons of motoneurons and proprioceptive and vestibular sensory neurons.

NEURONS PARTICIPATE IN PATHWAYS

No neuron is an island, and no neuron functions in isolation. In the human and, indeed, in all mammals, the activity of a single neuron does not produce behavior, but groups of neurons can. Neurons that share similar physiological and anatomical characteristics, receive and make similar connections, and contribute to similar functions are grouped into neighborhoods. Somata in the PNS group together within *ganglia*. In the CNS, neuronal somata are gathered into spheroidal collections called *nuclei*; into layers, termed *laminae*; or scattered in a *tegmental* or *reticulated* pattern. Laminae that are organized along the outer rind of the brain form a *cortex* (from Latin for "bark"). There are two cortices: in the cerebellum and in the cerebrum. When not otherwise specified, the term "cortex" invariably refers to *cerebral* cortex. A distinction is made between the three-layered cerebral cortex (e.g., hippocampus) found in both reptiles and mammals and the six-layered *neocortex* found only in mammals.

When neurons connected by synaptic contacts produce a certain outcome, such as visual perception or voluntary movement, we talk of a *pathway*. Most of this book concerns pathways. We follow voluntary motor and autonomic motor pathways from the CNS to the PNS, and we follow sensory pathways from the PNS to the CNS.

A major distinction between central and peripheral neurons derives from their different developmental lineages. Peripheral neurons derive from either neural crest or placodes, whereas central neurons derive from neural tube. Because the developmental history of central and peripheral neurons differs, so do the disorders that affect either central (e.g., autism, intellectual disability) or peripheral (e.g., hereditary sensory autonomic neuropathies) neurons. Neurons are deemed central or peripheral based on the location of their cell body (Fig. 2-4). For example, *a neuron in a sensory ganglion is a peripheral neuron because its soma is located in the periphery; this holds true even though the cell's axon enters the CNS.* By the same rule, motoneurons that have their cell bodies in the CNS are considered central neurons even though they send their axons into the periphery.

A second distinction between the central and peripheral nervous systems is an anatomical one. The CNS is surrounded by the three meningeal layers: the dura, arachnoid, and pia mater. The integrity of these membranes is essential for the mechanical and chemical protection of the CNS. Yet the meninges have a weakness, which is exploited by *polio* and *rabies viruses* as well as by *tetanus toxin*. None of these pathogens can cross the meninges, and yet all can gain access to central neurons. This access is accomplished by using a "Trojan horse" strategy (see Box 2-3). Motoneurons pick up the virus or toxin at their synaptic terminal and transport it through the meninges inside of the motoneuronal axon. Thus, central neurons have vulnerabilities to peripheral substances.

Pathways are multineuronal, multisynaptic chains of connections between batches of neurons that are located at some distance from each other. Axons are the means by which neurons communicate from one location to another within a pathway. The axons form bundles, which are termed *tracts* in the CNS and *nerves* in the PNS. Although not all axons are myelinated, virtually all tracts have at least some myelinated axons, and, since myelin is white, most tracts have an overall white appearance. In contrast, nuclei and cortices that are dominated by cells and dendrites appear gray in unstained brains. Thus, regions of cells are termed *gray matter*, and areas containing axonal tracts are termed *white matter*. It should be remembered that various histological stains can alter the appearance of gray matter, white matter, or both. For example, application of myelin stains renders white matter blue or black and makes the unstained gray matter appear white. Indeed, many of the photomicrographs in this book, particularly those in Section 2, are of

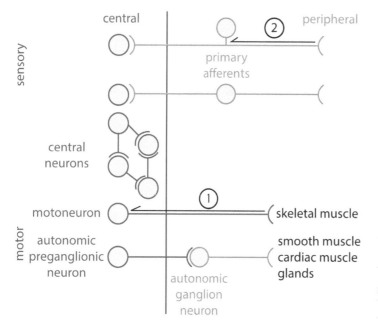

central   peripheral

sensory

primary
afferents

central
neurons

motor

motoneuron   skeletal muscle

autonomic
preganglionic   smooth muscle
neuron   cardiac muscle
                                            glands
autonomic
ganglion
neuron

Figure 2-4 The distinction between central and peripheral cells is based on the location of the soma. Most neurons of the brain and spinal cord are contained entirely within the central nervous system (central neurons), within the meninges. However, whereas the dendrites and somata of motoneurons and autonomic preganglionic neurons are within the central nervous system, the axons of these cells exit the meninges to access the periphery. Cells of the enteric nervous system and autonomic ganglion cells (also termed postganglionic neurons) are contained entirely within the periphery. In contrast, sensory afferents send an axon into the central nervous system and thereby cross the meninges. Retrograde transport through motoneuronal axons provides the main route through which substances may access the central nervous system from the periphery (*half arrow marked 1*). Herpes virus may travel through primary afferent processes to access peripheral sensory ganglia (*half arrow marked 2*) but does not typically enter the central nervous system. In this and other diagrammatic representations, cells are not represented to scale.

myelin-stained tissue in which "white matter" appears dark and "gray matter" appears light.

GLIAL CELL TYPES

Most glial cells arise from ectoderm and are termed *macroglia*, whereas fewer than 5% are thought to arise from the hematopoietic line and are termed *microglia*. There are four main types of macroglia. Two types of macroglia are part of the PNS:

- *Schwann cells* provide myelin to peripheral axons.

- *Satellite cells* support peripheral neurons in sensory and autonomic ganglia.

The other two types reside in the CNS:

- *Oligodendrocytes* provide myelin to central axons and comprise roughly 75% of central glia.

- *Astrocytes* support central neurons and synapses and are critical for normal development; they comprise roughly 20% of central glia.

Schwann cells and oligodendrocytes provide myelin. Many things can go wrong with mature myelin. For example, the myelin wrapping can loosen, the immune system may attack and break down myelin, or a mutation may prevent production of a molecule critical to myelination.

When myelin is compromised for any reason, we term this *demyelination*. Demyelination inevitably impairs neuronal communication by altering the timing of action potentials (see Chapter 10).

Schwann cells provide myelin for axons in the periphery and oligodendrocytes do the same for axons within the CNS. Associated with that difference, the molecular vulnerabilities of peripheral and central myelin are distinct. As a result, *demyelinating diseases affect myelinated axons in either the CNS or PNS but not in both* (see more in Chapter 10). In the quintessential central demyelinating disease, *multiple sclerosis*, myelin provided by oligodendrocytes is disrupted, but myelination provided by Schwann cells is unaffected. Conversely, a peripheral demyelinating disease such *Charcot-Marie-Tooth disease* involves damage to peripheral myelin only, leaving central myelin intact.

Astrocytes are the workhorses of the glial family despite comprising only about 20% of CNS glia. Astrocytes maintain ionic homeostasis in the extracellular fluid that surrounds neurons, playing a particularly important role in regulating potassium ion levels. Astrocytes rapidly clear some neurotransmitters, the nervous system's chemical communication agents, from synapses and thereby terminate many interneuronal dialogues. Astrocytes metabolize neurotransmitters and release the metabolites into the synaptic space, allowing neurons to retrieve metabolites that can be used to synthesize new neurotransmitter molecules. Beyond their importance to recycling certain neurotransmitters, astrocytes appear to stabilize synapses and modulate communication between neurons in important ways that are only recently beginning to be identified and understood. Astrocytes also contribute, sometimes in adverse ways, to many additional functions, including the response to injury. Finally, the astrocytic lineage is critical to development, as explored after a brief detour into microglia.

Microglia appear to derive embryologically from the same lineage that gives rise to blood cells, making them the only cells in the vertebrate nervous system that do not develop from ectoderm. Microglia resemble the peripheral immune cells known as macrophages. The function of microglia under healthy conditions is unclear. However, it is clear that microglia react to damage, even extremely slight injury, and disease. They sense substances indicative of damage or disease, including viruses, bacteria, and elevated extracellular levels of potassium ions, and they respond by becoming *reactive*. For example, microglia become reactive in response to human immunodeficiency virus (HIV); *prions*, the infectious agent that causes *Creutzfeldt-Jakob disease*; and *β-amyloid*, a protein that accumulates in the brains of patients with *Alzheimer's disease*. Reactive microglia are also found in the brains of patients with *Parkinson's disease* and in the spinal cord of animals with persistent pain. Once in the reactive state, microglia promote inflammation and phagocytose damaged tissue and foreign matter. Although inflammation may be beneficial at early stages of nervous system injury, it appears to be largely detrimental at later stages and is therefore the target of anti-inflammatory therapeutic efforts.

Glial cells are critical to the developmental processes that result in the mature nervous system. Glial cells direct axons to their targets, promote the survival of nascent neurons, and are needed for synapse formation. Many newborn neurons destined for the cerebral cortex migrate to their final destination along a scaffold composed of *radial glial cells*. In addition to serving as neuronal scaffolds, radial glial cells divide to give rise to neurons as well as glial cells; this role in cell proliferation is further explored in the following section.

PROGENITOR CELLS IN THE NERVOUS SYSTEM

One of the challenges of development is to generate the enormous number of cells in the adult nervous system, 170 billion cells in the (human) brain alone. This job falls to *neural progenitor cells*, a type of stem cell. Stem cells are cells that are not terminally differentiated and are capable of proliferation. Whereas embryonic stem cells are pluripotent and can divide into cells of every tissue type, stem cells in the nervous system are multipotent, able to follow only a select few potential routes of differentiation to become either neurons or glia. At each division, progenitor cells can give rise to two more progenitor cells—this is called *symmetric division*, or to a progenitor cell and a differentiated cell, termed *asymmetric division*. In the nervous system, asymmetric division of progenitor cells during development gives rise to another progenitor cell and a cell that will become a neuron, oligodendrocyte, or astrocyte.

Neurons are born and mature during development and thereafter cannot and do not divide. *When mature neurons die in the adult, their number is not replenished because there is no sizable population of neuronal progenitor cells.* Naturally, there has been great interest in the possibility that stem cells exist in the adult human brain and that these cells could be the source of new neurons. Part of the excitement around this possibility stems from findings in rodents. Rodents have two regions where neural progenitor cells, cells that can divide into neurons, are present in the adult brain: the *subventricular zone (SVZ)* and the *dentate gyrus* of the hippocampus. Stem cells in the SVZ move through the rostral migratory stream into the olfactory bulb. Unfortunately, the situation in the adult human is quite different. Neural progenitors in the olfactory bulb are only found in humans under the age of 18 months. Neural progenitor cells in the hippocampus that persist into adulthood are few in number and have limited proliferative potential. Thus, there is little realistic possibility that neural progenitor cells can repopulate the severely injured adult brain with new neurons.

Despite the limited potential for neuronal regeneration within the adult brain, stem cells hold great promise for elucidating the pathophysiology of neurological disease and designing novel treatments. In particular, *induced pluripotential stem (iPS) cells* can now be engineered from adult cells. The adult cells are de-differentiated through directed expression of a suite of transcription factors and then differentiated into neurons by a different set of factors. Using iPS cells from patients, the mechanisms by which, for example, a mutation in α-synuclein leads to the death of dopamine-producing neurons, and consequently to Parkinson's disease, can be interrogated. Furthermore, the efficacy of potential treatments can be tested on differentiated iPS cells from patients afflicted with neurological disease.

The vast majority of progenitor cells in the adult brain are competent to divide into either astrocytes or oligodendrocytes. Glial progenitor cells are present throughout the CNS. In response to damage caused by either trauma or disease, glial cells undergo reactive changes that are collectively termed *gliosis*. Glial progenitor cells divide, resulting in more glia, and may produce a *glial scar*. Mature astrocytes may also react and contribute to gliosis. Because glial progenitor cells are widespread in the CNS, this reaction occurs in response to diversely located insults. Glial scars severely hamper recovery by promoting inflammation and serving as physical roadblocks to cut or crushed axons trying to regrow. Efforts aimed at providing a molecular environment that antagonizes inflammation and favors regrowth of injured axons are generating excitement for the possible treatment of spinal cord injury and other central damage.

MOST BRAIN TUMORS ARE METASTASES FROM OUTSIDE THE NERVOUS SYSTEM

The most common form of intracranial tumor is a metastasis from a primary lung or breast tumor or a melanoma. Two factors are in play here. First, the incidence of primary lung, breast, and skin cancers combined is high, with nearly two new cases (1.7) per 1,000 in the United States in 2015 (see Table 2-2). Second, the population of dividing cells in the cranium that is at risk for transformation is relatively small (more on this later). Correspondingly, the incidence of primary intracranial tumors is about 0.07 per 1,000 in the United States. The likelihood of rogue cancer cells entering the brain at any one time is low, but the metastasizing cells keep on "trying" because neoplasms repeatedly shed cells

Table 2-2 **THE ESTIMATED NUMBERS OF NEW CASES AND DEATHS FOR SELECTED CANCERS ARE LISTED**

PRIMARY SITE	NEW CASES	DEATHS	CASE FATALITY (%)
Breast	234,190	40,730	17
Lung	221,200	158,040	71
Skin (melanoma)	73,870	9,940	13
Brain	22,850	15,320	67
Eye and orbit	2,580	270	10

These estimates are for the United States in 2015 and are published in the American Cancer Society's Cancer Facts & Figures 2015. For reference, the American population is roughly 315 million. Notably, only a small proportion of cancers of the eye and orbit involves the retina.

into the circulation. In the end, about 40% of patients with "the big three neoplasms" (lung, breast, melanoma) develop a brain metastasis. Thus, intracranial tumors from metastases outnumber primary intracranial tumors in adults. As one would expect from the low incidence of lung and breast neoplasms and melanoma in children, metastatic brain cancer is rare in children.

Metastatic tumors enter the brain from the blood stream, slipping through the blood–brain barrier (BBB) by mechanisms that are under active investigation. Metastases can form at locations throughout the brain, and the presenting symptoms are the result of this *location* rather than, for example, primary tumor type. Available treatments include surgery, chemotherapy, and local or whole-brain radiation therapy. The presence of multiple metastases, which occurs in about half of patients, bears on a patient's treatment choice. The occurrence of a metastasis in the brain is a "turning point . . . because it indicates that death is almost inevitable" (Taillibert and Delattre 2005). Even with treatment, median survival time is less than a year and 5-year survival is an exceptional occurrence.

PRIMARY INTRACRANIAL TUMORS ARE NOT NEURONAL

Primary brain tumors (from a tissue type found within the cranium) are not of neuronal origin. The absence of primary neuronal tumors is likely due to two factors:

- Mature neurons are terminally differentiated and do not divide; and

- There is a paucity of neuronal progenitor cells in adult humans.

The situation is different in children and consequently the types and locations of pediatric primary tumors are different. In children, progenitor cells are actively dividing in the hindbrain of children because the cerebellum continues to develop for years after birth. Progenitor cells continue to generate neurons and glia that populate the cerebellum. It is therefore not surprising that most childhood primary brain tumors are located in the cerebellum. The primary cell type involved is neuron-like in the case medulloblastomas that arise from progenitors that give rise to neurons, or astrocytic in the case of astrocytomas that arise from astrocyte progenitors.

In adults, gliomas represent the most common primary intracranial tumor. These tumors are thought to arise from progenitor cells that are competent to make new glia in the adult brain. *Astrocytomas*, neoplasms of astrocytes, account for roughly 30% of intracranial tumors. Unfortunately, many astrocytomas are malignant and spread diffusely along white matter tracts, precluding surgery as an effective treatment option. The most severe grade of astrocytoma is *glioblastoma multiforme*, which typically results in death within a year of diagnosis (Fig. 2-5). Effective chemotherapeutic treatment of malignant gliomas is complicated by the presence of tumorigenic progenitor cells that may not respond to drugs that successfully kill nondividing tumor cells.

Less common forms of gliomas include *Schwannomas* and *oligodendrogliomas*. The most common Schwannoma is a *vestibular schwannoma*, which develops at the root of the cranial nerve innervating the inner ear; these relatively common tumors are typically treatable. Note that axons in nerve roots are myelinated by Schwann cells despite their location inside the dural sac. Neoplasms can also stem from an overproliferation of nonglial neuroepithelial cells. Common examples of this include *meningiomas*, which contain cells of arachnoid origin, and *pituitary adenomas*, which contain pituitary cells, and, far more rarely, *pinealomas* that contain pineal gland cells.

Many primary intracranial tumors are benign, meaning that they do not metastasize within the nervous system. (As a rule, intracranial tumors do not metastasize to extracranial sites.) However, it is important to remember that benign brain tumors that cannot be surgically removed can be, and often are, lethal. This is because if benign tumors grow to occupy enough space within the cranium, the resulting increase in intracranial pressure will shut down brain function and, if unchecked, lead to death (see more in Chapter 8). In other words, *the benign oncological classification of a primary intracranial neoplasm does not in any way imply that the tumor is benign in a clinical or vernacular sense*, a point that patients and their loved ones need to understand.

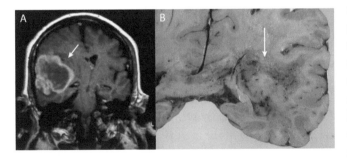

Figure 2-5 A: A large glioblastoma (*white arrow*) is shown in a CT scan. B: Invasion of the white matter by a glioblastoma multiforme (*white arrow*) is shown. Scan (A) kindly provided by Javad Hekmat-Panah, MD, and photograph (B) kindly provided by Peter Pytel, MD, both of University of Chicago.

PARANEOPLASTIC AND AUTOIMMUNE DISEASES OF THE BRAIN

Uncommonly, neurological disease can occur as an indirect result of a neoplasm located outside of the nervous system. In paraneoplastic disease, a tumor located outside the nervous system releases a substance that negatively affects neural function or elicits an autoimmune reaction that in turn negatively affects neural function. An example of the former type of paraneoplastic disease is *Cushing's syndrome* resulting from the release of either adrenocorticotropic hormone (ACTH) or a substance that mimics ACTH (see Chapter 27). Patients with Cushing's syndrome typically have upper body obesity, excess hair growth, hypertension, and increased thirst coupled with excess micturition reflective of impaired fluid homeostasis. (Note that Cushing's syndrome is named after *Cushing's disease*, which involves the same symptoms as the result of an adenoma of ACTH-releasing pituitary cells.) The paraneoplastic version of Cushing's syndrome is secondary to a tumor such as a small-cell lung carcinoma that secretes ACTH. Cushing's syndrome can also result from prescribed steroid medications, which is in fact the most common cause.

Lambert-Eaton syndrome is an example of an autoimmune paraneoplastic disease in which antibodies are formed in response to antigens produced by a tumor, typically a small-cell lung carcinoma. The antibodies impair synaptic transmission (see Chapter 11), and the most affected type of synapse is that between a motoneuron and skeletal muscle. As a result, patients with Lambert-Eaton syndrome are weak.

Recently (in the past 10 years), a group of diseases termed *autoimmune encephalitis* has come to light. The first member of this disease family to be discovered was *anti-NMDA-receptor antibody encephalopathy*, which occurs when antibodies against the N-methyl-D-aspartate (NMDA) receptor, a widespread receptor for the neurotransmitter glutamate, gain access to the brain. Anti-NMDA receptor antibodies can be made in response to an ovarian tumor called a *teratoma*, a weird type of tumor that contains derivatives from two or three germ layers rather than only a single tissue type as is true of most tumors. Some teratomas have teeth, hair, bone, or miniature portions of an organ. Other patients with anti-NMDA receptor encephalitis do not have a tumor and start making anti-NMDA receptor antibodies idiopathically, or for no discernible reason. The proportion of patients with and without a teratoma is not yet clear. Whether through stimulation of receptor endocytosis or competitive antagonism, the antibodies reduce the number of NMDA receptors available for glutamate binding and thereby work against and depress glutamatergic transmission at the NMDA receptor. The effect is similar to that produced by ketamine, an abused substance often called "special K," in that a psychotic break from reality can be produced.

How do antibodies gain access to the brain, which is normally protected by a barrier made up of tight junctions between epithelial cells lining brain capillaries, a barrier known as the *blood–brain barrier*? As it turns out, antibody-producing immune cells regularly enter the brain by *transcellular diapedesis*, which is a process in which one cell actually tunnels through another cell. Essentially, a leukocyte puts out a cellular protrusion that progressively invades a barrier cell until the protrusion reaches all the way across the barrier cell. Eventually, the leukocyte migrates across the pioneering path and, in this way, crosses the barrier cell and enters the brain. In several diseases, diapedesis into the brain is upregulated. Whether this upregulation causes disease or is the result of disease is unclear at present. It may be that disease starts with a few immune cells that invade the brain through normal diapedesis and that only after the production of autoimmune antibodies begins does diapedesis get upregulated.

The role of a compromised BBB in central autoimmune diseases such as the autoimmune encephalitis diseases, stiff-person syndrome, *Sydenham's chorea* (consequent to rheumatic fever), and multiple sclerosis remains to be fully elucidated. Even beyond these obvious suspects, neurodegenerative diseases such as Alzheimer's and Parkinson's are also thought to involve a breakdown in the BBB. Again, whether this breakdown represents the chicken or the egg is not clear. Inflammation, which occurs for many reasons including as a result of an ischemic or hemorrhagic stroke, leads to an upregulation in diapedesis. As tissue swells, the spaces between cells are stretched, and so at least some of this increase may occur through an increase in *paracellular diapedesis* in which invading cells pass through actual physical gaps *between* barrier cells.

DIVERSE NEURODEGENERATIVE DISEASES SHARE COMMON MECHANISMS OF PATHOGENESIS

Neurodegenerative diseases are marked by a strong dependence on age, occurring with increasing frequency in older individuals. Thus, neurons may live for decades before dying in association with a neurodegenerative disease. The neurons that eventually die actually survive and function normally for a remarkably long time, often the better part of a century. Yet, once cell death begins, an inexorable snowballing effect begins with more and more vulnerable neurons dying. Tragically, as of the early 21st century, no way exists to prevent neurodegeneration or even to decelerate the pace of neuronal death once the disease process starts. More hopefully, recent research advances reveal commonalities in the neurodegenerative process across a number of different diseases and offer the promise that prevention and treatment may yet yield to scientists' efforts. These commonalities in molecular, cellular, and systems-level mechanisms provide confidence that neurodegenerative diseases form a biologically meaningful group of disorders worthy of examination as a group.

Diverse neurodegenerative diseases share a disease process that was first identified in *prion disease*. Prions are *pro*teinacious *in*fectious agents; prion rolls off the tongue more easily than *proin* and also parallels the phonetics of *virion*, the term for an infectious virus particle. Prions are proteins with the same amino acid sequence as cellular proteins that are not pathogenic. However, prions (PrP^{Sc} for *pri*on *p*rotein *sc*rapie, the latter is a prion disease in sheep) and their normal cellular counterparts (PrP^{C} for *pri*on *p*rotein *c*ellular) differ in their three-dimensional conformations. Prions *infect* through seeding a conformational change in PrP^{C} which, you recall, has the same sequence as PrP^{Sc}. In other words, upon exposure to a pathological scrapie prion, normal cellular prion proteins change their folding. They form insoluble fibrils. The fibrils accumulate into larger and larger aggregates. In humans, aggregates of PrP^{Sc} are responsible for *Creutzfeldt-Jacob Disease* (CJD), an aggressive and uniformly lethal disease characterized by rapidly progressing dementia. Patients typically die within 6 months of diagnosis, and there is no treatment. The brains of patients with CJD are spongy, or *spongiform*, because of widespread neuronal death that produces actual holes in the brain.

Aggregations of insoluble fibrils made of pathological proteins also occur in neurodegenerative diseases that do not involve prions. Diseases that involve pathological protein aggregations include *Alzheimer's, Parkinson's,* and *Huntington's* diseases; *amytrophic lateral sclerosis* (*ALS*), and *spinocerebellar ataxias*. A diverse set of proteins capable of pathological aggregation includes tau (a microtubule-associated protein; see earlier discussion), *β-amyloid, α-synuclein, TDP-43,* and *huntingtin*. The latter is noteworthy because it exemplifies a polyglutamine protein that results from an excess of *tri-nucleotide repeats*, in this case in the gene coding for the huntingtin protein. The CAG repeats found in patients with Huntington's disease and several forms of inherited spinocerebellar ataxia result in proteins with an excessively long chain of glutamines at the N-terminus, giving rise to the term *polyglutamine disorder*. The connection between excessively long sequences of glutamines and neurodegeneration appears to be the propensity for polyglutamine-proteins to adopt a pathological conformation and form insoluble fibrils.

The proteins that form pathological aggregates differ across different neurodegenerative diseases as well as between patients with the same disease. For example, accumulations of α-synuclein, β-amyloid, and huntingtin are most common in Parkinson's, Alzheimer's, and Huntington's disease, respectively. Yet, one patient with Alzheimer's disease may have aggregates of α-synuclein as well as β-amyloid and another only the latter. Probably the most common protein aggregate across all of the neurodegenerative diseases is one of tau fibrils, which are found in patients with Parkinson's, Alzheimer's, and Huntington's disease as well as in brains from patients with *chronic traumatic encephalopathy (CTE)*, *progressive supranuclear palsy (PSP)*, and *frontotemporal dementia* (Fig. 2-6).

The involvement of tau in multiple neurodegenerative diseases highlights the importance of axonal transport to neurodegeneration. As discussed earlier, fresh synaptic proteins made in the soma need to make their way to the synaptic terminal, and used-up, damaged proteins as well as protein aggregates must make the reverse trip to be cleared by lysosomes in the cell body. Imagine that this process is impaired or slowed by only an infinitesimal amount. After years and years and decades of accumulated damage,

a neuron may reach a breaking point that sends that neuron to its demise. In support of this idea, mutated and variant forms of proteins that impact intracellular protein trafficking—such as kinesins involved in anterograde transport and dynactin, a component of the retrograde transport machinery—are associated with an increased risk for several neurodegenerative diseases.

Protein aggregation and subsequent death of one, ten, or even a thousand neurons would not produce the devastating results that come with neurodegenerative disease. The *devastation results from cell death that follows synaptically connected neurons, eventually destroying entire pathways*. As with prions, pathological aggregates of tau, for example, can travel trans-synaptically to infect the next neuron in a pathway. In this way, cell loss progressively visits successive brain regions. Different neurodegenerative diseases are associated with the loss of different pathways, which in turn results in disease-specific symptoms. For example, Parkinson's disease is associated with the loss of midbrain neurons that project to the striatum. This loss produces a poverty of movement. On the other hand, Alzheimer's disease involves loss of neurons in the medial temporal lobe and consequently the loss of declarative memory formation.

In sum, neurodegenerative disease, a modern scourge that tempers enthusiasm over medical advances to prolong life, is slowly yielding to focused scientific investigation that mixes basic exploration with translational inquiry.

ADDITIONAL READING

Cahalan S. *Brain on Fire: My Month of Madness*. New York: Simon & Schuster; 2013.

Carman CV. Mechanisms for transcellular diapedesis: Probing and pathfinding by 'invadosome-like protrusions'. *J Cell Sci.* 122: 3025–3035, 2009.

Crawford AH, Stockley JH, Tripathi RB, Richardson WD, Franklin RJ. Oligodendrocyte progenitors: Adult stem cells of the central nervous system? *Exp Neurol.* 260: 50–55, 2014.

Dheen ST, Kaur C, Ling EA. Microglial activation and its implications in the brain diseases. *Curr Med Chem.* 14: 1189–1197, 2007.

El Waly B, Macchi M, Cayre M, Durbec P. Oligodendrogenesis in the normal and pathological central nervous system. *Front Neurosci.* 8: 145, 2014.

Gavrilovic IT, Posner JB. Brain metastases: Epidemiology and pathophysiology. *J Neurooncol.* 75: 5–14, 2005.

Herculano-Houzel S. The glia/neuron ratio: How it varies uniformly across brain structures and species and what that means for brain physiology and evolution. *Glia.* 62:1377–1391, 2014.

Herrup K, Yang Y. Cell cycle regulation in the postmitotic neuron: Oxymoron or new biology? *Nat Rev Neurosci.* 8: 368–378, 2007.

Holmes BB, Diamond MI. Prion-like properties of Tau protein: The importance of extracellular Tau as a therapeutic target. *J Biol Chem.* 289: 19855–19861, 2014.

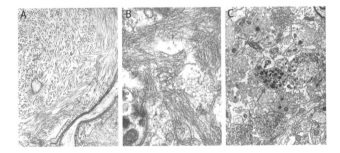

Figure 2-6 Electromicrographs from an Alzheimer's disease patient showing neurofibrillary tangles and plaques. A: Aggregations of tau, termed paired helical filaments, form insoluble neurofibrillary tangles. B: Aggregates of amyloid form fibrils. C: Amyloid collects to form plaques in the brains of affected individuals (*red arrow*). Photomicrographs kindly provided by Eliezer Masliah, MD, University of California, San Diego.

Hunn BH, Cragg SJ, Bolam JP, Spillantini MG, Wade-Martins R. Impaired intracellular trafficking defines early Parkinson's disease. *Trends Neurosci*. 38: 178–188, 2015.

Langley RR, Fidler IJ. The seed and soil hypothesis revisited—the role of tumor-stroma interactions in metastasis to different organs. *Int J Cancer*. 128: 2527–2535, 2011.

Mota B, Herculano-Houzel S. All brains are made of this: A fundamental building block of brain matter with matching neuronal and glial masses. *Front Neuroanat*. 8: 127, 2014. doi:10.3389/fnana.2014.00127.

Peters A. Golgi, Cajal, and the fine structure of the nervous system. *Brain Res Rev*. 55: 256–263, 2007.

Sanai N, Nguyen T, Ihrie RA, et al. Corridors of migrating neurons in the human brain and their decline during infancy. *Nature*. 478: 382–386, 2011.

Seeley WW, Crawford RK, Zhou J, Miller BL, Greicius MD. Neurodegenerative diseases target large-scale human brain networks. *Neuron*. 62: 42–52, 2009.

Sotelo C. Viewing the brain through the master hand of Ramón y Cajal. *Nature Reviews Neuroscience*. 4: 71–77, 2003.

Taillibert S, Delattre JY. Metastatic tumors of the nervous system. *J Neurooncol*. 75: 1–3, 2005.

Wolfe MS. Tau mutations in neurodegenerative diseases. *J Biol Chem*. 284: 6021–6025, 2009.

SECTION 2

NEUROANATOMY

Neuroanatomy forms the link between physical structure and the sweet mystery of animal life. Neuroanatomy is challenging, presenting two obstacles to the beginner: vocabulary and spatial visualization. Concerning vocabulary, there are hundreds of common neuroanatomical terms, at least a few hundred of which you will learn here. The only approach to take is to dive in, engage, touch a human brain, and repeat. Regarding spatial visualization, the central nervous system (CNS) develops twists and turns, including a couple of impressive "comb-overs," that obscure the brain's underlying simplicity. Even as we follow its developmental gyrations, we maintain our fixation on the brain's fundamental geometry.

There is one more trick that eases the path to understanding neuroanatomy. Instead of learning a map of locations and connections, the essentials of neuroanatomy, here, metaphors will be used liberally to build a story of *functional neuroanatomy*. Consider that the brain is a major urban center. In this analogy, neuroanatomy would simply be the information contained in a detailed city map. Such an encyclopedic approach places equal importance upon the one-block alley lined with car garages and the central square occupied by city hall. A livelier approach is to start by learning the location and character of the city's major divisions— downtown, south side, west side, near north, and so on—before moving on to a more granular knowledge of individual neighborhoods.

Just as important as brain regions are the connections between locations. The brain uses major and minor tracts and projections just as city inhabitants move either speedily or at a leisurely pace from one place to another, employing highways, boulevards, roads, bike paths, and sidewalks. Finally, the specific weaknesses of different city areas to power outages, flooding, and bus strikes are needed for a deep understanding of how a city works and how it breaks down. In the same vein, we will examine the brain's major divisions, neighborhoods, highways, and geographical vulnerabilities.

3

DEVELOPMENTAL OVERVIEW OF CENTRAL NEUROANATOMY

THE TUBE WITHIN THE BRAIN

The early embryo contains a homogeneous sheet of dividing cells that develop into a complex, patterned nervous system containing billions of neurons in the human. This phenomenal transformation from a simple sheet of cells to a complex structure serves as a roadmap to understand the basic anatomical organization of the brain. In this chapter, we follow as a small number of ectodermal cells proliferate and fold up into a tube of neural progenitor cells, termed the *neural tube*. The adult central nervous system (CNS) retains the organization of the embryonic neural tube. This gestalt of brain neuroanatomy endures, and, for all its complexity, the adult human brain is still a tubular structure, albeit with many distracting features. Neural development is a framework for understanding brain structure and introducing central neuroanatomy. Developmental concepts such as proliferation, stem cells, patterning, and signaling centers are covered only cursorily.

PRIMARY AND SECONDARY NEURULATION FORM THE NEURAL TUBE

Neural plate cells proliferate and invaginate to form a neural fold or groove within three weeks of gestation (Fig. 3-1). During the fourth week of human gestation, the neural fold closes off to form a tube around a central lumen, the future ventricular space (Fig. 3-1B). Ectodermal cells then proliferate and, along with invading mesenchyme, cover the neural tube dorsally (Fig. 3-1C). Thus, the developed CNS is located deep to overlying skin, protected by the bony vault of the skull and the perforated bony enclosure of the vertebral column.

Neural tube closure, termed *primary neurulation*, starts at the junction of the hindbrain and the spinal cord, a site in the future neck, and proceeds in both directions. Later, neural tube closure initiates at a second site, located at the very rostral end of the neural tube, and proceeds caudally. The anterior end of the neural tube closes first because closure converges at the anterior end, which is near to both initiation sites. After the anterior opening or *neuropore* closes, the neural tube continues to zip up in the caudal direction until the *posterior neuropore* closes (Fig. 3-1A). When the neural tube between the anterior and posterior neuropores is closed, usually around day 28, neural tube closure is complete.

The anterior neuropore ends up within the forebrain, but the posterior neuropore is located in mid-sacral segments of the spinal cord. Subsequent to primary neurulation, secondary neurulation leads to the formation of the caudal portion of the sacral spinal cord. *The end result of primary and secondary neurulation is a long tube of cells destined to be central neurons and glia surrounding a central ventricle.*

A FAILURE OF THE NEURAL TUBE TO CLOSE IS A COMMON BIRTH DEFECT

Failures of neuroectoderm to properly close into a neural tube are termed *neural tube defects*, commonly abbreviated as *NTDs* (Fig. 3-1A). Some embryos with NTDs never come to term, being naturally aborted, often early in the first trimester when neural tube closure occurs. In other cases, a neural tube forms but remains open in a spot, either in the front or the back. A failure of the neural tube to close completely during the fourth week of human gestation is a severe birth defect.

The most severe NTD occurs when closure fails to initiate, resulting in an open neural tube and a condition called *craniorachischisis* that is lethal (Fig. 3-1A). Failure of the anterior neuropore to close produces *exencephaly*, another lethal condition in which neuroectoderm destined to become brain does not form a closed tube. As a result,

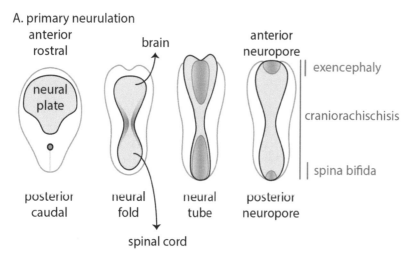

A. primary neurulation

anterior
rostral

neural
plate

posterior
caudal

brain

neural
fold

neural
tube

anterior
neuropore

exencephaly

craniorachischisis

spina bifida

posterior
neuropore

spinal cord

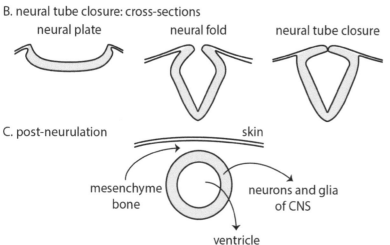

B. neural tube closure: cross-sections

neural plate   neural fold   neural tube closure

C. post-neurulation   skin

mesenchyme
bone

neurons and glia
of CNS

ventricle

Figure 3-1 A: During the third week of gestation, the dorsal ectoderm forms the neural plate anterior to the node (*dark circle*). By the end of the third week, the neural plate has invaginated to make a neural fold, which then closes up to form a neural tube. Neural tube closure proceeds both rostrally and caudally from a starting point near the location of the future neck. Two openings, the anterior and posterior neuropores, are the last areas of the neural tube to close. Failure to initiate closure results in craniorachischisis, whereas failure of the anterior or posterior neuropores to close results in exencephaly or spina bifida, respectively. B: Cross-sectional views of neuroectoderm are diagrammed from a stage after neural plate formation through to neural tube fusion. C: After neural tube closure, the overlying ectoderm separates from the neural tube. In the region of the spinal cord, bone and muscle invade the space between nervous tissue and the skin.

the future brain is externalized in the embryo. Over the course of the remaining fetal term, the exencephalic tissue that is exposed degenerates. Over time, surviving exencephalic embryos lose more and more brain tissue so that those embryos that come to term have very little brain left, a condition termed *anencephaly*. Slightly more than 50% of anencephalic cases die before or within 1 hour of birth, and less than 25% live for more than 1 day.

Failure of the posterior neuropore to close results in *open spina bifida*, in which the caudal spinal cord is uncovered, open to the outside (Fig. 3-1A). The degree of disability caused by open spina bifida depends on the spinal level at which neural tube closure stops. Patients may be weak or paralyzed in their lower extremities and unable to void. Additional potential problems stem from the additional trajectory traveled by the spinal cord, which may render the cord length insufficient for the length of the vertebral column and may lead to the spinal cord tugging on the brain. Indeed, individuals with open spina bifida often have an abnormality termed *Chiari* malformation in which the cerebellum herniates out of the foramen magnum and

into the spinal canal. They may also suffer from *hydrocephalus*, a condition of fluid accumulation in the brain resulting in increased intracranial pressure. The initial treatment for spina bifida, surgery shortly after birth, comes months after the initial insult as well as after further damage has occurred. Therefore, an innovative new strategy is to perform surgery on the fetus to ameliorate the severity of open spina bifida.

Craniorachischisis, open spina bifida, and exencephaly are defects of neural tube closure. Other types of defects may occur *after neurulation* if the correctly closed neural tube is incompletely covered by bone and skin (Fig. 3-1C). For example, an *encephalocele* is an externalized sac attached to the cranium. The sac is covered by skin and lined with meninges. Treatment is early surgery, and prognosis depends in part on the sac's contents, which can be either fluid or brain tissue, with the former associated with a better outcome than the latter. In the most fortunate cases, surgery can allow a patient with an encephalocele to live a relatively normal life. Another post-neurulation "defect" is *spina bifida occulta*, a common condition in which the vertebral bones at the mid sacral level are abnormal. The spinal cord is unaffected and therefore spina bifida occulta is an asymptomatic condition that typically goes undiscovered unless found incidentally during an imaging study.

An epidemiological connection between low socioeconomic status and the incidence of NTDs pointed to a possible role for nutrition in the pathogenesis of NTDs. We now know that proper neural tube closure requires *folic acid* and that folate supplements decrease the incidence of NTDs. Since primary neurulation completes by the end of the fourth week of gestation, at a time when many women do not yet know they are pregnant, folate supplements directed at the prenatal market would be largely ineffective. As a result, several countries, including the United States and Canada, have required folic acid supplementation of grain products such as breakfast cereals since the 1990s. This approach of ensuring sufficient folate intake among child-bearing women and the general population alike has resulted in a decline in the prevalence of NTDs, particularly in areas that previously had a high prevalence. In the United States, inadequate consumption of folate-supplemented foods and the lack of supplements in gluten-free foods may portend a future increase in NTDs.

The mechanisms by which folate prevents NTDs are not fully understood. Furthermore, this dietary factor does not act alone but rather interacts with multiple gene products so that two individuals with the same folate levels can have different clinical outcomes. Roughly 30% of NTDs are not sensitive to folate. Recent evidence suggests that, at least in some cases, these defects may be rescued by supplemental inositol.

THE NEURAL TUBE GROWS, BULGES, AND CONTRACTS TO FORM THE FIVE MAJOR DIVISIONS OF THE CNS

Post-neurulation, the neural tube reaches from a caudal point that will eventually become the *conus medullaris*, or caudal end of the spinal cord, rostrally to the *lamina terminalis*, the rostral end of the neural tube (Fig. 3-2). The lamina terminalis, at the very front of the neural tube on day 28 ends up located *deep* within the adult human brain. A major goal of this chapter is to understand how the lamina terminalis becomes buried within the cerebrum and thereby enable a gestalt perspective on brain anatomy. If we accomplish this mission, the reader will be able to orient to any image of a brain, regardless of whether that image is an

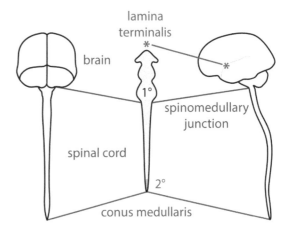

Figure 3-2 Immediately after neural tube closure, the embryonic central nervous system (*middle*) consists of the developing spinal cord and three vesicles that will comprise the adult brain. Almost all of the neural tube is formed by primary neurulation (*stippled area marked 1°*). Secondary neurulation (2°) forms the spinal cord from mid-sacral levels to the conus medullaris, the caudal tip of the spinal cord. The rostral end of the neural tube, the lamina terminalis (*), ends up at a site that is buried deep within the adult brain (left from a posterior view and right from a side view). The junction between the developing spinal cord and brain is the spinomedullary junction. Note that drawings are schematic and not to scale.

unstained slice, computed tomography (CT) scan, or magnetic resonance imaging (MRI) image.

Let's get started. At the end of the fourth gestational week, the closed neural tube contains three bulges or *vesicles* at its rostral end (Fig. 3-3A). The three vesicles destined to become the brain are, from front to back:

- *Prosencephalon*, which will develop into the forebrain
- *Mesencephalon*, which will develop into the midbrain
- *Rhombencephalon*, which will develop into the hindbrain

The most caudal portion of the neural tube develops into the spinal cord. The level at which the rhombencephalon and spinal cord meet develops into the *spinomedullary junction*, which is located at the *foramen magnum*.

At about the fifth week of gestation, the prosencephalon divides into the *telencephalon* and the *diencephalon* (Fig. 3-3B). Almost immediately after forming, the single telencephalic vesicle invaginates at the midline to become two telencephalic hemispheres. Since the points of attachment for the hemispheres are off the midline, the lamina terminalis, representing the front end of the neural tube, is now located at the front end of the diencephalon (Fig. 3-3C).

The vesicles are the embryonic progenitors of brain regions in the adult. This means that the embryonic rhombencephalon is properly termed the hindbrain at birth. Adult structures retain their developmental origins in the sense

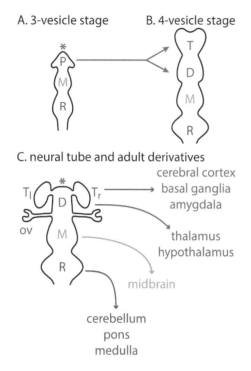

A. 3-vesicle stage

B. 4-vesicle stage

C. neural tube and adult derivatives

cerebral cortex
basal ganglia
amygdala

thalamus
hypothalamus

midbrain

cerebellum
pons
medulla

Figure 3-3 In the three-vesicle stage of neural development, the embryonic brain (A) consists of the prosencephalon (P), mesencephalon (M), and rhombencephalon (R). B: The prosencephalon divides into a caudally located diencephalon (D) and rostrally situated telencephalon (T), which together with the mesencephalon and rhombencephalon, comprise the four-vesicle stage. C: The single telencephalic vesicle invaginates along the midline to form the laterally displaced left (Tl) and right (Tr) cerebral hemispheres. The rostral end of the neural tube, the lamina terminalis (* in A and C), ends up deep within the adult brain. From the diencephalon emerges the optic vesicle (ov), which will develop into the optic nerve and retina. The derivatives of the telencephalon, diencephalon, mesencephalon, and rhombencephalon are listed.

that the hindbrain is rhombencephalic. Yet, as mentioned in Chapter 1, there are no commonly used terms for the telencephalon and diencephalon. Therefore, we continue to use the embryonic vesicle terms even when referring to the fully developed brain.

In the adult, the telencephalon includes both hemispheres of cerebral cortex, the core components of the basal ganglia, and the amygdala. The diencephalon contains the thalamus and hypothalamus. The mesencephalon develops into the adult midbrain, and the rhombencephalon develops into the adult pons, medulla, and cerebellum (Fig. 3-3C). The anterior third or so of the rhombencephalon gives rise to the pons and cerebellum, whereas the posterior portion develops into the medulla.

Beyond yielding the thalamus and hypothalamus, the diencephalon gives rise to bilateral outpouchings called the *optic vesicles*. The stalks of the optic vesicles become the *optic nerves*, and the cups at the end of the outpouchings become the two *retinas*. The retina is composed of the *neural retina* and the non-neural *pigment epithelium* (see Chapter 15).

Because it develops from the neural tube, the retina is part of the CNS. This is of great consequence because the retina is accessible without any invasive procedures. As the most accessible part of the CNS, by far, the retina is considered a "window to the brain." In essence, the CNS can be readily and noninvasively visualized by looking through an ophthalmoscope at the *fundus*, or back, of the eye (Fig. 3-4). Insults that profoundly impact brain function globally, such as increased cranial pressure, will cause changes in the appearance of the retina. In sum, ophthalmoscopy is a quick, important, and very inexpensive diagnostic tool.

In summary, by the end of the fifth week, the embryonic human brain contains four vesicles. From rostral to caudal:

- Telencephalon ≈ cerebral cortex, basal ganglia, amygdala

- Diencephalon ≈ thalamus, hypothalamus + retina and optic nerves

- Mesencephalon = midbrain

- Rhombencephalon = hindbrain = pons, medulla, and cerebellum

The spinal cord and the four regions of the brain comprise the five divisions of the adult CNS.

THE TERRITORY ALLOTTED TO THE DORSAL TELENCEPHALON IS GREATLY EXPANDED IN THE HUMAN

At five weeks, the CNS of a human fetus resembles a long tube with two Mickey Mouse ears, representing the telencephalic hemispheres, at the front end (Fig. 3-3C). For inflexible, reflex-driven sea creatures, such an anatomy might suffice. On the other hand, mammals have evolved from terrestrial vertebrates who must combat gravity at every moment and modify behavior based on social interactions (see Box 3-1). The social complexity and interdependence of mammals has further fueled the need for more neurons, particularly in the cerebral cortex, to power evolutionary success.

The increase in the number of cortical neurons is not matched by proportional increases of neuronal numbers in other brain areas. As a result, derivatives of the neural tube caudal to the telencephalon line up in an orderly sequence from spinal cord to hindbrain, midbrain, and diencephalon. This orderliness breaks down completely upon reaching the greatly expanded cerebral cortex. The cerebral cortex extends in all directions in what can be thought of as the "great cortical comb-over." The opportunistic expansion of

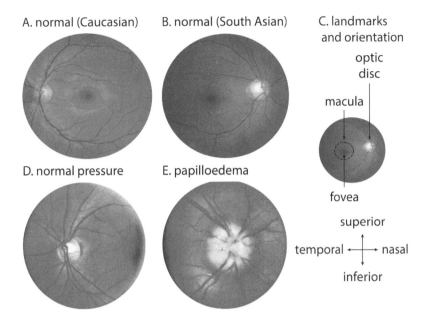

A. normal (Caucasian)   B. normal (South Asian)   C. landmarks and orientation

optic disc

macula

fovea

superior

temporal ←——→ nasal

inferior

D. normal pressure   E. papilloedema

Figure 3-4 Using an ophthalmoscope, also called a funduscope, a trained person may visualize the retina, which is the most accessible part of the central nervous system. Such access allows physicians to visualize not only retinal disease but also increases in intracranial pressure. A–B: The normal pigmentation of the retina varies across people, with the retina of Caucasians appearing red, orange, and pink (A) whereas that of south Asians (B) and Africans (not shown) has a darker appearance. C: As a sentinel of brain health, the most important landmark is the optic disc where fibers leaving the retina gather to form the optic nerve and where retinal blood vessels access the retina. The optic disc is located nasal to the fovea and macula (region in dashed circle), the regions of the retina serving central vision. Thus, the retina in A is from the left eye and that in B from the right. D–E: Magnified views show the optic disc from a healthy individual (D) and from a person with papilledema (swelling of the optic disc) due to elevated intracranial pressure (E). Photographs in A and B are reprinted with permission from Quant L, Anatomy of the eye and the healthy fundus, in *Diabetic retinopathy: Screening to treatment* (P Dodson, ed.). New York: Oxford University Press, 2008. Photographs in C and D are reprinted with permission from Kennard C, Abnormal vision, in *Brain's diseases of the nervous system* (12th ed., M Donaghy, ed.). New York: Oxford University Press, 2009.

the cerebral cortex within the cranial vault produces juxtapositions that, although initially difficult to understand, are fundamentally straightforward, as we shall now see.

To accommodate the 15 billion cells of the cerebral cortex, the territory of the human dorsal telencephalon grows in every direction. It extends rostrally, ventrally, laterally, and caudally (Fig. 3-5). The volume of dorsal telencephalic tissue is

---

Box 3-1 **THE SIZE OF THE HUMAN BRAIN IS TYPICAL FOR A PRIMATE OF HUMAN BODY SIZE**

When comparing the size of brains across species, a common approach has been to express brain size in relation to body size. Indeed, within each mammalian order, there is a fairly tight correlation between brain and body size. Humans are prototypical primates with a brain-to-body ratio that allows for relatively small brains in a relatively small cranium to contain a huge number of neurons. In contrast, a typical rodent would need a 77-pound (35 kg) brain to house the average number of neurons in a human brain (86 billion).

Unlike body size, cellular scaling rules strongly and consistently influence the number of neurons in a brain. What this means is that the number of glial cells per neuronal volume, the density of glial cells, is highly conserved across mammals

as well as across brain regions. Compare the brainstem and thalamus, with relatively few neurons per unit volume, to the cerebellum where, thanks to the enormous number of granule cells, neurons are packed at very high density. The *number* of glia per neuron is nearly 50 times higher in the brainstem and thalamus than in the cerebellum. Yet the number of glia per volume of tissue is the same. The phylogenetic and regional constancy of glial number serving brain tissue suggests that glial cells serve similar neuronal processes in dendrites, somata, and axons alike. In other words, glial cells serve the same volume of brain tissue regardless of the mix of axons, small neurons, large neurons, and dendrites contained therein.

so great that the cerebral cortex covers the tops and sides of the diencephalon, midbrain, and much of the hindbrain. It is this radical "comb-over" that obscures the fundamentally tubular structure of the brain. Yet, even the cap of brain tissue formed by telencephalic expansion yields insufficient territory for the human cerebral cortex. In the human and several other mammals, cortical neurons populate a bulge of tissue that curves around and out, as a ram's horn does, to form the temporal lobe (Fig. 3-5B). The temporal lobe further hides the diencephalon, midbrain, and much of the hindbrain from view.

A. top-down view of telencephalic expansion

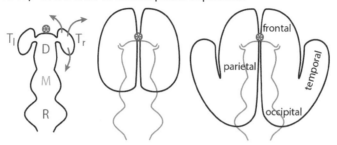

B. side view of telencephalic expansion

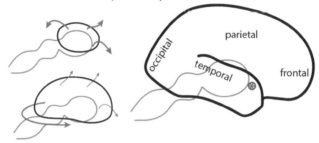

C. midsagittal cartoon of embryonic brain   D. midsagittal view of adult brain

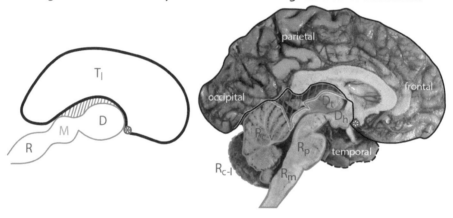

Figure 3-5 In the human, the cerebral cortex is greatly expanded. A–B: Top-down (A) and side (B) views illustrate the expansion of embryonic dorsal telencephalic tissue from its point of attachment to the diencephalon at the lamina terminalis (*red star*). The dorsal telencephalon extends in all directions until it covers the diencephalon and mesencephalon completely and also reaches the midline. Temporalization, the expansion of cerebral cortex to form a temporal lobe allows for more neural tissue devoted to language, face recognition, and factual memory. C–D: When viewed from the midsagittal plane (see Fig. 1-3), the frontal lobe remains connected to the diencephalon at the lamina terminalis. In both the embryonic (C) and adult brains (D), the parietal lobe sits atop the diencephalon from which it is separated by the velum interpositum (*red hatching*). In the adult brain (D), the visible derivatives of the diencephalic vesicle are the thalamus (D_t) and hypothalamus (D_h). The mesencephalic vesicle becomes the midbrain (M), and the rhombencephalic vesicle gives rise to the medulla (R_m), pons (R_p), cerebellar vermis (R_{c-v}), and cerebellar lobes or hemispheres (R_{c-l}).

Even as the cerebral cortex extends backward over the caudal divisions of the brain, it remains distinct from them. In other words, *there is no cellular bridge between the bottom of the cerebral cortex and the top of the diencephalon or midbrain* (Fig. 3-5C, D). There exists a space between the cortex on the top and the thalamus and midbrain below that is outside of the brain. This space is outside of the brain even though it is located deep within the cranium! This region or cavity, termed the *velum interpositum*, lies above the roof of the diencephalon and rostral midbrain (Fig. 3-5C). The velum interpositum houses large blood vessels including the internal cerebral veins,

as well as the (non-neural) *pineal gland*. Most importantly for the purpose of this chapter, if you can visualize that the velum interpositum is a space outside of the brain, even though it is located deep inside of the brain, then you have conquered the most difficult part of neuroanatomy. In this way, the velum interpositum serves as a great litmus test for understanding the three-dimensional anatomy of the brain.

The cerebral cortex is a thin sheet of laminated cells comprising only the outer few millimeters of tissue (Fig. 3-6). *Cortex* comes from the Latin word for "bark." Indeed cerebral cortex forms the outer rind of telencephalic tissue.

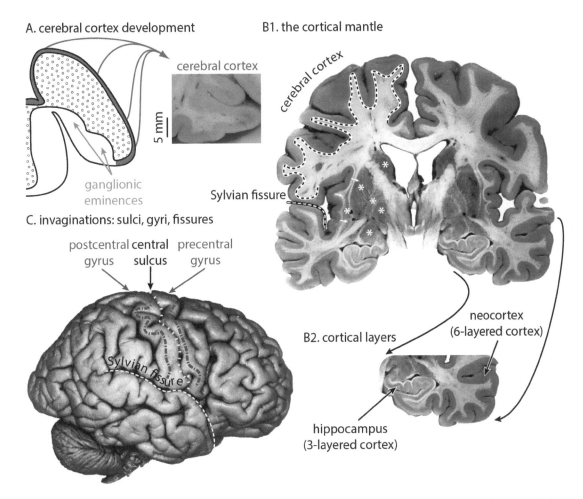

Figure 3-6 Cortex is a laminated neuronal structure (inset) on the surface of the brain that arises from the dorsal part of the telencephalic vesicle (A). Structures deep to the cortex, termed subcortical, arise from a pair of ganglionic eminences in the ventral telencephalic vesicle. B1: The cerebral cortex forms a mantle or rind on the surface of the cerebral hemispheres. Subcortical structures (*white asterisks*) are present deep to the cerebral cortex (*white arrows*). Most of the cerebrum is covered by six-layered neocortex (B2). The hippocampus, sometimes called archicortex, has three layers (B2). B–C: The surface area of the cerebral cortex is greatly increased by the Sylvian fissure and by gyrification, which produces sulci (*yellow*) and gyri (*blue*). The central sulcus runs from the dorsal midline to the Sylvian fissure and divides the precentral gyrus in the frontal lobe from the postcentral gyrus in the parietal lobe. Most of the cerebral cortex is deep within the sulci rather than decorating the surface of the brain.   Photographs in B1, B2, and C are reprinted by permission of deArmond S et al., *Structure of the human brain: A photographic atlas.* New York: Oxford University Press, 1989.

Embryologically, the cerebral cortex develops from the dorsal portion of the telencephalic vesicle (Fig. 3-6A). The ventral telencephalon gives rise to two *ganglionic eminences*, which will develop into the subcortical *striatum, globus pallidus*, and *amygdala* in the adult. In the adult, these subcortical structures are tucked within the confines of the cerebral cortical mantle (Fig. 3-6B).

Expansion of the space-hungry cerebral cortex within the limited confines of the skull requires more brain surface area. Cortical surface area is increased by formation of the *Sylvian fissure* that demarcates the temporal lobe (Fig. 3-6C). In addition, the cerebral hemispheres invaginate to form *sulci* (*sulcus* is the singular form), or chasms, and *gyri* (*gyrus* is the singular form), or ridges. Such *gyrification*, which is extensive in many mammals including

humans, greatly increases the surface area of the cortex. *In the human, only about a third of the cerebral cortex is exposed on the outer surface, with the remainder buried within the sulci* (Fig. 3-6B, C). The ultimate result of the dorsal telencephalic expansion is that if the human cerebral cortex were removed from the cranium, unfolded, and flattened out, it would occupy the area of a 22-inch (56 cm) diameter pizza.

THE LUMEN OF THE NEURAL TUBE DEVELOPS INTO THE ADULT VENTRICULAR SYSTEM

Tubes have an inner lumen, and the neural tube is no exception. The fluid-filled lumen of the embryonic neural tube is lined with neural progenitor cells that proliferate to form the brain *parenchyma* or matter (Fig. 3-7A). It is the embryonic lumen that develops into the *cerebrospinal fluid* (*CSF*)-filled ventricular system of the adult (Fig. 3-7B). Here, we fast-forward from the embryonic neural tube to the adult brain to learn the eventual fate of the embryonic lumen at different points along the neuraxis (Fig. 3-7B–H).

The spinal cord surrounds a central lumen called the *central canal*. The central canal, patent in the embryo (Fig. 3-7D), is clogged with ependymal cells and debris in the adult human, yet it still serves as a landmark. Just rostral to the spinomedullary junction, the central canal opens into the *fourth ventricle*, the ventricle present in the hindbrain (Fig. 3-7E). The fourth ventricle occupies the space between the medulla and pons ventrally and the cerebellum dorsally. If we removed the cerebellum and viewed the fourth ventricle from above, we would see a depression, or fossa, shaped like a diamond or rhombus. Consequently, the space occupied by the fourth ventricle is often referred to as the *rhomboid fossa*.

At the junction of the rhombencephalon and mesencephalon, the fourth ventricle narrows into a thin channel. This channel, present in the midbrain only, is called the *cerebral aqueduct* (Fig. 3-7F). The narrow cerebral aqueduct links the fourth ventricle to the *third ventricle* present on the midline of the diencephalon. From the diencephalic third ventricle, the lumen splits to form a Y shape with a pair of ventricles serving the two cerebral hemispheres. The invagination of the telencephalic vesicle (Fig. 3-3C) not only splits the cerebrum into two hemispheres but also splits the lumen into two distinct ventricles. Thus, each hemisphere has its own lumen, which develops into a *lateral ventricle* connected to the third ventricle through a short, narrow strait called the *foramen of Monro* (Fig. 3-7H). To accommodate the expanded cerebral cortex, the lateral ventricle in each hemisphere extends along every axis of telencephalic growth. This means that each lateral ventricle extends rostrally to form the *frontal horn* and caudally to form the *occipital horn* (Fig. 3-7C). Furthermore, the lateral ventricle curves around from an enlargement in the parietal lobe, the *atrium*, to enter the temporal lobe and form the *temporal horn*. Thus, the lateral ventricle resembles the logo of the University of Chicago, Chicago Bears, and Cincinnati Reds with the backward spur representing the occipital horn.

To reap all that we can from knowing the anatomy of the ventricular system, we need to understand CSF production. CSF is essentially blood that has been filtered through *choroid epithelium*, a specialized type of cuboidal epithelium located at specific spots in the ventricular system. Blood is delivered to the choroid epithelium from a rich supply of capillaries in the pia. Choroid epithelium, capillaries, and pia are tightly invested tissues that comprise the *choroid plexus* (Fig. 3-8A). The plexus is an intricate system of tiny branches with protuberances called *villi*. Now think about this: CSF is inside the brain and capillaries are part of the cardiovascular system, definitely outside of the brain. Thus, the choroid plexus straddles the barrier between the inside and outside of the brain. Consequently, wherever you see choroid plexus, you know that the side opposite to the ventricle is outside of the brain. This simple rule helps orient even the most experienced neuroanatomist to forebrain anatomy.

Since choroid plexus must border on the periphery, it is not present in either the central canal or the cerebral aqueduct, both of which are tubes surrounded on all sides by parenchyma. Choroid plexus is present in the fourth ventricle, third ventricle, and lateral ventricles, but only in specific places. For example, the third ventricle is surrounded by parenchyma everywhere except along the roof of the diencephalon. Recall that the velum interpositum sits in the space above the diencephalon and below the telencephalic hemispheres. Capillaries arising from blood vessels in the velum interpositum dive down into the roof of the third ventricle, are invested in choroidal epithelium, and form the third ventricle's complement of choroid plexus. Thus, choroid plexus is present in the roof of the third ventricle but not along its sides or floor.

The location of choroid plexus in the lateral ventricles is slightly more complicated. Remember that the telencephalic hemispheres expand as though traversing a ram's horn from the base to the tip. Choroid plexus runs long the inside of the ram's horn, lining all parts of the lateral ventricles except the frontal and occipital horns, two places where parenchyma completely surrounds the ventricular lumen (Fig. 3-8B, C).

Three anatomical structures follow the shape of the lateral ventricle (Fig. 3-9). As we saw earlier, the lateral ventricle in each hemisphere follows the general outline of the cerebral hemispheres and thus resembles a C (Fig. 3-7). Telencephalic structures that follow the lateral ventricle include:

- choroid plexus

- *caudate*, a part of the *striatum*

- *fimbria-fornix*, an important axonal pathway between the hippocampus—a cortical region required for memory formation—and the *mammillary bodies* on the ventral surface of the hypothalamus, also critical for memory

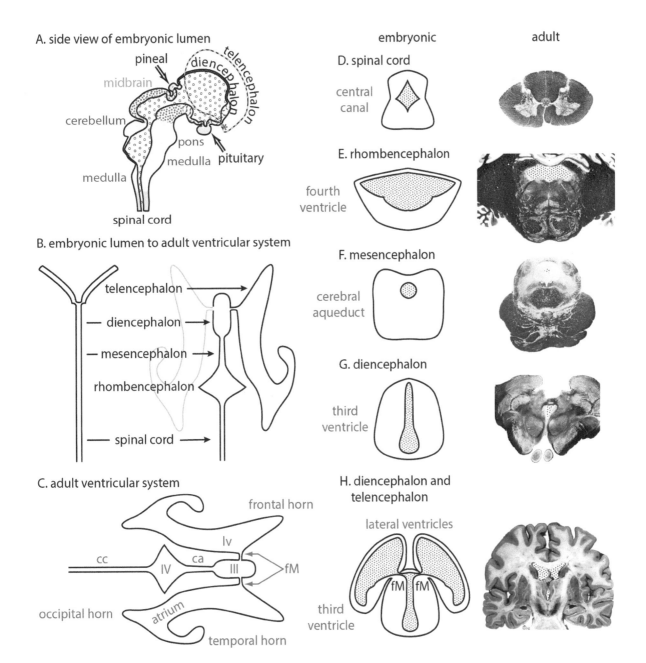

A. side view of embryonic lumen

pineal

telencephalon

diencephalon

midbrain

cerebellum

pons

medulla   pituitary

medulla

spinal cord

embryonic

D. spinal cord

central
canal

adult

E. rhombencephalon

fourth
ventricle

F. mesencephalon

cerebral
aqueduct

B. embryonic lumen to adult ventricular system

telencephalon

diencephalon

mesencephalon

rhombencephalon

spinal cord

G. diencephalon

third
ventricle

C. adult ventricular system

frontal horn

lv

cc   ca

IV   III   fM

occipital horn   atrium

temporal horn

H. diencephalon and
telencephalon

lateral ventricles

fM fM

third
ventricle

Figure 3-7 The embryonic lumen of the neural tube becomes the adult ventricular system. A: A mid-sagittal view of the embryonic brain shows the lumen of the neural tube lined by proliferating cells. B: The embryonic lumen begins simply and remains fundamentally simple in the fully developed brain. C: A cartoon of the ventricular system, viewed from above, shows the adult fate of the lumen at each level of the embryonic neural tube. The lumen of the embryonic spinal cord becomes the central canal (*cc*), which is not patent in the adult mammal. The lumen of the rhombencephalon becomes the fourth ventricle (*IV*) and that of the mesencephalon becomes the narrow cerebral aqueduct (*ca*). The lumen of the diencephalon becomes the third ventricle (*III*), and the lumen in each adult telencephalic hemisphere is a lateral ventricle (*lv*), connected to the third ventricle by the foramen of Monro (*fM*). In humans, the lateral ventricle is greatly expanded to accommodate the extensive cerebral cortex and stretches rostrally into the frontal lobe (frontal horn), caudally into the occipital lobe (occipital horn), and also curves around into the temporal lobe (temporal horn). The atrium is situated at the intersection of the parietal, occipital, and temporal portions of the lateral ventricle. D–H: Transverse cartoons (*left*) through the embryonic spinal cord (D), hindbrain (E), midbrain (F), diencephalon (G, H), and telencephalon (H) are arranged next to photomicrographs of brain slices from the same regions in the adult (*right*). The central lumen (*red stipple; red asterisk in D*) at every level of the neuraxis is marked. Note that the brain slices in D–G are stained for myelin so that white matter is dark and gray matter is light; the slice in H is unstained. Although the lumen adopts different shapes, it is located on the midline in the spinal cord, hindbrain, midbrain, and diencephalon. However, the telencephalic hemispheres are located lateral to the diencephalon, and, consequently, the lumen divides and courses laterally into each telencephalic hemisphere. The narrow foramina of Monro (*fM*) connect the lumen of the diencephalon to the lumen of each telencephalic hemisphere.   Photographs in D–H are reprinted by permission of deArmond S et al. *Structure of the human brain: A photographic atlas.* New York: Oxford University Press, 1989.

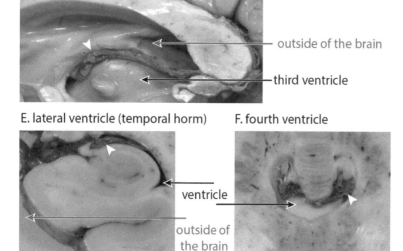

A. choroid plexus is a brain boundary

choroid
epithelium

pia

outside of the brain

pial surface

blood

basal lamina

ventricle (inside brain)

c s f

choroid plexus

B. locations of choroid plexus

C. lateral ventricles (body)

— lateral ventricle

— outside of the brain

D. third ventricle

— outside of the brain

— third ventricle

E. lateral ventricle (temporal horm)

ventricle

outside of
the brain

F. fourth ventricle

Figure 3-8 **A:** The choroid plexus is comprised of outpouchings of vascularized pia lined with choroid epithelium. Choroid epithelial cells have small protuberances called microvilli on their apical surface. Due to hydrostatic pressure, blood from the capillaries of the pia traverses the basal lamina and is filtered by the choroid epithelium to produce cerebrospinal fluid (CSF). The outside of the brain is located on the pial side of choroid plexus, and the ventricle is located on the choroidal side. **B:** Choroid plexus develops in specific areas of the developing neural tube (*red lines*). **C–F:** The choroid plexus (*white arrowheads*) is always located at the border between a ventricular space and a region that is outside of the pia and thus outside of the brain. In the hindbrain, arteries enter into the space between the cerebellum above and the pons and medulla below.

Photographs in C–F kindly provided by Peter Pytel, MD, University of Chicago.

It is worth remembering that the choroid plexus lining the lateral ventricle is actually sandwiched between the ventricle and the outside of the brain. This arrangement can be visualized as the choroid plexus wraps around the inside of the ram's horn shape of the hemispheres.

In the rhombencephalon or hindbrain, the roof of the neural tube opens up and is covered by pia. However the roof does not remain open. Along the edge of the hindbrain roof plate is the *rhombic lip* that houses

the progenitor cells that generate the cells that populate the cerebellum. Cells in the rostral rhombic lip give rise to the cerebellum (Fig. 3-10A). As the number of cerebellar cells increases, the cerebellum expands from the rostral part of the rhombencephalon, destined to become the pons. The expanding cerebellum grows back over the caudal part of the rhombencephalon, destined to become the medulla (Fig. 3-10B). As a result, the cerebellum is attached to the rest of the brain only at two sites on either

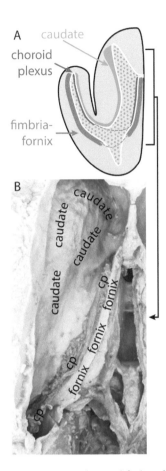

Figure 3-9 A: The choroid plexus, caudate, and fimbria-fornix all follow the C-shape of the lateral ventricle. A: A cartoon view from above shows the orientation of the three structures along the lateral ventricle (*outlined in white*). The scale of the fimbria-fornix in particular has been exaggerated for illustrative purposes. B: In this dissection of the human brain, the dorsal cerebral cortex, corpus callosum, and roof of the lateral ventricles have been removed. This photograph shows the view as one looks down on the brain and *through the lateral ventricle*. Rostral is located at the top of the figure and caudal at the bottom. The caudate, choroid plexus (*cp*), and fornix all follow the curvature of the lateral ventricles. Photograph in B reprinted by permission of Bruni JE, Montemurro D, *Human neuroanatomy: A text, brain atlas, and laboratory dissection guide.* New York: Oxford University Press, 2009.

side of the fourth ventricle. The attachments are called *cerebellar peduncles* (Fig. 3-10C). In an arrangement reminiscent of the cerebral hemispheres arcing back over the diencephalon, the cerebellum overhangs the entire fourth ventricle. Blood vessels enter between the roof of the fourth ventricle and the cerebellum and decorate the roof of the fourth ventricle with choroid plexus.

FROM AN ORDERLY NEURAL TUBE TO THE ADULT HUMAN BRAIN

Our picture of brain anatomy is almost complete but not quite. To recap, immediately after neural tube closure,

the divisions of the embryonic brain line up in a row: hindbrain-to-midbrain-to-diencephalon-to-telencephalic-hemispheres. Moreover, the two telencephalic hemispheres are physically separate, and each is linked to the diencephalon at only one place, near the lamina terminalis. Weeks later, the *comb-over* portion of the still-expanding telencephalon surrounds the underlying diencephalon on three sides without connecting to it.

The adult brain differs from the early embryonic brain in several important and prominent ways. Our erect posture places our brain at a right angle to our spinal cord. In fact, the human hindbrain is oriented just off the vertical, and most of the forebrain is oriented in the horizontal plane. Thus, the turn in orientation is primarily accomplished by a wedge-shaped midbrain (Fig. 3-5D). The other prominent differences between early embryonic and adult brains are two major fiber tracts in the forebrain. As illustrated in Figure 3-11, the fiber tracts join the telencephalic hemispheres to each other and to the diencephalon:

- *Corpus callosum*: A large fiber bundle containing connections between cortical neurons in the left and right cerebral hemispheres

- *Internal capsule*: Two large fiber bundles containing axons descending from the cerebral cortex that traverse the space between the cerebral hemispheres and the diencephalon, and, in so doing, form a physical connection

The axons in the corpus callosum and internal capsule are myelinated, rendering these structures white in appearance in unstained tissue (Fig. 3-11A). Moreover, these white matter structures contain axons and glia but are neuron-free. Although growth of both tracts begins during gestation, myelination of these tracts, and of axons throughout the nervous system, is not complete until years after birth.

Most of the axons, or fibers, in the internal capsule descend from the cerebral cortex to lower parts of the CNS. The remaining axons in the internal capsule travel from the thalamus to the cerebral cortex. Fibers of the internal capsule travel along a course that passes between the medial edge of the ventral telencephalon and the lateral edge of the diencephalon. These fibers physically link the telencephalon and diencephalon (Fig. 3-11). In fact, beyond the small attachments surrounding the foramina of Monro, the internal capsules are the only connection between the telencephalon and diencephalon. Thus, cutting the internal capsule on either side allows the telencephalic cap to be removed from the underlying diencephalon and brainstem.

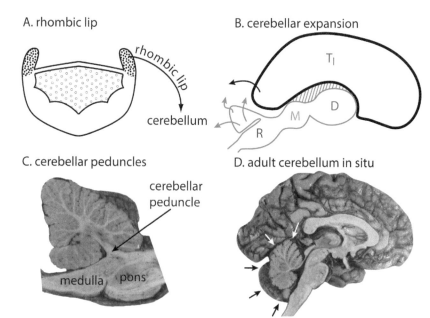

A. rhombic lip

B. cerebellar expansion

C. cerebellar peduncles

D. adult cerebellum in situ

Figure 3-10 **A:** The cerebellum develops from the rhombic lip, located in the anterior portion of the rhombencephalic vesicle. **B:** The cerebellum grows caudally back from the rhombic lip, eventually covering most of the medulla as well as all of the pons in the adult (D). **C:** The cerebellum is attached to the hindbrain only through the cerebellar peduncles. Photographs in C–D kindly provided by Peter Pytel, MD, University of Chicago.

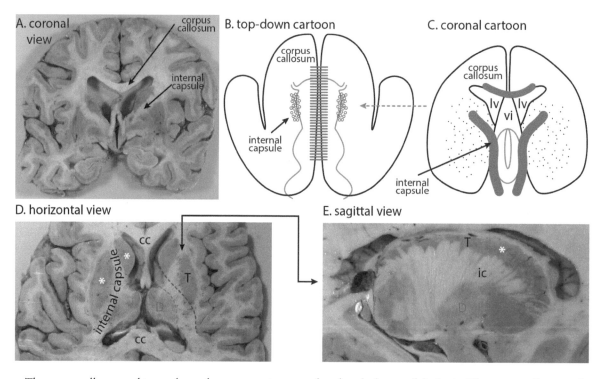

Figure 3-11 The corpus callosum and internal capsule are two major tracts that alter the layout of the brain. The corpus callosum is the major commissural tract that carries axons linking the two cerebral hemispheres and the internal capsule forms a physical join between each cerebral hemisphere and the thalamus. **A:** A coronal section through the brain shows both major tracts. **B:** A top-down cartoon shows the corpus callosum joining the two hemispheres. The internal capsule runs between the lateral edge of the diencephalon and the medial edge of each cerebral hemisphere. From the top-down perspective, the axons of the internal capsule run in and out of the page and are therefore depicted as transversely cut. **C:** A coronal cartoon through the brain (at the level indicated by the dotted arrow) shows that the velum interpositum (*vi*) is situated between the corpus callosum and the roof of the diencephalon. The internal capsule runs through the subcortical portion of the telencephalon (*stippled area*) and outlines the lateral edge of the diencephalon. **D–E:** Horizontal (D) and sagittal (E) sections through the brain show the internal capsule running between the diencephalon (*D*) and the subcortical structures (*white asterisks*) of the telencephalon (*T*). Abbreviations: corpus callosum, *cc*; internal capsule, *ic*; lateral ventricle, *lv*. Photographs in A, D, and E kindly provided by Peter Pytel, MD, University of Chicago.

THE CORPUS CALLOSUM CONNECTS THE LEFT AND RIGHT CEREBRAL HEMISPHERES

The corpus callosum contains axons originating in the cerebral cortex on one side destined for the *corresponding* area of cortex in the opposite hemisphere. It is the largest of the brain's *commissures*, white matter tracts that connect the two sides of the nervous system. The corpus callosum serves the full anterior-to-posterior length of the brain. Thus, neurons in frontal cortex send axons through anterior portions of the corpus callosum (*genu, rostrum*) to the frontal cortex in the contralateral, or opposite, frontal cortex, whereas the axons of neurons in the occipital cortex traverse the most posterior portion of the corpus callosum (*splenium*). Intermediate cortical regions are connected by the *body* of the corpus callosum. In sum, the corpus callosum allows the two cerebral hemispheres to share information and to seamlessly function with an apparent common purpose.

The corpus callosum is the major conduit for interhemispheric communication but not the only one. The *hippocampal* and *anterior commissures* connect the hippocampus and other parts of the temporal lobe, respectively. Additional commissures that connect subcortical regions include the diencephalic *optic chiasm*, the *posterior commissure* in the midbrain, and the *anterior white commissure* of the spinal cord.

People or animals with a severed corpus callosum are termed "split-brain." Some individuals are born without a corpus callosum due to *agenesis of the corpus callosum*. Others receive a callosotomy at the hands of a neurosurgeon in order to treat intractable generalized epileptic seizures. Interestingly, cutting the corpus callosum does not simply reduce the bilateral spread of seizures but actually reduces the incidence of seizure activity, suggesting a role for callosal fibers in facilitating activity in both hemispheres. According to this idea, callosal fibers excite neurons in the two hemispheres, taking them above threshold for epileptiform discharge at the same moment. Recent recordings support the finding that seizures begin simultaneously in both cortices. Cutting the corpus callosum would then block the facilitatory input, which may be just enough to take the excitatory input below threshold and thereby reduce the incidence of seizures.

In work that earned him the 1981 Nobel Prize in Physiology or Medicine, Roger Sperry studied split-brain individuals with his student, Michael Gazzaniga, who has greatly extended this work since Sperry's death. Split-brain patients appear normal upon casual observation and even upon examination. Yet, functional deficits readily become apparent using tests that restrict input and output to opposite hemispheres. For example, if you ask a split-brain patient to view an object located in his left *visual field* (i.e., to the left of where the patient is looking), the patient will be unable to name the object. This is because the left visual scene is represented in the right occipital cortex, which, without the corpus callosum, has no access to the left hemisphere needed for verbal language. Despite being unable to say the name of the object, the patient can correctly pick out the object with the left hand (controlled by the right cortex). Moreover, the patient can only pick out an object from the left visual field with the left hand that is controlled by the right hemisphere. The left hemisphere, which controls the right hand, has no clue that anything happened in the left visual world.

Let's take this one step further and consider a patient who was shown two pictures, a snow scene and a chicken claw, with the snow scene flashed to the left visual field and chicken claw to the right. When asked to point to the picture that best matched what he had just seen, the patient preformed perfectly: with his left hand, he pointed to a chicken and with his right hand to a snow shovel. So far, so good. Next, the patient was asked to explain his choices. He says, "Oh, that's simple. The chicken claw goes with the chicken. And you need a shovel to clean out the chicken shed" (p. 82, Gazzaniga, 2011). No mention of snow! Moreover, neither this nor similarly challenged patients say, "I have no idea why I did that," which would be the truth. Instead, a narrative is made up by the left hemisphere. Making up a sensible explanation or justification for our actions, telling a plausible story for why we do what we do, arises out of the left hemisphere playing the role of *interpreter*. The left hemisphere interpreter is not bound by truth and, in fact, is often responsible for confabulation.

Critical to understanding ourselves is understanding that *the interpreter works its confabulatory magic in all of us*, not just in split-brain patients. In a classic experiment by the American psychologist Norman Maier, people were asked to tie two hanging cords together. The cords were too far apart to make this a simple task. After subjects struggled with the task for a while, Maier nonchalantly set another cord into pendulum motion. Immediately thereafter, the subjects swung one cord as they would a pendulum and were able to grab both cords and accomplish the task. When asked how they came up with the solution, no subject offered that Maier's action had influenced them. One subject who was a psychology professor reported an elaborate image of monkeys swinging across a river that appeared to him out-of-the-blue as his motivation. Even when specifically told about the cue, subjects averred that they could see that others may have used the clue but were sure that they had not. Maier's experiment from the early 20th century has been repeated over and over with simple and sophisticated ruses and methods alike. The answer is always the same. We may report reasons for our actions, but, more often than not, these reasons have a sketchy relationship to actuality.

In the chicken–shovel example, the patient saw both of his hands with both hemispheres. In this way, the left hand's action of pointing to the snow shovel was seen by the left hemisphere, which was enough to spur the interpreter to come up with the shoveling-out-the-chicken-shed idea. But, if the left hemisphere is needed for fully understanding and expertly producing verbal language—which it is (see Chapter 16)—how was the split-brain patient able to use verbal instructions to point to the snow shovel with his left hand to begin with? The simple answer is that the right hemisphere has some capacity for language comprehension and is able to understand syntactically simple instructions and to even produce simple words nonverbally by, for example, arranging letter blocks with the left hand. It even appears that the right hemisphere's language capacities are improved by damage to the left hemisphere, suggesting some degree of ongoing suppression of the right hemisphere by the left.

Because the right hemisphere can understand simple instructions, it has been possible to test each hemisphere independently in split-brain patients. The picture that has emerged is that the hemispheres are not duplicates, with identical abilities and only differing with respect to the side involved. Instead, the left and right cerebral hemispheres each have particular propensities or talents that are not fully shared by the other. The left hemisphere, beyond housing critical regions involved in language, is particularly well suited to logical, mathematical, and sequential thoughts. In contrast, the right hemisphere possesses a more global perspective and is particularly good for non-sequential image-derived reasoning independent of language. For example, when asked to put blocks together to match a pattern, the right hemisphere controlling the left hand succeeds quickly, and the left hemisphere fails miserably in directing the right hand to accomplish the same task.

Both hemispheres may be able to accomplish similar endpoints but will do so differently. For example, to commit a list of words to memory, the left brain–dominated individual may string the words into a semantic mnemonic, whereas the right brain–dominated individual may imagine a picture that incorporates images reminiscent of the words. There is support for the idea that *dyslexia*, marked by a difficulty in learning to read, a left hemisphere–dominated function, is accompanied by enhanced spatial abilities rooted primarily in the right hemisphere.

DEVELOPMENTAL TERRITORIES CONFER A BASIC FUNCTIONAL ORGANIZATION TO THE BRAIN AND SPINAL CORD

Before beginning a spinal-cord-to-forebrain anatomical march through the nervous system, we glean one more point from the development of the CNS. Within each division of the CNS, areas with different functions in the adult arise from different embryonic territories. This is most simply illustrated in the spinal cord. In the embryonic cord, the central lumen has a bilateral inflection point or indentation. The inflection point, termed *sulcus limitans* (Fig. 3-12), separates the embryonic spinal cord into dorsal and ventral halves (see Box 3-2). Cells in the dorsal *alar plate* are destined to serve largely sensory functions, and those in the ventral *basal plate* serve motor functions in the adult (Fig. 3-12A). Thus, primary sensory afferents enter the spinal cord from the dorsal side, bringing information to the dorsal part of the spinal gray matter. Motoneurons innervating skeletal muscles have somata in the ventral portion of the spinal gray and send an axon out from the ventral spinal surface. Sandwiched between the sulcus limitans and the motoneurons are the autonomic preganglionic neurons, the nervous system's motor neurons for autonomic targets.

The dorsal covering of the neural tube opens up in the hindbrain as the fourth ventricle replaces the central canal. At this point, the sulcus limitans is still visible as an inflection point in the hindbrain (hollow arrowhead in Fig. 3-12B). Furthermore, the sulcus limitans in the hindbrain still separates the alar plate, giving rise to cells serving sensory functions, from the basal plate serving motor functions. The only difference is that, because of the opening of the fourth ventricle, *dorsal* within the spinal cord corresponds to *lateral* in the hindbrain, and *ventral* in the spinal cord corresponds to *medial* in the hindbrain. Thus, brainstem cells with a sensory function are lateral, rather than dorsal, to cells with a motor function.

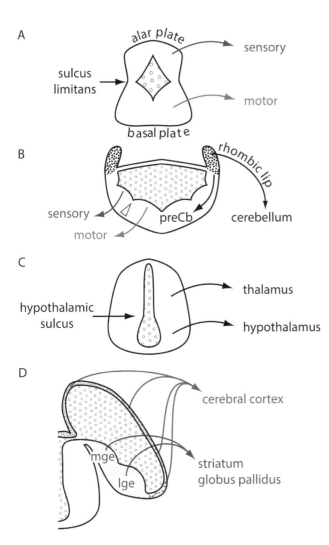

A

Figure 3-12 In the spinal cord (A), a distinct inflection point, the sulcus limitans, separates the alar plate, destined to give rise to neurons that receive input from primary sensory afferents, from the basal plate that gives rise to motoneurons, autonomic motor neurons, and motor interneurons. In the hindbrain (B), the sulcus limitans (*arrowhead*) again separates cells destined for a sensory role from those destined to become motor-related. Cells in the rhombic lip give rise to the cerebellum and to hindbrain nuclei that provide direct input to the cerebellum (*preCb*). In the diencephalon (C), the hypothalamic sulcus separates the territories of cells destined to become hypothalamus and thalamus. In each telencephalic hemisphere (D), the thin rind of the dorsal telencephalon becomes the cerebral cortex, whereas the lateral and medial ganglionic eminences (*lge, mge*) develop into the striatum, pallidum, and portions of the amygdala.

Within the embryonic diencephalon, the inflection point in the lumen corresponds to the hypothalamic sulcus (Fig. 3-12C). Dorsal to the hypothalamic sulcus, cells are destined to become thalamus—also called dorsal thalamus—and ventral to the sulcus, cells give rise to hypothalamus.

As we learned earlier, the embryonic telencephalon has distinct dorsal and ventral territories (Fig. 3-12D). Dorsally, the thin rind of tissue is destined to become the

To accommodate our upright posture, the human brain and spinal cord are oriented at right angles to each other. This difference in orientation is accomplished through a gradual change in orientation that occurs primarily in the midbrain but also in the hindbrain. Because of the right angle between the spinal cord and forebrain, there is also a difference in the meaning of directional terms within the brain and spinal cord of humans relative to quadrupeds. In essence, our forebrain has the same orientation as that of the quadruped but our spinal cord and also our hindbrain are oriented in a vertical rather than horizontal plane. For example, within the human spinal cord, the terms "posterior" and "dorsal" mean the same thing. Similarly, "anterior" and "ventral" are synonyms when applied to the human spinal cord but not when used with reference to the spinal cord of a quadruped. Basic scientists use directional terms appropriate for quadrupeds even when discussing the human spinal cord. On the other hand, clinicians typically employ "posterior" and "anterior" in place of "dorsal" and "ventral." In this book, basic terminology is employed and clinical terms are mentioned, an approach that prepares the reader to both understand the scientific literature and converse with clinicians.

Within the brain, orientation gradually changes from nearly vertical in the hindbrain to horizontal in the forebrain. Here, too, we employ the same directional terms that would be used for the brain of a sheep or donkey or rat. Thus, moving up the *neuraxis*, from hindbrain to the telencephalon, will be viewed as movement in both the rostral and anterior directions.

cerebral cortex. Ventrally, telencephalic tissue is amassed into bulges called ganglionic eminences. The territory occupied by the medial and lateral ganglionic eminences becomes striatum and pallidum, the two core structures of the basal ganglia. Within the telencephalon, there is some migration from cells' place of origin and their final location in the mature brain. For example, a population of cells in the medial ganglionic eminence ends up as interneurons in the cerebral cortex. As another example, at least one group of amygdala cells migrates in from the dorsal telencephalon. Despite these examples, most cells in the dorsal telencephalon stay in the cerebral cortex, and most cells in the ganglionic eminences stay *subcortical*, or deep to the cerebral cortex.

DEVELOPMENT CONTINUES POSTNATALLY

Development does not stop at birth. In fact, most of the neurons in the cerebellum are born during the first several postnatal years of human life. Axons are not fully myelinated until years after birth. The number of synaptic connections peaks within the first year of life and then steadily declines through *synaptic pruning* of unused or rarely used synapses. Pruning continues into the teenage years. More subtle changes than pruning also occur with adjustments of synaptic strength. Thus, connections are made, pruned, and fine-tuned at a steady rate throughout childhood and adolescence.

Learning to use our brain, learning how to interpret the neural signals evoked by external and internal stimuli, and learning the effect of activity in our brain on our muscles, is a process that occupies our infancy and childhood. As will be discussed in later chapters, the ability to develop certain capabilities is optimal during the early years of life. For example, animals, including humans, need to *learn how to see*, meaning how to convert neural signals arriving from the retina into the recognition and interpretation of visual scenes. If a cat or a human or other mammal does not see early during its life because of congenital cataracts, severe myopia, or the like, that animal will never see well. Even if perfect optics are restored to the individual during adulthood, the person will be unable to understand and interpret what he or she sees. The window of time when we must train our brain for vision occurs during early life. Missing that window means that vision will never be normal. Once adulthood is reached, the brain remains somewhat plastic although far less so than is the case during childhood. Beyond allowing adults to grow and change, learning in adults allows for partial recovery from brain injuries including strokes.

A DEVELOPMENTALLY INSPIRED VIEW OF ADULT BRAIN ANATOMY

Now we are ready to look at the adult brain and *see* the tube, present since the nervous system's earliest embryonic hours, within. A first step in achieving this perspective is the production of a two-dimensional representation of the three-dimensional brain. As with all map projections, flattening the CNS offers advantages and disadvantages. The advantages are that the fundamental organization of the CNS is revealed, serving to highlight the fundamental features of each part of the brain and spinal cord. The disadvantages, the loss of several juxtapositions that occur in the brain, will be corrected for elsewhere.

Figure 3-13A shows a developmentally inspired cartoon of the CNS. The spinal cord, midbrain, and diencephalon are lined up as they were in the earliest neural tube. In the hindbrain, the cerebellum sits *above* the pons and medulla while being connected only to the pons. To illustrate this, we cut the cerebellum down the midline and then unfold the cerebellar halves outward to each side. The telencephalic hemispheres are illustrated in isolation through virtual cuts of the internal capsule. Additionally, each hemisphere is spread out along the trajectory of the ram's horn so that the temporal lobe is shown lying to the side of the parietal lobe (Fig. 3-13A).

MAPPING FUNCTIONS ONTO THE SPINAL CORD, BRAINSTEM, AND FOREBRAIN

With our two-dimensional cartoon of the CNS in hand, we can now create a neuroanatomical map for the four functions of the nervous system introduced in Chapter 1: perception, voluntary movement, homeostasis, and abstract or higher function. The four functions will be mapped onto the three major parts of the CNS: spinal cord, brainstem, and forebrain. Moreover, since the spinal cord and brainstem work in concert with associated portions of the peripheral nervous system, spinal nerves will be considered along with the spinal cord, and cranial nerves will be considered along with the brainstem. Finally, differences between the midbrain and hindbrain, two CNS divisions that collectively make up the brainstem, will be noted. Let's get started.

Sensory pathways enter the CNS through the spinal cord, brainstem, and forebrain (Fig. 3-13B). The spinal cord receives all the somatosensory input from the body and a great portion of the viscerosensory input from deeper structures. This input arrives via *spinal nerves*. Spinal cord or nerve damage can impair the perception of touch, vibration, temperature, pain, and the position of the body from the legs, trunk, arms, neck, and back of the head. The brainstem receives a wide variety of sensory input via cranial nerves:

- Somatosensory input from the face, oral cavity, and anterior fossa

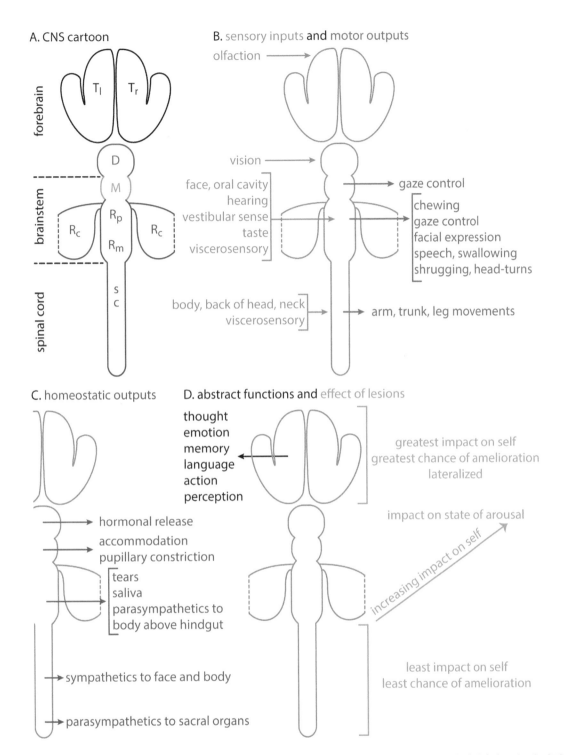

A. CNS cartoon

forebrain

T_l T_r

brainstem

D
M
R_p
R_c R_c
R_m

spinal cord

s
c

B. sensory inputs and motor outputs

olfaction

vision

face, oral cavity
hearing
vestibular sense
taste
viscerosensory

gaze control

chewing
gaze control
facial expression
speech, swallowing
shrugging, head-turns

body, back of head, neck
viscerosensory

arm, trunk, leg movements

C. homeostatic outputs

hormonal release
accommodation
pupillary constriction

tears
saliva
parasympathetics to
body above hindgut

sympathetics to face and body

parasympathetics to sacral organs

D. abstract functions and effect of lesions

thought
emotion
memory
language
action
perception

greatest impact on self
greatest chance of amelioration
lateralized

impact on state of arousal

increasing impact on self

least impact on self
least chance of amelioration

Figure 3-13 A developmentally inspired cartoon of the human brain and spinal cord (sc). For illustrative purposes, the left (T_l) and right (T_r) telencephalic hemispheres are shown unconnected to the diencephalon (D) and the rhombencephalic cerebellum (R_c) is filleted down the middle and splayed out. The brainstem consists of the hindbrain and the midbrain (M). The adult derivatives of the rhombencephalon include the pons (R_p), medulla (R_m), and cerebellum (R_c). B: The sources and modalities of sensory inputs to the spinal cord, hindbrain, diencephalon, and telencephalon are illustrated on the left. The skeletal muscle targets of motoneurons in the spinal cord, hindbrain, and midbrain are illustrated on the right. C: The autonomic targets of autonomic preganglionic neurons in the spinal cord, hindbrain, and midbrain are illustrated. D: A non-exhaustive catalog of abstract functions served by the telencephalon is listed on the left. As illustrated on the right, damage to different levels of the neuraxis impacts an individual's sense of self to varying degrees. The chance for improvement following injury also varies with the level of damage.

- Viscerosensory input from viscera above the hindgut

- Special sensory inputs from the inner ear, which supports hearing and the vestibular sense

- Special sensory input from the oral and pharyngeal cavities that support taste

All of the sensory input received by the brainstem enters into the hindbrain; the midbrain does not receive any sensory input. The final two sensory systems, vision and olfaction, depend on inputs that enter the forebrain. Optical information from the retina arrives in the diencephalon, and information about odorants enters the telencephalic olfactory bulbs.

Although the ports of entry for sensory inputs are distributed across the CNS, perception ultimately depends on the neocortex. Thus, sensory inputs must reach the neocortex for perception to occur. From the point of entry into the CNS, sensory information must traverse successively more rostral parts of the CNS en route to the forebrain. Consequently, damage to the brainstem can have adverse affects on hearing, for example, but may also disrupt somatosensory perception from the body. The all-roads-lead-to-Rome metaphor is apt, with the neocortex playing the role of Rome and sensory pathways serving as "all roads." It then follows that damage to the neocortex may alter any of the perceptual modalities.

The points of CNS exit for pathways involved in producing voluntary actions are restricted to the brainstem, both midbrain and hindbrain, and spinal cord (Fig. 3-13B). There are no motoneurons in the forebrain. Movements of the body, from the shoulders down, depend on spinal motoneurons and spinal nerves. Movements controlled by brainstem motoneurons and cranial nerves include:

- Shrugging and shaking the head in a "No" gesture

- Tongue movements important in chewing and speaking

- Movements of the upper airway musculature important to swallowing, speaking, coughing, and the like

- Facial expression

- Movements of the eyes to enable gaze control

- Jaw movements used in chewing

In the case of pathways critical to motor control, all roads lead *from* Rome, the metaphorical neocortex. Thus, motor control information travels down the neuraxis, traversing progressively more caudal parts of the nervous system. Thus, damage to the CNS impacts movements that depend

on motoneurons leaving the CNS from points caudal to the site of damage. Yet, all *volitional actions* are initiated by neocortex. Thus, voluntary motor control of any part of the head or body may be affected by forebrain damage.

Regarding homeostasis, we restrict ourselves to autonomic control pathways, output from the CNS that influences glands and cardiac and smooth muscle through an autonomic ganglionic intermediary. The forebrain, midbrain, hindbrain, and spinal cord all participate in autonomic control (Fig. 3-13C). The forebrain, specifically the diencephalic hypothalamus, controls the pituitary gland from which a wide variety of hormones is secreted. Pituitary hormones play critical roles in growth, fluid and electrolyte balance, thermoregulation, metabolism, mating and reproduction, and arousal evoked by stress. The hypothalamus is also important in setting the circadian rhythm through its influence on both the pituitary and pineal glands.

Brainstem and spinal cord contributions to autonomic control are many and varied but fall into two categories: parasympathetic and sympathetic. As introduced in Chapter 1, the sympathetic system enlists the body's energy resources to support action coupled to alert vigilance, whereas the parasympathetic system promotes rest, inactivity, digestion, and recuperation. The entire sympathetic output of the CNS arises from the thoracic spinal cord (actually T1–L2) and travels in spinal nerves (Fig. 3-13C). The output is topographic, so that sympathetic control of the pupil and facial sweat glands arises from high thoracic segments and sympathetic outputs to the bladder and colon come from more caudal spinal segments. Parasympathetic outflow destined to influence structures in the eyes, oral cavity, and most of the body emanates from the brainstem and travels in cranial nerves. Parasympathetic outflow destined for the bladder, hindgut, and sexual organs of the pelvic floor arises from the sacral spinal cord and travels in spinal nerves.

The control of autonomic function does not require neocortex as perception and voluntary movement do. Instead, the control of autonomic outflow is a distributed process with both local and distant brain regions playing important roles. In addition, autonomic control pathways are not as well-delineated as are the pathways for perception and voluntary movement. With few guiding principles on how CNS damage affects autonomic control, clinically relevant anatomical features will be described as they arise in our caudal to rostral tour of the nervous system.

Abstract or higher function, also called cognition, depends on the forebrain (Fig. 3-13D). The cerebral cortex, including both the hippocampus and the neocortex, are the stars of cognition. Although both cerebral hemispheres produce cognition, the left and right hemispheres are not simply mirror images of each other, as is thought to be the case in the rest of the CNS. As discussed earlier, the cerebral cortices in the right and left hemispheres have lateralized functions.

The cerebral cortex does not work in isolation, but requires the thalamus and basal ganglia for proper function. The midbrain and hypothalamus also lend a hand by controlling arousal state (Fig. 3-13D). Clearly, a person needs to be awake, responsive, and alert to fully express emotions and thoughts, learn from experiences, and recall past events. In contrast to the midbrain and forebrain, the spinal cord is not involved in cognition. In other words, a person possesses the same cognitive capacity before and after damage to the spinal cord.

AN OVERVIEW OF THE OUTCOMES OF NERVOUS SYSTEM TRAUMA

With an understanding of how functions map onto neural regions, we now examine the alignment between function and neuroanatomy from the perspective of each part of the nervous system. What deficits or consequences could result from damage to the spinal cord, brainstem, or forebrain? What are the possibilities for recovery? What is the impact of damage on the person's everyday mode of life? How does damage alter a person's sense of self?

The spinal cord is critical to movement of the body, sensory feelings from the body, and much, but not all, of the autonomic control of the body. Spinal cord damage, through trauma or disease, can produce profound losses such as the inability to voluntarily move part of the body or to control voiding. These losses require major changes in how one lives, such as adapting to using a wheelchair. The likelihood of symptom amelioration is low; the clinical picture 1 year after a spinal cord injury is likely to be not dramatically different from the picture at 1 week. Yet, spinal cord and spinal nerve dysfunction do not directly alter an individual's sense of self (Fig. 3-13D).

Forebrain damage produces, in most respects, directly opposite consequences from spinal cord injury. Forebrain damage is very likely to affect an individual's personhood through changes in personality, emotionality, mood, likes, and dislikes. It may in addition cause devastating losses such as *aphasia*, an inability to understand or produce spoken language, that diminish a person's ability to interact with others.

The good news is that in a sizable proportion of people with damage to the forebrain, such as that produced by stroke, the symptoms ameliorate with time (Fig. 3-13D). After a few years, acquaintances or even close friends and family may not be able to detect persistent changes. Yet, even such clinical success is almost invariably accompanied by a sense of change to the self by the *patient*. For example, 2 years after removal of a meningioma, one patient says that she is "a new person. My friends still think I'm the same but I know I'm different." Despite a clinical assessment that they have recovered, patients often view life as divided into "before" and "after," a testament to the inexorable link between the forebrain and the nuanced sense of self.

Damage to the brainstem can impair far more functions than are affected by spinal cord injury. Problems with balance and equilibrium, gaze control, speech, and swallowing commonly result after brainstem trauma or disease. Moreover, all motor information from the forebrain destined for the spinal cord and all sensory information traveling in the other direction pass through the brainstem. Therefore, brainstem damage can produce all of the losses of a complete spinal cord transection and then more. Amelioration of symptoms after brainstem damage is often intermediate, neither as dramatic as after forebrain damage nor as unlikely as after spinal cord injury. For example, Jean-Dominique Bauby's suffered a pontine stroke on December 8 and "did not fully awake until the end of January." Following this return to alert consciousness, there was little amelioration of Bauby's incapacitation.

As with spinal cord injury, brainstem damage leaves cognition intact. Yet the changes produced by damage in either region are unrelenting. Every moment of one's life with locked-in syndrome or as a quadriplegic is a radical departure from any moment prior, unimaginable to the previously healthy person. As Bauby eloquently subtitled his book, locked-in syndrome can be experienced as a *life in death*. In the end, there is exactly one expert on the experience of neurological impairment and that is the patient.

ADDITIONAL READING

Baker CVH, Bronner-Fraser M. Vertebrate cranial placodes: Embryonic induction. *Dev Biol.* 232: 1–61, 2001.

Bedeschi MF, Bonaglia MC, Grasso R, et al. Agenesis of the corpus callosum: Clinical and genetic study in 63 young patients. *Pediatr Neurol.* 34: 186–193, 2006.

Brugmann SA, Moody SA. Induction and specification of the vertebrate ectodermal placodes: Precursors of the cranial sensory organs. *Biol Cell.* 97: 303–319, 2005.

Copp AJ. Neurulation in the cranial region—normal and abnormal. *J Anat.* 207: 623–635, 2005.

Gazzaniga MS. *Who's in Charge?* New York: HarperCollins Publishers, 2011.

Greene ND, Copp AJ. Neural tube defects. *Annu Rev Neurosci.* 37: 221–242, 2014.

Matsuo A, Ono T, Baba H, Ono K. Callosal role in generation of epileptiform discharges: Quantitative analysis of EEGs recorded in patients undergoing corpus callosotomy. *Clin Neurophysiol.* 114: 2165–2171, 2003.

Nakatsu T, Uwabe C, Shiota K. Neural tube closure in humans initiates at multiple sites: Evidence from human embryos and implications for the pathogenesis of neural tube defects. *Anat Embryol.* 201: 455–466, 2001.

Nisbett R, Wilson T. Telling more than we can know: Verbal reports on mental processes. *Psychol Rev.* 84: 231–259, 1977.

Pearse II, RV, Tabin CJ. Twists of fate in the brain. *Nature.* 439: 404–405, 2006.

Sherman C. Right brain-left brain–A primer. *Cerebrum.* Jan 10, 2013. http://www.dana.org/News/Details.aspx?id=43539

Sperry RW. Cerebral organization and behavior: The split brain behaves in many respects like two separate brains, providing new research possibilities. *Science.* 133: 1749–1757, 1961.

Sperry RW. Some effects of disconnecting the cerebral hemispheres. Nobel Lecture, Karolinska Institutet; December 8, 1981; Stockholm.

Wingate RJ. The rhombic lip and early cerebellar development. *Curr Opin Neurobiol.* 11: 82–88, 2001.

4.

CONDUIT BETWEEN BODY AND BRAIN

PATHWAYS FOR MOVING AND FEELING THE BODY TRAVERSE THE LENGTH OF THE NEURAXIS

Just as major thoroughfares provide a better framework than one-block, dead-end alleys for learning the layout of a city, long "highways" are key to navigating through the nervous system. As we embark on our toe-to-nose journey through the nervous system, we closely follow the three longest pathways that traverse the length of the central nervous system (CNS) between the spinal cord and cerebral cortex:

- *Lemniscal pathway*: Information about light touch, vibration, and proprioception (the position of the body) is carried through the *dorsal column-medial lemniscus pathway.*

- *Spinothalamic pathway:* Information about pain and temperature is carried through the *spinothalamic tract,* also known as the anterolateral system.

- *Corticospinal pathway:* Information about voluntary movements is carried from cortex through the *corticospinal tract* to spinal motoneurons innervating muscles of the body.

The lemniscal and spinothalamic pathways are sensory pathways, communicating sensory information from the body and into the CNS, through the spinal cord and brainstem to the forebrain (Fig. 4-1). The corticospinal tract is a motor pathway that carries information from the cerebral cortex, *down* the neuraxis, to motoneurons that control contraction of the body's skeletal or voluntary muscles.

As we make our way through the nervous system from the periphery to the spinal cord, brainstem, and eventually the forebrain, we will always note the location of the lemniscal, spinothalamic, and corticospinal pathways.

PATHWAYS FOR SENSATION AND VOLUNTARY MOVEMENT CROSS FROM ONE SIDE TO THE OTHER

The lemniscal, spinothalamic, and corticospinal pathways begin on one side and end on the opposite or contralateral side (see red asterisks in Fig. 4-1). As a result, the cerebral cortex on one side is responsible for both voluntary movement and somatosensory perception of the other side of the body. Because knowing where each pathway crosses is essential to deciphering the location of damage responsible for any given set of symptoms, we start with an overview of the pathways, including the locations of their crossings.

Information that gives rise to perceptions of light touch, vibration, or proprioception—the sense of the body's position in space—stimulates primary afferent neurons that have a cell body in the *dorsal root ganglia (DRG)*. Primary afferents send an axon into the spinal cord that ascends through the *dorsal columns* of the spinal cord to the *dorsal column nuclei* in the medulla. In the medulla, primary afferents synapse on—thereby passing information onto—neurons in a dorsal column nucleus. *Dorsal column nuclear neurons send axons across the midline within the caudal medulla.* These axons then ascend, on the side contralateral to the pathway origin, through a tract called the *medial lemniscus* to the thalamus. Because it crosses or decussates, the lemniscal pathway ends in the brain on the opposite side from the part of the body served. The crossing of dorsal column nuclear cells is often referred to as the *sensory decussation.* Thalamic neurons receive information from dorsal column nuclear neurons, via synapses, and then send out an axon that ascends through the *somatosensory radiation* to the *primary somatosensory cortex.*

In total, the lemniscal pathway involves a minimum of four neurons—primary afferent, dorsal column nuclear cell, thalamic neuron, and cortical neuron—and three synapses. The crossing in the lemniscal pathway is accomplished by

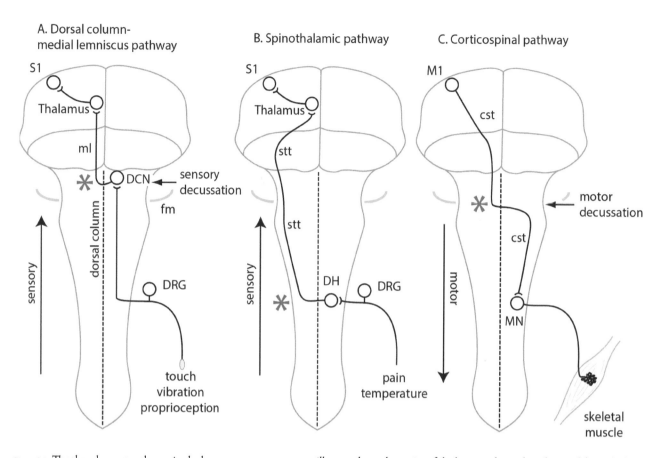

A. Dorsal column-medial lemniscus pathway

B. Spinothalamic pathway

C. Corticospinal pathway

Figure 4-1 The three longest pathways in the human nervous system are illustrated on schematics of the brain and spinal cord viewed from the back. Note that the schematics are stretched horizontally for illustrative purposes. The dotted line in the spinal cord and caudal medulla marks the midline. The foramen magnum (*fm*) separating the spinal cord, below, from the brain, above, is indicated by the blue arcs. A: The lemniscal pathway carries information about touch, vibration, and proprioception from the body to the contralateral cerebral cortex. Primary afferents with somata located in dorsal root ganglia (*DRG*) transmit tactile information from the periphery all the way to the dorsal column nuclei (*DCN*) in the caudal medulla. Within the spinal cord, these primary afferents travel in the ipsilateral dorsal column. Cells in the dorsal column nuclei that receive input from primary afferents in turn project to the contralateral thalamus. To reach the thalamus, dorsal column nuclear cells send their axons across the midline. The crossing of dorsal column nuclear axons marks the sensory decussation. When the dorsal column nuclear axons reach the contralateral side, they take a turn to travel rostrally through the brainstem as the medial lemniscus (*ml*). Thalamic cells project to primary somatosensory cortex (*S1*). B: The spinothalamic pathway carries information about pain and temperature from the body to the contralateral cerebral cortex. Primary afferents that innervate the periphery have cell bodies located in the dorsal root ganglia and transmit information from the periphery to the dorsal horn (*DH*) of the spinal cord. Cells in the dorsal horn send an axon across the midline to travel rostrally in the spinothalamic tract (*stt*) all the way to the contralateral thalamus. Thalamic cells receiving input from the spinothalamic tract project to primary somatosensory cortex. C: The corticospinal pathway originates from cells in the primary motor cortex (*M1*) that send an axon through the corticospinal tract (*cst*) to contralateral motoneurons (*MN*) in the spinal cord. At the spinomedullary junction, corticospinal tract fibers cross the midline, marking the motor decussation. Motoneurons that receive input from the corticospinal tract innervate skeletal muscle, required for voluntary movement. Red asterisks mark where each pathway crosses the midline.

the axon of the dorsal column nuclear cell, the secondary (the neuron receiving input from the primary afferent) sensory neuron in the pathway. Upon reaching the neocortical primary somatosensory cortex, information carried through this pathway can lead to perceptions of touch, vibration, or body position.

Information that gives rise to perceptions of pain or temperature is carried in the spinothalamic pathway. As with the lemniscal pathway, the spinothalamic pathway involves four neurons and three synapses. Primary afferents that respond to potentially injurious stimuli or to temperature

changes are *nociceptors* and *thermoreceptors*, respectively; these primary afferents are distinct from those that feed the lemniscal pathway carrying tactile, vibratory, or proprioceptive information. Nociceptors and thermoreceptors carry information from the body surface, muscles, bones, internal viscera, and other deep structures into the spinal cord where they synapse on a spinal cord neuron in the *dorsal horn*. The dorsal horn cell involved is a *spinothalamic tract* cell that sends its axon across the midline to ascend through the spinothalamic tract to the thalamus. Spinothalamic tract axons travel in the ventrolateral quadrant of the spinal cord.

Recall that, in the human spinal cord, the terms "anterolateral" and "ventrolateral" are synonymous. Therefore, the spinothalamic pathway is frequently termed the *anterolateral system* in the clinical literature. Thalamic neurons that receive synaptic input from spinothalamic tract cells in turn send information to the primary somatosensory cortex.

Pain perception involves components of both sensory-discrimination—the what, where, and when of a stimulus—and affect—the emotional and motivational reaction evoked by a stimulus. The spinothalamic pathway, which ultimately reaches primary somatosensory cortex, is primarily involved in the sensory-discriminative rather than the affective component of pain. The affective component of pain is carried through indirect channels into regions of the cerebral cortex that include but extend beyond the somatosensory cortex. The clinical import of this is that central lesions may exert differential effects on sensory-discriminative and affective aspects of pain.

The *corticospinal pathway* starts with neurons in the *primary motor cortex* of the frontal lobe. These cortical neurons project all the way down to the spinal cord through the *corticospinal tract*. The axons of the corticospinal tract travel through the forebrain, midbrain, and pons and then form the *pyramids*, two parallel columns that run down either side of the ventral medullary midline. For this reason, the corticospinal tract is also termed the *pyramidal tract*. Corticospinal tract axons cross the midline at the junction of the spinal cord and the medulla and travel down the spinal cord, where they contact motoneurons that control voluntary movements of the legs and arms. Because it decussates, *the corticospinal tract starts in the brain on the opposite side from the muscles whose movement it ultimately influences.* The point where the corticospinal tract fibers cross is often termed the *motor* or *pyramidal decussation*.

The *corticobulbar tract* forms an analogous pathway to the corticospinal tract, controlling voluntary movement of the face, jaw, tongue, and upper airway along with selected shoulder and neck movements. Because motor centers targeted by the corticobulbar tract are located in the brainstem, the corticobulbar tract traverses a much shorter distance and correspondingly is affected by lesions in a far more restricted area than the corticospinal tract. As detailed further in Chapter 23, the corticobulbar tract differs from the corticospinal tract in another respect: it does not uniformly cross, so that motoneurons controlled by the tract may be located ipsilateral, contralateral, or both, to the site of corticobulbar tract origin.

One final point is worthy of mention. About 90% of all the axons that are present in the medullary pyramids cross at the motor decussation and the remainder do not. The axons that cross form the *lateral corticospinal tract*, which is commonly called simply the corticospinal tract as is done throughout this chapter. The remaining corticospinal tract axons do not cross the midline and instead travel down the ipsilateral spinal cord in the *ventral corticospinal tract*. The ventral corticospinal tract is important in the bilateral control of axial and proximal limb muscles for postural adjustments.

Even this simple overview provides enough information to use deductive reasoning to estimate the likeliest location of a lesion when presented with symptoms. We consider two examples. First, consider someone who cannot feel anything—pain, temperature, or touch—on the right side of her body, nor can she move the muscles on the right side of her body. One possibility is that all of the peripheral nerve conduits for sensory and motor information of the body on the right have suddenly failed altogether. This is possible, and yet it is exceedingly unlikely. Thus, one who can neither feel nor move one side of the body has a *central* rather than a peripheral lesion. Now, we narrow down the potential location of the lesion to (1) either brain or spinal cord and (2) to either left or right. Try to solve this problem before reading the spoiler below.

The spinothalamic and lemniscal pathways serving each side of the body only travel together above the sensory decussation located in the caudal medulla. Therefore, the lesion must be in the brain, above the caudal medulla. Since both sensory pathways carrying information about the right side of the body and the corticospinal tract carrying motor information destined for muscles on the right all travel through the *left* brainstem and forebrain, the lesion must be on the left, at a point above the sensory and motor decussations.

In a second example, consider someone who shows a loss of temperature sensation and a diminution of tactile sensitivity throughout the body bilaterally while having intact motor function. No single lesion could produce this constellation of symptoms since temperature information from the left body and temperature information from the right body travel on opposite sides of the spinal cord and on opposite sides of the brain. The same is true for tactile information from the left and right. Although it is formally possible that the brain suffers perfectly symmetrical damage, we can exclude this possibility. Bilateral impairment of sensory or motor function usually results from a *systemic disease* rather than a focal anatomical lesion. In fact, patients with *Hansen disease*, commonly known as leprosy, often present, or first seek medical attention, with a loss of temperature and touch sensation caused by a systemic loss of sensory nerve function.

THE SPINAL CORD AND SPINAL NERVES SERVE THE BODY

The spinal cord, contained within the vertebral column, is the conduit for sensory information from the body and motor directives ultimately bound for the body's skeletal muscles. Spinal cord communication with the body is accomplished through axon highways in the form of *roots* and *nerves* (Fig. 4-2). Nerves are *peripheral* bundles of axons. Roots are *central* bundles of axons that carry axons between the CNS and the exit point from the dural envelope. Thus, the same axons pass through roots and nerves. Motor axons

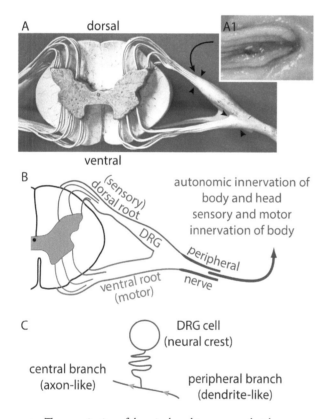

arise from spinal cord neurons and travel through roots before exiting the dura and entering the nerves. Sensory information from the periphery passes through a spinal nerve before entering a spinal root and then the spinal cord. Thus, spinal nerves are *mixed*, carrying both sensory fibers that terminate in the spinal cord and motor axons that arise from the spinal cord, whereas roots are not.

Nerves that exit from the vertebral column are called *spinal nerves*; nerves that exit through holes in the skull are termed *cranial nerves*. For the most part, the cranial nerves carry sensory information into and motor information out of the brainstem. However, there is one exception to this rule. Motoneurons that innervate two neck muscles (trapezius, sternocleidomastoid) are located in the spinal cord and send their axons into the skull and then out of the skull as cranial nerve XI, which is also known as the *spinal accessory nerve* (see Chapter 5). This case highlights that nerves are deemed spinal or cranial depending on their point of exit rather than the site of their origin.

The spinal cord and spinal nerves serve sensory and motor functions involving the *body*. However, the spinal cord serves slightly different areas of the body for sensory and motor purposes. Sensory information arising from the limbs, trunk, shoulders, neck, back of the head, and even part of the ears travels through spinal nerves. Sensory input from the face, top of the head, oral and nasal cavities, and upper airway enters the brainstem via cranial nerves. Spinal motoneurons that send their axons out through spinal nerves control muscles of the limbs and trunk and most but not all neck muscles. Obviously, there is no motor control of the scalp. Motoneurons that send their axons through cranial nerves control muscles involved in producing facial expressions, chewing and swallowing, speech articulation, shrugging, and turning the head from side to side. Thus, sensory input from the neck is carried by spinal nerves, but the motor innervation of neck muscles is shared between cranial and spinal nerves.

Both spinal and cranial nerves carry sensory information from and autonomic motor information to internal organs such as the heart, pancreas, and colon. Consequently, both the spinal cord and brainstem are involved in visceral sensation and autonomic motor control.

Figure 4-2 The organization of the spinal cord is stereotyped with sensory inputs arriving dorsally and motor outputs exiting ventrally. A: A spinal cord segment has a bilateral pair of dorsal and ventral roots. Roots are contained within the dural sheath (*located at arrowheads*). A1: The dorsal rootlets from one side of one spinal segment exit the dura as a single group and become a peripheral nerve on the peripheral side of the dura. B: Primary afferent neurons whose cell bodies are in the dorsal root ganglia (DRG) collect information from the skin, muscles, joints, bone, tendons, and viscera of the body and then carry this information into the spinal cord through the dorsal root. Motor output, both somatomotor and autonomic, exits the spinal cord through the ventral root to reach targets in the head and body. Because peripheral nerves contain both sensory fibers en route to the dorsal roots and motor fibers emanating from the ventral roots, they serve a mixture of motor, sensory, and autonomic functions. C: Dorsal root ganglion neurons send out a single process that bifurcates into peripheral, dendrite-like, and central, axon-like, processes. Sensory information flows from the periphery to the spinal cord (*orange arrowheads*).   Photograph in A reprinted by permission of Bruni JE, Montemurro D, *Human neuroanatomy: A text, brain atlas, and laboratory dissection guide.* New York: Oxford University Press, 2009.

SPINAL NERVES CONTAIN A MIX OF AXONS WITH SENSORY, SKELETAL MOTOR, AND AUTONOMIC MOTOR FUNCTIONS

As should be evident by now, spinal nerves contain axons serving a very limited number of functions: somatosensory, autonomic motor, and somatomotor.

Somatosensory inputs enter the spinal cord through *dorsal roots*. Motor outputs, both somatomotor (destined for skeletal muscle) and autonomic, exit the spinal cord via *ventral roots*. *A dorsal root and a ventral root join to form a mixed peripheral nerve.* All spinal nerves are mixed (i.e., they contain sensory, motor, and, in some cases, preganglionic autonomic fibers; Fig. 4-2).

Somatosensory afferents bring information from the skin, muscles, bones, and internal organs to the spinal cord. The dorsal root ganglia contain the somata of all spinal afferents, are derived from neural crest, and comprise part of the peripheral nervous system. Thus, neurons in the dorsal root ganglia sit just outside the dural envelope and are susceptible to external damage from toxins, viruses, and the like. The cell body of a dorsal root ganglion neuron sends out only one process that, after an initially torturous route, bifurcates into central and peripheral branches (Fig. 4-2C). The central branch enters the spinal cord as part of the dorsal root, and the peripheral branch travels to a target tissue such as skin, muscle, bone, or tendon. The central branch of a dorsal root ganglion axon is axon-like in function, and the peripheral branch is dendrite-like in function, an arrangement that supports information transfer from the periphery (dendrites) to the CNS (axon). Importantly, the dorsal root ganglion cell provides biochemical and nutritive support to the entire process, which can be more than a meter in length (see Chapter 2).

Information from one region of skin reaches several segments (Fig. 4-3). Therefore, a lesion to a single dorsal root ganglion or dorsal root causes only a narrow strip of *anesthesia* (i.e., insensitivity to any form of somatosensory stimulation). In contrast, a nerve lesion may cause a wider region of anesthesia. Beyond anesthesia, which is a negative symptom, damage to somatosensory pathways also typically produces positive symptoms, perceptions that are inappropriate for the stimulus (see Chapter 1). Abnormal somatosensory perceptions are *paresthesias*, or are *dysesthesias* when associated with an unpleasant reaction. Bauby, introduced in Chapter 1, experienced relatively innocuous paresthesias (e.g., numbness) as well as distressing dysesthesias (pins and needles, burning pain). These perceptions are abnormal in that they are not the normal perception for the stimulus, which was no stimulus in Bauby's case. In other words, a perception of pins and needles (or anything else) is inappropriate when there is no stimulus present, as is the case with spontaneous paresthesias. Paresthesias often occur after a loss of sensation. Thus, a somatosensory paresthesia may be accompanied by anesthesia, a total loss of somatosensory sensation, or by some deficit (but not complete loss) in somatosensation as happens when sensory fibers are damaged but not severed completely. Nerve damage often produces paresthesias, including dysesthesias, whereas root damage tends to produce painful dysesthesias (Fig. 4-3).

Because of these arrangements, the consequences of nerve lesions are more severe than those of root lesions. Nerve lesions may cause anesthesia in a wide area of peripheral tissue along with the complete inability to use a skeletal muscle, termed *paralysis*. In contrast, a root lesion results in motor weakness and a very limited region, if any, of anesthesia. Damage to sensory axons anywhere along the line typically produces paresthesias, including dysesthesias.

The ventral root carries motor information from spinal motoneurons bound for somatic muscles. Motoneurons that innervate a single skeletal muscle sit together in cylindrical collections called *pools* that stretch longitudinally across several spinal segments (Fig. 4-3). Therefore, *motoneuron axons from one pool and destined for one skeletal muscle exit through several adjacent roots.* Axons from multiple roots but arising from a single motoneuron pool join together within a nerve that innervates one muscle. The convergence of input from several roots onto one muscle-bound nerve means that a nerve injury causes greater motor impairment than a root injury. Thus, nerve lesions or *neuropathies*, particularly distal ones, can cause a complete inability to use a muscle, termed *paralysis*, whereas root lesions or *radiculopathies* typically cause weakness or *paresis*.

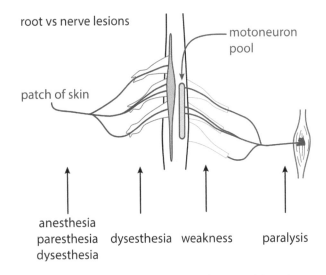

Figure 4-3 Sensory axons from a single region of skin travel through a single nerve and then enter the spinal cord through multiple roots to reach several spinal segments. Similarly, motor axons arising in multiple segments exit through multiple roots before eventually converging onto one nerve to reach the target muscle. Because of these arrangements, the consequences of nerve lesions are more severe than those of root lesions. Nerve lesions may cause anesthesia in a wide area of peripheral tissue along with the complete inability to use a skeletal muscle, termed *paralysis*. In contrast, a root lesion results in motor weakness and a very limited region, if any, of anesthesia. Damage to sensory axons anywhere along the line typically produces paresthesias, including dysesthesias.

The suffix *-plegia* is synonymous with paralysis and is typically used with a prefix denoting the location of the problem. For example, the inability to move one side of the body is referred to as *hemiplegia*. Paresis is also used as a suffix, so that weakness on one side of the body is referred to as *hemiparesis*. *Palsy* is an ambiguous term used to refer to either weakness or paralysis. Palsy is a useful term for conditions that, depending on severity, are associated with either weakness or paralysis.

THE SPINAL CORD IS TOPOGRAPHICALLY ORGANIZED

In the embryo, the caudal portion of the neural tube that will develop into the spinal cord is flanked by *somites*, repeating collections of mesodermal tissue that will become dermis, skeletal muscle, and axial bones. Because they differentiate from somites, skin, skeletal muscle, and bone are considered somatic tissues. Even though somites are not the source of all skin, skeletal muscle, and bone in the body, we use the term *somatic* to refer to all such tissues. The term *viscerosensory* refers to sensory pathways from the viscera. Finally, *somatosensory system* is an umbrella term that encompasses both somatic and visceral sensation from the head and body.

The spinal cord is a segmented structure, with each segment consisting of the region of spinal cord connected to bilateral pairs of roots that connect with a bilateral pair of spinal nerves. During embryonic development, the segments of the spinal cord line up with the somites so that roots from the nascent cord travel straight laterally to innervate the tissues derived from the adjacent somite. Thus, it is the somites that confer segmentation onto the spinal cord through the arrangement of roots and nerves.

Each spinal nerve provides sensory and motor innervation to a restricted portion of the body, and there is a topographical mapping of the represented part of the body across spinal cord segments. Thus, cervical segments innervate structures closer to the head, and sacral segments innervate tissues closer to the tail or, in our case, tailbone. In between, neighboring spinal cord segments innervate topographically sequential body structures. However, there is an important wrinkle in the topographical map. The spinal cord of humans retains the gross organization of our quadrupedal ancestors from whom we recently evolved (Fig. 4-4). Since the perineum and tail are behind the hind legs in quadrupeds, the topographic sequence of the spinal cord is the quadrupedal sequence: neck—arms—trunk—legs—sacrum. Even on a more granular level, the order of dermatomes clearly

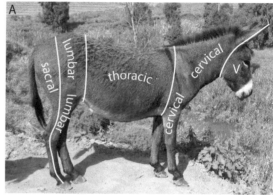

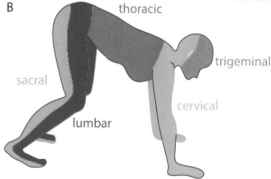

Figure 4-4 The organization of the human spinal cord (B) has the topography of the quadrupedal spinal cord (A). In quadrupeds, the perineum and genitalia, and the coccyx or tail in some species, are the most caudal structures, *not* the hind limbs. Due to this evolutionary inheritance, the spinal representations of the upper and lower limbs are interposed at the sites representative of where the limbs join the body axis.

evolved from a quadrupedal body plan. For example, the shoulder dermatome of C5 abuts the dermatome of T1 with the intervening dermatomes serving the forelimb (Fig. 4-5). Thus, our evolution from quadrupedal predecessors trumps our current bipedal appearance with respect to spinal organization.

The segments of the spinal cord are divided into divisions, which are from rostral to caudal (Fig. 4-5):

- *Cervical (C)*: Eight segments innervating the back of the head, neck, shoulders, and arms

- *Thoracic (T)*: Twelve segments innervating the thorax and upper abdomen and providing sympathetic outflow to the body

- *Lumbar (L)*: Five segments innervating the hips and most of the legs and feet

- *Sacral (S)*: Five segments innervating the back of the legs and the *saddle* region, including urogenital and perianal structures, and providing parasympathetic outflow to the hindgut and pelvic organs

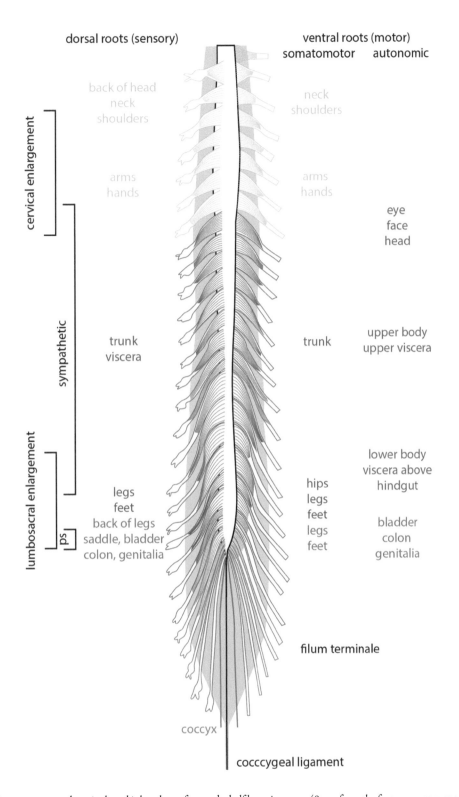

dorsal roots (sensory)   ventral roots (motor)

somatomotor   autonomic

cervical enlargement

back of head
neck
shoulders

neck
shoulders

arms
hands

arms
hands

eye
face
head

sympathetic

trunk
viscera

trunk

upper body
upper viscera

lumbosacral enlargement

lower body
viscera above
hindgut

ps

legs
feet
back of legs
saddle, bladder
colon, genitalia

hips
legs
feet
legs
feet

bladder
colon
genitalia

filum terminale

coccyx

cocccygeal ligament

Figure 4-5 In humans of average stature, the spinal cord is less than a foot and a half long, just over 40 cm, from the foramen magnum to the conus medullaris. Each spinal cord segment has a stereotyped structure with dorsal roots, leading to dorsal root ganglia, emanating from the dorsal side of the cord (*left side*) and ventral roots emanating from the ventral side of the cord (*right side*). Dorsal and ventral roots travel through the dural sleeve (*gray region*) containing the spinal cord to exit from the vertebral column, often at a location far more caudal than the segment's location, where rootlets emerge from the cord. The innervations provided by sensory, somatomotor, and autonomic motor neurons in cervical (*light blue*), thoracic (*red*), lumbar (*dark blue*), and sacral (*green*) segments are listed. The cervical enlargement that serves the arms is located from C4 to T1, and the lumbosacral enlargement that serves the legs includes segments from L1 to S3. The locations of preganglionic sympathetic and parasympathetic (*ps*) neurons are marked on the left. Since the vertebral column lengthens far more than the spinal cord during development, all roots save the most rostral ones must travel caudally to reach the appropriate exit point from the vertebral column. As a consequence, the most caudal portion of the vertebral column contains a large number of spinal roots but no cord, an area termed the cauda equina (see Fig. 4-6). Attaching the spinal cord at the caudal end is accomplished by the filum terminale, a condensation of pia that is invested with dura to form the coccygeal ligament as it leaves the dural sleeve. The coccygeal ligament attaches to the coccyx. In this way, the conus medullaris is anchored to the coccyx by the filum terminale/coccygeal ligament.   Modified with permission from deArmond S et al. *Structure of the human brain: A photographic atlas.* New York: Oxford University Press, 1989.

- *Coccygeal (Co)*: One segment innervating the coccyx or tailbone; not of great clinical significance and not discussed further

Cervical to sacral spinal divisions are abbreviated as C, T, L, and S. The segments are numbered from rostral to caudal, so that C1, the first cervical segment, abuts the medulla, C8 abuts T1, T12 is sandwiched between T11 and L1, and so on.

The number and diversity of tissues, as well as the number and diversity of fine movements possible, are far greater with the arms and legs than with the trunk. Correspondingly, cervical and lumbosacral segments that support arm (C4–T1) and leg (L1–S3) sensation and movement are enlarged (Fig. 4-5). The widest portion of each enlargement serves the most distal parts of the limbs: the hands and fingers (C7–C8) in the case of the cervical enlargement and the feet and toes (L5–S1) in the case of the lumbosacral enlargement. As one might expect, the cervical enlargement is larger than the lumbosacral one.

The level of a spinal cord injury is critical to understanding the clinical consequences. Damage at high cervical levels may impair movement of both limbs as well as sensation from the entire body, but damage to the thoracic cord will leave both sensation and movement of the arms and hands unaltered.

ROOTS FROM PROGRESSIVELY MORE CAUDAL SEGMENTS TRAVEL PROGRESSIVELY LONGER TO EXIT THE VERTEBRAL COLUMN

The C1 ventral roots (there are no C1 dorsal roots) exit the vertebral column from between the skull and the first cervical vertebral bone. Roots from successively more caudal segments exit from between successively more caudal pairs of vertebrae (i.e., C2 roots exit between C1 and C2 vertebrae, C3 from between C2 and C3 and so on). However, a wrinkle in this layout arises because there are only seven cervical *vertebrae* to the eight cervical *cord segments*. Therefore, C8 roots exit between C7 and T1 vertebrae. Thereafter, all thoracic, lumbar, and sacral segments exit between the eponymous vertebral bone and its caudal neighbor.

As mentioned earlier, the segments of the embryonic spinal cord line up with somites. They also line up with the vertebrae so that roots travel laterally out of the vertebral column to innervate target tissues. However, the vertebral column and body then grow far more than does the spinal

cord. This differential growth renders the mature spinal cord and vertebral column out of register. In the adult, the spinal cord occupies only the top two-thirds or so of the vertebral column. Because of this, spinal roots, at least those exiting from segments caudal to mid-cervical levels, must travel caudally within the dural sac to exit through the appropriate pair of vertebrae and reach the tissues they are destined to innervate. For example, the L5 segment of the cord sits at roughly the level of the final thoracic vertebral segment (T12). Yet, the roots from the L5 segment exit five vertebral segments away, from just below the L5 vertebral bone.

As a result of the far greater growth of the vertebral column than of the spinal cord, the conus medullaris is located at about the second lumbar vertebral bone in the adult and at roughly the fourth lumbar vertebra in a young child. Caudal to the conus medullaris, the CSF-filled meninges house spinal roots but no spinal cord. The collection of roots caudal to the conus medullaris is called the *cauda equina*, Latin for "horse's tail," which it resembles in appearance (Fig. 4-6).

The cauda equina is clinically significant for two reasons. First, physicians access the *lumbar cistern*, the pool of

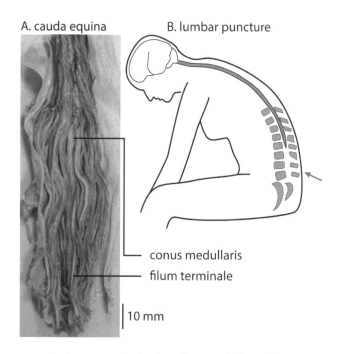

A. cauda equina   B. lumbar puncture

conus medullaris
filum terminale

10 mm

Figure 4-6 A: Opening up the dural envelope reveals the cauda equina, consisting of roots from lumbar and sacral segments of the cord that travel beyond the conus medullaris. B: Because the cauda equina contains roots but does not contain any spinal cord tissue, accessing the subarachnoid space here is relatively safe. Therefore, clinicians may insert a needle through the dura and into the cauda equina at lower lumbar levels (*red arrow*) in order either to measure the pressure of the subarachnoid space or to sample cerebrospinal fluid (CSF). This procedure is called a lumbar puncture.

CSF surrounding the cauda equina, by inserting a needle into the cauda equina at lower lumbar levels (*red arrow* in Fig. 4-6), a procedure known as a *lumbar puncture* or, more colloquially, a spinal tap. Lumbar punctures are used to obtain a sample of CSF or to measure central pressure as diagnostic tools for meningitis, hemorrhage, hydrocephalus, cancerous growth, and the like. Less frequently, drugs may be introduced directly into the CNS via a lumbar puncture. Because the roots of the cauda equina move aside easily, a needle can enter the cistern without risking damage, as would be likely at more rostral levels where the cord is present (Fig. 4-6). Lumbar punctures are typically performed at vertebral level L4–L5, where the cauda equina is present, and well below the danger zone where the spinal cord is present.

The second clinically significant point regarding the cauda equina relates to the potentially lethal symptoms that result from cauda equina damage. *Cauda equina syndrome* involves damage to the roots of the cauda equina. It can arise from a number of causes including trauma from a hard fall. Typically, this syndrome produces anesthesia within a saddle distribution. The most worrisome features of the cauda equina syndrome are urinary retention and constipation, with the former being potentially fatal if untreated.

AUTONOMIC NEURONS BELONG TO EITHER THE SYMPATHETIC OR PARASYMPATHETIC DIVISION

As introduced in Chapter 2, autonomic motor control is achieved through a two-neuron pathway (see Fig. 2-4). Spinal autonomic motor neurons, termed *preganglionic*, form the first neuron in the chain. The second neuron in the chain is a motor neuron in an autonomic ganglion, which we call the *postganglionic neuron*. The soma of the preganglionic neuron is within the CNS, in either the spinal cord or brainstem. Preganglionic neurons send their axons through the ventral roots, just as motoneurons do. However, preganglionic autonomic neurons synapse on neurons in autonomic ganglia rather than on the final target muscle, as is the case for motoneurons. A neuron in an autonomic ganglion is the second neuron in the autonomic control chain, and it sends its postganglionic axon to an autonomic target of the body or head. There are three types of autonomic target tissues:

- *Smooth muscle* forms a layer around many internal organs, such as blood vessels, the bladder, bronchi, and intestines. Smooth muscle also is present in the eye,

around the pupil and lens, eyelid, and skin, where it is attached to hair follicles.

- *Cardiac muscle* is the striated muscle that makes up the heart.

- *Glands* are organs that secrete substances such as tears, mucus, sweat, saliva, cerumen (ear wax), and so on.

There is one exception to the two-neuron chain rule of autonomic motor control. The adrenal medulla, which releases epinephrine and norepinephrine during periods of stress or arousal, receives direct innervation from preganglionic neurons. Notably, adrenal chromaffin cells are similar to sympathetic ganglion cells in developmental origin (neural crest) and neurotransmitter class (catecholamine, see Chapter 12).

As the reader knows, the autonomic nervous system has sympathetic and parasympathetic divisions. Whereas both sympathetic and parasympathetic function depend on a two-neuron chain from the CNS to peripheral target tissues, the anatomy of the divisions differs in several ways (Table 4-1). Preganglionic sympathetic neurons are

Table 4-1 THE SYMPATHETIC AND PARASYMPATHETIC BRANCHES OF THE AUTONOMIC NERVOUS SYSTEM DIFFER IN THEIR ORGANIZATION, NEUROCHEMISTRY, AND FUNCTION

PROPERTY	SYMPATHETIC	PARASYMPATHETIC
Location of preganglionic somata	Thoracic and upper lumbar (T1–L3) cord	Brainstem and sacral cord (S2–S4), thus "craniosacral"
Axonal anatomy	Preganglionic axon shorter than postganglionic axon	Preganglionic axon much longer than postganglionic axon
Location of autonomic ganglia	Paravertebral and prevertebral sympathetic ganglia arranged in chains and located at some distance from targeted tissue	Ganglia located in or very near targeted tissue
Ganglionic neuronal transmitter	Mostly norepinephrine, except for sympathetic ganglionic neurons innervating sweat glands, which use acetylcholine	Acetylcholine
Circumstances of maximal activation	Engaged maximally during periods of high arousal and excitement, including during fights and escapes	Engaged maximally during rest and sleep to promote, growth, digestion, and recuperation

only present in the thoracic and upper lumbar cord. They send their preganglionic axons out through spinal ventral roots to terminate in either *paravertebral ganglia* that hug the spinal cord or *prevertebral ganglia* found closer to abdominal target tissues. The ganglia lie in a line called the *sympathetic chain* or trunk, situated just ventrolateral to the vertebral column. The chain has a beaded appearance because it consists of sympathetic ganglia connected by bundles of preganglionic axons en route to the appropriate ganglia. The most anterior portions of the sympathetic chain are merged within the large *superior cervical ganglion.* From sympathetic ganglia, postganglionic axons travel relatively long distances to target tissues. Targets of the sympathetic system include the eyelid, pupillary dilator, and lacrimal and salivary glands within the head and the viscera of the body. Beyond these targets, the sympathetic system also innervates sweat glands and cutaneous blood vessels all over the body and head.

Preganglionic parasympathetic neurons are found both in the brainstem and in the sacral spinal cord, giving rise to the term *craniosacral* as a synonym for parasympathetic. Preganglionic parasympathetic neurons send out long axons that travel to parasympathetic ganglia, which are located in or near the final target tissue. Targets of the sacral

parasympathetic system include the hindgut and organs of the pelvic floor, such as the bladder, colon, rectum, and sexual organs. The cranial contribution to the parasympathetic system reaches the lens, pupillary constrictor, and lacrimal and salivary glands within the head and the viscera of the body above the hindgut.

When we consider spinal cord anatomy, the sympathetic innervation of the eye and face is of particular clinical importance (Table 4-2). The *oculosympathetic pathway* starts with hypothalamic neurons that send axons to descend through the brainstem and spinal cord and synapse on preganglionic sympathetic neurons in T1 and T2 (Fig. 4-7). Preganglionic axons exit through the T1 root, travel close to the apex of the lung, through the sympathetic chain, and ultimately synapse in the superior cervical ganglion. Ganglionic neurons that innervate the *superior tarsal* muscle, which lifts the eyelid, and the pupillary dilator muscle that dilates the pupil send postganglionic axons along the internal carotid artery, through the cavernous sinus, and ultimately to the eye. Sympathetic nerves supplying facial blood vessels and sweat glands travel along the external carotid. Interruption of the sympathetic pathway to the eye at any point causes *Horner syndrome,* which consists principally of *miosis,* or pupillary constriction, and may be accompanied by *ptosis,* or

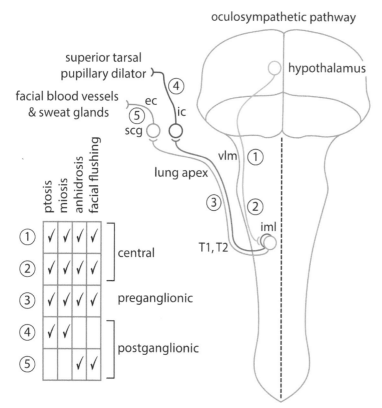

Figure 4-7 The oculosympathetic pathway involves three neurons. A hypothalamic neuron projects through the ventrolateral medulla (*vlm*) to preganglionic sympathetic neurons in the intermediolateral cell column (*iml*) of the upper thoracic cord (*T1, T2*). Preganglionic sympathetic neurons send axons through the sympathetic chain to the superior cervical ganglion (*scg*), passing by the apex of the lung along the way. Distinct populations of ganglionic sympathetic neurons project along the external and internal carotids (*ec, ic*) to the facial skin and eye, respectively. Central (*1, 2*), preganglionic (*3*), and postganglionic (*4, 5*) lesions produce different combinations of symptoms as shown in the table inset.

drooping eyelid. Miosis and ptosis result from disruption of the tonic sympathetic excitation of the pupillary dilator and superior tarsal muscles. Facial *anhidrosis*, or lack of sweating, along with facial *flushing* indicative of vasodilation, occur when the sympathetic innervation to facial sweat glands and blood vessels is interrupted.

Horner syndrome can result from central lesions but more commonly arises because of a lesion of pre- or postganglionic nerve fibers. A *Pancoast lung tumor* or neck malignancy can impinge on sympathetic nerves as they emerge from the thoracic cord and course toward the superior cervical ganglion. Disruption of postganglionic fibers often accompanies carotid artery dissection.

The particular constellation of symptoms observed depends on the level of the lesion or impairment of the oculosympathetic pathway (Fig. 4-7). For example, facial anhidrosis and flushing are associated with central and preganglionic lesions but less commonly with postganglionic lesions since the fibers to the eye and to the facial skin take postganglionic different routes. As another example, impingement on the exiting preganglionic fibers is likely to cause arm and shoulder pain through effects on somatosensory fibers of the brachial plexus; isolated arm pain rarely accompanies Horner syndrome due to central or postganglionic causes. These examples show the logic associated with using neuroanatomy to understand the causative agent of a clinical presentation.

A second clinically important autonomic consequence of spinal cord or nerve damage is the isolation of sacral parasympathetic neurons from the brain (Table 4-2). Damage to axons descending from the brain to the sacral cord may impair micturition, sexual function, and defecation. Moving food through the gastrointestinal tract is largely dependent on the peripheral enteric nervous system, which can operate independently of the CNS. Therefore, defecation is

typically not the most urgent medical concern after spinal cord injury. The motor and sensory components of sexual function include arousal, climax, and the perceptual experience of orgasm; all involve the sacral spinal cord and therefore may be drastically altered by spinal cord injury in both men and women. Nonetheless, disorders of sexual function are not life-threatening.

The most urgent medical concern following from interruption of the brain's connection to the sacral cord is bladder control. *Micturition*, the medical term for urination, depends on parasympathetically mediated contraction of the bladder (*detrusor* muscle) along with relaxation of the *external urethral sphincter*, a voluntary muscle. The message that initiates sphincter relaxation arises in the brain and is sent down to the sacral cord (S2–S4) where sphincter motoneurons and preganglionic neurons that target the detrusor are located. Therefore, spinal cord damage above sacral levels may interrupt the command for sphincter relaxation. Since most spinal cord injury is above S2, micturition is often affected in spinal cord-injured patients. The urinary retention that results from interrupting this message is potentially lethal and must be treated, typically with catheterization, with some urgency.

PERIPHERAL NERVES CONTAIN LARGE AND SMALL CALIBER FIBERS

Axons within a peripheral nerve, often referred to as *fibers*, belong to more than a dozen functionally and molecularly distinct neuronal types. However, for our current purposes, we simply consider large and small caliber, or diameter, fibers.

Skeletal motor function is critically dependent on large diameter fibers. It is of great advantage that *all* movement-serving fibers are myelinated and conduct action potentials very rapidly. Rapid conduction of action potentials in motoneuron axons innervating skeletal muscles enables quick execution of movement commands. Moreover, immediate motor corrections in the face of unexpected obstacles are enabled by fast-conducting sensory fibers, such as those serving proprioception. Any delay in either muscle control or sensory feedback would inevitably impair movement. Another group of large diameter fibers are sensory axons that support the perception of touch and contribute to the sensory feedback necessary for voluntary movements.

Small caliber fibers serve a range of varied functions that can be broadly categorized as sensory and autonomic. Small

Table 4-2 **KEY SPINAL CORD SEGMENTS, ROOTS, AND NERVES**

SPINAL SEGMENTS	KEY COMPONENT	POTENTIAL DEFICIT
C3–C5	Phrenic motoneurons	Breathing
C6–C8	Motoneurons serving hand muscles	Hand dexterity
C8–T2	Preganglionic sympathetic innervation of the eye	Horner syndrome
L5–S2	Motoneurons serving foot muscles	Foot dexterity
S2–S4	Preganglionic parasympathetic innervation of the bladder	Bladder sphincter dyssynergia

diameter primary afferent fibers carry sensory information that may lead to perceptions of pain or temperature. Other small diameter primary afferent fibers carry information about pleasurable touch. Still other small caliber fibers are *efferents*, postganglionic axons from autonomic ganglion neurons that target heterogeneous tissues and produce a wide variety of homeostatic effects.

Neuropathies are one of the most common neurological conditions. They are a heterogeneous group of syndromes caused by diverse etiologies that result in damage to peripheral nerve fibers, their myelin sheaths, or both. The symptoms of neuropathies depend on the type or types of peripheral fibers damaged, which in turn differ across etiologies. *Traumatic injury*, meaning damage due to physical impact, cutting, tearing, or crushing, of a peripheral nerve causes indiscriminate damage to both large and small nerve fibers and therefore has motor and sensory consequences. Compression neuropathies, such as the common *carpal tunnel syndrome*, arise from trauma, repetitive use, ischemia, and likely from factors yet to be discovered. Several metabolic and autoimmune diseases target peripheral nerve fibers that have a particular molecular signature or metabolic vulnerability. For example, the hyperglycemia and plasma hyperosmolality present in diabetic patients tend to selectively damage large diameter sensory fibers serving touch and cause mostly sensory clinical symptoms. *Guillain-Barré syndrome* is an autoimmune condition that causes an acute and, in most people, transient demyelination of large diameter fibers, thereby causing primarily motor symptoms. Finally, diverse inherited neuropathies target developmental programs critical to the development of specific subsets of nerve fibers, causing correspondingly diverse sets of symptoms.

The longest nerves are most vulnerable to neuropathies caused by trauma or environmental exposure (e.g., to glucose or antibodies). Furthermore, since all tissues distal to the site of damage may be affected, the most common neuropathies involve the feet, located at the distal end of our longest nerves. Because the hands also are vulnerable to long-nerve damage, patients frequently present with symptoms in a *glove and stocking* distribution. For reasons that are also related to nerve length, neuropathies produce sympathetic dysfunction far more frequently than parasympathetic dysfunction. Recall that parasympathetic ganglia are very close to their targets; thus, parasympathetic postganglionic axons are short. In contrast, sympathetic postganglionic axons that innervate sweat glands and cutaneous blood vessels, including vessels supplying the nail beds, are long and widely distributed. Therefore, sympathetic postganglionic axons are frequently affected by damage.

In sum, the predominant fiber types affected in most neuropathies are (1) large diameter motor-serving axons, (2) large diameter sensory fibers involved in touch, (3) small diameter sensory fibers involved in signaling pain and temperature, and (4) small diameter sympathetic fibers innervating cutaneous blood vessels and sweat glands.

Damage to each category of fiber type produces predictable symptoms. Damage to large diameter fibers produces weakness by interfering with motoneuronal innervation of skeletal muscle. For example, a neuropathy may cause foot drop, or it may result in an inadequate grip. Deficits in proprioception, which depends on large diameter proprioceptive fibers, can exacerbate motor symptoms, leading to "clumsiness." For example, without normal sensory feedback, a person may fall rather than recovering from a stumble or fail to detect that a held object is slipping from her grasp and end up dropping the object. In contrast to the negative signs resulting from damage to fibers involved in motor control, sensory fiber damage typically results in paresthesias and positive signs, as explained earlier.

Damage to small caliber fibers produces sensory and autonomic consequences. The sensory consequences, resulting from damage to fibers supporting pain and temperature perception, are typically dysesthesias. Dysesthesias vary greatly, ranging from an unpleasant sensation of pins and needles to an intolerable burning pain. An extreme version of a dysesthesia is *phantom limb pain*, in which pain is perceived from a body part that does not exist and has no innervation. Autonomic motor symptoms are primarily negative so that small diameter neuropathies may be accompanied by flushed and dry skin due to a loss of vasoconstriction and sweating. Changes in the appearance of nails due to interruption of the vascular supply to the nail bed are also a common symptom.

EACH SPINAL SEGMENT IS ASSOCIATED WITH A DERMATOME AND MYOTOME

The region of skin from which sensory information reaches a spinal segment is termed a *dermatome*. Throughout the body and parts of the limbs, dermatomes appear as horizontal slices across the body and longitudinal slices of the limbs (Fig. 4-8). This arrangement is another evolutionary inheritance from our quadrupedal ancestors.

One way to visualize a dermatome is to map the effects of the *varicella zoster virus* that can live in a dormant form in dorsal root ganglion cells and eventually re-erupt to cause

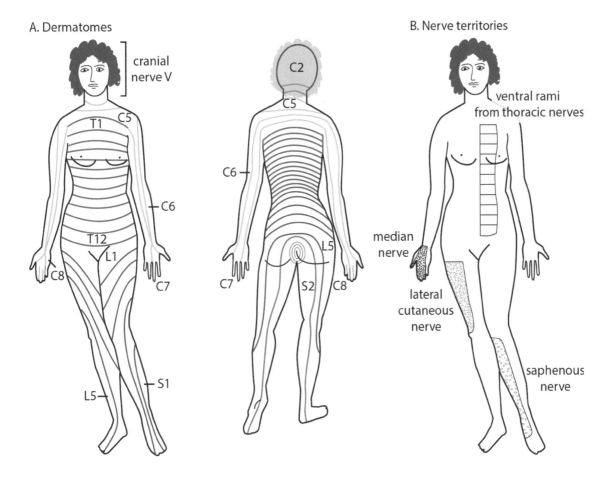

A. Dermatomes

cranial nerve V

C5
T1
C6
T12
L1
C8
C7
L5
S1

B. Nerve territories

C2
C5
C6
C7
S2
C8
L5

ventral rami from thoracic nerves

median nerve

lateral cutaneous nerve

saphenous nerve

Figure 4-8 A: Spinal dermatomes are the cutaneous regions innervated by the sensory fibers of each spinal segment. Note that these territories appear primarily as horizontal slices through the trunk but as longitudinal slices in the limbs. Limb dermatomes actually share the same orientation as trunk dermatomes in a quadruped. Thus, in a person on all fours, the orientations of the dermatomes in trunk and limbs are roughly parallel. Note that there is no sensory root in the first cervical segment. The top of the head, face, and oral cavity are innervated by the fifth cranial nerve (see Chapter 5). The innervation of the ear (not shown) is shared by the C2 spinal nerve and several cranial nerves. B: Nerve territories differ substantially from dermatomes in shape and orientation. The few examples illustrated here show that nerve territories can cut across dermatomes. For example, the territory supplied by the median nerve includes parts of dermatomes from segments C6 to C8. The territory of the lateral cutaneous nerve includes parts of several lumbar dermatomes. In other cases, particularly in the trunk, nerve territories are substantially smaller than dermatomes. For example, the ventral rami from the thoracic nerves innervate no more than a quarter of the corresponding thoracic dermatome.

a very painful condition called *herpes zoster* or *shingles* (Fig. 4-9). The varicella zoster virus initially causes chickenpox, usually in young children. At the time of the initial infection, virus particles may be taken up by sensory neuron terminals and retrogradely transported back to the sensory afferent somata. The virus can remain latent in the dorsal root (or trigeminal) ganglion neurons for a lifetime. Alternatively, latent varicella zoster virus particles can reactivate. When the virus particles present in a peripheral ganglion reactivate, they produce a blistering and exquisitely painful rash. A herpes zoster rash covers the dermatome innervated by the infected ganglion cells and is thus contained within a single, unilateral spinal dermatome or a single division of the trigeminal dermatome (see Chapter 5).

The skeletal muscles controlled by each spinal segment are the *myotome*. The topographical mapping of myotomes does not closely align to the dermatomal map. For example, C7 receives sensory information from the middle finger and carries motoneuronal output to the triceps. Furthermore, because of the convergence of roots from several segments onto the nerve serving each muscle, the myotomes are spread over several segments. For example, hip movements depend primarily on nerves from L2 and L3 but also involve motoneurons located in L4, L5, and S1.

Of critical importance to life is the innervation of the diaphragm, which stems from *phrenic* motoneurons in C3–C5 (Table 4-2). Phrenic motoneurons, required for breathing, need *instructions*. The instructions come from medullary neurons that communicate a respiratory rhythm

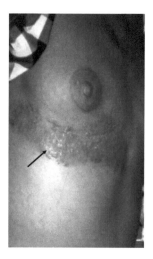

Figure 4-9 An acute shingles rash occupying the right T5 dermatome is shown. Photograph is reprinted with permission from Davis LE, King MK., Shingles and postherpetic neuralgia, in *Clinical neurology of aging* (3rd ed., M Albert and J Knoefel, eds.). New York: Oxford University Press, 2010.

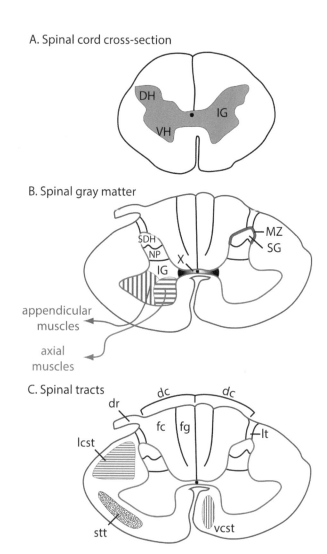

Figure 4-10 A: The spinal cord is divided into a central region of gray matter and a surrounding region of white matter. The gray matter contains the dorsal horn (*DH*), ventral horn (*VH*), and intermediate gray (*IG*) on each side and a midline region around the central canal (*X* marked in B). B: The dorsal horn contains a superficial region (*SDH*) that processes pain and temperature information, and a deeper area called nucleus proprius (*NP*), where tactile information is processed. The superficial dorsal horn is further subdivided into the marginal zone (*MZ*), which contains neurons that project to the brain and the substantia gelatinosa (*SG*), where interneurons are concentrated. In the ventral horn, motoneurons are topographically arranged. Motoneurons innervating appendicular, or limb, muscles are present in a lateral extension to the ventral horn, whereas the medial portion of the ventral horn contains motoneurons that innervate axial muscles. C: The white matter of the spinal cord is divided into sections called funiculi (funiculus is the singular form). The dorsal root (*dr*) carries afferent axons into the spinal cord. Those afferent axons enter either the dorsal horn or the dorsal columns (*dc*), which make up the dorsal funiculus. The dorsal columns contain axons carrying information about touch, vibration, and proprioception. Tactile information arising from the legs travels medially in the fasciculus gracilis (*fg*) and that from the arms travels more laterally in the fasciculus cuneatus (*fc*). The lateral funiculus contains the lateral corticospinal tract (*lcst*) dorsally and the spinothalamic tract (*stt*) ventrally. The ventral funiculus contains tracts primarily related to axial motor function, such as the ventral corticospinal tract (*vcst*). Section drawings are adapted with permission of deArmond S et al., *Structure of the human brain: A photographic atlas*. New York: Oxford University Press, 1989.

to phrenic motoneurons and thereby support breathing. Any damage to the connection from the medulla to phrenic motoneurons will impair breathing to one degree or another. An individual with a complete spinal transection above C3 only survives if placed on a ventilator. Depending on the extent of their lesions, patients with spinal cord injuries affecting the upper cervical cord may require continuous or primarily nighttime breathing support. Key sensory and motor territories of the spinal cord are listed in Table 4-2.

THE SPINAL CORD CONTAINS AN INNER BUTTERFLY OF GRAY MATTER SURROUNDED BY WHITE MATTER

Neurons occupy the central portion of the spinal cord and are surrounded by axonal tracts, traveling up or down the neuraxis, on all sides (Fig. 4-10A). Sensory-related neurons occupy the *dorsal horn*, the dorsal portion of the spinal gray matter, whereas motor-related neurons occupy the *ventral horn* (Fig. 4-10B). Primary afferents carrying information about touch, proprioception, and vibration enter the dorsal columns bound for the dorsal column nuclei in the medulla. Primary afferents that carry pain and temperature information synapse in the superficial part of the dorsal horn. Motoneurons in the ventral horn send axons out the ventral roots to skeletal muscles.

Beyond the dorsal and ventral horns, there is an *intermediate gray* and a central canal region (Fig. 4-10B). The intermediate gray contains preganglionic autonomic neurons but only in two regions:

- T1–L2 segments contain sympathetic preganglionic neurons;
- S2–S4 segments contain parasympathetic preganglionic neurons.

In both cases, the preganglionic neurons are located in the intermediate gray. Sympathetic preganglionic neurons occupy the intermediate gray in a column of cells known of as the *intermediolateral cell column*, which is often abbreviated as *IML*. The IML juts out laterally into the lateral funiculus and is so pronounced that it is also termed the *intermediate horn* (Fig. 4-11). The intermediate horn provides an easily recognizable marker for thoracic segments. Additional preganglionic sympathetic neurons are found more medially, near the central canal, in an area known of as the *intermediomedial cell column*. In segments S2–S4, the intermediate gray contains preganglionic parasympathetic neurons in a region that is sometimes called the *sacral autonomic nucleus* (Fig. 4-11). Preganglionic parasympathetic neurons send their axons out the ventral roots to parasympathetic ganglia typically located in or very near the ultimate target organ.

The spinal white matter that surrounds the spinal gray on all sides is divided up into anatomical chimneys called *funiculi* (singular form is *funiculus*). We recognize dorsal, lateral, and ventral funiculi. The dorsal portion of the lateral funiculus is typically termed *dorsolateral*, and the ventral portion termed *ventrolateral*. All long-distance connections between the spinal cord and brain or between spinal segments travel in the funiculi surrounding the spinal gray.

THE APPEARANCE OF THE SPINAL SEGMENTS DIFFERS GROSSLY ALONG THE LENGTH OF THE CORD

The different functions of the sacral, lumbar, thoracic, and cervical spinal cord are reflected in markedly different appearances in respective cord segments (Fig. 4-11). The dorsal and ventral horns within the lumbar and cervical enlargements dwarf those of the thoracic cord. This follows naturally from the far greater sensory innervation density and the greater number of muscles in the hands and feet relative to the thorax and abdomen. Corresponding to the greater sensory density in the hands and feet, the dorsal horn in the cervical and lumbosacral enlargments is extensive, whereas that in the thoracic cord, where sensory function is most rudimentary, is far smaller.

Within the ventral horn, *motoneurons that control axial or trunk musculature are located close to the midline*. To accommodate motoneurons innervating limb or appendicular muscles, there is an actual lateral extension to the ventral horn. This lateral extension is only present in the cervical and lumbosacral enlargements (Fig. 4-11). Thus, thoracic segments contain a narrow ventral horn, located close to the midline, which contains motoneurons innervating axial muscles exclusively.

The relative amount of white and gray matter also changes across the segments of the spinal cord. Since all motor tracts descend into the spinal cord from the brain and all sensory tracts ascend from the spinal cord to the brain, the greatest amount of white matter is located most rostrally, in cervical segments. Essentially, all roads lead to Rome, and the brain is the neural version of Rome. The least amount of white matter is present in the sacral cord and the coccygeal segment. Because of the sensory and motor complexity of the limbs, particularly the arms, relative to the trunk, the largest area of gray matter is found in the cervical enlargement and the smallest gray area is found in the thoracic cord. Finally, the outer shape of the cord changes along its rostral to caudal length. Sections from the cervical enlargement have an elongated oblong shape, thoracic sections appear almost diamond-shaped, and lumbar sections appear squat and roundish in shape. Sacral sections are almost square in shape and are instantly recognizable for having almost no white matter.

THE ORGANIZATION OF THE SPINAL GRAY

Superficial, middle, and deep regions of the dorsal horn contribute to different somatosensory functions. The *superficial dorsal horn*, consisting of a thin *marginal zone* overlying the thicker *substantia gelatinosa*, is critical to processing pain and temperature information (Fig. 4-10B). The marginal zone contains most of the neurons critical to the perception of pain and temperature, and these project from the spinal cord to the brain. The substantia gelatinosa is home to interneurons involved in the processing of somatosensory information, especially that resulting from noxious and thermal stimulation. Deep to the superficial dorsal horn, the *nucleus proprius* processes light touch information. Finally, the deep dorsal horn serves heterogeneous purposes including processing pain, temperature, and viscerosensory input.

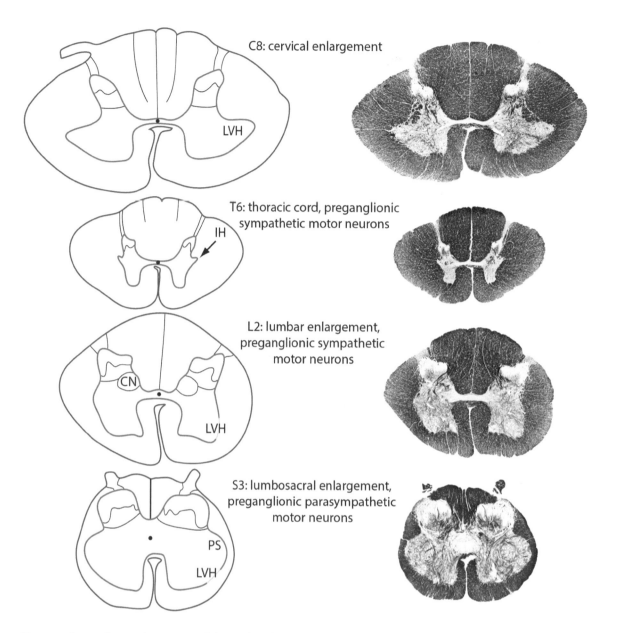

Figure 4-11 The outer shape and internal appearance of the spinal cord differ along the cord's length. Sections from the cervical enlargement (C8) have an elongated oblong shape, a large dorsal horn, a lateral ventral horn (*LVH*), and a large amount of white matter. Thoracic sections (T6) are small and have spindly dorsal and ventral horns, with a pronounced intermediate horn (*IH*) containing preganglionic sympathetic neurons. Lumbar sections, L2 is shown here, are roundish in shape, have a large dorsal horn, a lateral ventral horn, and relatively little white matter. In addition, Clarke's nucleus (*CN*), which processes proprioceptive information from the legs bound for the cerebellum, forms a prominent medial bulge in the dorsal horn of segments T12 to L3. The sacral section shown here, S3, is the most caudal part of the lumbosacral enlargement. It is almost square in shape, has a large dorsal horn, a bulging intermediate gray area, a lateral ventral horn, and almost no white matter. Preganglionic parasympathetic neurons (*PS*) are present in segments S2 to S4 in the intermediate gray. In sum, a few cues can be used to identify the level of a spinal cord section. The cervical cord has the greatest proportion of white matter and the lumbosacral cord the least. Segments from the lumbosacral and cervical enlargements, but not from thoracic cord, contain a lateral ventral horn, reflective of motoneurons that innervate muscles in the distal limb. An intermediate horn marks the thoracic cord.   Photographs reprinted and sections modified with permission from deArmond S et al., *Structure of the human brain: A photographic atlas.* New York: Oxford University Press, 1989.

Within the ventral horn there are pools of motoneurons containing motoneurons innervating a single muscle. Pools are rostrocaudally oriented and cylindrically shaped neuronal collections that cross spinal segmental boundaries. Motor interneurons fill the ventral horn in the space surrounding the motoneuron pools. In addition to the intermediomedial and intermediolateral cell columns that contain autonomic preganglionic neurons, the intermediate gray contains a number of interneurons with important roles in transforming sensory input into skeletal motor output.

THE THREE LONG PATHWAYS TAKE THREE DIFFERENT COURSES THROUGH THE SPINAL CORD

Now that we understand the basic anatomy of the spinal cord, we are ready to follow the routes traveled by the three long pathways (Fig. 4-12). We start with the lemniscal pathway (Fig. 4-12A). Axons from dorsal root ganglion cells that respond to light touch, vibration, and proprioception travel through the dorsal roots and enter the ipsilateral dorsal funiculus, or dorsal column, to travel rostrally. Axons enter the dorsal column from the lateral edge. Therefore, at the level of the cervical cord, axons from the most caudal sacral ganglia, carrying input from the perineum, are located most medially within the ipsilateral dorsal column. This is because axons of progressively rostral dorsal root ganglia, carrying input from the legs, trunks, and arms, take up positions progressively more and more lateral to that of the afferents from the perineum.

There is a gross division within the dorsal columns so that axons carrying tactile information from the legs and most of the trunk travel in the slender *fasciculus gracilis* (from the Latin word for "slender"), whereas axons carrying input from the arms and upper trunk travel in the laterally adjacent, wedge-shaped *fasciculus cuneatus* (from the Latin word for "wedge," Fig. 4-10C). Together, the fasciculus gracilis and the fasciculus cuneatus comprise a dorsal column. *In sum, each dorsal column carries information about light touch, vibration, and proprioception from the ipsilateral body.*

Axons from dorsal root ganglion cells that respond to noxious and thermal stimuli travel through the dorsal roots to synapse in the superficial dorsal horn (Fig. 4-12B). Spinothalamic cells located in the marginal zone carry pain and temperature information across the midline through the *ventral spinal commissure*, just ventral of the central canal gray. *The axons of spinothalamic cells cross in the same segment in which they are located and enter the contralateral ventrolateral funiculus.* Spinothalamic axons travel rostrally

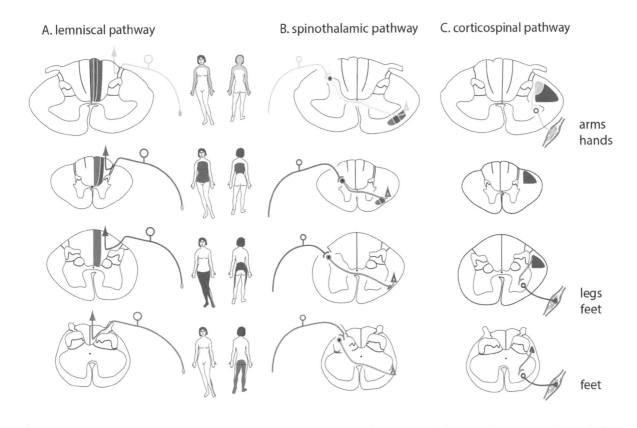

A. lemniscal pathway   **B. spinothalamic pathway**   **C. corticospinal pathway**

arms
hands

legs
feet

feet

Figure 4-12 A: Dorsal root ganglion cells that code for light touch, proprioception, and vibration send their central process into the dorsal columns. Since afferent input always joins the dorsal columns from the lateral side, legs are represented most medially and arms most laterally. B: Dorsal root ganglion cells that code for pain and temperature send their central process into the dorsal horn to the marginal zone. Cells in the marginal zone send an axon across the midline in the ventral spinal commissure to the contralateral spinothalamic tract, located in the ventrolateral funiculus. C: Corticospinal tract axons that control fine voluntary movements travel in the dorsolateral funiculus as the lateral corticospinal tract. Lateral corticospinal axons leave the dorsolateral funiculus and contact motoneurons in the ventral horn of the cervical and lumbosacral enlargements.   Section drawings are adapted with permission from deArmond S et al., *Structure of the human brain: A photographic atlas.* New York: Oxford University Press, 1989.

within the spinothalamic tract of the ventrolateral funiculus to reach the thalamus. In sum, each ventrolateral funiculus contains information about pain and temperature from the contralateral side of the body.

Finally, we consider the corticospinal pathway, which, unlike the two sensory pathways, travels *down* the neuraxis from the cerebral cortex to the spinal cord (Fig. 4-12C). We pick up the pathway in the cervical spinal cord. Recall that the motor decussation is located at the spinomedullary junction, which means that, within the spinal cord, the corticospinal pathway travels contralateral to its point of origin in the cerebral cortex and *ipsilateral to the muscles that it ultimately influences*. When the corticospinal tract divides into two unequal parts at the motor decussation, the smaller portion does not cross the midline and forms the ventral corticospinal tract (*vcst* in Fig. 4-10C). The ventral corticospinal tract supports bilateral postural adjustments of the trunk and proximal limbs but is not involved in controlling fine movements of the hands or feet.

The majority of axons from motor cortex cross at the motor decussation and descend in the dorsolateral funiculus as the lateral corticospinal tract (*lcst* in Fig. 4-10C). At the level of the targeted motoneurons, corticospinal axons leave the dorsolateral funiculus to enter the ipsilateral ventral horn, where they contact motoneurons and motor interneurons (Fig. 4-12C). The lateral corticospinal tract is primarily involved in signaling voluntary movements of the limbs. *In sum, each dorsolateral funiculus contains axons critical to the voluntary movement of ipsilateral limb muscles.*

TEST YOUR UNDERSTANDING OF SPINAL CORD FUNCTION BY DEDUCING THE CLINICAL EFFECTS OF THREE LESIONS

Now is the time to realize how much clinically applicable information you have learned in this chapter. We consider the effect of three lesions, starting with a spinal hemisection, a lesion that has been used as a teaching tool for more than 150 years. Although a perfect hemisection rarely happens, it is of such traditional importance that the lesion has a name: the *Brown-Séquard syndrome* (Fig. 4-13A). So, what symptoms would we expect if half the spinal cord were cut?

In a left hemisection of the spinal cord, the spinal cord is cut completely from the midline to the left edge of the cord. There are three major consequences:

- Perception of all light touch, vibration, and proprioceptive stimuli arising from the same or

ipsilateral side as the lesion—the left side—would be impaired for dermatomes at the level of and caudal to the lesion.

- Pain and temperature sensation would be impaired on the opposite or contralateral side—the right side—for dermatomes at the level of and caudal to the lesion. At the level of the lesion, pain and temperature would be impaired bilaterally due to damage of the crossing spinothalamic tract axons (see more later).

- Voluntary movements would be impaired on the side ipsilateral to the lesion—the left side—for myotomes at the level of and caudal to the lesion.

The deficits caused by spinal disease or injury depend critically on the level of the lesion. Deficits stem from the interruption of long axonal tracts and therefore only apply to tissues innervated by segments at and caudal to the lesion. Clearly, a hemisection in the lumbar cord will result in impaired movement of and sensation from the leg, but the movement of and sensation from the arm will be unaffected. In addition to the obvious topographical effects of lesions at different spinal levels, there are three key syndromes to consider:

- Damage above the sacral cord may adversely affect micturition, sexual function, and defecation.

- Damage above thoracic levels may result in an ipsilateral Horner syndrome.

- Damage above mid-cervical levels may produce breathing insufficiency either all the time or at night.

Next, we consider a lesion affecting the central canal region (Fig. 4-13B). A lesion of the central canal region has no effect on voluntary movements because it does not reach the dorsolateral funiculus. Second, the dorsal columns are not affected. Consequently, a lesion in the central canal region produces no change in voluntary movement or in the sensations of touch, vibration, and proprioception. However, the spinothalamic pathway is affected by a lesion around the central canal because the axons of spinothalamic tract cells cross the midline just ventral to the central canal. These axons, which cross at the level of the primary afferent input, are interrupted by a lesion of the central canal. Therefore, pain and temperature sensations in the dermatome or dermatomes at the level of the lesion are impaired *bilaterally*.

A lesion of the central canal is more than theoretical. The most common cause is *syringomyelia*, which occurs

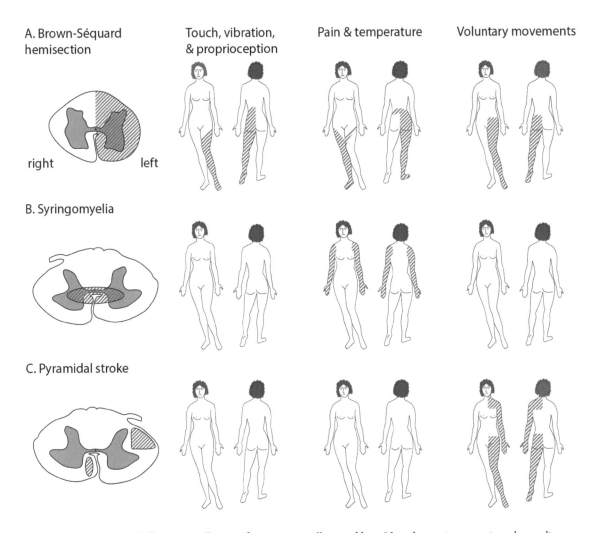

| A. Brown-Séquard hemisection | Touch, vibration, & proprioception | Pain & temperature | Voluntary movements |

| B. Syringomyelia | | | |

| C. Pyramidal stroke | | | |

right   left

Figure 4-13 Three lesions that produce different constellations of symptoms are illustrated here. Note that sections are oriented according to radiological convention with the right side on the left and the left side on the right. A: A hemisection causes Brown-Séquard syndrome, which includes ipsilateral (to the lesion) loss of tactile, vibratory, and proprioceptive sensation, contralateral loss of pain and temperature sensations, and ipsilateral loss of voluntary movements. In addition, pain and temperature sensations are lost bilaterally at the level of the hemisection. Illustrated here is the pattern of deficits after a left L2 hemisection. B: In its early stages, syringomyelia causes a lesion localized to the central canal region. This lesion affects only one of the three long pathways: the spinothalamic tract pathway. Axons crossing through the ventral spinal commissure are interrupted, causing a bilateral loss of pain and temperature sensations. Syringomyelia most commonly affects lower cervical segments; shown here are the deficits expected from a lesion affecting segments C6–C8. C: After a right pyramidal stroke, the axons in the left lateral corticospinal tract are no longer connected to the motor cortex. Therefore, voluntary movement of the left side will be severely impaired. The motor impairment due to unilateral, or one-sided, corticospinal tract damage is most severely apparent in limb movement. Voluntary movements of the trunk are far less impaired in part because the ventral corticospinal tract on the unaffected side can largely compensate. No sensory deficits are associated with damage to the corticospinal tract.   Section drawings are adapted with permission from deArmond S et al., *Structure of the human brain: A photographic atlas.* New York: Oxford University Press, 1989.

when either a cyst, or a cavity termed a *syrinx* (Greek for "pipe" or "channel"), forms around the central canal. The earliest symptom is usually a *bilateral* loss of pain and temperature sensation without any diminution in tactile or proprioceptive sensations. This selective loss of pain and temperature sensation bilaterally results from the interruption of crossing spinothalamic tract axons. The distribution of sensory loss is dermatomal, from the dermatome of the segment where the damage is located. Syringomyelia most frequently affects cervical segments, giving rise to a

bilateral loss of pain and temperature in a glove distribution bilaterally.

Most commonly, syrinxes are congenital and are associated with *Chiari malformations*. Individuals with a Chiari malformation have an abnormally formed fourth ventricle that pushes out of the cranium and into the spinal column. In many affected individuals, the pressure of the fourth ventricle forms a syrinx around the central canal. Other cases of syringomyelia result when a syrinx forms in reaction to trauma, infection, or tumor. Neurosurgical treatment is tailored to the cause of syringomyelia. Typically, the aim of surgery is to either relieve the pressure feeding a syrinx or to remove a cyst or tumor.

Finally, we consider a stroke affecting the right pyramidal tract (Fig. 4-13C). Remember that the corticospinal tract travels in the medullary pyramids *above the motor decussation*. Therefore, a lesion of the right medullary pyramid would affect the left lateral corticospinal tract, which would impair voluntary movements of the left arm and right leg. The ventral corticospinal tract is also lesioned by a pyramidal stroke. However, since the ventral corticospinal tract influences motoneurons innervating axial muscles *bilaterally*, voluntary movements of the trunk are far less impaired than are voluntary limb movements. Pyramidal lesions do not affect either the lemniscal or spinothalamic pathways, and, consequently, no sensory symptoms are present.

ADDITIONAL READING

Edwards A, Andrews R. A case of Brown-Sequard syndrome with associated Horner's syndrome after blunt injury to the cervical spine. *Emerg Med J.* 18: 512–513, 2001.

Burnett C, Day M. Recent advancements in the treatment of lumbar radicular pain. *Curr Opin Anaesthesiol.* 21: 452–456, 2008.

Cuellar JM, Montesano PX, Antognini JF, Carstens E. Application of nucleus pulposus to L5 dorsal root ganglion in rats enhances nociceptive dorsal horn neuronal windup. *J Neurophysiol.* 94: 35–48, 2005.

Dartt DA. Neural regulation of lacrimal gland secretory processes: Relevance in dry eye diseases. *Prog Retinal Eye Res.* 28: 155–177, 2009.

Jensen MC, Brant-Zawadzki MN, Obuchowski N, Modic MT, Malkasian D, Ross JS. Magnetic resonance imaging of the lumbar spine in people without back pain. *N Engl J Med.* 331: 69–73, 1994.

Kiba T. Relationships between the autonomic nervous system and the pancreas including regulation of regeneration and apoptosis: Recent developments. *Pancreas.* 29: e51–58, 2004.

Malpas SC. Sympathetic nervous system overactivity and its role in the development of cardiovascular disease. *Physiol Rev.* 90: 513–557, 2010.

Matsuka Y, Spigelman I. Hyperosmolar solutions selectively block action potentials in rat myelinated sensory fibers: Implications for diabetic neuropathy. *J Neurophysiol.* 91: 48–56, 2004.

Proctor, GB, Carpenter GH. Regulation of salivary gland function by autonomic nerves. *Autonom Neurosci.* 133: 3–18, 2007.

Shibasaki M, Wilson TE, Crandall CG. Neural control and mechanisms of eccrine sweating during heat stress and exercise. *J Applied Physiol.* 100: 1692–701, 2006.

Tai CF, Barniuk JN. Upper airway neurogenic mechanisms. *Curr Opin Allergy Clin Immunol.* 2: 11–19, 2002.

Wilhelm H. The pupil. *Curr Opin Neurol.* 21: 36–42, 2008.

5

CRANIAL NERVES AND CRANIAL NERVE NUCLEI

ranial nerves connect the brain to organs located outside of the cranium. For the clinician, they serve as sentries, well situated to provide the first indication of a serious brain problem and offer observable clues as to the location of a vascular or traumatic mishap. Yet the functions of our cranial nerves are not part of our vernacular language. No one seeks medical help, saying, "Gee, the strangest thing happened last night; my right glossopharyngeal nerve went on the fritz," or "I don't understand it. My stylopharyngeus muscle is just not working right." Therefore, although learning the names of the nerves and structures targeted by nerves aids in conversations with medical professionals, it does not facilitate effective communication with lay people including friends, family, and patients. To understand a patient's concerns, we need to understand cranial nerve function in *lay* terms and then be able to translate a patient's complaint back into "cranial nerve-speak" as well. Therefore, in this chapter, we concentrate on how the cranial nerves support everyday life and on what goes wrong—in both everyday and medical terms—when they do not work correctly.

Were it not for the 12 cranial nerves, the brain and the body would be unconnected islands, a reality explored in numerous works from the *brain-in-a-vat* science fiction genre. Cranial nerves are nothing more special than the ferries, trains. and buses that provide for communication between intra- and extracranial organs (Fig. 5-1). Each cranial nerve leaves the cranium through a *foramen*, a hole in the skull. Cranial nerves can be either one- or two-way conduits with sensory information entering the brain, motor information exiting the brain, or both. In total, five cranial nerves are entirely motor, three are exclusively sensory, and four contain both sensory and motor components.

The cranial nerves connect up to the brainstem on one side and the periphery on the other. This principle is well illustrated by the facial nerve, a mixed cranial nerve containing somatosensory, gustatory, motor, and autonomic components (Fig. 5-2). On the brainstem side are *cranial nerve nuclei*. Motor cranial nerve nuclei contain *efferents*, axons from the brain en route to the periphery, and *afferents*,

axons arising from peripheral neurons that enter the brain to synapse in sensory cranial nerve nuclei. Efferents may be motoneurons or preganglionic parasympathetic neurons. Afferents support somatosensation as well as the special senses of hearing, taste, and the vestibular sense.

Peripherally, cranial nerves split into smaller nerves that traverse diverse pathways to reach target organs located primarily in the head. Centrally, the organization is functional, meaning that *each cranial nerve nucleus serves one function*, such as somatosensation from a particular region or controlling the movement of specific muscles. *Peripheral organization is topographical* with sensory, autonomic, and skeletomotor targets sharing space in the face, eye, oral cavity, upper airway, and so on. Whereas eight of the cranial

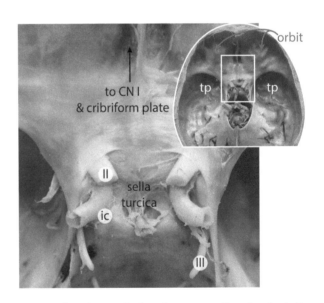

Figure 5-1 Looking down at the dura that remains adhered to the skull with the brain removed, the optic (*II*) and oculomotor (*III*) nerves can be seen leaving the dural sac of the cranium. The optic nerves join together in a midline structure called the optic chiasm (*not shown*) that sits just over the sella turcica where the pituitary is housed. The olfactory nerve (CN I) consists of small unmyelinated fibers that enter the cranium through the cribriform plate (*labeled arrow at top*). The inset shows the location of the magnified area (*white box*) within the anterior fossa from which the forebrain has been removed. The depressions on either side hold the temporal lobes with the temporal poles (tp) located rostrally. The roof of the orbits indent into the cranium at the site of the orbitofrontal cortex. ic, internal carotid.

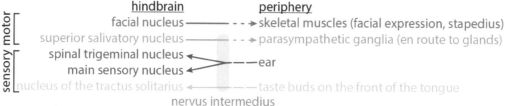

A. central and peripheral connections of the facial nerve

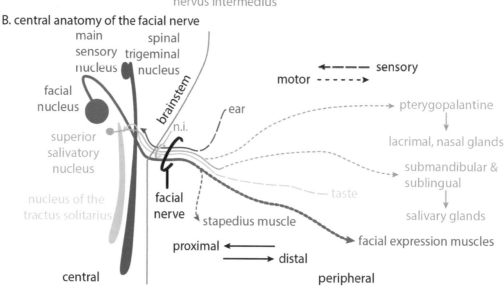

B. central anatomy of the facial nerve

Figure 5-2 The facial nerve is a mixed cranial nerve that connects to multiple cranial nerve nuclei. A: Motor (branchial) axons arising from the facial nucleus form the main portion of the facial nerve whereas axons from the superior salivatory nucleus (preganglionic parasympathetic) gather with sensory axons destined for the main sensory nucleus and spinal trigeminal nucleus (somatosensory) and nucleus of the tractus solitarius (special sensory) in a separate bundle (*gray*) that is sometimes called the nervus intermedius. B: The cranial nerve nuclei of the facial nerve are illustrated in a top-down cartoon of the hindbrain. The courses of peripheral nerves (not drawn to scale) are shown on the right. Axons connected to cranial nerve nuclei, five of which are shown here, exit from the pontomedullary junction as the facial nerve, consisting of a main root and the nervus intermedius (n.i.). They leave the cranium and thread through the petrous temporal bone, eventually splitting up into smaller peripheral nerves to reach target organs. Thus, axons from several brainstem regions join together into the facial nerve, which exists as an entity only for a short stretch and then diverges again to reach many peripheral targets. Consequently, injuries to the facial nerve pathway cause very different complements of symptoms depending on the site of the lesion. A lesion of the facial nerve trunk will impair all of the sensory, autonomic, and motor functions served by the facial nerve. Peripheral lesions that are progressively more distal, or far from the central nervous system, cause progressively more limited impairments that a discerning physician can identify. Central lesions cause impairments that are limited in terms of facial nerve function but typically cause additional, unrelated symptoms due to damage of neighboring areas that serve other roles.

nerves serve one or a few related functions, four serve multiple, unrelated functions for organs of the head and internal viscera.

Due to the requisite partnerships among cranial nerve nuclei, cranial nerves, and peripheral organs to produce function, damage in any of these locales can produce the same symptom. However, the *collection of symptoms* will differ in logical and diagnostically invaluable ways. For example, consider a person who has difficulty in making facial expressions. The problem could be in cranial nerve VII, which carries motor axons to the muscles of facial expression; this occurs in *Bell's palsy*, an important condition that we consider later. Alternatively, the problem could be central. The facial nucleus, the cranial nerve nucleus that contains the motoneurons that innervate muscles of facial

expression, could be damaged by stroke. The inability to make facial expressions could also result from a lesion of the descending (corticobulbar) inputs that target facial nucleus motoneurons. Finally, the disease could be in the muscle or the neuromuscular junction, as occurs in *myasthenia gravis* for example.

How is it possible to distinguish between a neuromuscular junction problem, a nerve problem, and a brain problem? Essentially, by considering the *ensemble of symptoms* exhibited. A collection of symptoms that matches the particular components of one cranial nerve probably results from damage to that cranial nerve. On the other hand, central damage caused by trauma, stroke, or tumor is seldom so tidy as to affect only one brain locus or one cranial nerve nucleus. Therefore, although central and cranial nerve damage can cause the same symptom, they do so in conjunction with different sets of accompanying symptoms. Knowing the anatomy of cranial nerves with respect to other cranial nerves and underlying brain structures permits you to accurately estimate whether a cranial nerve lesion could be the source of a given set of symptoms, as well as to predict—and therefore look for—additional signs likely to accompany the presenting issue.

After completing this chapter, the potential contributions of individual cranial nerves to patients' complaints will be clear. Armed with a solid knowledge of cranial nerve function and anatomy, the potential causes of impairments such as difficulty with swallowing, smiling, or maintaining a steady gaze can be narrowed down. All cranial nerves, including the forebrain ones, are discussed because testing them forms a core part of the neurological exam and is invaluable in diagnosis and lesion localization. In fact, easily observed signs in combination with a good patient history can allow you to finely localize lesions with accuracy and economy that rivals or even exceeds that afforded by a modern radiological image.

THERE ARE 12 CRANIAL NERVES

The cranial nerves are grouped and numbered through historical convention. They are labeled by Roman numerals from I to XII, with I entering the olfactory bulb at the rostral tip of the brain and IX, X, and XII exiting from the caudal medulla (Fig. 5-3). Each cranial nerve has a common name. The common names of all cranial nerves, the nature of their components, and the part of the brain from where the root exits are listed in Table 5-1. This information should be memorized.

Cranial nerves I and II, which enter the forebrain, will be discussed briefly here, with more detail on the optic nerve (CN II) provided in Chapter 7. The remaining cranial nerves, which exit from either the brainstem (III–X, XII) or the spinal cord (XI), are the focus of this chapter. Cranial nerves differ from spinal nerves in that they exit from the cranium rather than from the vertebral column. In another dissimilarity from spinal nerves, cranial nerves can contain only sensory fibers or only motor fibers, as well as a mixture of sensory and motor fibers. In contrast, recall that spinal nerves are mixed because they carry both sensory and motor axons, or fibers. In this chapter, you will learn the target of each cranial nerve and, more importantly, the symptoms associated with dysfunction of each cranial nerve.

Eight of the 12 cranial nerves serve one or a few related functions and are therefore fairly easy to learn and

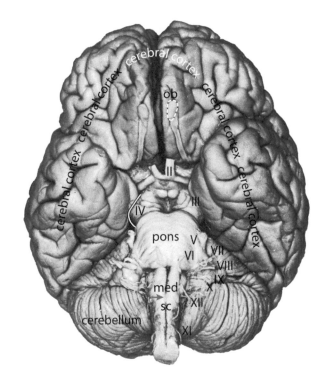

Figure 5-3 The brain from the ventral surface. The pyramidal decussation (*red arrow*) marks the junction between the spinal cord (*sc*) and medulla (*med*) and the location of the foramen magnum. Rostral to the medulla is the pons, marked by a bulbous base, and rostral to the pons is the midbrain (unlabeled). The roots of the cranial nerves are labeled except for the olfactory nerves, which have been sheared off. The olfactory nerve consists of a large number of tiny axons that connect the nasal epithelium to the olfactory bulb (*ob*). These tiny axons are not visible, but the bulb is clearly seen at the base of the frontal lobes. The roots of cranial nerves II, III, V, VI, VII, VIII, and X are visible and marked. The root of cranial nerve IV exits from the dorsal side of the midbrain and snakes around to the ventral surface of the brainstem near the junction of the pons and midbrain (*yellow nerve marked IV*). Photograph reprinted with permission from deArmond S et al., *Structure of the human brain: A photographic atlas.* New York: Oxford University Press, 1989.

remember. The olfactory nerve (I) carries olfactory information, the optic nerve (II) carries visual information, and the vestibulocochlear nerve (VIII) carries auditory and vestibular information from the inner ear. The abducens (VI) and trochlear (IV) nerves each innervate a single extraocular muscle capable of moving the eye. The spinal accessory (XI) and hypoglossal (XII) nerves carry motor output to muscles of the neck and tongue, respectively. The oculomotor nerve (III) is more complex but nonetheless serves related functions: eyeball and eyelid movements, lens accommodation, and pupillary constriction.

Four cranial nerves with both sensory and motor components—V, VII, IX, X—are more challenging to learn and remember. Yet damage to each of these has a dominant clinical consequence. The trigeminal nerve (V) carries the vast majority of the somatosensory input from the face and oral cavity and serves the dominant role in facial and oral

Table 5-1 **CRANIAL NERVES ARE NUMBERED FROM ROSTRAL TO CAUDAL AND ROMAN NUMERALS ARE TRADITIONALLY USED**

CRANIAL NERVE #	COMMON NAME	COMPONENTS (CLINICALLY MOST IMPORTANT COMPONENT/S IN ITALICS)	EXIT/ENTRY POINT
I	Olfactory	*Special sensory (olfaction)*	Telencephalon (olfactory bulbs)
II	Optic	*Special sensory (vision)*	Thalamus
III	Oculomotor	*Somatic motor (eye and eyelid movements)* Autonomic motor (*pupillary constriction*, lens accommodation)	Mid-midbrain
IV	Trochlear	*Somatic motor (eye movement)*	Pons-midbrain junction (dorsum)
V	Trigeminal	*Somatosensory (from face, oral cavity, meninges of the anterior cranial fossa)* Branchial motor (chewing muscles, one middle ear muscle)	Mid-pons
VI	Abducens	*Somatic motor (lateral eye movement)*	Pontomedullary junction (midline)
VII	Facial	*Branchial motor (facial expression muscles, one middle ear muscle)* *Autonomic motor (salivation, tearing)* Special sensory (taste from front 2/3 of tongue) Somatosensory (part of ear)	Pontomedullary junction (lateral)
VIII	Vestibulocochlear	*Special sensory (hearing, vestibular sense)*	Pontomedullary junction (far lateral)
IX	Glossopharyngeal	*Branchial motor (swallowing, speech, gag reflex)* Autonomic motor (parotid salivation) Special sensory (taste from back 1/3 of tongue, soft palate) Viscerosensory (carotid body input) Somatosensory (tympanic membrane, parts of ear, posterior tongue, pharynx)	Rostral medulla
X	Vagus	*Branchial motor (swallowing, speech including laryngeal muscles, gag and cough reflexes)* Autonomic motor (body viscera above the hindgut) Special sensory (taste from pharynx) Viscerosensory (aortic arch, thoracic and abdominal viscera above the hindgut) Somatosensory (meninges of the posterior fossa, parts of ear, pharynx)	Rostral medulla
XI	Spinal accessory	*Branchial motor (shrugging, turning head)*	Cervical spinal cord
XII	Hypoglossal	*Somatic motor (tongue muscles)*	Caudal medulla (lateral to inferior olives)

sensation. The dominant roles of the facial nerve (VII) are motor control of muscles involved in making facial expressions along with providing the parasympathetic drive for salivation, lacrimation, and nasal secretions. Disruption of facial somatic motor axons results in facial paralysis, whereas lesions of the parasympathetic axons in the facial nerve produces dryness of the eyes, nose, and mouth. The bulk of the fibers in the vagus nerve (X) are parasympathetic fibers destined for viscera above the hindgut. However, *the dominant clinical consequence of vagus damage arises from disruption of motor fibers to the upper airway, resulting in difficulties in speech (dysarthria) and swallowing (dysphagia), hoarseness, and impairment of the gag and cough reflexes* that prevent airborne irritants, liquids, and solids from entering the throat and airway, respectively. The glossopharyngeal nerve (IX) carries a hodge-podge of sensory, motor, and autonomic information. As with the vagus nerve, the clinical consequences of glossopharyngeal nerve damage are dominated by the motor innervation of the upper airway. Thus, glossopharyngeal nerve damage may produce dysphagia and impairment of the cough reflex.

As is true of the symptoms that result from spinal neuropathy or radiculopathy, damage to cranial nerves typically produces negative motor and sensory symptoms along with positive sensory symptoms (Table 5-2). Disruption of motor fibers to skeletal muscle results in paralysis or weakness;

Table 5-2 COMMON CLINICAL SYMPTOMS ASSOCIATED WITH CRANIAL NERVE DAMAGE

CRANIAL NERVE	NEGATIVE SYMPTOM	POSITIVE SYMPTOM
I (typically only if damage is bilateral)	Anosmia	Phantom smells
II	Blindness	Phosphenes (rare)
III	Diplopia (extraocular muscle paralysis), ptosis, loss of near vision, loss of pupillary reflexes in affected eye	
IV	Diplopia (superior oblique muscle paralysis)	
V	Anesthesia of face and oral cavity, loss of corneal reflex	Facial, oral paresthesias and dysesthesias
VI	Diplopia (lateral rectus muscle paralysis)	
VII	Facial paralysis (throughout affected side), loss of corneal reflex, xerostomia (dry mouth), dry nose and eyes	Paresthesias and dysesthesias of the ear
VIII	Deafness, vertigo and disequilibrium (loss of sense of balance)	Tinnitus
IX	Stylopharyngeal muscle paralysis (dysphagia, impaired gag reflex)	
X	Upper airway paralysis (dysphagia, dysarthria, hoarseness, impaired gag and cough reflexes)	
XI	Sternocleidomastoid muscle paralysis (loss of head turning), trapezius muscle paralysis (loss of shrugging), winged scapula	
XII	Tongue muscle paralysis	

positive signs such as excess movements are not observed with nerve lesions. Similarly, lesions of autonomic output to parasympathetic ganglia in the head result in a loss of salivation, lacrimation, pupillary constriction, or accommodation. Interestingly, even a complete lesion of the vagus nerve with its large number of parasympathetic fibers destined for the body viscera has no dramatic consequences on visceral function.

Negative sensory symptoms resulting from cranial nerve damage include blindness, deafness, facial and oral anesthesia, *anosmia* (inability to smell), and *ageusia* (inability to taste). With respect to somatosensation, hearing, olfaction, and taste, interruption of sensory fibers, either partial or complete, often produces positive signs such as spontaneous paresthesias, *tinnitus* (ringing in the ear), and phantom smells or tastes. Vision is different from the other sensory systems because damage to the optic nerves often produces loss of vision without the positive sign of *phosphenes*, spontaneously perceived light flashes that occur independently of optical input. One final point regarding positive sensory signs is worth noting. Individuals who lack a sense from birth do not experience positive signs of that sense. For example, a congenitally deaf person does not experience tinnitus and a congenitally anosmic individual (rare) does not perceive phantom smells. Thus, positive signs require past perceptual experience with a sensory modality along with acquired damage to the sensory pathways involved.

CRANIAL NERVE EXIT POINTS AND NUCLEI FOLLOW A MIDLINE-MOTOR TO LATERAL-SENSORY RULE

Remember from Chapter 3 that, in the developing spinal cord, a dorsally located alar plate gives rise to sensory neurons and a ventrally located basal plate gives rise to motoneurons and preganglionic autonomic neurons (Fig. 5-4A). Recall that an indentation in the embryonic central canal, the sulcus limitans, marks the border between alar and basal plates and thus between dorsal sensory and ventral motor territories. Corresponding to the dorsal sensory and ventral motor gray areas, spinal roots carrying sensory information enter dorsally, and roots carrying motor information into the periphery exit the spinal cord ventrally. The same sensory–motor separation principle applies in the hindbrain but with a topographical relationship that runs from sensory functions *laterally* to motor functions *medially* (Fig. 5-4B). The sulcus limitans, still present as a shallow groove on the floor of the fourth ventricle, remains the dividing point between sensory and motor territories. Thus, regions medial to the sulcus limitans serve motor functions, and cranial nerve nuclei located lateral to the sulcus limitans serve sensory functions. Since the division between sensory and motor territories is diagonally oriented, sensory and motor territories

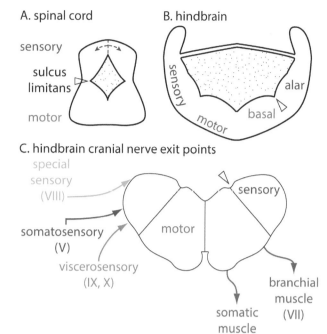

A. spinal cord

sensory

sulcus
limitans

motor

B. hindbrain

sensory

motor

alar

basal

C. hindbrain cranial nerve exit points

special
sensory
(VIII)

sensory

somatosensory
(V)

motor

viscerosensory
(IX, X)

branchial
muscle
(VII)

somatic
muscle
(III, IV, VI, XII)

Figure 5-4 A: The same sensory-motor topography present in the developing spinal cord (A) is present in the developing hindbrain (B), but shifts due to the opening of the fourth ventricle (*dashed purple lines at the top of A*). The regions devoted to each type of neuron are oriented from lateral to medial in the brainstem instead of from dorsal to ventral as in the spinal cord. C: To understand this organization, imagine a diagonal line from the sulcus limitans to the ventrolateral surface of the brainstem. Nuclei medial to this line send axons out to serve motor functions and nuclei lateral to the line receive input from sensory afferents. The exit points for brainstem cranial nerves can be mapped onto the pie-slice organization. In the five cranial nerves with mixed functions (III, V, VII, IX, X), exit points are best predicted by the territory serving the nerve's greatest number of fibers. As will be further detailed in the next chapter, visceral serving efferents and afferents hug the sensory-motor boundary while somatic motor efferents exit most medially and somatosensory afferents enter more laterally.

- Motor types:
  - *Somatomotor*: Skeletal muscles derived from somites
  - *Branchial motor*: Branchiomeric muscles (skeletal muscles derived from branchial arches; see later discussion)
  - *Autonomic motor*: Preganglionic parasympathetic neurons

- Sensory types:
  - *Somatosensory*: Somatosensory from the face and oral cavity
  - *Viscerosensory*: Somatosensory from the body viscera; taste
  - *Special sensory*: Hearing, vestibular sense, olfaction, vision

Before explaining the utility of learning this organization, we take a detour to understand the meaning of the branchial motor category.

The subcategory of *branchial motor* refers to muscles derived from *branchial arches*, also known as *pharyngeal arches*, which are transient developmental structures of the vertebrate embryo that give rise to some but not all of the muscles in the head. The remaining muscles of the head, along with muscles of the body, derive from somites. In fish, branchial arches develop into the gills; in mammals, they complement rostral somites to become the source of bones, cartilage, and muscles in the head region. In the human, five arches give rise to muscles used for chewing (innervated by cranial nerve V) and facial expression (VII) along with muscles found in the middle ear (V, VII), upper airway (IX, X), and neck (XI). Muscles arising from branchial arches are termed *branchiomeric muscles*, and the motoneurons that innervate them are *branchial motoneurons*. There are no known differences in the functional properties of *adult* branchiomeric and somite-driven muscles. Nonetheless, the distinction is helpful to learning the anatomy of cranial nerve nuclei and exit points. Additionally, learning the terms enables you to read the human and nonhuman research literature. The term *skeletomotor* will be used to refer to all skeletal muscles, including both branchiomeric and somatic motor (referred to as *somatomotor* here) ones.

Within each pie slice, subtypes of sensory and motor functions occupy specific regions. The most medial region of the medial motor pie slice contains somatic motoneurons. Lateral to this most medial region, but still medial to the sulcus limitans, visceromotor neurons (i.e., preganglionic parasympathetic neurons) and branchial motoneurons reside. Pie slices lateral to the sulcus limitans contain secondary sensory neurons that receive input from visceral afferents and taste inputs medially

in the hindbrain can be imagined as modified pie slices (Fig. 5-4C).

The exit points for brainstem cranial nerves can be mapped onto the pie slice organization. In the five cranial nerves with mixed functions (III, V, VII, IX, X), exit points are best predicted by the territory serving the nerve's greatest number of fibers. As will be further detailed in the next chapter, visceral-serving efferents and afferents hug the sensory–motor boundary, whereas somatic motor efferents exit most medially and somatosensory afferents enter more laterally.

The pie slice organization of the brainstem does not simply distinguish between motor and sensory. Instead, there are characteristic locations for subtypes of motor and sensory functions. The functions served by cranial nerves include three motor and three sensory types (Fig. 5-4C):

and somatosensory and special afferents more laterally. For the purposes of cranial nerve exits, considering four slices of the brainstem suffices. From medial to lateral, the regions are involved in:

- Somatomotor output to somatic muscles

- Output to parasympathetic ganglia and branchiomeric muscles

- Receiving afferents from the viscera and from taste buds

- Receiving somatosensory and special afferents

It is this four-part-organization that aligns with cranial nerve exits (Fig. 5-4C). Brainstem cranial nerves that contain only one type of fiber (IV, VI, VIII, XI, XII) exit from the appropriate pie slice. Thus, the vestibulocochlear nerve (VIII), exclusively serving a special sensory function, exits the hindbrain at the far lateral margin.

Cranial nerves with an exclusive (IV, VI, XII) somatic motor component exit the brainstem from points very close to the midline (Fig. 5-5). The trochlear nerve (IV) is an exception because it exits from the dorsal midline of the caudal midbrain (Fig. 5-6), the only cranial nerve that does not exit from the base of the brain. It then wends its way around the side of the brainstem to emerge on the ventral side (Fig. 5-3).

For the remaining (brainstem) cranial nerves that contain more than one fiber subtype (III, V, VII, IX, X), there is a twist. The exit points for the mixed cranial nerves align to the region that represents the nerve's *anatomically* most predominant component. Thus, the oculomotor nerve (III), containing mostly somatic motor axons, exits along the midline of the midbrain (Fig. 5-5). The facial nerve (VII), which contains primarily branchial motor fibers, exits more laterally, but still medial to the sensory pie slices. The remaining mixed cranial nerves (V, IX, X) are

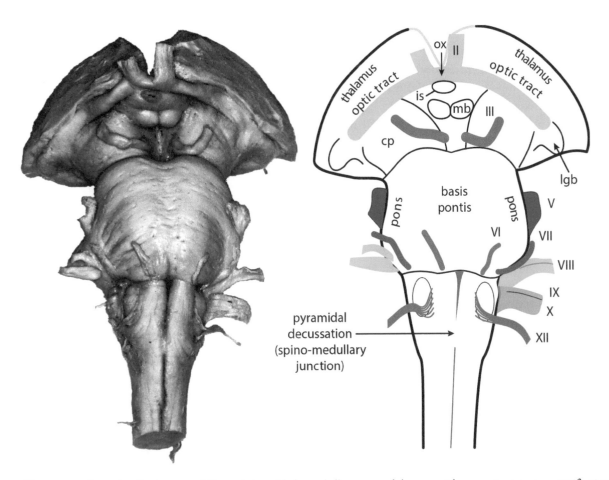

Figure 5-5 The ventrum of an isolated brainstem and diencephalon with the cerebellum removed shows cranial nerve exits at greater magnification. The roots of cranial nerves II, III, V, VI, VII, VIII, IX, X, and XII are visible in the photograph and labeled in the diagram on the right. Additional landmarks are provided for orientation. The bulbous base of the pons is termed the basis pontis. The oculomotor nerves exit from the medial margin of the cerebral peduncles (*cp*) that mark the midbrain ventrum. Diencephalic structures include the mammillary bodies (*mb*), infundibular stalk (*is*), optic tract and chiasm (*ox*), lateral geniculate body (*lgb*), and thalamus.   Photograph reprinted with permission from deArmond S et al., *Structure of the human brain: A photographic atlas.* New York: Oxford University Press, 1989.

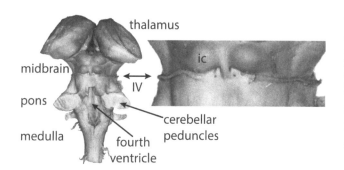

thalamus

midbrain

pons

medulla

IV

ic

cerebellar peduncles

fourth ventricle

Figure 5-6 The trochlear nerve (*IV*) exits from the dorsal surface of the brainstem, the only cranial nerve to do so. A magnified view, shown at right, shows the exit of the trochlear nerve near the junction between the pons and midbrain, just caudal to the inferior colliculus (*ic*), an auditory processing region in the caudal midbrain. For orientation, the medulla, pons, midbrain, and thalamus are labeled on the brainstem, illustrated at left, and viewed from the dorsal side. The cerebellum has been removed by cutting the cerebellar peduncles. Without the cerebellum, the dorsal surface of the hindbrain is revealed, exposing the floor of the fourth ventricle. Photograph reprinted with permission from deArmond S et al., *Structure of the human brain: A photographic atlas*. New York: Oxford University Press, 1989.

dominated by sensory fibers and enter the ventrum of the brainstem through the lateral pie slice. In the case of the vagus nerve (X), the exit point aligns to the *anatomically dominant* component (viscerosensory) rather than to the foremost clinical component (branchial motor). The exit points for the trigeminal (V; somatosensory-dominated) and vestibulocochlear (VIII; exclusively special sensory) nerves are lateral to the exit of the vagus nerve (viscerosensory). The glossopharyngeal nerve (IX) contains a mélange of fiber types that enter the medulla in line with fibers of the vagus nerve.

Finally, there is a rostro-caudal order to the exit points of the nine brainstem cranial nerves, with the higher numbers exiting more caudally (Fig. 5-3). The abducens, facial, and vestibulocochlear nerves (VI–VIII) exit at the pontomedullary junction where the pons and medulla meet (Fig. 5-5). All higher numbered cranial nerves (IX–XII) exit from the medulla, or the spinal cord in the case of cranial nerve XI. Cranial nerves III, IV, and V exit from the midbrain, ponto-mesencephalic (pons-midbrain) junction, and pons, respectively.

THE BRAINSTEM CRANIAL NERVE NUCLEI ARE THE SOURCE OR TARGET OF THE NINE BRAINSTEM CRANIAL NERVES

Cranial nerve nuclei, brainstem collections of neurons that connect with cranial nerves, are a diverse group. Because the correspondence between cranial nerves and cranial nerve nuclei is far from one-to-one, the symptoms that arise from peripheral (cranial nerve) and central (cranial nerve nucleus) lesions are different. In order to appreciate how certain collections of symptoms could only arise from cranial nerve damage, the cranial nerve nuclei are introduced here (Table 5-3); further detail is provided in Chapter 6. The sensory cranial nerve nuclei are listed here:

- The *main* or *principal sensory nucleus* and the *spinal trigeminal nucleus* are two somatosensory nuclei that process somatosensory information from the face and oral cavity. Input to the trigeminal nuclei travels primarily through the trigeminal nerve (V) with far smaller contributions from VII, IX, and X.

- The *nucleus of the solitary tract* or *nucleus tractus solitarius* (viscerosensory) processes both taste and viscerosensory information, the latter from the viscera above the hindgut. Virtually all of the viscerosensory input travels in the vagus nerve (X), with input from the carotid body arriving via IX. Taste input travels in cranial nerves VII, IX, and X.

- The *vestibular nuclei* (special sense) process vestibular input that provides information about the movement and position of the head. All input arises from the vestibular portion of the vestibulocochlear nerve (VIII).

- The *cochlear nuclei* (special sense) process sound-related input and are critical to speech perception and other auditory functions such as the auditory startle reflex. All input arises from the cochlear portion of the vestibulocochlear nerve (VIII).

Cranial motor nuclei can be divided roughly into three groups:

- Somatomotor nuclei contain motoneurons innervating the tongue and extraocular muscles:
  - Motoneurons in the *hypoglossal nucleus* send axons through the hypoglossal nerve (XII) to innervate tongue muscles.
  - Motoneurons in the *abducens* nucleus send axons through the abducens nerve (VI) to innervate one extraocular muscle, the lateral rectus.
  - Motoneurons in the *trochlear* nucleus send axons through the trochlear nerve (IV) to innervate one extraocular muscle, the superior oblique.

CRANIAL NERVE NUCLEUS	CRANIAL NERVES	FUNCTION SERVED
Edinger-Westphal	Oculomotor (III)	Pupillary constriction, accommodation (lens rounding)
Oculomotor	Oculomotor (III)	Motor control of four extraocular muscles and levator palpebrae superioris
Trochlear	Trochlear (IV)	Motor control of one extraocular muscle
Motor trigeminal	Trigeminal (V)	Motor control of chewing muscles, tensor tympani
Main sensory	Principally trigeminal (V) with small contributions from VII, IX, X	Tactile sensation from the face
Spinal trigeminal	Principally trigeminal (V) with small contributions from VII, IX, X	Pain and temperature sensation from the face and oral cavity
Abducens	Abducens (VI)	Motor control of one extraocular muscle
Facial	Facial (VII)	Motor control of facial expression muscles, stapedius muscle
Cochlear*	Vestibulocochlear (VIII)	Hearing
Vestibular*	Vestibulocochlear (VIII)	Sense of balance and equilibrium
Nucleus of the solitary tract	Principally vagus (X) with contributions from VII, IX	Taste and viscerosensation
Ambiguus	Vagus (X) and glossopharyngeal (IX)	Motor control of upper airway
Dorsal motor nucleus of the vagus	Vagus (X)	Parasympathetic control of the viscera above the hindgut
Hypoglossal	Hypoglossal (XII)	Motor control of tongue muscles

- Motoneurons in the *oculomotor* nucleus send axons through the oculomotor nerve (III) to four extraocular muscles and the levator palpebrae superioris (eyelid).

- Nuclei containing branchial motoneurons innervating muscles derived from branchial arches:
  - Motoneurons in the *motor trigeminal nucleus* send axons through the trigeminal nerve (V) to chewing muscles and to the tensor tympani, a middle ear muscle that stretches the tympanic membrane.
  - Motoneurons in the *facial nucleus* send axons through the facial nerve (VII) to muscles of facial expression and to one middle ear muscle, the stapedius, which pulls the stapes away from the cochlea.
  - Motoneurons in *nucleus ambiguus* send axons through the glossopharyngeal (IX) and vagus (X) nerves to muscles of the upper airway, including those of the pharynx and larynx.
  - Motoneurons in the ventral horn of the cervical cord send axons through the spinal accessory nerve (XI) to innervate two neck muscles, the sternocleidomastoid and the trapezius, which support shrugging and head-turning.

- Visceromotor cranial nerve nuclei contain preganglionic parasympathetic neurons that project to parasympathetic ganglia controlling autonomic functions of the head and the body above the hindgut:
  - The *Edinger-Westphal nucleus* contains preganglionic parasympathetic neurons that produce pupillary constriction and lens accommodation. The nucleus' output travels exclusively in the oculomotor nerve (III). Since the Edinger-Westphal nucleus is a close neighbor of the oculomotor nucleus, damage to one of these often damages the other as well.
  - The *salivatory nuclei* control the production of tears, nasal secretions, and saliva. There are two nuclei, which send their output through the facial (VII) and glossopharyngeal (IX) nerves. These nuclei are not of great clinical import because they are not injured in isolation, and, when lesioned, they account for the most minor of the resulting problems. They are not discussed further.
  - The *dorsal motor nucleus of the vagus* provides parasympathetic control of the heart and other viscera and of the digestive tract above the hindgut. Output is through the vagus (X) nerve.

The remainder of this chapter details the function of each cranial nerve, including the forebrain ones, along with the potential clinical consequences of damage to each nerve.

The olfactory nerve consists of very thin, unmyelinated, short axons that arise from olfactory sensory neurons in the nasal (or olfactory) epithelium and project into the olfactory bulbs at the very rostral tip of the brain. The olfactory nerve carries the entire output of the olfactory epithelium into the brain. No other route exists by which chemosensory information regarding airborne chemicals (aka odors) can reach the brain.

The delicate, thin axons of the olfactory nerve thread the skull's cribriform plate and are vulnerable to horizontal shearing action. Indeed, a common cause of olfactory nerve damage is *whiplash* from a car crash or sports injury. The quick back-and-forth movement clips the thin olfactory axons as they pass through the cribriform plate. Since the nasal epithelium contains neural progenitor cells that continue to make new olfactory neurons throughout an individual's lifetime, one may surmise that anosmia due to whiplash would resolve once new olfactory sensory neurons are born. However, typically this is *not* the case, perhaps because scar tissue blocks the nascent sensory axons from entering into the olfactory bulb.

The appearance of *anosmia*, the inability to smell, or *hyposmia*, a reduction in smell detection and discrimination, in young people is usually due to a peripheral lesion acquired through trauma, viral infection, or chemical injury from smoke, nasal sprays, or the like. A smaller number of anosmic patients have a congenital condition. Since olfactory testing is not common, congenital patients may not become aware of their sensory deficit until reaching their teens or early twenties. In older individuals, the loss of smell or reduction in the ability to discriminate between smells may be an early sign of a neurodegenerative condition such as Alzheimer's or Parkinson's disease. Central changes to the modulatory control of olfactory bulb processing appear to be responsible for the impairment of olfaction in neurodegenerative diseases.

In *Kallmann syndrome*, congenital anosmia is coupled with a failure to enter puberty and therefore reach sexual maturity. In this syndrome, the axons of olfactory sensory cells fail to cross the cribriform plate to reach the olfactory bulb. Furthermore, hypothalamic neurons that make and release *gonadotropin releasing hormone* (*GnRH*) are born in the olfactory epithelium, a highly unusual, perhaps unique, example of central neurons that are not of neural tube origin. GnRH neurons normally migrate along the axons of the olfactory sensory cells (the developing olfactory nerve) into the olfactory bulb and then on to the hypothalamus. If the olfactory nerve fails to develop, GnRH-containing neurons cannot reach the hypothalamus. As a result, puberty is not initiated in these patients! Hormonal therapy allows patients with Kallmann syndrome to mature sexually but they will remain unable to smell. Mutations in a number of different genes involved in the development of olfactory sensory neurons and axon guidance of olfactory nerve fibers may cause Kallmann syndrome.

Patients with acquired anosmia rarely present with the complaint that they cannot smell. Instead, they are more likely to complain that everything tastes bland; this follows from flavor's heavy dependence, estimated at roughly 80%, on smell more so than on taste. *Flavor* is a compound sensation that integrates the primary senses of taste, smell, texture, and temperature. Flavor is even heavily influenced by vision—hence the garnish that adorns plates presented by top chefs—and contextual cues such as lighting, music, conversation, and the social milieu. The extreme dependence of flavor on non-oral cues has been used to successfully fool food critics into raving about fast food presented as fine, organic food. Even though taste plays a smaller role than smell in flavor, people commonly refer to a food's flavor as its "taste."

The *loss of smell* can be an emotionally devastating experience and is typically accompanied by depression. It can cause weight loss—without smell, food becomes far less appetizing—or weight gain—eating more is required to reach a sensation of fullness—and even alternating weight loss and gain. Food preferences may also shift to involve hot and spicy ingredients that contribute to flavor by engaging somatosensory (trigeminal) rather than olfactory pathways. The pleasure of intimate relations may also be diminished by a loss of smell. Finally, patients with acquired anosmia may experience *phantom smells*, which are typically unpleasant.

The emotional toll exacted by anosmia on congenital patients is usually less than it is for those with acquired anosmia. From one perspective, we don't miss what we have never had. As a rule, humans don't pine for the electric eel's ability to sense electric fields or the ability to hear a bat's ultrasonic calls. However, missing a sensory modality that everyone else has can be challenging both socially and medically. Failure to appreciate that one's clothes have an unpleasant odor can be socially awkward and failing to smell smoke, spoiled milk, or rotten food is potentially dangerous. Moreover, the condition is sufficiently rare that awareness is low and patients often encounter disbelief and even hostility from teachers, friends, and strangers. The reader can participate in creating a more understanding and compassionate future for anosmic patients.

THE OPTIC NERVE CARRIES VISUAL INPUT FROM THE VISUAL FIELDS

The second cranial nerve, the optic nerve, exits the cranium, and yet is part of the central nervous system. Recall that the retina and optic nerve develop from the optic vesicle, itself an outpouching of the diencephalon (see Chapter 3). Therefore, the optic "nerve" is actually an axon bundle contained entirely within the CNS, typically termed a tract. Nonetheless, *the optic nerve leaves the cranium* and therefore meets the most critical criterion for a cranial nerve. The nomenclature involving these axons is peculiar as the very same axons from the retina are called by two different names at different parts of their trajectory. Between the retina and the optic chiasm, retinal axons form the optic nerves (Fig. 5-7). As these same axons continue past the chiasm to the thalamus, they are called the *optic tracts*.

Each optic nerve carries all of the information from one eye. Thus, a complete lesion of an optic nerve causes blindness of one eye. Since the bulk of the visible world is viewed binocularly, through both eyes, vision may remain largely intact with loss of only a small monocular crescent on the side of the lesion (see Chapter 15). Optic nerve damage, such as that caused by *optic neuritis*, an inflammation of the nerve often found in patients who either have or go on to develop multiple sclerosis, may cause blurred or reduced vision of the eye—and sometimes blindness—on the affected side.

Optic nerve lesions do not cause double vision or diplopia. Instead diplopia results from a misalignment of the eyes due to a problem with the motor control of eye position (see more later). Conversely, visual loss that persists, even when viewing the world monocularly through one or the other eye, is due to a problem in the optic nerve, retina, or eye (Fig. 5-7). As will be explored in more detail in Chapter 7, visual loss that affects the ability to see part of the world, or *visual field*, with *either eye* results from a retrochiasmal lesion distal to the optic chiasm.

The optic nerve carries optical information that serves functions beyond visual perception. Such nonvisual

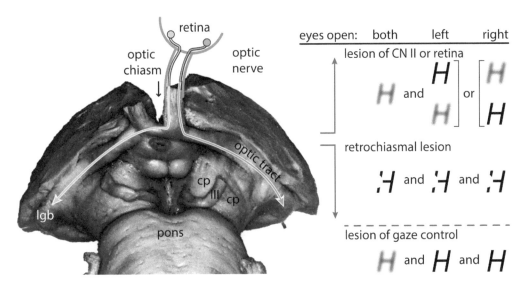

Figure 5-7 The route traveled by retinal axons that form the optic nerve is diagrammed on the ventral surface of the brain. Retinal axons leave the retina via the optic nerve. At the optic chiasm, axons from the nasal hemiretina (*gray*) cross the midline while temporal retinal axons (*blue*) bypass the optic chiasm, destined for the lateral geniculate body (*lgb*) on the same side. Between the optic chiasm and the lateral geniculate, retinal axons continue into the optic tracts, which travel next to the cerebral peduncles (*cp*), a major fiber tract at the base of the midbrain. Despite the different names, the optic nerves and optic tracts contain the same retinal axons. Additional structures labeled for orientation include the pons and the oculomotor nerve (*III*). On the right, the visual consequences of damage to either visual or gaze control pathways are diagrammed for a person looking at an italicized H. Moderate to severe damage to the retina or optic nerve may impair vision when both eyes are open. The same impairment will occur when the affected eye is open alone but not when the affected eye is closed. Visual losses that affect one part of the world, viewed through either eye, are due to retrochiasmal damage. A common example of this is a scotoma, a small region of visual loss, illustrated here as a chunk missing from the *H*. A scotoma is present when either eye is open alone as well as when both eyes are open together. Visual problems that do not appear when either the left or right eye is open alone are due to a problem with gaze pathways; these problems produce double vision or diplopia. Note that patients may not report their symptoms in medically accurate terms, for example referring to diplopia as blurry vision. Photograph reprinted with permission from deArmond S et al., *Structure of the human brain: A photographic atlas.* New York: Oxford University Press, 1989.

functions include the entrainment of the circadian rhythm. Of great clinical import, the optic nerve carries sensory information that drives the *pupillary light reflex*. This reflex links changes in ambient *luminance*, the overall level of light, to pupillary diameter: increasing the pupil size when light levels dim and decreasing pupillary diameter when the amount of light increases. The pupillary light reflex is very easy to test clinically by dimming the room lights and flashing a light onto a person's eye. After some minutes in dim lighting, a healthy person's pupils will be large. Flashing a light onto the eyes in this condition will elicit pupillary constriction. The reflex depends on the optic and oculomotor cranial nerves, along with midbrain circuitry. After introducing the oculomotor nerve, the logic of pupillary light reflex testing will be explained.

EYE MOVEMENTS ARE ACCOMPLISHED BY SIX EXTRAOCULAR MUSCLES

We use *gaze* to visually explore the environment, either maintaining gaze on an object of interest or shifting gaze from one location to another. The direction of gaze is tightly controlled by the brain through a process known as *fixation*. Light emanating from every spot in our visual field is refracted topographically onto spots on the retina. The topographic arrival of light rays from the world on the retina is accomplished by the eye's refractive power (plus glasses if needed) and represents *focus*.

Before diving into gaze control, it is critical that the reader understands the precise meanings of *fixate* and *focus*. Unfortunately, *focus* is often used incorrectly and *fixate* is not in the common vernacular, although it should be. The correct usages are:

- Light is focused onto the retina; eyes are not focused. An image is *in focus*. Eyes are not in focus.

- We fixate objects when we look at or turn our gaze upon those objects. We do not focus our gaze.

Thus, when an individual fixates on an object, light from that object is focused onto the retina. We can now move on.

At rest, the eye sits in the *neutral position*, looking straight ahead with the pupil located in the center of the *palpebral fissure*, the visible part of the eye. Extraocular muscles move the eye in the *horizontal, vertical,* and *torsional* planes. Horizontal eye movements move the eye side to side, and vertical eye movements move the eye up and down (Fig. 5-8). A horizontal movement of the eye toward the temple is called *abduction*,

and one toward the nose is *adduction*. Up and down vertical eye movements are termed *elevation* and *depression*, respectively. Torsional movements are rotations of the eyes around the anterior-posterior axis that goes through the eye; *intorsion* is a rotation of the top of the eye toward the nose and *extorsion*, away from the nose.

Gaze depends on the position of both the head and the eyes within the head. Even so, eye movements do more of

A. Vertical movements about a horizontal axis

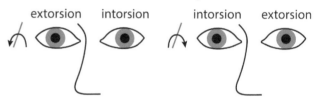

B. Torsional movements about the optic axis

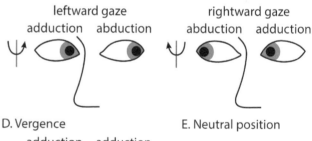

C. Conjugate horizontal movements about a vertical axis

D. Vergence

E. Neutral position

Figure 5-8 There are three axes about which the eyes move—horizontal, vertical, and the optic axis that runs through the eye. A: Moving the eyes up and down, termed elevation and depression, involves rotation of the eyes around a horizontal axis. B: Rotating the eyes around the optic axis that goes through the pupil is called torsion, with rotating the top of the eye toward the nose termed intorsion and away from the nose, extorsion. C: Moving an eye in the horizontal plane is accomplished by rotating the eye around a vertical axis. Movement of the eye toward the nose is termed adduction, and moving it toward the temple is abduction. D: When viewing near objects, the two eyes converge. This vergence, or convergence, is disconjugate (the two eyes move in different directions) with the left eye moving right and the right eye moving left. Vertical (A) and torsional (B) movements are always conjugate, meaning that the two eyes invariably move in the same direction. Horizontal movements can either be conjugate (C) or disconjugate in the case of vergence (D). E: For viewing far objects located straight ahead, the eyes relax back to the neutral position.

the work in determining gaze than do head movements. Small gaze shifts are accomplished using eye movements almost exclusively, and even large gaze shifts depend primarily on eye movements (see Chapter 19). Six *extraocular* muscles, muscles that attach to the eyeball, are responsible for moving the eyes and directing gaze. All extraocular muscles are innervated by three cranial nerves: oculomotor (III), trochlear (IV), and abducens (VI). Before delving into the functions of these cranial nerves, a detour into how the extraocular muscles produce eye movements is warranted.

The six extraocular muscles include four rectus and two oblique muscles; their pulling directions are illustrated in Figure 5-9. The simplest extraocular muscles are the *medial* and *lateral recti* (singular is *rectus*), which adduct and abduct the eye, respectively (Fig. 5-8C). The medial and lateral recti not only have one action each, but they accomplish that action solo. The remaining four extraocular muscles—*inferior oblique, superior rectus, superior oblique, inferior rectus*—are more complicated because they all have secondary actions as well as a primary action. Furthermore, the actions of each of these muscles depend on eye position.

To understand the actions of the inferior oblique, superior rectus, superior oblique, and inferior rectus muscles, we need to look at the anatomy of the orbit (Fig 5-10A–E). The four rectus muscles all arise at the annulus of Zinn located at the back vertex of the bony orbit (Fig. 5-10A). Since the recti insert at sites anterior to the equator of the globe, their pulling directions are relatively straightforward, true to the etymology of rectus (Latin for "straight"). The superior

rectus elevates the eye, and the inferior rectus depresses. The only wrinkle to this comes from the fact that the axes of the superior and inferior recti muscles are not parallel to the axis of the eye (in the neutral position), the line through the center of the cornea and lens (Fig. 5-10B). Therefore, when the eye is in the neutral position, the superior and inferior recti muscles adduct the eyeball as well as elevate or depress it (Fig. 5-10D). They also cause a torsional rotation; for example, the superior rectus intorts the eye, rotating the top of the eye toward the nose around both the optic and vertical axes, along with causing elevation and adduction (Fig. 5-10D, G). However, when the eye is abducted, the optic axis lines up with the axis of the superior and inferior recti muscles (Fig. 5-10E). Consequently, the recti muscles produce a pure vertical movement: an elevation in the case of the superior rectus and a depression in the case of the inferior rectus (Fig. 5-10E, H).

The oblique muscles differ substantially from the rectus muscles in both anatomy and action. The inferior oblique muscle arises medially at the front of the bony orbit and inserts on the back of the globe, posterior to the equator (Fig. 5-10C). The superior oblique muscle passes through the trochlea, a loop in the medial wall of the orbit, and then transitions into a tendon that inserts on the globe, posterior to the equator (Fig. 5-10I). The upshot of this is that the superior oblique rotates the eye forward around the horizontal axis. The forward rotation around the horizontal axis is responsible for the counterintuitive inversion whereby the superior oblique muscle depresses the eye and the

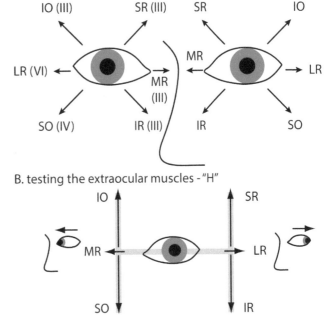

Figure 5-9 A: The primary action of each extraocular muscle when the eyes are in the neutral position is illustrated with the innervating cranial nerve listed in parentheses. This diagram makes evident that conjugate vertical and torsional movements depend on the pairings of the superior rectus (SR) with the contralateral inferior oblique (IO) and the inferior rectus (IR) with the contralateral superior oblique (SO). B: Testing the cranial nerves innervating extraocular muscles can be accomplished by having a person trace an "H" with his gaze. The required muscle activations to reach the six points of the H are listed. Note that medial is to the left and lateral to the right in this illustration. In the adducted eye, the oblique muscles serve as the elevators and depressors whereas in the abducted eye, the recti muscles do so.

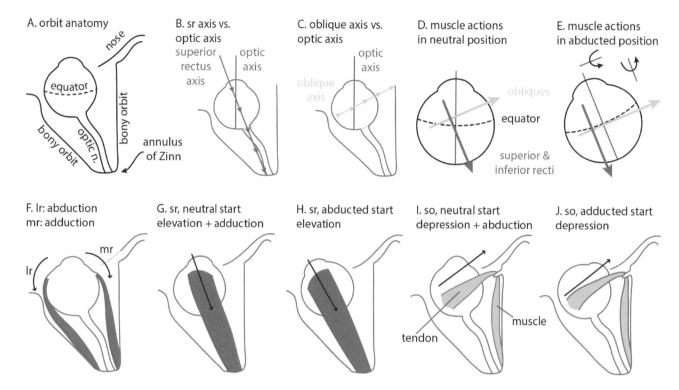

A. orbit anatomy

B. sr axis vs. optic axis

C. oblique axis vs. optic axis

D. muscle actions in neutral position

E. muscle actions in abducted position

F. lr: abduction mr: adduction

G. sr, neutral start elevation + adduction

H. sr, abducted start elevation

I. so, neutral start depression + abduction

J. so, adducted start depression

Figure 5-10 The logic behind the pulling directions of the rectus and oblique muscles is illustrated on a cartoon of the left orbit viewed from above. A: The rectus muscles arise at the annulus of Zinn and insert at sites that are anterior to the globe equator. The oblique muscles arise medially at the front of the bony orbit. The inferior oblique inserts posterior to the equator as does the tendon connected to the superior oblique (I). B–E: The pulling directions of the inferior and superior rectus muscles are angled with respect to the axis of the eye and are at a right angle to the pulling directions of the inferior and superior oblique muscles. D: When the eye is in the neutral position, rotation of the inferior and superior rectus muscles results in adduction as well as depression or elevation. Conversely, the inferior and superior oblique muscles abduct the eye in addition to their primary action of shifting eye position vertically. There are also torsional consequences, with superior oblique muscle contraction causing intorsion and inferior oblique muscle contraction causing extorsion. E: When the eye is abducted, the inferior and superior rectus muscles rotate the eye purely around a horizontal axis, whereas the inferior and superior oblique muscles cannot contribute to depression or elevation because their pulling directions are parallel to the horizontal axis of the eye. F: The medial and lateral recti cause simple adduction and abduction, respectively. G: The superior rectus elevates, adducts, and intorts the neutrally positioned eye. H: When the eye is abducted, the superior rectus is a strong elevator of the eye. I–J: The superior oblique depresses, abducts, and intorts the neutrally positioned eye but is a strong depressor of the eye in the far adducted position.

inferior oblique elevates the eye. Furthermore, although the oblique muscles pull toward the midline, they abduct the eye (a secondary action) because of their insertion posterior to the equator of the globe (Fig. 5-10C, D). This secondary action disappears, and the oblique muscles become strong elevators and depressors when the eye is fully adducted (Fig. 5-10J). Notably, when the eye is adducted, the rectus muscles are nearly parallel with the horizontal axis and therefore cannot contribute to elevation or depression, which are accomplished by the superior and inferior oblique muscles (Fig. 5-10J).

The eyes move together, in *conjugate*, during all vertical (and torsional) eye movements and most horizontal eye movements. This means that if one eye moves up, the other eye also moves up; when one eye *abducts* to the right, the other also moves to the right but *adducts* to do so. Conjugate eye movements employ pairing an extraocular muscle on one side with a different extraocular muscle on the other side. To accomplish a horizontal gaze shift, the lateral rectus muscle on one side and medial rectus on the opposite side are paired together. We can thus consider that each lateral rectus muscle is yoked to the contralateral medial rectus muscle. The other two muscle pairings are less obvious. They are:

• superior rectus + contralateral inferior oblique

• inferior rectus + contralateral superior oblique

For example, when looking down and to the left, the left superior oblique and the right inferior rectus are contracted together. The yoked movements of the three pairs of extraocular muscles support all conjugate eye movements.

As should be evident by now, positioning the eye so that two muscles are parallel to the horizontal axis (Fig. 5-10D, E) isolates the function of a single extraocular muscle (beyond the medial and lateral recti). For example, in the adducted position, the superior and inferior rectus muscles cannot rotate the globe about a horizontal axis because their line of action is parallel with the horizontal axis. Therefore, the inferior oblique elevates the adducted eye and the superior oblique depresses the adducted eye. By similar logic, the superior and inferior rectus muscles elevate and depress the abducted eye, respectively. Figure 5-9B illustrates the use of these principles in a valuable clinical test of extraocular function that involves a person using gaze to trace the shape of an H.

Not *all* eye movements are conjugate. *Vergence*, a disconjugate eye movement, occurs automatically when one switches from looking at a far object to viewing a near object in the horizontal plane (Fig. 5-8D). During vergence, both eyes adduct in toward the nose. This is accomplished by contraction of both medial rectus muscles. When switching from near to far viewing, both eyes return from an adducted position to the neutral position. This latter movement occurs through passive relaxation of the adducting muscles and does not involve active muscle contraction.

DEFICITS IN GAZE CONTROL CAN LEAD TO DOUBLE VISION

Gaze is special, very special. The position of no other part of the body, including the hands, digits, or mouth, is controlled as precisely as is gaze. Because of the brain's tight control of gaze, light from an object hits corresponding points on the left and right retinas (Figure 5-11; see more on this in Chapter 7). Corresponding points are always judged relative to the fovea so that, for a person gazing straight ahead and viewing an object on the left, the corresponding points will be in the nasal retina on the left and temporal retina on the right (Fig. 5-11A). A gaze shift to fixate on the object will then result in light from that object hitting the fovea of both retinas (Fig. 5-11B).

If the two eyes are misaligned by even the minutest amount, double vision or *diplopia* will result. The problem is that light from an object is focused onto different locations in retinal coordinates, termed *retinotopic*, in the two eyes. In other words, the retinotopic locations hit by one object upon the two retinas will be shifted with respect to each other. For example, if the fixation point of the right eye is on the target but the left eye is fixated to the right of the target, the scene viewed by the two eyes will be different, displaced in the horizontal direction (Fig. 5-11C). The result will be a *horizontal diplopia*, with the right eye's image displaced to the right of the left eye's image. When the images viewed by the two eyes are displaced in the vertical

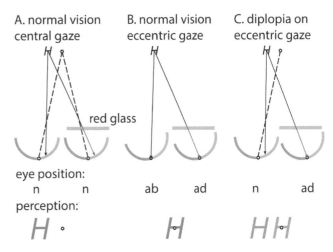

eye position:
n   n   ab   ad   n   ad

perception:

Figure 5-11 Normally, light from peripherally located objects in the world (H at the top of each panel) hits corresponding points on the left and right retinas regardless of whether eye position is neutral (A) or eccentric (B). In cases of diplopia (C), light from a single target hits non-corresponding points on the two retinas. The cause of diplopia can be diagnosed by using "red-glass testing" in which a red glass or filter is placed over one eye (right as illustrated here), thereby distinguishing the images viewed by the two eyes. A: When looking straight ahead with the eyes in the neutral position (n), light from a peripheral target hits the peripheral retina on either side. In the case illustrated, light from a target in the left visual field (left of the fixation point marked by the empty circle) hits the left retina at a site nasal to the fovea and hits the right retina, temporal to the fovea. A single overlapping image is perceived (*bottom*) with that image located to the left of the point of fixation (*empty circle*). Light from the point of fixation is refracted so that it reaches the fovea of each eye (*dashed lines*). B: Abduction (*ab*) of the left eye and adduction (*ad*) of the right eye shifts gaze to the left. This gaze shift brings the point of fixation to an eccentric, or off center, eye position where light from the target hits the fovea of each retina. Consequently, a single image is perceived in the center of the visual field. C: In a patient with a left abducens palsy, the left eye does not abduct and remains in the neutral position (*n*) while the right eye adducts. As a result, light from the target hits the fovea of the right eye but hits a spot nasal to the left fovea. The perception arising from the input from the right eye, colored red by the filter, will therefore be perceived at the point of fixation whereas the perception arising from input to the left eye will be located to the left of the point of fixation (*dashed line*). Thus, the red target image will be perceived as located to the right of the uncolored image.

direction, we call this a *vertical diplopia*. The fact that diplopia occurs with even tiny misalignments of only a degree is a testament to the incredible level of control that is normally exerted over gaze.

Not surprisingly, people rarely report their symptoms using medical terminology, often complaining of blurry vision when the problem is in fact diplopia. Thus, the first step in analyzing a vision problem is to determine if the issue is one of gaze control or of visual processing (Fig. 5-7). Luckily, there is an easy way to determine whether poor vision results from mispositioning of the eyes, as is often the case, or from a problem with the visual system. The patient must simply close each eye in turn and report whether the visual disturbance persists (Fig 5-7). If the problem does not occur when either eye is open alone and only occurs when the two eyes are open, then gaze control is to blame.

One consequence of tight gaze control is that the world appears steady as we move through the world. *Oscillopsia* is a devastating failure of gaze control that results in visual inconstancy. Images are perceived as moving or oscillating as they would if you viewed the world through a hand-held camera rather than through your rock-steady gaze. To understand what this looks like, twirl yourself around a few times and then stop. Your eyes will beat back and forth in a pattern called *post-rotatory nystagmus*. This oscillation in eye position—and therefore in the visual scene—is perfectly healthy but mimics oscillopsia, the condition that represents the polar opposite of our normally steady and controlled gaze.

DAMAGE TO CN III, IV, OR VI LEADS TO SPECIFIC FORMS OF DIPLOPIA

As you know by now, the oculomotor nerve innervates four of the six extraocular muscles, whereas the trochlear and abducens nerves innervate one extraocular muscle each. The muscles innervated by the oculomotor nerve are:

- *Medial rectus*: Adducts the eye toward the nose

- *Superior rectus*: Elevates and adducts the eye

- *Inferior oblique*: Elevates and abducts the eye

- *Inferior rectus*: Depresses and adducts the eye

The trochlear nerve innervates the superior oblique, and the abducens nerve innervates the lateral rectus muscle. Right away, one important fact is evident. *Upward gaze depends solely on the oculomotor nerve.* Thus, impairment of upward gaze necessarily involves the oculomotor nerve or the upstream pathways that control it.

Deducing the symptoms of oculomotor, trochlear, and abducens palsies is straightforward and the effects entirely logical. As we shall now see, the diplopia resulting from damage to a cranial nerve involved in extraocular motor control may occur in the neutral position and be exacerbated in particular eye positions and mitigated in others. For some types of diplopia, a compensatory head posture that returns gaze to the neutral position may occur.

A lesion of the oculomotor nerve negates the actions of four of the six muscles controlling the ipsilateral eye. The only muscles that remain operative are the superior oblique

and the lateral rectus, innervated by cranial nerves IV and VI, which pull the eye down plus laterally (IV) and laterally (VI), respectively. Therefore, oculomotor nerve damage can produce an eye that is "down and out" at rest, during what would normally be a straight-ahead gaze. In fact, the eye on the side of a complete oculomotor nerve lesion cannot *fully* reach any other position besides the down and out position. Therefore, diplopia will be pervasive, present in virtually all gaze locations and in all directions, but worse during upward gaze and medial eye movement with the affected eye. Diplopia is only one of several symptoms that occur after oculomotor nerve damage.

Remember that after exiting from the dorsal surface of the brainstem, the tiny trochlear nerve wends its way around to the ventral side of the brainstem (Fig. 5-6). Perhaps because of this perilous journey, the cranial nerve most commonly damaged by head trauma is the trochlear. Trochlear nerve palsy, while not devastating, happens. It has more restricted effects than does oculomotor nerve damage, causing vertical diplopia particularly during downward gaze, rendering descending stairs or reading a book in one's lap particularly challenging. Because the superior oblique's depressing action is most apparent when the eye is in the adducted position, the effects of trochlear nerve palsy are most severe during ipsilateral gaze—meaning while looking toward the side of the lesion. When fixating straight ahead, there is a small deviation in the desired eye position that patients can, and often do, mitigate with a downward tuck of the chin away from the side of the lesion. In this way, patients use head position to make up for a deficit in eye movement control and thereby maintain relatively normal gaze.

The sixth cranial nerve, which innervates the lateral rectus muscle, is of great clinical importance because it is absolutely required for lateral eye movements, which are critical for reading (among other functions). As they exit from the pontomedullary junction near the midline, abducens nerve roots straddle the basilar artery (a large artery at the base of the pons, see Chapter 8). A number of paths lead to abducens nerve dysfunction including tumors, aneurysms, and even sinus infections.

As with oculomotor and trochlear nerve palsies, *abducens palsy* involves diplopia, which is most severe when looking to the side of the affected nerve (Fig 5-11C). During horizontal gaze to the affected side, the eye on the affected side fails to abduct even as the contralateral eye adducts. For example, if a person with a left abducens palsy makes a leftward eye movement, the right eye adducts while the left eye remains looking forward (Fig. 5-11C). Two different scenes instead of one shared scene hit the two eyes, and diplopia results. During straight-ahead gaze, the eye on the affected side may be slightly adducted due to the medial rectus muscle acting unopposed by the lateral rectus muscle. A slight turn of the head toward the affected side moves the eye's proper position medially and can correct the diplopia during straight-ahead gaze. In this way, a head movement can compensate for an eye movement deficit.

A SUDDEN HEADACHE, DOUBLE VISION, AND PTOSIS ARE CAUSE FOR SERIOUS CONCERN AND IMMEDIATE ACTION

The oculomotor nerve exits from the base of the midbrain (Figs. 5-3 and 5-5), a location that is particularly vulnerable to any increase in intracranial pressure. As we shall see in Chapter 8, a stroke may increase pressure so that the forebrain pushes down on the midbrain, resulting in a sudden loss of oculomotor nerve function on one or both sides. Increased pressure on the forebrain as well as pressure on the midbrain compromises consciousness or creates a clinical state of confusion. Therefore, when associated with a sudden-onset headache along with confusion or any degree of unresponsiveness, acute signs of oculomotor nerve impairment should be interpreted as a sign of a cerebrovascular accident and treated as a medical emergency.

Damage of the oculomotor nerve produces several gaze issues, as discussed earlier:

- Down and out eye (visible in an unconscious patient)

- Inability to look up (requires an alert and cooperative patient)

- Diplopia (requires an alert and communicative patient)

Oculomotor damage has additional consequences because, beyond carrying the motor innervation to four extraocular muscles, the third cranial nerve also innervates one skeletal muscle in the eyelid and provides all parasympathetic innervation to the eye. Therefore, a lesion of the oculomotor nerve also results in:

- Ptosis (most obvious in an alert patient)

- Loss of the *pupillary light reflex* (testable in an unconscious patient)

- A failure of near vision (requires an alert and cooperative patient)

Each of these clinical issues is discussed in turn.

The oculomotor nerve innervates the *levator palpebrae superioris*, a skeletal muscle in the eyelid. The levator palpebrae superioris is not an extraocular muscle since it does not attach to the globe. It is the only muscle that supports *voluntary* eyelid elevation. Therefore, interruption of levator palpebrae superioris innervation results in a droopy eyelid, or ptosis. However, in the absence of levator palpebrae superioris contraction, the eyelids may not close completely during waking because the superior tarsal muscle, a smooth muscle under sympathetic control, remains active and attaches to the levator palpebrae superioris. As you learned in Chapter 4, the superior tarsal muscle is innervated by the sympathetic system so that the eyes are open during waking and the eyelid increasingly elevated during periods of progressive arousal. Because of the two eyelid muscles, ptosis can result either from damage to the oculomotor nerve or from Horner's syndrome. These two causes can be distinguished because voluntary eyelid elevation ameliorates the ptosis due to Horner's but not that caused by oculomotor palsy.

The oculomotor nerve, in concert with the optic nerve, is critical to the pupillary light reflex, a reflex that opposes changes in overall luminance or brightness. Testing the pupillary light reflex arc provides a reliable tool to query the health of both cranial nerves involved (II, III). The reflex arc starts with sensory information regarding luminance that arises in the retina and travels through the optic nerve to reach the ipsilateral midbrain (Fig. 5-12A). This information is processed within the midbrain and transformed into a parasympathetic motor signal that travels back to the eye. Preganglionic parasympathetic axons of the oculomotor nerve reach the ciliary ganglion, where they contact parasympathetic neurons that innervate the pupillary sphincter muscle, a smooth muscle.

Luminance information crosses in the midbrain so that the pupils of both eyes react to luminance changes presented to either eye. For example, an increase in the light level hitting the right eye triggers left as well as right pupillary constriction. The pupillary reflex evoked on the same side as the change in luminance is *direct*, whereas the pupillary reflex in the contralateral eye is termed *consensual*. The end result is that the pupils on both the same and opposite side as the original stimulus constrict (Fig 5-12A). Given this circuitry, consider the following three scenarios, which are summarized in Figure 5-12B:

- *Optic nerve (CN II) lesion*: Flashing a penlight into the eye on the affected side elicits neither a direct nor

A. pupillary light reflex circuit

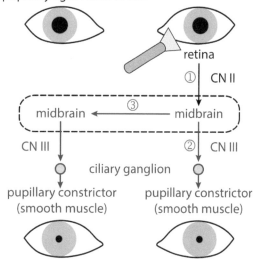

consensual pupillary reflex   direct pupillary reflex

B. lesions affecting pupillary light reflex

	(unilateral) lesion site		
			midbrain
	CN II	CN III	(midline)
	①	②	③
ipsilateral stimulus			
direct response	X	X	√
consensual response	X	√	X
contrateral stimulus			
direct response	√	√	√
consensual response	√	X	X

Figure 5-12 The pupillary light reflex is a simple reflex that is of great clinical utility. A: Information regarding a change in luminance travels from the retina to the midbrain through the optic nerve. Within the midbrain, luminance information is processed by the pretectal nucleus and then passed on to the Edinger-Westphal nucleus, which contains preganglionic parasympathetic neurons that travel in the oculomotor nerve and ultimately control the pupillary constrictor muscle. Importantly, information crosses the midline within the midbrain so that a luminance change in one eye affects the pupils of both eyes. B: The effects of three common lesions on the direct and consensual pupillary reflexes evoked by light flashed into each eye are illustrated. Check marks represent responses that are intact and "X" marks represent responses that are impaired or absent, depending on the extent of the lesion. The location of each lesion site (*circled numbers*) is marked in panel A.

a consensual response. In contrast, a penlight flashed into the unaffected eye elicits normal responses on both sides.

- *Oculomotor nerve (CN III) lesion*: Flashing a penlight into the eye on the affected side will elicit a consensual response but not a direct one. A penlight flashed on the unaffected side will elicit a direct response but not a consensual one. Thus, no response will occur on the affected side although stimulation of either eye will

elicit a response on the unaffected side. Additionally, interruption of the parasympathetic input to the pupil results in an absence of any constriction to oppose the tonic pupillary dilation driven by sympathetic activity. Therefore, a large or "blown" (and nonreactive, as above) pupil (in common parlance) results. The medical term for a blown pupil is *mydriasis*.

- *A midline lesion in the midbrain*: A midline midbrain lesion interrupts the crossing of reflex information and therefore prevents the consensual response on either side. The direct responses remain intact on both sides. Increased intracranial pressure that presses down on the midbrain dorsum caused by a pineal tumor, for example, is a common source of midbrain crossing lesions.

The clinical utility of the pupillary light reflex is enormous. This simple, noninvasive test reliably assesses the health of two pairs of cranial nerves. Moreover, the pupillary light reflex does not require a patient's participation, making it appropriate for unconscious, uncooperative, confused, and preverbal individuals. All that is required is a dim room to maximize the evoked change in pupillary diameter, a penlight, and a trained observer.

THE OCULOMOTOR NERVE IS NECESSARY AND SUFFICIENT FOR THE NEAR TRIAD

The final function of the oculomotor nerve is the *near triad*, a collection of three adjustments that allow for fixation on close objects. The near triad is important to everyday life, particularly in the modern literary world. Failure of the near triad means trouble with reading and using a computer, problems that are highly likely to motivate one to seek help.

The near triad consists of one skeletomotor and two parasympathetic components:

- Vergence of the eyes changes the angle of incident light and thereby increases the eye's refractive power (skeletomotor)

- *Accommodation* adjusts the eye's refractive power by modifying the shape of the lens (parasympathetic)

- Pupillary constriction narrows the pupil and thereby reduces the *cone of blur* (parasympathetic)

How each of the components of the near triad contributes to near vision will be elaborated in Chapter 15. Here, we focus on the cranial nerve requirements of the near triad. As you already know, vergence depends on medial rectus muscles. The other two components of the near triad depend on preganglionic parasympathetic neurons that travel in the oculomotor nerve and control ciliary and pupillary constrictor muscles. Thus, *the oculomotor nerves are wholly responsible for all three components of the near triad.*

Vergence is the only component of the near triad under voluntary control. A person adducts both eyes in order to fixate on a near object. Pupillary constriction and accommodation then occur automatically, outside of conscious control. You can see two of the three reactions by watching someone as he switches his gaze from the horizon to a finger held in front of his face. Most obviously, you will see that the two eyes converge. Also observable, but more difficult to see, is constriction of the pupils. The third component of the near triad, rounding up of the lens, is not visible.

When switching from viewing a near to a far object, the near triad is reversed through passive mechanisms. In other words, the medial rectus muscles relax, but the lateral recti are not actively contracted. Similarly, contraction of the pupillary sphincter and ciliary muscles is terminated, allowing the pupil to slowly open and the lens to flatten.

Accommodation inevitably fails with age, a failure that stems from an increasing inelasticity of the lens rather than through any neural inadequacy. Progressive lens stiffness with age is unavoidable, up there with gravity and taxes, and fuels the need for "reading glasses" among individuals in their fifth decade and beyond. The age-related failure of the near triad, termed *presbyopia*, or old-man-vision, is a consequence of accommodative failure. As such, it allows affected individuals to appreciate, through its absence, the fine-tuning provided by the lens's refractive power.

In sum, impairment of the oculomotor nerve will lead to any, some, or all of the following symptoms:

- Diplopia, down and out eye at rest
- Ptosis
- A blown and nonreactive pupil
- Failure of the near triad

Oculomotor nerve axons that innervate skeletal muscles arise from the oculomotor nucleus, whereas preganglionic parasympathetic axons that innervate the ciliary ganglion arise from the neighboring, but not overlapping, Edinger-Westphal nucleus. Therefore, *a single lesion that impairs both skeletomotor and parasympathetic oculomotor functions is more likely to arise from an injury to the oculomotor nerve than to the brain*. In contrast to the multiple deficits caused by oculomotor nerve damage, only diplopia results from damage to the trochlear or abducens nerves.

THE TRIGEMINAL NERVE CARRIES SOMATOSENSORY INFORMATION FROM THE FACE AND ORAL CAVITY

The large trigeminal nerve exits from the lateral edge of the pontine base, the *basis pontis* (Figs. 5-3, 5-5). The largest of the cranial nerves, the trigeminal nerve has two components, a large sensory one and a modest motor one. Sensory-wise, the trigeminal nerve comprises fibers from cells in the trigeminal ganglion, also known as the Gasserian or semilunar ganglion, that carry somatosensory information—touch, vibration, pressure, pain, temperature, proprioception—from the face and oral cavity. The trigeminal ganglion is essentially the face's version of a dorsal root ganglion because it contains almost all of the primary somatosensory neurons that innervate the face and oral cavity.

The trigeminal dermatome is larger and more complex than the typical spinal dermatome. The trigeminal nerve splits into three bundles as it leaves the trigeminal ganglion. These three bundles form the *ophthalmic, maxillary,* and *mandibular* branches of the trigeminal nerve, carrying information from eponymous regions of the face (Fig. 5-13). The trigeminal nerve does not carry sensory input from a region of skin around the ear, the outer ear canal, the pharynx, and the back of the tongue, and a few other small areas, all of which are innervated by other cranial nerves (VII, IX, X). Regardless of which cranial nerve carries the sensory information from the periphery to the brainstem, the central targets are the same. In other words, somatosensory afferents in the trigeminal, facial, glossopharyngeal, and vagus nerves all end in the spinal trigeminal nucleus and main sensory nucleus. Cervical spinal nerves, rather than the trigeminal nerve, innervate the back of the head, most of the back side of the ear, and the neck.

The face and oral cavity have an unusual number of special structures that are associated with exquisite pain but not with other somatic perceptions such as vibration, coolness, warmth, or touch. For example, any stimulation of an exposed tooth root elicits an expression of pain and an imploration to stop, consequences that are evoked regardless of the type of stimulus: air puff, cool or warm probe, vibration, and so on. Such all-roads-lead-to-pain organs are concentrated in the head and include the meninges, nasal sinuses, cornea, and teeth.

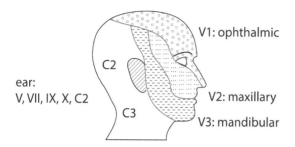

V1: ophthalmic

C2

ear:
V, VII, IX, X, C2

C3

V2: maxillary

V3: mandibular

Figure 5-13 Fibers exit the trigeminal ganglion in three bundles, or branches, destined for three different regions of the face. Each region of the face is innervated by one branch of the trigeminal nerve. The cutaneous areas supplied by the ophthalmic (also termed V₁), maxillary (V₂), and mandibular (V₃) branches of the trigeminal nerve are shown. As their names would suggest, the maxillary and mandibular branches of the trigeminal nerve innervate the upper and lower parts of the oral cavity, respectively. Unlike the case with spinal dermatomes, the regions supplied by the three branches of the trigeminal nerve do not overlap. The skin of the ear is innervated by cranial nerves V, VII, IX, and X and spinal nerve C2 (C1 is peculiar in having no sensory root). The back of the head and neck is innervated by spinal nerves C2 and C3.

Dural afferents travel in the trigeminal and high cervical nerves; the trigeminal nerve innervates the meninges of most of the forebrain, and cervical dorsal roots innervate the dura covering the brainstem. Intracranial inflammation or damage is sensed by dural afferents, which carry this information into the brainstem. Within the medulla, sensory afferents from dura and skin converge onto the same neurons, which "cannot tell the difference" between the two inputs (see more in Chapter 17). Thus, headache can be viewed as "dura-pain" that is *referred* more superficially, often to the skin of the ophthalmic division. Many effective headache treatments are designed to block the initial excitation by inflammatory chemicals of sensory afferents that innervate the dura.

Recall the important difference between the clinical consequences of motor and sensory lesions. Motor nerve lesions lead to negative symptoms, most notably weakness and paralysis. In contrast, *impairment of sensory nerves, including the trigeminal nerve, typically leads to positive signs as well as negative signs.* Thus, a sensory nerve lesion typically produces paresthesias that may or may not be accompanied by *anesthesia* (i.e., an absence of any sensation). The trigeminal nerve is host to two notable painful dysesthesias: *trigeminal neuralgia* and *burning mouth syndrome*. Patients with trigeminal neuralgia, also called *tic douloureux*, feel electric and excruciating pain that shoots down the face, typically down the jaw. The jolts of pain can be triggered by the lightest touch or can occur spontaneously. Trigeminal neuralgia is difficult to treat and, when ineffectively managed, can drive its sufferers to suicide. Less common and less understood is burning mouth syndrome, which, as its name suggests, involves a perception that one's mouth is ablaze.

A small component of the trigeminal nerve carries motor axons to muscles of mastication such as the masseter and digastric muscles that close and open the jaw, respectively. The exit of the *motor root* is discernibly separate from that of the larger sensory root. Clinical difficulties with chewing are not debilitating because central control is bilaterally distributed, and the jaw is obviously joined. Nonetheless, a trigeminal nerve lesion will lead to muscle atrophy on the affected side. Furthermore, the jaw may deviate to the affective side upon opening.

The motor root of the trigeminal nerve also controls the tensor tympani, a middle ear muscle that can tighten the tympanic membrane. Unlike most skeletal muscles, the tensor tympani contracts *automatically* and cannot be willfully controlled. Tensor tympani contraction occurs during chewing and enhances the frequency difference between airborne sounds and the bone-conducted sounds that occur during food mastication and speech (see more in Chapter 16). The contraction of the tensor tympani that accompanies self-generated actions is not reflexive but rather an example of a centrally controlled, anticipatory adjustment that is hard-wired to occur during a motor action. As with the oculomotor nerve's sufficiency for the near triad, the trigeminal nerve contains fibers needed for both chewing and adjusting hearing during chewing.

FACIAL EXPRESSION DEPENDS ENTIRELY ON THE FACIAL NERVE

The facial nerve exits from the lateral edge of the ponto-medullary junction and weaves through to a bony canal in the petrous temporal bone to reach the face. A major function of the facial nerve is controlling the muscles of facial expression (Fig. 5-2). The facial nerve allows us to smile, frown, wrinkle our nose, raise an eyebrow, wince in pain, and pucker our lips. When the facial nerve is inoperative, the lips and eyelids droop so that drooling and leaking tears, with resulting dry eyes, may occur. The forehead may smoothe out, demonstrating the contribution of the facial nerve to our appearance, even to our wrinkles and even at so-called rest.

The facial nerve innervates the orbicularis oculi muscle, which encircles the entire eye. Contraction of the *orbicularis oculi* pulls the skin surrounding the eye inward toward the pupil and supports voluntary movements such as squinting and winking, as well as eye-widening expressions of fear and startle. The orbicularis oculi also supports deliberate eye closure, which is easy to test in the clinic. From a clinical perspective, the facial nerve's role in reflexive blinking is critical. Reflexive blinking protects the eye from damage. Stimulation of the cornea elicits a blink through the *corneal reflex*. The corneal reflex depends on sensory information carried by the ophthalmic division of the trigeminal nerve and a motor command that travels through the facial nerve to the orbicularis oculi. Consequently, the cornea must be protected in individuals without a functioning facial (or trigeminal) nerve. Recall that movements of the upper eyelid that are associated with vertical gaze shifts are not dependent on the facial nerve because they are accomplished using the levator palpebrae superioris innervated by the oculomotor nerve.

The effects of a facial nerve lesion depend on the location of the lesion along the nerve's long and branching course. Of some clinical importance, a distal lesion can damage the somatomotor efferents to the orbicularis oculi palpebrae while leaving intact the parasympathetic efferents to the lacrimal glands. As a result, the lower eyelid droops away from the cornea and tears spill out onto the face without being drained through the lacrimal puncta. To guard against damage to the cornea (due to dry, tearless eyes), care must be taken in dry environments such as airplane cabins and while sleeping.

The facial nerve innervates one skeletal muscle that is not involved in making facial expressions. This is the stapedius, a middle ear muscle that, as with the tensor tympani, modifies sound transmission. The stapedius also resembles the tensor tympani in that it is controlled automatically and cannot be contracted by conscious volition. However, stapedius activation is *reflexive*, occurring in response to loud sounds. When the stapedius contracts, the stapes is pulled away from the cochlea, which results in a decrease in the intensity of subsequent sounds (see Chapter 16). Without the stapedius reflex, loud sounds arrive to the inner ear at full volume, resulting in great discomfort; this symptom is termed *hyperacusis*.

As discussed at the outset of this chapter, the facial nerve is multifaceted and contains more than skeletomotor output. The axons of preganglionic parasympathetic neurons support tear production, nasal secretions, and salivation, reaching their targets via the facial nerve. Preganglionic parasympathetic neurons of the facial nerve target the *pterygopalatine ganglion*, leading to control of tear production in the lacrimal gland and nasal secretions from the nasal mucosa, for crying and nasal lubrication, respectively (Fig. 5-2). Facial nerve regulation of salivation derives from connections to parasympathetic neurons in the submandibular and sublingual ganglions that control secretions of saliva from the submandibular and sublingual glands.

Because of the parasympathetic components of the facial nerve, *facial nerve dysfunction can cause dryness of the eyes, mouth, and nose.*

Despite the dryness that results from interrupting the preganglionic parasympathetic fibers of the facial nerve, the parasympathetic system is not solely responsible for producing lubricating fluids. This principle can be illustrated by examining the varied influences on tear production. The lacrimal gland (parasympathetic) is most critical for the aqueous layer of tears, which is sandwiched between a hormone-sensitive mucus layer secreted by the conjunctiva and a thin superficial lipid layer. While parasympathetic innervation (from the facial nerve) primarily determines the rate of tear production, tear composition is under the influence of both parasympathetic and sympathetic (recall that sympathetic outflow emanates from cells in the thoracic spinal cord) inputs, as well as hormones. When working correctly, irritation of the cornea, sensed by trigeminal neurons, stimulates lacrimal tear production in addition to reflexive blinking. As the offending irritation increases in intensity, tear production increases. Should tear production fail to match need, the cornea is insufficiently protected and can become inflamed. Corneal inflammation can, in turn, overstimulate sympathetic innervation of the lacrimal glands, producing excessively watery tears and giving the rheumy appearance to eyes that is sometimes present among the elderly. In postmenopausal women, decreased levels of estrogen lead to a decline in production of the mucus layer. If lacrimal gland tear production is not sufficiently boosted to compensate, dry eye results. In fact, dry eye is a common complaint among postmenopausal women.

There are two final components contained in the facial nerve. Special sensory information arrives from sensory neurons in the geniculate ganglion that innervate taste buds located in the front two-thirds of the tongue. Somatosensory information from a small region around the opening of the ear travels through the facial nerve to central trigeminal nuclei.

The cumulative functions of the facial nerve are reflected in the diverse symptoms that result from a lesion of the facial nerve (Fig. 5-2). Loss of skeletomotor fibers leads to loss of facial expression, loss of the corneal reflex, and hyperacusis. A lesion of preganglionic parasympathetic fibers leads to dry eye and dry mouth. Damage to the somatosensory fibers of the facial nerve often results in pain around the ear canal; remember that dysfunction of sensory nerves usually gives rise to paresthesia or dysesthesia. Finally, loss of the special sensory fibers contained in the facial nerve will lead to a loss of taste in the front two-thirds of the tongue. All of the symptoms resulting from facial nerve damage are on the same side as the lesion.

As it turns out, facial nerve dysfunction is relatively common and luckily is also usually transient. *Bell's palsy* is an infection or inflammation of the facial nerve (Fig. 5-14). A person may wake up one day and find that she is unable to make expressions on one side of the face. Given the importance of facial expressions to social communication, individuals with Bell's palsy readily seek medical help. One of the cardinal signs of facial nerve paralysis is an absent or decreased *nasolabial fold* on the side of the lesion. The nasolabial fold is a deep wrinkle or fold that runs from the lateral edge of the nose to the lateral edge of the mouth. Since Bell's palsy affects all branches of the facial nerve, not just the motor control of the muscles of facial expression, symptoms may include:

• Weakness or paralysis of muscles of facial expression (with loss of corneal reflex)

• Hyperacusis due to paralysis of the stapedius muscle

• Dry eye and dry mouth due to impairment of preganglionic parasympathetic nerves to lacrimal and salivary glands

• Pain radiating from the external ear through effects on the small number of sensory afferents carried in the facial nerve

Patients with Bell's palsy rarely complain of a loss in taste since only a minority of the taste buds in the oral cavity are affected. Furthermore, as mentioned earlier, smell dominates taste in determining *flavor*, which is critical to the experience of eating. Yet, if Bell's palsy is suspected, testing for taste can be accomplished by placing salt or sugar on the front of the tongue on the affected side.

Bell's palsy typically remits spontaneously within some months. However, while the facial muscles are paralyzed or weakened, care must be taken to keep the eye on the affected side protected from either drying out or being injured by a foreign object, dangers that are present due to the patient's loss of the corneal reflex.

HEARING AND BALANCE DEPEND ON THE VESTIBULOCOCHLEAR NERVE

The vestibulocochlear nerve exits the brainstem at the *cerebellopontine angle* just lateral to the facial nerve (Fig. 5-15). It has two components: one for hearing and one for sensing the head's orientation and acceleration in space. *Hair cells*, non-neural sensory cells derived from placodes, are located in both the cochlea and the vestibulum. Those in the cochlea respond to sound, and those in the vestibulum respond to accelerating forces, including gravity, that act on the head. Full considerations of auditory and vestibular function are presented in Chapters 16 and 18, respectively.

The cochlear portion of the eighth cranial nerve contains fibers from the *spiral ganglion* that innervate the cochlea, our auditory sensor. Impairment of the cochlear

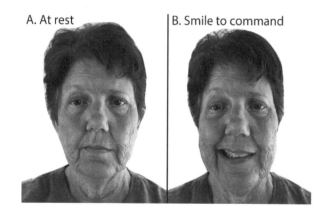

A. At rest | B. Smile to command

Figure 5-14 A person with Bell's palsy cannot contract muscles on the affected side of the face. A: In older individuals such as the woman shown here, wrinkles are present at rest but are less pronounced on the affected side (compare the right and left forehead wrinkles). At rest, the face on the affected side sags, unable to oppose gravity. The mouth droops, the eyebrow is lax so that it is less elevated than the unaffected side, and the lower eyelid is everted. This latter symptom can lead to overflowing tears. B: No facial expression muscles on the affected side participate in a volitional smile, resulting in an asymmetric expression. Photographs kindly provided by Julie Altenau and Carolyn Pearce.

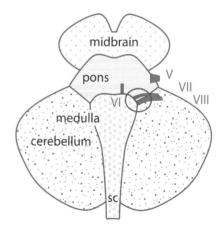

Figure 5-15 A cartoon of the base of the brain illustrates the location of the cerebellopontine angle (blue circle) at the convergence of the cerebellum, pons, and medulla. The smallest tumors at the cerebellopontine angle cause vestibular and hearing problems. With progressively larger tumors, symptoms attributable to impairment of the facial, trigeminal, and abducens nerves can also occur.

nerve causes hearing loss in the ear on the same side. Since hearing loss is easier to treat when it is mild, and since many causes of hearing loss are progressive, the cause of hearing loss, even a minor one, should be aggressively pursued. Hearing loss is often accompanied by tinnitus, a positive sign that ranges from mildly bothersome to severe and debilitating (Table 5-2).

The vestibular portion of the eighth cranial nerve contains fibers from *Scarpa's ganglion* that innervate the vestibular apparatus. The vestibular apparatus contains sensory hair cells that are sensitive to angular or linear head acceleration. Vestibular signals are critical to maintaining posture and balance. Thus, a lesion of the vestibular nerve may produce a sense of *vertigo* or *disequilibrium* that is typically reported as "dizziness." Vertigo refers to a sense of rotatory motion so that, to an affected individual, either the room or the self may appear to be spinning even when sitting still. Disequilibrium refers to a sense of unsteadiness or imbalance. Both vertigo and disequilibrium are often accompanied by nausea. Dizziness is the colloquial term used by most people to refer to a wide range of symptoms including vertigo and disequilibrium. However, a patient may use the word dizziness to describe lightheadedness, which usually stems from a cardiac problem. Therefore, the clinician should interrogate further to understand the experience of a patient reporting dizziness. After some recovery time, vestibular symptoms usually subside, but a person may continue to feel unsure and unsteady, particularly in reduced light conditions when visual information is minimal.

One of the most common intracranial tumors is a *vestibular schwannoma*, historically termed an *acoustic neuroma*, which usually stems from an overproduction of Schwann cells in the vestibular portion of the nerve. These tumors are relatively common, occurring in 1 in 100,000 people. Vestibular schwannomas form in the Schwann cell lining at the root–nerve junction of the vestibular portion of the eighth cranial nerve. Vestibular schwannomas cause problems with equilibrium first and foremost. However, since they form at a point near the cerebellopontine angle, progressively larger tumors eventually impair function of the cochlear component of cranial nerve VIII and may progress to involve facial, glossopharyngeal, and even trigeminal nerves (Fig. 5-15). Surgical removal is typically the preferred treatment although targeted radiation is becoming more common.

The majority of vestibular schwannomas are idiopathic or sporadic, meaning that they happen to individuals "out of the blue" for no known reason. Most idiopathic vestibular schwannomas are also benign. A notable exception to the benign and idiopathic nature of most of these tumors occurs in patients with either of two types of *von Recklinghausen neurofibromatosis*, a pair of distinct dominant autosomal genetic diseases in which cell cycle control proteins are absent or defective. Patients with both types of neurofibromatosis are vulnerable to the development of a variety of tumors primarily in the skin and nervous system. Patients with neurofibromatosis type II most often present with *bilateral* vestibular schwannomas that are quite rare under any other circumstance.

THE GLOSSOPHARYNGEAL AND VAGUS NERVES PROTECT AND CONTROL THE UPPER AIRWAY

The ninth and tenth cranial nerves—glossopharyngeal and vagus—emerge from the ventrolateral edge of the medulla, with the glossopharyngeal rootlets lying immediately rostral to vagus rootlets (Fig. 5-5). In fact, the rootlets of cranial nerves IX and X form a continuous row with no clear demarcation between their exit points. The glossopharyngeal nerve serves a hodgepodge of functions, with no single one of them dominating. The vagus nerve is the visceral colossus, carrying preganglionic parasympathetic fibers to and sensory fibers from viscera in the thorax and abdomen including the lungs, larynx, heart, digestive tract from esophagus through midgut, and pancreas. The vagus also innervates skeletal muscles of the pharynx and larynx.

Sensory fibers carried in the vagus and glossopharyngeal nerves serve the following functions:

- Somatosensory input from parts of the external ear (IX, X), tympanic membrane (IX), middle ear (IX), pharynx (IX, X), posterior tongue (IX), and meninges of the posterior fossa (X)

- Taste information from the posterior third of the tongue, soft palate (IX), and pharynx (X)

- Viscerosensory information about blood chemistry— oxygen levels, presence of nasty chemicals, pH, and the like—and blood pressure from the carotid body (IX) and aortic arch (X); trachea, esophagus, epiglottis, lungs, heart, stomach, intestines, and other thoracic and abdominal viscera (X)

Note that much of the sensory information carried by the glossopharyngeal and vagus nerves does not reach conscious perception. For example, blood chemistry information such as blood oxygenation is not consciously perceived. Furthermore, when perception does occur, it is not discriminative in nature. In other words, the texture, shape, and even size of a kidney stone are not perceived even as that same stone causes intense pain.

The glossopharyngeal nerve carries motor innervation to the stylopharyngeus muscle, a skeletal muscle that elevates the pharynx during talking, swallowing, and vomiting or *emesis*. Depending on the severity, impairment of glossopharyngeal innervation of the stylopharyngeus can have little effect or can result in difficulty swallowing, termed *dysphagia*, or talking, termed *dysarthria*. The glossopharyngeal nerve also contributes to salivation by targeting postganglionic parasympathetic neurons in the otic ganglion that control parotid gland secretions of saliva.

Two very important reflexes of the throat depend on the ninth and tenth cranial nerves. The *pharyngeal reflex*, commonly known as the *gag reflex*, closes the throat in response to a foreign body touching the oropharynx or back of the mouth or the posterior tongue. Rotten-tasting food or emetic chemicals in the blood stream can also elicit a gag reflex. Roughly a third of healthy people do not have a gag reflex, demonstrating that this reflex is not critical to life. On the other end of the spectrum, some people show a conditioned gag reflex in response to non-threatening stimuli such as a pill placed on the anterior tongue or even a nauseating image. The *laryngeal adductor reflex*, or *cough reflex*, protects the lungs from food bits, saliva, and irritants such as pollutants or capsaicin. Mechanical or chemical stimuli of the trachea or bronchi elicit a reflexive inspiration followed by an explosive expiration of air, known as a cough. *The cough reflex is critical to a long life because it excludes anything besides air from entering the lungs.*

Since rootlets of the glossopharyngeal and vagus nerves exit at adjacent sites, lesions that affect one of these nerves commonly also affect the other one and may thus compromise the gag and/or the cough reflex. For the gag reflex, sensory information arrives primarily through the glossopharyngeal nerve, and the motor arm of the gag reflex is carried primarily by the vagus nerve. In contrast, the vagus works without the glossopharyngeal nerve to protect the upper airway from undesirable foreign matter entering from above, as well as from aspiration of vomitus emerging from below. In both the gag and cough reflexes, participation of additional skeletal muscles is also required. Most notably, the diaphragm, innervated by the phrenic nerve, is critical to producing the cough reflex.

Despite the diaspora-like parasympathetic projections of the vagus, *symptoms arising from vagus (or glossopharyngeal) lesions are largely restricted to hoarseness, breathy speech, dysphagia, dysarthria, and compromised gag and cough reflexes, all of which depend on a relatively limited number of skeletomotor axons.* Thus, despite viscerosensory and preganglionic parasympathetic fibers greatly outnumbering skeletomotor fiber types in the vagus and glossopharyngeal, the primary clinical function of these nerves is to control skeletal musculature of the throat and upper airway. Consequently, lesions of these nerves lead to problems with speech, swallowing, and choking or aspiration.

THE SPINAL ACCESSORY NERVE SUPPORTS HEAD GESTURES

The spinal accessory nerve emerges from the cervical spinal cord, but, rather than exiting from the vertebral column, it climbs up into the cranium, within the CSF-filled subarachnoid space, and then exits from the skull through the jugular foramen. This nerve provides motor innervation to two muscles: the trapezius, involved in shrugging, and the sternocleidomastoid. Contraction of the sternocleidomastoid muscle rotates the head to the contralateral side. It also can tilt the head down and ipsilaterally; note that balanced bilateral activity yields a downward glance that is not skewed to either side. Asking a patient to shake her head to indicate "no" and to look down tests both of the sternocleidomastoid muscle's actions.

Iatrogenic damage of the spinal accessory nerve can occur during medical procedures on the neck such as cervical lymph node biopsies. One sign of damage to the innervation of the trapezius muscles is a *winged scapula* in which the shoulder blade juts out from the rib cage, a condition that limits the ability to perform everyday actions.

THE HYPOGLOSSAL NERVE CONTROLS TONGUE MOVEMENT

Hypoglossal rootlets exit from the base of the ventral medulla, close to the midline. The hypoglossal nerve innervates the muscles of the tongue, which are critical to breathing, eating, swallowing, speech, emesis, and a myriad of other functions such as communicating anger through a particularly immature gesture. Isolated hypoglossal nerve injury or dysfunction is not a common occurrence.

DEDUCTIVE REASONING
ALLOWS YOU TO NARROW
DOWN POSSIBLE CAUSES
OF SYMPTOMS INVOLVING
CRANIAL NERVE FUNCTIONS

How does knowledge about the projections and functions of the cranial nerves help you figure out what is wrong with someone? Consider someone who complains that "everything is blurry." As you know by now, this complaint could stem from damage to the optic nerve carrying visual signals or from an impaired oculomotor, abducens, or trochlear nerve. Testing reveals that the patient sees normally out of each eye when the other eye is covered. Now you know that the problem is with gaze control rather than with visual processing. Of the three cranial nerves that could give rise to misalignment of the eyes, oculomotor is the most likely culprit because it innervates four muscles compared to the one apiece innervated by the abducens and trochlear nerves. Upon examination of the person's eye movements as she traces an H, you may see, for example, that the right eye moves laterally and downward but does not move medially, toward the nose, or upward, adding to your suspicion that the oculomotor nerve, on the right side, is causing diplopia. Such a finding provides impetus to test the remaining functions of the oculomotor nerve: eyelid elevation while looking up, the pupillary light reflex, and near vision, any or all of which may be affected.

Peripheral lesions wreak their havoc regardless of context. An individual with a lesioned facial nerve is unable to make a facial expression on the affected side under any circumstance. In other words, cranial nerves *cannot distinguish between different contexts*. The CNS is very different. As we shall see throughout this book, the CNS contains multiple circuits that influence a common motor output. For example, imagine a person who cannot voluntarily look to the left but can reflexively move her eye to the left. Could this presentation result from an abducens nerve lesion? No, certainly not. An abducens nerve lesion would prevent any movement, for any reason, of the eye to the side. In contrast, a central lesion may impair lateral gaze shifts but not reflexive lateral eye movements; this is a common problem among individuals with multiple sclerosis, a central demyelinating disease (much more on this in Chapter 19). Because the CNS molds behavior to subtle differences in circumstances, *context-specific impairments are always a result of CNS damage and not peripheral damage.*

Conglomerations of symptoms that could not arise from injury of a single site in the brain are often due to a disease process. Some diseases produce anatomical lesions of neural elements that share a specific molecular vulnerability. An example of this is multiple sclerosis in which a myelin-related molecule fails to function properly. Other diseases may target functional pathways. For example, *amyotrophic lateral sclerosis* leads to the death of neurons within select pathways supporting voluntary movement. Finally, disease may not act on the nervous system. For example, weakness in all skeletal muscles of both eyes, extraocular and levator palpebrae superioris alike, could only result if the oculomotor, trochlear, and abducens nerves on both sides were damaged. Such damage would be expected to also produce blown and unreactive pupils. However, no parasympathetic symptoms are observed in *chronic progressive external ophthalmoplegia*, a mitochondrial *muscle disorder* that, over time, produces a paralysis of all skeletal muscles around the eye without any autonomic symptoms. This unfortunate disease eventually affects the long muscles of the limbs and torso, causing the patient great difficulty in standing and walking, as well as in eye movements.

ADDITIONAL READING

Dartt DA. Regulation of mucin and fluid secretion by conjunctival epithelial cells. *Prog Retinal Eye Res.* 21: 555–576, 2002.

Evinger C, Manning KA, Sibony PA. Eyelid movements. Mechanisms and normal data. *Invest Ophthalmol Vis Sci.* 32: 387–400, 1991.

Hawkes C, Shah M. Why bother testing the sense of smell? *Pract Neurol.* 5: 224–229, 2005.

Miller RJ. Oral and pharyngeal reflexes in the mammalian nervous system: Their diverse range in complexity and the pivotal role of the tongue. *Crit Rev Oral Biol Med.* 13: 409–425, 2002.

Walker HK. Cranial nerve XI: The spinal accessory nerve. In: Walker HK, Hall WD, Hurst JW, eds. *Clinical Methods: The History, Physical, and Laboratory Examinations.* 3rd ed. Boston: Butterworths; 1990. http://www.ncbi.nlm.nih.gov/books/NBK387/#top

6.

THE VERSATILE BRAINSTEM

Throughout the millennia of human existence, cardiac death has defined death. However, most of the modern world now views people without brain function as dead as well. The switch from exclusive cardiac death to cardiac-or-brain-death came about in the second half of the 20th century as a response to two medical advancements. First, the development of respirators and other palliative technology allowed patients without brain function to continue to beat their hearts. Second, the development of organ transplantation led to the realization that organs from people without brain function who would never recover could be put to use, saving others' lives. Thus was born the concept that people with a beating heart but no brain function are dead.

According to US law, brain death only applies to individuals with *no intracranial nervous function*. In other words, both the brainstem and forebrain must be beyond repair. The legal requirements for brain death in the United States are that a patient must stop breathing, termed *apnea*; show no intact brainstem reflexes, such as the corneal and pupillary light reflexes; and not react to painful stimuli. The final legal requirement is peculiar from a strictly neurobiological perspective because the spinal cord supports reactions to noxious stimulation of the hands, feet, and other parts of the body.

The *persistent vegetative state* stands in a markedly different legal category from brain death. In persistent vegetative state, an intact brainstem supports physiological life, but a lack of any forebrain function means that that life is without meaning. Patients in a persistent vegetative state do not recover and will never return to their former selves. Nonetheless, the United States classifies the persistent vegetative state as a living state; these patients are not legally dead.

The behavior of individuals in a persistent vegetative state stems entirely from the brainstem and spinal cord.

Essentially, the persistent vegetative state isolates and brings to the fore the capabilities of the brainstem. We see that the brainstem can coordinate breathing and, when combined with medical support, can maintain a minimally hospitable physiological state that supports cardiac life. In fact, the body may persist functioning for a very long time as long as critical supports such as feeding, hydration, and ventilation are provided. In addition, brainstem reflexes support movement of the eyes, swallowing, grasping, and the like. Yet the patient is without awareness of self or surroundings.

The outward facade of life enabled by the brainstem is so compelling that loved ones can find the inner vacancy difficult to accept. Brainstem-supported reflexes appear tantalizingly close to meaningful behavior and are often interpreted by emotionally distraught family and friends as momentous signs that a loved one is on the verge of returning to life. Accepting that the body's residual functions are not a sign of brain life is extremely difficult for some. Consequently, a number of people choose to maintain "life" support for loved ones who have neither brain activity nor the hope of regaining meaningful brain function. Even so, an increasing number of people have adopted the opposite tack, choosing proactively to legally decline future life support should the circumstances arise.

It is critical to understand the experience of loved ones suddenly caught up in an unwanted and unanticipated life-and-death drama. Incapacitation always happens quickly. It yanks family and friends from their regular routine into an overwhelming maelstrom of medical terms, interventions, technology, and choices. Medical activity is directed at the patient and continues on, independent of family's and friends' emotions. In this context, observing reflexive movements combined with the desperate emotions of despair and hope engendered by the sight of an incapacitated loved one can fuel disbelief in the poor prognosis that is inevitable in a person in a persistent vegetative state. Family and friends frantically desire for loved ones to return to the way they were on *the preceding day.* The physician can play an important role by showing compassion for the extraordinary position that friends and family find themselves in when faced with a suddenly incapacitated loved one. Patient, clear, and repeated explanations of the biological realities of a brainstem-supported life can go a long way to leading family and friends to reluctant acceptance.

Individuals with a working brainstem and at least some telencephalic capacity may enter a *minimally conscious state.* At a minimum, this state involves intermittent signs of awareness evidenced by a patient's tracking or fixating on a loved one. However, since such signs typically occur infrequently at unpredictable times, they may not be present during brief visits from medical professionals. Moreover, it may take weeks or months for a patient in a vegetative state to show signs of the minimally conscious state. The period of time after which the vegetative state should be considered permanent remains unclear. Of critical importance is the fact that patients *may emerge from a minimally conscious state to a frequently or fully conscious state, either accompanied by motor limitations or not.* The very real possibility of improvement and even recovery from a minimally conscious state raises profoundly emotional ethical issues for a patient, the patient's loved ones, and the physicians involved in the patient's care. For those interested in this topic, a recent book by Joseph Fins, *Rights Come to Mind,* is highly recommended.

BRAINSTEM FUNCTIONS CHANGE FROM LIFE-SUPPORT CAUDALLY TO EXPRESSION ROSTRALLY

As you know, the medulla, pons, and cerebellum of the hindbrain along with the midbrain comprise the four major components of the adult brainstem. In addition to cranial nerves using the brainstem as a conduit between the periphery and the forebrain, tracts that shuttle information between the spinal cord and forebrain traverse the brainstem en route to their destinations. As we move through the brainstem, we keep track of our three major pathways: lemniscal, spinothalamic, and corticospinal. We also note the locations of cranial nerve nuclei and the course of axons arriving at or departing from these nuclei. Finally, we focus on several structures too large and obvious to be ignored and, more importantly, so visually remarkable as to provide easily recognizable landmarks.

The brainstem divides up the fundamental processes of human life, with the most automatic and basic ones supported most caudally and progressively more complex, even luxurious, functions depending on more rostral brainstem regions. Painting with a broad brush, neurons of the medulla, pons, and midbrain are largely responsible for different physiological processes:

- Medulla:
  - Blood pressure
  - Breathing
  - Gastrointestinal motility
  - Ingestion
  - Equilibrium
- Pons:
  - Horizontal gaze
  - Reflexive eye movements
  - Posture
  - Rapid eye movement (REM) sleep
  - Facial expressions
- Cerebellum:
  - Motor coordination
  - Postural balance, gait, speech, eye movements, reaching, grasping
- Midbrain:
  - Vertical eye movements
  - Near vision
  - Pupillary control
  - Posture and locomotion
  - Non-REM sleep
  - Level of arousal

This division of labor greatly oversimplifies the overlapping roles and multiple contributions of each brainstem region. For example, the medulla, pons, and midbrain all contribute to the maintenance of an upright posture against gravity. Yet, medullary lesions are most likely to disturb the sense of equilibrium, resulting in vertigo or disequilibrium, whereas midbrain lesions preferentially result in a person's adopting a fixed and abnormal posture. In addition to impairing normal functions such as eye movements, damage to the brainstem also can give rise to a number of positive signs such as hiccups, nausea, or dysesthesias.

The functions of many neurons in the medulla, pons, and midbrain are associated with cranial nerves. For example, the vagal nerve's exit from the medulla dictates the medulla's involvement in controlling the upper airway as well as blood pressure, gastrointestinal motility, and other homeostatic processes. The midbrain's roles in vertical eye movements, vergence, and pupillary control follow from the oculomotor nerve's exit from the midbrain.

Superimposed on the different functions of nuclei in each brainstem region are functions provided by *tracts*. Damage to any part of the brainstem can impair motor or sensory function by interrupting corticospinal, corticobulbar, or spinothalamic tracts; the medial lemniscus; or any number of additional axonal highways that traverse the brainstem. In fact, the reason a pontine stroke can produce locked-in syndrome is that it can disrupt connections traversing the pons (Latin for "bridge"). In this chapter, we start by looking from the outside and then proceed to view selected brainstem cross-sections.

In continuing our caudal-to-rostral trip up the neuraxis, we move from medulla to pons to midbrain, noting the locations of the three longest pathways, the cranial nerve nuclei, and remarkable brainstem structures. The medulla contains the densest concentration of areas of interest and therefore we dwell more on medullary sections than on pontine or midbrain ones.

MAJOR STRUCTURES INVOLVED IN MOVEMENT AND LIGHT TOUCH SENSATION ARE PRESENT IN THE MEDULLA

The medulla, the most caudal part of the brainstem, emerges from the spinal cord at the foramen magnum. At this spinomedullary junction, the pyramidal decussation—synonymous with motor decussation—marks where lateral corticospinal tract axons cross the midline. The pyramidal decussation appears as a blurring, or fusion, of the otherwise well-marked midline fissure (Fig. 6-1). Corticospinal tract fibers cross from the side of their origin in motor cortex to the side of their destination in the ventral horn. *Above or rostral to the pyramidal decussation, voluntary motor commands travel contralateral to the muscles that they ultimately control. In contrast, caudal to the pyramidal decussation, voluntary motor commands travel ipsilateral to the targeted muscles.*

Just lateral to the pyramids at the base of the medulla, bumps called the *olivary tubercles* indicate the location of the *inferior olivary nuclei* or *inferior olives* (Fig. 6-2). The inferior olives, unrelated to any cranial nerve, are highly distinctive landmarks of the caudal medulla. They provide an important signal that teaches the cerebellum how to

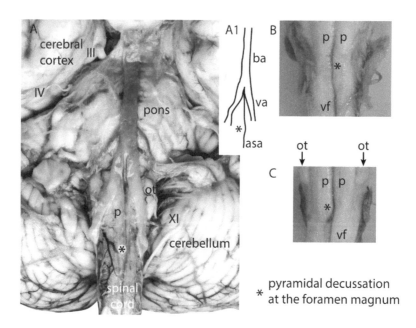

Figure 6-1 A: The pyramids (*p*) and pyramidal decussation (*) are seen on the ventrum of the spinomedullary junction where the brain joins the spinal cord and where the foramen magnum is situated. At the pyramidal decussation, most corticospinal fibers cross the midline to travel in the lateral corticospinal tract of the spinal cord. Within the spinal cord the ventral midline is taken up with the ventral funiculi (*vf*). The olivary tubercles (*ot*) are located just lateral to the pyramids in the rostral medulla (in A and C). As labeled in the inset (A1), the basilar artery (*ba*) forms from the two vertebral arteries (*va*) at the caudal end of the pons. The anterior spinal artery (*asa*) runs down the midline of the medulla, and jogs to the side at the pyramidal decussation. B–C: Magnified views from two additional brains, shorn of blood vessels, show the variability in the appearance of the pyramidal decussation. For example, the midline is nudged to the right in some cases (B) and to the left in others (C). Abbreviations: III, oculomotor nerve; IV, trochlear nerve (sweet); XI, spinal accessory nerve.

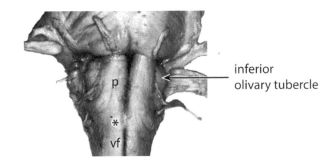

inferior
olivary tubercle

Figure 6-2 The olivary tubercles straddle the pyramids (*p*) on the ventral surface of the rostral medulla. Underneath these bumps are the inferior olivary nuclei, important pre-cerebellar nuclei of the medulla. Caudal to the pyramidal decussation (*) the ventral midline is occupied by the ventral funiculi (*vf*) and rostral to the decussation by the pyramids. Photograph reprinted with permission from deArmond S et al., *Structure of the human brain: A photographic atlas*. New York: Oxford University Press, 1989.

make an intended movement correctly and smoothly (see Chapter 24). Of note, rootlets of the hypoglossal nerve (XII) emerge along the border between the olivary tubercles and the pyramids. Farther laterally, rootlets of the vagus (X) and glossopharyngeal (IX) nerves emerge.

Upon viewing the brainstem from above, one sees that the dorsal columns of the spinal cord continue seamlessly into bumps called the *tubercle gracilis*, located medially, and the *tubercle cuneatus*, located laterally and a bit rostrally (Fig. 6-3). These tubercles contain the dorsal column nuclei, where primary afferents carrying information about ipsilateral light touch, vibration, and proprioception terminate. Each of the tubercles represents the external manifestation of the underlying eponymous nucleus, receiving its input from the fasciculus of the same name. Thus, light

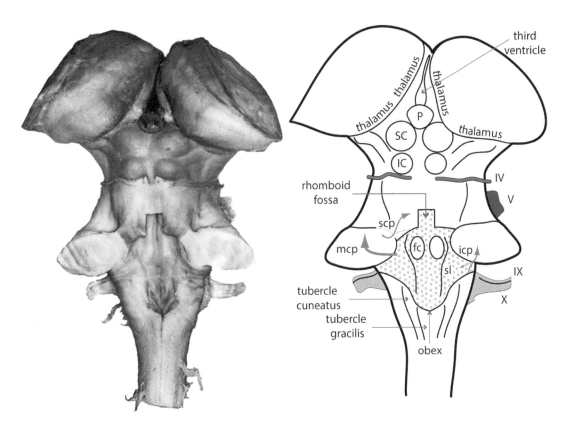

Figure 6-3 Major landmarks on the dorsum of the brainstem and diencephalon are shown in photographic and diagrammatic forms. The brainstem was isolated by removing the telencephalon and the cerebellum. None of the surfaces illustrated is open to view in the intact brain. The medulla is marked by the tubercles cuneatus and gracilis, which are bumps overlying the dorsal column nuclei. Recall that the nuclei cuneatus and gracilis are the site of the first synapse in the dorsal column-medial lemniscus pathway, which carries tactile information from the same side of the body. The obex is the caudal-most point in the rhomboid fossa (*patterned area*), the cavity of the fourth ventricle. Note that the anterior portion of the rhomboid fossa is obscured in the photograph at left by the overlying medullary velum or veil, a thin non-neural tissue that forms the roof of the fourth ventricle. The facial colliculi (*fc*), where facial motoneuron axons make a hairpin turn around abducens motoneurons, are located on either side of the pontine midline. Lateral to the facial colliculi are the sulci limitans (*sl*), small indentations in the floor of the fourth ventricle that demarcate the border between sensory and motor nuclei. The pons is delimited by the cerebellar peduncles, which were cut transversely to prepare this isolated brainstem. The middle cerebellar peduncles (*mcp*), containing axons from the basis pontis destined for the cerebellum, occupy most of the cut surface. The inferior cerebellar peduncles (*icp*) contain primarily axons entering the cerebellum from the medulla and the spinal cord and a smaller number of cerebellar efferents bound for hindbrain targets. The superior cerebellar peduncles (*scp*) primarily consist of axons leaving the cerebellum for the midbrain and diencephalon. The dorsal surface of the midbrain is marked by four prominent bumps: pairs of inferior and superior colliculi (*IC, SC*). The meso-diencephalic junction is marked by the pineal gland (*P*), while the third ventricle marks the thalamus. The roots of cranial nerves IV, V, IX, and X are prominent in this preparation and are marked. Photograph reprinted with permission from deArmond S et al., *Structure of the human brain: A photographic atlas*. New York: Oxford University Press, 1989.

touch, vibration, and proprioceptive information from the ipsilateral leg and lower trunk travel through the fasciculus gracilis to the *nucleus gracilis*, also termed the gracile nucleus, which is viewed from the outside as the tubercle gracilis. Similarly, tactile and other low-threshold information arising from the upper trunk and arms travels in the fasciculus cuneatus to reach the *nucleus cuneatus* or cuneate nucleus, which is visible from the outside as the tubercle cuneatus. Within the lemniscal pathway, *the dorsal column nuclei represent the first central synapse for information about light touch, vibration, and proprioception from the same side of the body (and destined for the contralateral cortex).*

The central canal, patent in fetal life but occluded after birth, moves to a progressively more dorsal position within the cervical spinal cord until it reaches the dorsal surface and opens up into the fourth ventricle. The point where the fourth ventricle emerges from the central canal opening is termed the *obex* (Fig. 6-3). The fourth ventricle forms the ventricular space of the hindbrain. From above, the floor of the fourth ventricle appears diamond-shaped and is therefore called the *rhomboid fossa* (Fig. 6-3).

External structures rostral to the obex follow the margins of the rhomboid fossa rather than aligning purely along straight rostral–caudal lines. For example, the tubercles gracilis and cuneatus veer laterally as they extend rostrally, hugging the outline of the widening rhomboid fossa. Within the rhomboid fossa, two small bumps straddle the midline (Fig. 6-3). These bumps are the *facial colliculi*. They mark the *facial genu* (from the Latin word for "knee") where facial nerve axons bend around the abducens nucleus (discussed in greater detail later).

MOTOR STRUCTURES DOMINATE THE EXTERNAL LANDSCAPE OF THE PONS AND CEREBELLUM

The cerebellum itself consists of a midline *vermis* flanked by two laterally situated *hemispheres* or *lobes* (Fig. 6-4A). The most medial portion of each cerebellar hemisphere is termed the *paravermis*, and the lateral portions of the lobes are simply called the lateral lobes or hemispheres. The vermis

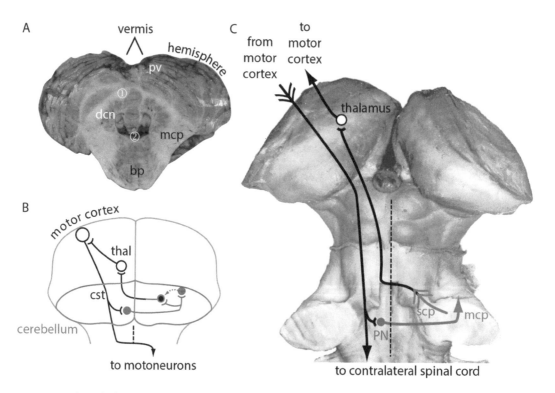

Figure 6-4 A: A cross-section through the mid-pons and attached cerebellum shows the three divisions of the cerebellum: the narrow vermis, a strip of paravermis (*pv*), and the lateral hemispheres. At this level, the large size of the middle cerebellar peduncles (*mcp*), which carry axons from neurons in the contralateral basis pontis (*bp*), is evident. Also present are the deep cerebellar nuclei (*dcn*), cerebellar white matter (*1*), and fourth ventricle (*2*). B-C: The circuit that connects the corticospinal tract (*cst*) with the cerebellum is illustrated. Collaterals from corticospinal axons contact neurons in the pontine nuclei (*pn*), which in turn send a projection across the midline and into the cerebellum through the middle cerebellar peduncle. After processing within the cerebellum, the output from the cerebellum travels through the superior cerebellar peduncle (*scp*) to the contralateral thalamus and thence back to motor cortex. It should be evident from this circuit that the cerebellum modulates ipsilateral movements. Photograph in C reprinted with permission from deArmond S et al., *Structure of the human brain: A photographic atlas.* New York: Oxford University Press, 1989.

and paravermis together are critical to the orchestration of motor actions, ensuring that the movements are smooth and finish on target. The lateral lobes are critical to coordinating visually guided movements and to learning complex new movements. For example, when learning to play a new sport or a new instrument, we repeat and repeat and repeat. Our initial attempts are uncoordinated and slow, but, after more repetition, a sequence of awkward movements is transformed into smooth, fluid action. The lateral lobes are critical to that magical transformation. Finally, there is a *flocculonodular lobe* tucked in on the underside of the cerebellum; this is critical to the coordination of balance, eye movements, and visually guided movements. For example, adjusting to eyeglasses with a new prescription requires adjustments performed by the flocculonodular lobe. Damage to the flocculonodular lobe can have devastating effects on a person's ability maintaining steady balance and gaze (see Chapter 19).

The convexity of the base of the pons, termed the *basis pontis*, contains resident *pontine nuclei* that receive messages about intended movements from corticospinal tract axons (Fig. 6-4B). Neurons in the pontine nuclei in turn send this message *across the midline* and into the cerebellum. In this way, the cerebellum receives information about all movements that the contralateral cortex is commanding,

planning to initiate, or even just considering. After processing the information from motor cortex, the cerebellum sends out its verdict to the *contralateral* thalamus to ultimately reach the motor cortex. Thus, the motor cortex connects with the contralateral cerebellum via two midline crossings (pontine nucleus to cerebellum, cerebellum to thalamus). Now remember that motor cortex controls movements on the opposite side of the body. Thus, *cerebellar modulation affects ipsilateral movements* (controlled by contralateral cerebral cortex).

Recall from Chapter 3 that the cerebellum is attached to the brainstem only through the *cerebellar peduncles*. Three individually named peduncles (Latin for "stalk") collectively consist of millions of fibers that connect the cerebellum to the pons:

- The *inferior cerebellar peduncle* contains fibers connecting the cerebellum with the spinal cord and medulla.

- The *middle cerebellar peduncle*, or *brachium pontis*, constitutes the bulk of the connection and carries fibers from neurons in the basis pontis destined for the cerebellum.

- Fibers exiting the cerebellum to reach midbrain and diencephalic targets make up the bulk of the *superior cerebellar peduncle* or *brachium conjunctivum*.

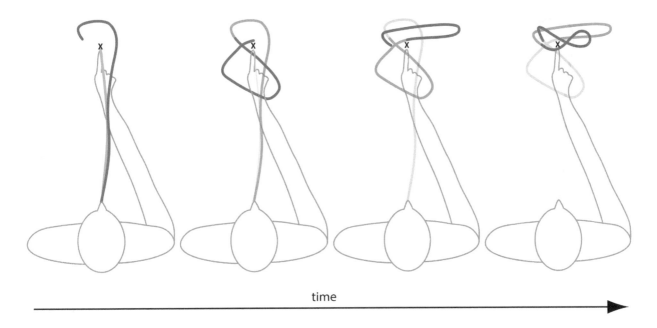

time

Figure 6-5 When asked to touch the nose and then a target (*X*), a neurologically normal individual makes a direct trajectory (*blue line*) to the target. When an individual with a cerebellar lesion is asked to perform the same task, the patient's finger traces a far more circuitous route to the target (*red line*). Lines in progressively darker shades of red depict successive moments in time. Deviations from a normal trajectory increase in frequency and magnitude as the finger approaches the end target. This type of uncoordinated movement is termed *ataxia* and is pathognomonic for cerebellar damage. In addition to traversing a roundabout path, ataxic movements are slower than normal ones. Whereas normally touching a target at arm's reach is accomplished in about a second, ataxic patients take well more than a second to just reach the vicinity of the target. They then require several more seconds to approach the target more closely and have great difficulty holding their finger stationary at the target.

Thus, the inferior and middle cerebellar peduncles carry information into the cerebellum, and the superior cerebellar peduncle carries information out of the cerebellum. The relative sizes of the peduncles—the superior cerebellar peduncle is far smaller than the middle cerebellar peduncle—reflect an important fact about the cerebellum; namely, that far more information goes into the cerebellum than comes out. The ratio of input to output is roughly 40:1.

As we will explore in Chapter 24, the cerebellum ensures that the movements we make are smooth and that they constitute the movements that we actually intend to make. The pathognomonic or defining characteristic of damage to the cerebellum is *ataxia*, a distinctive style of uncoordinated movement that uses successive corrections to reach a target (Fig. 6-5). Ataxic movements are slow. Ataxic movements are also decomposed into their component parts. In place of one smooth, fluid action, a series of overshooting or undershooting movements occurs with the errors increasing as a target is neared. The most common symptom to result from damage to the cerebellum *or to the cerebellar peduncles* is ataxia.

COLLICULI CAP THE MIDBRAIN AND CEREBRAL PEDUNCLES FLANK THE BASE OF THE MIDBRAIN

The basis pontis ends abruptly at the pontomesencephalic junction, where the midbrain's *cerebral peduncles* (entirely distinct from and not to be confused with cerebellar peduncles) take over the ventral surface (see Fig. 5-5). The cerebral peduncles carry axons descending from forebrain to the brainstem and/or the spinal cord. Fibers of the corticospinal pathway travel in the middle portion of each cerebral peduncle, ipsilateral to the cortex from which they arise and contralateral to the side of the muscles that they ultimately control.

At the anterior edge of the midbrain ventrum is the optic tract containing axons from the retina destined for the thalamus (see Fig. 5-5). The optic tract wraps around the anterior and lateral edges of the cerebral peduncles. Because of their anatomical proximity, these two elements—the cerebral peduncle and the optic tract—may be damaged by a single injury. The result is impairment of two very different functions: *contralateral voluntary movement* and *vision of the contralateral visual field*. As you recall from Chapter 5, the oculomotor nerve (III) emerges from the medial edge of the cerebral peduncles in the caudal midbrain. Just

rostral to the mesodiencephalic junction—the junction of the midbrain and diencephalon—are the mammillary bodies located at the caudal pole of the hypothalamus.

Four *colliculi* or hills occupy the dorsal surface of the midbrain (Fig. 6-3). Altogether, the four colliculi—bilateral pairs of inferior and superior colliculi—are sometimes referred to as the *corpora quadrigemina* (Latin for "four bodies"). The *inferior colliculi* are important to localizing sounds and are an essential way-station in the auditory pathway. Localizing sounds is a very important function for animals such as owls who must capture prey at night in order to survive. Sound localization is *not* a big part of modern human life, and clinical complaints regarding this faculty do not occur.

The *superior colliculi* are important for localizing stimuli, particularly visual stimuli, and for transforming sensory information into an orienting movement. The sensorimotor transformation accomplished by the superior colliculi coordinates orienting movements of the eyes and head toward unexpected sights and sounds. Whether the doorbell rings or someone waves frantically, you will use your superior colliculus to turn to the source of the greeting. Although the superior colliculi are not part of the pathway for conscious visual perception, they can contribute to subconscious perception. In fact, the superior colliculi contribute substantially to *blindsight*, in which people with a lesioned visual cortex can orient to objects with eye movements. For example, a person may orient toward an unexpected stimulus, such as a bolt of lightning, even though the lightning is not consciously *perceived* and cannot be described.

The midbrain gives way to the thalamus at the mesodiencephalic junction, marked by the optic tract ventrally and the pineal gland dorsally. The pineal gland, a non-neural gland that secretes melatonin and is important in biological rhythms, sits in a midline recess at the anterior pole of the superior colliculi and marks the caudal end of the velum interpositum (Fig. 6-3; see Chapter 3). The posterior commissure is also present at the mesodiencephalic junction and is sometimes visible as a white matter tract close to the dorsal surface of the brain just ventral to the pineal gland. Because it is easily visualized by noninvasive scanning techniques, the posterior commissure serves as an important landmark for brain imaging. The *AC–PC line* between the posterior commissure (PC) and the also easily imaged anterior commissure (or AC) forms the reference line for aligning magnetic resonance imaging (MRI) images of the brain.

Now we step inside the brainstem and learn our way around cross-sections.

The first section that we examine is one that contains the pyramidal decussation (Fig. 6-6). In cross-section, the pyramidal decussation looks like an "x" with fibers from the right cerebral cortex crossing from the right pyramid to the left side and those from the left cerebral cortex crossing to the right. Just caudal to the pyramidal decussation, the crossing fibers reach their destination in the spinal dorsolateral funiculus, where they form the lateral corticospinal tract (see Chapter 4).

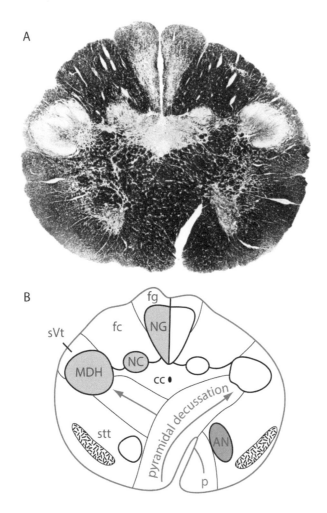

Figure 6-6 A photomicrograph (A) and diagram (B) of a section through the pyramidal decussation. The photomicrograph in A and all others in this chapter have been stained so that myelin is black. As a consequence, white matter is black and gray matter is white in appearance. The spinomedullary junction is marked by the pyramidal decussation where corticospinal tract fibers traveling in the pyramids (*p*) cross the midline to form the lateral corticospinal tract within the spinal cord. The pyramidal decussation is the motor decussation; above this level, the corticospinal pathway controls contralateral voluntary movements and below this level it controls ipsilateral voluntary movements. The spinothalamic tract (*stt*) is in roughly the same locale as in the spinal cord. At this level and throughout the brainstem, the spinothalamic tract carries pain and temperature information from the contralateral body. In this section, fibers from the dorsal columns have begun to terminate in the dorsal column nuclei. Many fibers from the fasciculus gracilis (*fg*) have terminated in nucleus gracilis (*NG*). As a consequence, the nucleus is large and the remaining fibers in the fasciculus gracilis are a minority. In contrast, only a small number of fibers in the fasciculus cuneatus (*fc*) have terminated in nucleus cuneatus (*NC*). Therefore, a large fasciculus cuneatus dominates a small nucleus cuneatus at this level. The fibers in the dorsal columns and the neurons in the dorsal column nuclei present in this section carry information about light touch, vibration, and proprioception from the ipsilateral body. The small solid circle in the center of the diagram in B represents the *approximate* location of the central canal (*cc*), which, although patent during embryogenesis, is occluded in the adult and therefore difficult to locate. The medullary dorsal horn (*MDH*), located dorsal and lateral to the central canal, is also called the *pars caudalis* of the spinal trigeminal nucleus. This portion of the spinal trigeminal nucleus receives primarily pain and temperature information from the ipsilateral face and oral cavity via the spinal trigeminal tract (*sVt*). The vast majority of the input to the medullary dorsal horn arises from the trigeminal nerve, with a minority of the input coming from cranial nerves VII, IX, and X. Motoneurons that innervate the sternocleidomastoid and trapezius muscles, muscles derived from branchial arches, originate in the ventral horn of the upper cervical cord, vestiges of which are present at this level. The cervical ventral horn containing sternocleidomastoid and trapezius motoneurons is sometimes referred to as the accessory nucleus (*AN*). Photomicrograph reprinted and drawing modified with permission from deArmond S et al., *Structure of the human brain: A photographic atlas*. New York: Oxford University Press, 1989.

The dorsal columns feed into the dorsal column nuclei starting at the spinomedullary junction and continuing more rostrally for several millimeters. Fibers in funiculus gracilis, carrying light touch, vibratory, and proprioceptive information from the legs and lower trunk, terminate in nucleus gracilis. Fasciculus gracilis fibers populate the dorsal columns more caudally than do fasciculus cuneatus fibers. At the level shown in Figure 6-6, nucleus gracilis is capped dorsally by a minority of funiculus gracilis fibers that have not yet reached their destinations. In contrast, the fasciculus cuneatus is large because only a small number of cuneatus fibers have terminated at or caudal to this level.

The spinothalamic tract, carrying pain and temperature information from the contralateral body, travels in the ventrolateral quadrant of the caudal medulla just as it did in the spinal cord.

As you recall from Chapter 5, the trigeminal nerve provides the bulk of the afferent input from the face and oral cavity. Trigeminal afferent fibers enter the pons and bifurcate or branch to reach the *main* or *principal sensory nucleus* located in the pons, and they also travel caudally in the *spinal trigeminal tract* (Fig. 6-7). Fibers in the spinal trigeminal tract terminate in the spinal trigeminal nucleus, which forms a long column that extends from the caudal pons through the full extent of the medulla. The most important part of the spinal trigeminal nucleus is the posterior portion, called the *pars caudalis*, which receives pain and temperature information from the face and oral cavity. Other parts of the spinal trigeminal nucleus serve nonperceptual functions such as proprioception and are of minor clinical relevance.

Because the pars caudalis is concerned with pain and temperature information, it is considered analogous to the superficial dorsal horn of the spinal cord. Moreover, it resembles the dorsal horn in appearance. Therefore, the caudal portion of the spinal trigeminal nucleus is often referred to as the *medullary dorsal horn*. Remember that the vagus, glossopharyngeal, and facial nerves innervate parts of the skin around the ear canal and ear. All somatic afferents from the face and mouth, regardless of their cranial nerve origin (V, VII, IX, X), terminate in the trigeminal nuclei (Fig. 6-7).

Neurons in the medullary dorsal horn that receive input from the trigeminal nerve send this information on to the thalamus. The secondary sensory neurons that form the *trigeminothalamic tract* send an axon across the midline to travel very near to the medial lemniscus, ultimately reaching the *ventral posteromedial (VPM thalamus)*. Thalamic neurons then send somatosensory

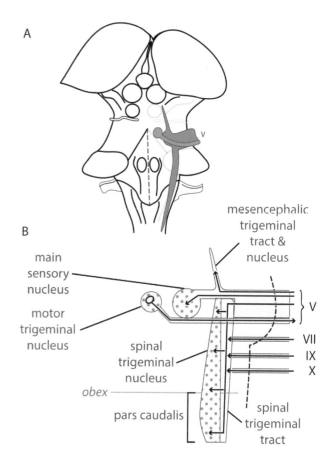

Figure 6-7 The central connections of the trigeminal nerve are diagrammed in anatomical relationship to brainstem landmarks (A) and in isolation (B). Panel A shows a cartoon of the dorsal view of an isolated brainstem. The trigeminal nerve consists of a large sensory root (*blue*) containing somatosensory information from the face, oral cavity, and nasopharynx, and a small motor root (*red*) containing the axons of motoneurons that innervate the muscles of mastication. The trigeminal sensory fibers enter the brainstem (*dotted line* in B) at the pons and terminate in three nuclei. First, trigeminal afferents that carry primarily tactile and vibratory information target the main sensory nucleus, located in the pons. Because it receives mostly low-threshold information, the main sensory nucleus is considered to be a rough trigeminal analog to the dorsal column nuclei. Second, trigeminal afferents descend in the spinal trigeminal tract to terminate in the long spinal trigeminal nucleus. The most caudal part of the spinal trigeminal nucleus, pars caudalis, is located caudal to the obex and receives mostly pain and temperature information. Thus, pars caudalis is considered to be a rough trigeminal analog to the superficial dorsal horn where pain and temperature afferents terminate. Third, the axons of a small number of proprioceptive afferents travel in the mesencephalic trigeminal tract to terminate in the nucleus of the same name. The mesencephalic trigeminal nucleus is considered to be a trigeminal analog to Clarke's nucleus in the thoracic cord (see Fig. 4-11). Both process proprioceptive information and project into the cerebellum. Since the mesencephalic trigeminal tract and nucleus are not involved in any common clinical syndromes, we do not consider these structures further. A small number of somatosensory afferents from cranial nerves VII, IX, and X enter the spinal trigeminal tract and terminate in both the spinal trigeminal nucleus and the main sensory nucleus. The motor trigeminal nucleus is located in the pons, in a pie slice that is medial to the sulcus limitans. The motoneurons in the motor trigeminal nucleus innervate the muscles of mastication, such as the masseter and anterior digastric muscles, as well as one middle ear muscle, the tensor tympani. All the muscles innervated by the trigeminal nucleus are derived from branchial arches.

SITE OF LESION	TACTILE INPUT FROM THE BODY	PAIN AND TEMPERATURE INPUT FROM THE BODY	PAIN AND TEMPERATURE INPUT FROM THE FACE
Spinal	Ipsilateral dermatomes at and below lesion	Contralateral dermatomes at and below lesion, ipsilateral dermatome at level of lesion	Not affected
Medial medulla*	Contralateral	Not affected	Contralateral
Lateral medulla*	Not affected	Contralateral	Ipsilateral
Midbrain & forebrain	Contralateral	Contralateral	Contralateral

* The medullary lesions are rostral to the sensory decussation.

information regarding the face on to the primary somatosensory cortex through the somatosensory radiation. Since blood vessels that supply the midline and lateral areas of the brainstem are distinct, strokes in the brainstem typically affect medial *or* lateral territories but not both (see Chapter 8).

A lateral medullary stroke typically lesions the laterally located spinal trigeminal tract, carrying pain and temperature input from the face and oral cavity, but it does not affect the medially located trigeminothalamic tract carrying somatosensory information from the contralateral face (Table 6-1). Thus, the somatosensory effects are:

- Loss of pain and temperature sensation from the contralateral (to the lesion) body

- Loss of pain and temperature sensation in the ipsilateral (to the lesion) face and oral cavity

- Paresthesias and dysesthesias in both territories affected by sensory loss

---

Box 6-1 **THE MOTOR DECUSSATION MARKS THE SPINOMEDULLARY JUNCTION**

Landmarks related to major tracts:
Pyramidal decussation: Corticospinal tract
Dorsal column nuclei (gracilis and cuneatus): Dorsal column-medial lemniscus pathway carrying ipsilateral tactile, vibratory, and proprioceptive information
Spinothalamic tract: Continues in ventrolateral quadrant, carrying contralateral pain and temperature information

Landmarks related to cranial nerves:
Accessory nucleus: Branchial motor through XI
Spinal trigeminal nucleus, pars caudalis, or medullary dorsal horn: Somatosensory from CN V, VII, IX, and X

A remnant of the spinal ventral horn combines with the medullary dorsal horn and the lack of a fourth ventricle to give a section through the spinomedullary junction a decidedly spinal appearance (Fig. 6-6). Motoneurons in the cervical ventral horn and adjacent accessory nucleus of the caudal medulla innervate the sternocleidomastoid and the trapezius, two neck muscles derived from branchial arches that are involved in head movements. The major landmarks of the spinomedullary junction (Fig. 6-6) are listed in Box 6-1.

THE CAUDAL MEDULLA IS MARKED BY THE INFERIOR OLIVES AND INTERNAL ARCUATE FIBERS

Cross-sections through the medulla rostral to the spinomedullary junction do not resemble the spinal cord, giving rise to a "Toto, we're not in Kansas anymore" feeling. Instead of the butterfly of gray matter surrounded by white matter that characterizes the spinal cord, the medulla contains interspersed nuclei and tracts. The nuclei and tracts mostly hug the outside of the brainstem, with the interior filled by a smattering of tracts, the occasional nucleus, and a region that looks like "filler," the *core reticular formation* or *tegmentum*. The reticular core of the brainstem serves fundamental, phylogenetically conserved homeostatic functions, such as the regulation of blood pressure and heart rate, modulation of gut motility, and generation of the breathing pattern.

In our next brainstem section, the pyramids appear ventrally as two tracts shaped as inverted "triangles" (hills really) located on either side of the ventral midline, just where we would expect them to be from their external appearance (Fig. 6-8). Remember that the pyramids carry voluntary movement commands to muscles on the opposite side of the body. The spinothalamic tract, carrying pain and temperature from the contralateral body, remains located ventrolaterally.

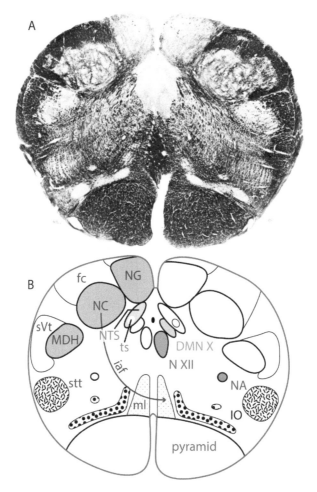

Figure 6-8 A photomicrograph (A) and diagram (B) of a section through the caudal pole of the sensory decussation. At this level, rostral to the pyramidal decussation, the corticospinal pathways travel in the pyramids. Each pyramid carries fibers that influence voluntary movement of muscles on the contralateral side. The spinothalamic tract, carrying pain and temperature information from the contralateral body, is still traveling in the ventrolateral quadrant. Virtually all of the fibers from the fasciculus gracilis have terminated in nucleus gracilis (*NG*) at or caudal to this level. Only a very small remnant of the fasciculus gracilis (unlabeled) is present capping the nucleus. Many but not all of the fibers in the fasciculus cuneatus (*fc*) have terminated in nucleus cuneatus (*NC*), which is more sizeable at this level than at the spinomedullary junction. Recall that neurons in the dorsal column nuclei project to the thalamus through the medial lemniscus (*ml*). The sensory decussation refers to axons from dorsal column nuclear neurons that arc around and cross the midline as internal arcuate fibers (*iaf*). The internal arcuate fibers can be clearly seen in the photomicrograph at top, and one arcuate trajectory is represented in the diagram at the bottom. Both the neurons in the dorsal column nuclei and the internal arcuate fibers carry information about light touch, vibration, and proprioception from the ipsilateral body. The same axon that is called an internal arcuate fiber prior to crossing the midline is part of the medial lemniscus after crossing the midline. Due to the decussation, medial lemniscus axons carry light touch, vibration, and proprioception from the *contralateral* body. Somatosensory fibers from cranial nerves V, VII, IX, and X travel in the spinal trigeminal tract (*sVt*) to reach the medullary dorsal horn (*MDH*). At this level, most of the somatosensory input to the medullary dorsal horn concerns pain and temperature from the ipsilateral face and oral cavity. The tractus solitarius contains primary afferents from cranial nerves VII, IX, and X, which carry viscerosensory and gustatory information into the nucleus of the solitary tract or nucleus tractus solitarius (*NTS*). Ventral to the nucleus of the solitary tract are three motor nuclei. The dorsal motor nucleus of the vagus (*DMN X*) contains preganglionic parasympathetic neurons that exit through the vagus nerve to innervate ganglia in the body's viscera above the hindgut. The nucleus ambiguus (*NA*) contains motoneurons that innervate the branchial arch–derived skeletal muscles of the upper airway. Nucleus ambiguus is so named because its borders are difficult to discern in sections prepared with most stains, including myelin stains. Ambiguus motoneurons project through both glossopharyngeal and vagal nerves to laryngeal and pharyngeal muscles critical to swallowing and speech. The hypoglossal nucleus (*N XII*) contains motoneurons that send axons through the hypoglossal nerve to innervate the various muscles of the tongue. The caudal beginnings of the large medullary precerebellar complex of inferior olivary (*IO*) nuclei (*regions with dots*) are present in this section. Although each cluster of cells constitutes a separate inferior olivary nucleus with a separate name, it is sufficient to refer to the conglomeration of nuclei as the inferior olivary complex or simply as the inferior olive (*IO*). Photomicrograph reprinted and drawing modified with permission from deArmond S et al., *Structure of the human brain: A photographic atlas*. New York: Oxford University Press, 1989.

The dorsal column nuclei are still present. At this level, very few gracilis fibers remain, and the nucleus gracilis is waning in size. In contrast, nucleus cuneatus is large. The output from the dorsal column nuclei is clearly visible as gracefully arcing fibers (Fig. 6-8) called *internal arcuate fibers* that decussate and then turn to ascend in the *medial lemniscus* destined for the somatosensory thalamus. This is the sensory decussation that was introduced in Chapter 4. Dorsal column nuclear neurons and internal arcuate fibers carry light touch, vibratory, and proprioceptive information from the ipsilateral side of the body. Just after crossing the midline, axons take a 90-degree turn to travel rostrally as the medial lemniscus. The medial lemnisci straddle the midline region just dorsal to the pyramids, with the right medial lemniscus carrying sensory information from the left side of the body and the left medial lemniscus carrying sensory information from the right side of the body.

In the section through the caudal medulla represented in Figure 6-8, several cranial nerve nuclei are apparent. The medullary dorsal horn, first seen at the level of the spinomedullary junction, is still present. The medullary dorsal horn receives mostly pain and temperature input, as well as some tactile input, from the ipsilateral mouth and face. Because of the relative locations of the medial lemniscus and spinothalamic tracts, midline medullary lesions impair perception of light touch, vibration, and proprioception while leaving pain and temperature pathways from the body unaffected (Table 6-1). Since the trigeminothalamic tract travels alongside the medial lemniscus, medial medullary lesions may interrupt pain and temperature pathways arising from the contralateral face.

The locations of nuclei in the central gray matter with respect to the imagined center, the site of the central canal, are useful clues to nuclear function. The *hypoglossal nuclei*, containing somatic motoneurons, appear as two discrete ovals located ventrally and medially, just off the midline (Fig. 6-8). The hypoglossal nuclei contain motoneurons that innervate tongue muscles via the hypoglossal nerve. Lateral and a bit dorsal to the hypoglossal nucleus is the *dorsal motor nucleus of the vagus*, a visceromotor nucleus. The dorsal motor nucleus of the vagus contains preganglionic parasympathetic motor neurons that influence thoracic and abdominal viscera above the hindgut via the vagus nerve's projections to parasympathetic ganglia. A third motor nucleus, *nucleus ambiguus*, contains motoneurons that innervate the skeletal muscles of the upper airway. Since the upper airway muscles are derived from branchial arches rather than somites, nucleus ambiguus is a branchial motor nucleus. Nucleus ambiguus is located ventrally within the pie slice that also contains the dorsal motor nucleus of the vagus more dorsally.

Lateral and dorsal to the motor nuclei, visceral afferents travel in a tight bundle of myelinated axons called the *tractus solitarius*, or *solitary tract*. The afferents in the solitary tract terminate in the gray matter immediately surrounding the solitary tract—the *nucleus of the solitary tract* or *nucleus tractus solitarius*—often abbreviated as

NTS. The solitary tract is an island of white matter located within the NTS. Sensory visceral information from the thoracic and abdominal viscera, larynx, pharynx, trachea, and esophagus, carried in the vagus and glossopharyngeal nerves, travels in the solitary tract and terminates in the caudal part of the nucleus of the solitary tract. Input from taste buds in the tongue, palate, and upper airway also travels in the solitary tract more rostrally and terminates in the rostral part of the nucleus of the solitary tract (see more on this later).

Ventrally, a distinctive nucleus that marks the caudal medulla makes its first appearance. This is the inferior olive, the nucleus under the bump that is the olivary tubercle and the source of a very important input to the cerebellum. Although not directly related to any cranial nerve or to any of the three long tracts, the inferior olives warrant our attention because they are so distinctive that they provide an easy way to recognize a medullary section.

THE CAUDAL MEDULLA IS DENSELY POPULATED BY CRANIAL NERVE NUCLEI

As we move rostrally in the medulla (Fig. 6-9), the same regions introduced in Figure 6-8 are present. Yet, this section features three structures—nucleus cuneatus, the internal arcuate fibers, and the inferior olive—more prominently than did the previous section. Here, we briefly review the long pathways, cranial nerve nuclei, and other remarkable medullary landmarks.

The pyramids and spinothalamic tract remain in the same positions that they occupied in the previous section. The dorsal column nuclei are more fully developed. No fibers remain in fasciculus gracilis, and the nucleus gracilis is waning in size. Nucleus cuneatus is now well formed. In addition, internal arcuate fibers from both dorsal column nuclei crowd the central portion of this section.

The same cranial nerve nuclei that were present in the last section are still present. The medullary dorsal horn is diminished in size but still visible. The hypoglossal nucleus, dorsal motor nucleus of the vagus, nucleus ambiguus, and nucleus tractus solitarius all remain in the same locations as they were in the previous section.

The inferior olives are more elaborate in this section. The inferior olives are actually a complex of multiple nuclei, more of which are present in the section illustrated in Figure 6-9 than that in Figure 6-8. Because of the larger inferior olivary territory, a noticeable bulge, the olivary tubercle, is noticeable.

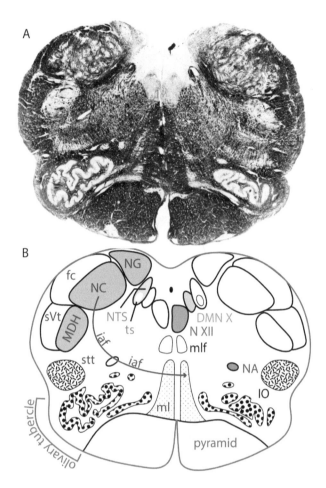

referred to as the MLF, is easily recognizable, it is a valuable navigational landmark, particularly in more rostral
sections.

The major landmarks of the caudal medulla (Figs. 6-8,
6-9,) are reviewed in Box 6-2.

Box 6-2 **NUCLEI CRITICAL TO FUNDAMENTAL
PHYSIOLOGICAL PROCESSES ARE FOUND IN THE
CAUDAL MEDULLA**

Landmarks related to major tracts:

Pyramids: Corticospinal tract carrying the commands for
voluntary movement destined for the contralateral side of
the body

Dorsal column nuclei (gracilis and cuneatus): Dorsal column
nuclear neurons send out axons that approach the midline
as internal arcuate fibers and then turn rostrally to form
the medial lemniscus. This is the caudal pole of the sensory
decussation

Medial lemniscus: Straddles the midline above the pyramids
and carries contralateral tactile and vibratory information

Spinothalamic tract: Continues in the ventrolateral
quadrant, carrying contralateral pain and temperature
information

Landmarks related to cranial nerves:

Hypoglossal nucleus: Somatomotor through CN XII

Dorsal motor nucleus of the vagus: Visceromotor through
IX and X

Nucleus ambiguus: Branchial motor to upper airway
muscles (IX, X)

Nucleus of the solitary tract: Viscerosensory from X and IX
and taste from VII (rostral two-thirds of the tongue), IX
(caudal third of the tongue and soft palate), and X (uvula
and pharynx)

*Spinal trigeminal nucleus, pars caudalis or medullary dorsal
horn*: Somatosensory from V, VII, IX, and X

Additional notable landmarks:

Inferior olive: Sends climbing fibers into the cerebellum

Medial longitudinal fasciculus: Carries axons critical to
coordination of eye and head movements

Reticular formation: Fills the core with neurons and
axons important to fundamental body processes, such as
regulation of breathing and blood pressure

Figure 6-9 A photomicrograph (A) and diagram (B) of a section through
the rostral sensory decussation. The structures present at this level
are similar to those in Figure 6-8 and will be described only briefly.
As is now familiar, the corticospinal pathways travel in the pyramids,
and the spinothalamic tract (*stt*) travels in the ventrolateral quadrant.
Nucleus cuneatus (*NC*) and the rostral pole of nucleus gracilis (*NG*)
are distinctive in this section. A minority of fasciculus cuneatus (*fc*)
remains; these fibers are destined to terminate just a bit rostrally.
Internal arcuate fibers (*iaf*) continue to leave the dorsal column nuclei
and trace an arcing path into the medial lemniscus. Medial lemniscus
axons carry light touch, vibration, and proprioception from the
contralateral body. The medial longitudinal fasciculus (*mlf*), a tract
involved in gaze coordination, straddles the midline just ventral to
the hypoglossal nuclei. Three cranial motor nuclei—the hypoglossal
nuclei (*N XII*), dorsal motor nuclei of the vagus (*DMN X*), and nuclei
ambiguus (*NA*)—are present in this section. Two sensory nuclei and
associated tracts are also present: the rostral pole of the medullary
dorsal horn (*MDH*), spinal trigeminal tract (*sVt*), nucleus tractus
solitarius (*NTS*), and solitary tract (*ts*). The inferior olivary complex is
larger and more elaborate in this section and forms a small bulge in the
ventrolateral medulla. This bulge is seen from the outside as the olivary
tubercle (see Fig. 6-2). Photomicrograph reprinted and drawing modified with permission
from deArmond S et al., *Structure of the human brain: A photographic atlas*. New York: Oxford University
Press, 1989.

One new feature makes its appearance in the section
illustrated in Figure 6-9. The *medial longitudinal fasciculus*
is a tract that runs between the upper cervical cord and the
midbrain. It coordinates conjugate eye and head movements. Because the medial longitudinal fasciculus, often

Progressing rostrally, the most remarkable transformation present in the mid-medulla, but not in the caudal medulla, is the opening of the fourth ventricle (Fig. 6-10). The floor of the fourth ventricle forms the dorsal border of the medulla at this level. This region of the fourth ventricle houses choroid plexus, which looks like irregular "crud" floating in the ventricle. As you recall from Chapter 3, choroid plexus in the roof of the fourth ventricle, along with that present in the third and lateral ventricles, produces cerebrospinal fluid (CSF). Visible on the floor of the fourth ventricle is the sulcus limitans, the indentation that marks the boundary between sensory and motor nuclei related to cranial nerves. Although not *attached* to the medulla, the cerebellum is located above the medulla and fourth ventricle at this level.

The mid-medulla (Fig. 6-10) contains most of the same regions present more caudally. Consequently, several structures may look familiar:

- The pyramids carrying messages for voluntary movement of contralateral muscles run the length of the medulla.

- The medial lemniscus carrying tactile, vibratory, and proprioceptive information from the contralateral body is in the same medial location, sandwiched between the inferior olives, and is still oriented in a dorsal-ventral direction. The dorsal column nuclei are notably absent.

- The spinothalamic tract still travels ventrolaterally, carrying pain and temperature information from the contralateral body.

- The inferior olives are large and elaborate at this level, bulging out to form the olivary tubercle.

- The medial longitudinal fasciculus, important in coordinating eye and head movements, is present as a discrete bundle of axons.

Five nuclei related to cranial nerves that were present more caudally, plus one additional cranial nerve nucleus, are visible. From medial to lateral, and thus motor to sensory, they are:

- The hypoglossal nucleus contains motoneurons that control tongue musculature.

- The dorsal motor nucleus of the vagus contains autonomic motor neurons bound for parasympathetic ganglia of the viscera above the hindgut.

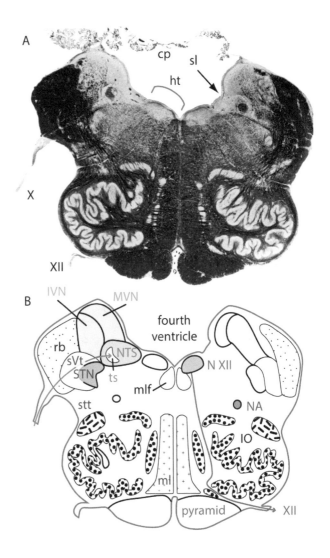

Figure 6-10 A photomicrograph (A) and diagram (B) of a section through the mid-medulla. The fourth ventricle has opened up and choroid plexus (*cp* in A) is visible. The pyramids, spinothalamic tract (*stt*), and medial lemniscus (*ml*) are in familiar locations. The elaborate inferior olives (*IO*) continue to bulge out, underlying the olivary tubercles. The medial longitudinal fasciculus (*mlf*) straddles the dorsal midline. Motor cranial nerve nuclei are present in pie slices medial to the sulcus limitans (*sl* in A), and sensory cranial nerve nuclei are present laterally. The hypoglossal nucleus (*N XII*) is still present and in fact forms a small bump, the hypoglossal trigone (*ht* in A), in the floor of the fourth ventricle. Hypoglossal motoneurons send their axons ventrally and then laterally to exit the medulla (rootlet labeled *XII* in A and *red line* in B). The rostral pole of the nucleus ambiguus (*NA*) is present, ventral to the hypoglossal nucleus and just dorsal to the inferior olives. The spinal trigeminal nucleus (*STN*) and spinal trigeminal tract (*sVt*) are diminished in size and less prominent at this level compared to levels caudal to the obex. Two vestibular nuclei make their first appearance in this section. The medial vestibular nucleus (*MVN*) is a homogenous-looking region located just lateral to the sulcus limitans. The inferior vestibular nucleus (*IVN*) is located lateral to the medial vestibular nucleus and has a distinctive checkerboard appearance. The restiform body (*rb*), located in the dorsolateral medulla, contains spinocerebellar fibers carrying somatosensory, proprioceptive, and viscerosensory information, which are destined to enter the cerebellum through the inferior cerebellar peduncle. Photomicrograph reprinted and drawing modified with permission from deArmond S et al., *Structure of the human brain: A photographic atlas.* New York: Oxford University Press, 1989.

- Nucleus ambiguus containing motoneurons that innervate muscles of the upper airway remains situated ventrally within the medullary reticular formation.

- The nucleus of the solitary tract and the solitary tract are clearly visible. At this level, the nucleus of the solitary tract is devoted to processing taste input from cranial nerves VII, IX, and X.

- Two of the four *vestibular nuclei*, all of which process input from the labyrinth related to head position and movement, appear in the mid-medulla (see more later).

- The spinal trigeminal tract carries somatosensory input from the face and oral cavity to a far less distinctive part of the spinal trigeminal nucleus than was present in more caudal sections.

The two vestibular nuclei, present at more caudal medullary levels, become more prominent in the mid-medulla. Vestibular afferents are excited by head acceleration, including that caused by Earth's gravity. They enter at the pontomedullary junction as the vestibular component of cranial nerve VIII and project to one or more of the four vestibular nuclei. The two vestibular nuclei present within the mid-medulla are important in keeping gaze steady through control of eye and head movements and in keeping an upright posture against the force of gravity.

A few additional structures demand our attention. The hypoglossal nerve emerges between the lateral edge of the pyramid and the medial edge of the olivary tubercle. In cross-section, one sees well-myelinated (and therefore darkly stained in myelin-stained tissue) hypoglossal axons traveling ventrally from the hypoglossal nucleus and then turning laterally at a point ventral to the inferior olives to emerge from the medullary ventrum. Vagal roots enter the medulla more laterally. Vagal axons travel dorsomedially to reach the nucleus of the solitary tract and the dorsal motor nucleus of the vagus. Just a bit more rostrally, glossopharyngeal nerve roots emerge from the same area as do the vagus nerve roots in this section. As mentioned in Chapter 5, no clear boundary divides vagal from glossopharyngeal rootlets. Only very small, pinpoint traumatic injuries would affect either the vagus or glossopharyngeal nerve rootlets without affecting the other. Therefore, it is rarely important to make the difficult determination whether any given fascicle emerging from the lateral medulla joins the vagus or the glossopharyngeal nerve.

The final structure that we recognize here is the *restiform body*, a tract that carries somatosensory and proprioceptive information from the spinal cord, as well as climbing fibers from the inferior olive into the cerebellum. The axons of inferior olivary neurons cross the midline, course through the contralateral inferior olive, and then arc into the restiform body. Moving rostrally through the medulla, the progressively larger restiform body foreshadows the appearance of the cerebellar peduncles into which it feeds. Ultimately, climbing fibers as well as axons from three spinocerebellar tracts enter the cerebellum through the restiform body. Because of the importance of the information carried in the restiform body to proper cerebellar function, injury to the restiform body results in ataxia (see Fig. 6-5) just as injury to the cerebellum itself does.

The major landmarks of the mid-medulla (Fig. 6-10) are listed in Box 6-3.

Box 6-3 **THE FOURTH VENTRICLE OPENS UP IN THE MID-MEDULLA**

Landmarks related to major tracts:

Pyramids: Corticospinal tract carrying the commands for voluntary movement destined for the contralateral side of the body

Medial lemniscus: Carrying tactile, vibratory, and proprioceptive information from the contralateral body

Spinothalamic tract: Carrying pain and temperature information from the contralateral body

Landmarks related to cranial nerves:

Hypoglossal nucleus: Somatomotor to tongue muscles through XII

Nucleus ambiguus: Branchial motor to upper airway muscles (IX, X)

Nucleus of the solitary tract: Viscerosensory from X and taste from VII (rostral two-thirds of the tongue), IX (caudal third of the tongue and soft palate), and X (uvula and pharynx)

Vestibular nuclei: Special sensory from VIII

Spinal trigeminal nucleus: Somatosensory from V, VII, IX, and X

Additional notable landmarks:

Inferior olive: Sends climbing fibers into the cerebellum

Medial longitudinal fasciculus: Carries axons critical to coordination of eye and head movements

Reticular formation: Fills the core with neurons and axons important to fundamental body processes such as ingestion

Restiform body: Carries spinal and inferior olivary input to the cerebellum

WALLENBERG SYNDROME RESULTS
FROM A LESION OF THE LATERAL
CAUDAL MEDULLA

IN THE ROSTRAL MEDULLA,
THE FACIAL AND COCHLEAR
NUCLEI APPEAR AS NUCLEI RELATED
TO VISCERAL FUNCTION FADE

For a quick test of your understanding of medullary anatomy, consider an interruption of the blood supply to the lateral medulla. This actually happens and is called either *Wallenberg* or *lateral medullary syndrome*. Which nuclei will be affected and what symptoms will result? Try to figure this out on your own before reading on.

Lateral lesions of the caudal medulla typically impair functioning of the caudal spinal trigeminal nucleus, spinothalamic tract, nucleus ambiguus, vestibular nuclei, and restiform body. As a result, common symptoms of Wallenberg syndrome include:

- Ipsilateral (to the lesion) anesthesia, or loss of sensation, in the face and oral cavity is due to damage to the caudal spinal trigeminal tract and nucleus. The most dangerous element of this symptom is the loss of corneal sensation and associated absence of the protective blink reflex. Corneal scarring can result if irritants are not blinked away.

- Impaired pain and temperature sensation on the contralateral side of the body results from damage of the spinothalamic tract.

- Dysphagia, impairment of swallowing, and dysarthria, impairment of speech articulation, occur because of damage to nucleus ambiguus.

- Vertigo, nausea, and ipsilateral ataxia (see Fig. 6-5) are consequences of damage to the vestibular nuclei and restiform body.

- Horner syndrome (see Chapter 4) develops because a tonic excitatory input to sympathetic neurons in the thoracic cord is interrupted. This excitatory input travels near the spinothalamic tract and is typically lesioned in Wallenberg syndrome.

The symptoms of the lateral medullary syndrome encapsulate a large number of medullary functions. Absent from the syndrome are problems with voluntary movements because the corticospinal tract travels so close to the midline of the medulla. Also typically absent are symptoms related to somatomotor and visceromotor functions of medial medullary nuclei: the hypoglossal nucleus and the dorsal motor nucleus of the vagus. Finally, the medial lemniscus is not affected by lateral medullary strokes. Consequently, light touch, proprioception, and vibration inputs from the body are unaffected.

Several of the now-familiar structures just listed are still present in the rostral medulla (Fig. 6-11). The pyramids occupy

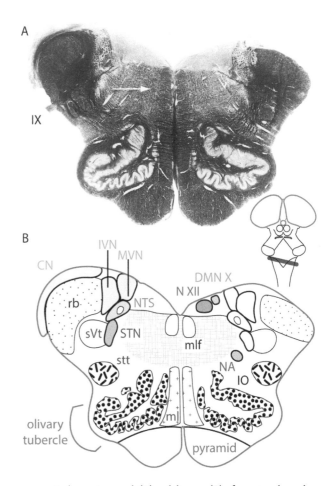

Figure 6-11 A photomicrograph (A) and diagram (B) of a section through the rostral medulla. Sections are often cut obliquely as is the case for this section. The left half of this section is from a more rostral level than is the right half of the section; the heavy brown line in the inset shows the approximate plane of section. Because we are interested in the rostral medulla, we focus on the left half of this section. The right half of the section contains mid-medullary structures as described in the caption for Figure 6-10. The pyramids, medial lemniscus (*ml*), and spinothalamic tract (*stt*) remain in the same relative locations as in previous sections. The inferior olives (*IO*) remain conspicuous medullary markers. The medial longitudinal fasciculi (*mlf*) straddle the dorsal midline as a pair of distinct tracts. The restiform body (*rb*) has swelled with more fibers as it nears the cerebellum. The hypoglossal nucleus is no longer present (on the left), and in fact, there is no motor cranial nerve nucleus at this level. The central core of the medulla is occupied by reticular formation (*white arrow* in A and *hatching* in B). Lateral to the motor region are the medial (*MVN*) and inferior (*IVN*) vestibular nuclei. The cochlear component of cranial nerve VIII projects into the cochlear nuclei (*CN*), which cap the restiform body. The rostral pole of the nucleus of the solitary tract (*NTS*), where taste is processed, is still present. Photomicrograph reprinted with permission from Bruni JE and Montemurro D, *Human neuroanatomy: A text, brain atlas, and laboratory dissection guide.* New York: Oxford University Press, 2009.

the base of the section. The medial lemniscus stands vertically between the large and elaborate inferior olives. The spinothalamic tract remains in the ventrolateral portion of the medulla. Other familiar landmarks still present are the medial longitudinal fasciculus and restiform body. The medullary reticular formation plays important roles in the regulation of heart rate, blood pressure, breathing, and ingestion.

Nucleus ambiguus, the dorsal motor nucleus of the vagus and the hypoglossal nuclei, and cranial nerve nuclei related to the glossopharyngeal, vagus, and hypoglossal nerves, are not present in the rostral medulla. The rostral pole of the nucleus of the solitary tract, a region concerned with processing taste input, is present. The caudal vestibular nuclei are still present, as is the spinal trigeminal nucleus and associated tract. Roots of the glossopharyngeal nerve emerge from the dorsolateral surface of the rostral medulla.

The hearing-related *cochlear nuclei*, which receive all input from the cochlea, form an outer cap on the restiform body that resembles a floppy dog's ear (see left side of Fig. 6-11). They appear in the rostral medulla in anticipation of the pontomedullary junction where the vestibulocochlear nerve enters. Although the cochlear nuclei receive monaural input, or input from a single ear, the *ventral cochlear nucleus* projects bilaterally to downstream auditory nuclei (Fig. 6-12). Therefore, *auditory pathways beyond the cochlear nuclei receive information about sound arriving at both ears.* Because of this early bilateralization of auditory information, the left and right sides of the brain process input from both the left and right ears. Therefore, the only traumatic injuries that can render a person deaf are in the cochlea, the vestibulocochlear nerve, or a cochlear nucleus. Injuries to central auditory pathways above the cochlear nuclei do not cause deafness.

The landmarks of the rostral medulla are listed in Box 6-4.

THE BASIS PONTIS AND THE MIDDLE CEREBELLAR PEDUNCLES MARK THE PONS

Because of its position midway between the spinal cord and cerebral cortex and its role as a requisite way-station for cerebral input to the cerebellum, the pons is like an air traffic hub, housing massive numbers of axons en route elsewhere, along with a local neuronal population large enough to provide support. The transition from medulla to pons is marked, without any trace of subtlety, by the appearance of the massive middle cerebellar peduncles and the basis pontis and the disappearance of medullary landmarks (Fig. 6-13).

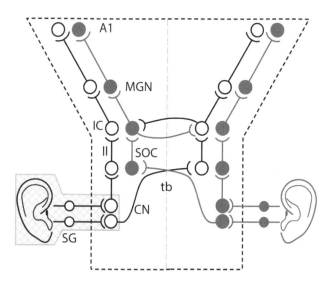

Figure 6-12 Information from the left ear (*black*) arrives in the left cochlear nucleus, and input from the right ear (*red*) reaches the right cochlear nucleus (*CN*). Cochlear nuclear neurons project to auditory nuclei on both ipsilateral and contralateral sides. Therefore, auditory pathways beyond the cochlear nuclei contain information about sounds arriving from both ears. For this reason, we skip over auditory tracts in this textbook except to briefly diagram them here. Cochlear nuclear neurons project to both the ipsilateral and contralateral superior olivary complex (*SOC*). The projection from the cochlear nucleus to the contralateral superior olivary complex travels across the midline (*blue dashed line*) in the trapezoid body (*tb*). Neurons in the superior olives project through the lateral lemniscus (*ll*) to the inferior colliculus (*IC*). Cells in the inferior colliculus are connected by a commissure. They project to the medial geniculate nucleus (*MGN*). Neurons in the medial geniculate nucleus in turn project to auditory cortex (*A1*). Since auditory information from both ears is present on both sides of the brain (*black dashed line*), a unilateral central lesion above the cochlear nuclei cannot produce deafness. Hearing problems are caused by damage in a restricted area (*tan hatched region*). Peripheral lesions of the ear, spiral ganglion (*SG*), or cranial nerve VIII (not labeled) are the typical causes of deafness. The only central lesion that can produce unilateral deafness is a complete lesion of the cochlear nuclei on one side.

The middle cerebellar peduncle forms the bulk of the attachment of the cerebellum to the brainstem as well as the lateral walls of the fourth ventricle. The superior cerebellar peduncles, visible in the dorsolateral roof of the fourth ventricle, carry the output of the cerebellum destined for midbrain and forebrain.

Just as the pyramids define the medulla, the basis pontis denotes pontine territory. The basis pontis contains three components:

- Neurons of the pontine nuclei, which are the resident cells of the basis pontis

- Axons of pontine neurons, which cross the midline and enter the middle cerebellar peduncle to provide a major input to the cerebellum; once in the cerebellum, these axons are known as *mossy fibers*

Landmarks related to major tracts:

Pyramids: Carrying commands for voluntary movement of the contralateral body

Medial lemniscus: Carrying low-threshold information from the contralateral body

Spinothalamic tract: Carrying pain and temperature information from the contralateral body

Nuclei related to cranial nerves:

Nucleus of the solitary tract: Taste from VII (rostral two-thirds of the tongue), IX (caudal third of the tongue and soft palate), and X (uvula and pharynx)

Spinal trigeminal nucleus: Processes somatosensory input from face and mouth

Vestibular nuclei: Process balance

Cochlear nuclei: Process auditory input

Additional notable landmarks:

Inferior olive: Source of climbing fibers, a critical input to the cerebellum

Medial longitudinal fasciculus: Carrying axons critical to orienting head and eye movements

Reticular formation: Fills the core with neurons and axons important to fundamental body processes such as salivation and ingestion

Restiform body: Carrying spinal and inferior olivary input to the cerebellum

• Corticospinal fibers en route from the cerebral cortex to the spinal cord with information related to voluntary movements of contralateral muscles

Corticospinal fibers, en route from the ipsilateral cerebral cortex to the contralateral spinal cord, are cut transversely and appear "on end" in a transverse section (circled x in Fig. 6-13A). As they pass through the pons, many corticospinal fibers give off collaterals that contact neurons in the pontine nuclei. Fibers that descend from cortex to reach pontine nuclear neurons either exclusively or as collaterals comprise a corticopontine tract. Pontine nuclear neurons, in turn, send axons across the midline and through the middle cerebellar peduncle into the cerebellum. As axons from

pontine nuclear cells cross the pons, they are cut longitudinally (white arrowhead in Fig. 6-13A). Pontine nuclear axons carry information about intended movements similar to the information that is sent to the spinal cord via the corticospinal tract.

The dorsal half of the pons contains the pontine tegmentum populated by cranial nerve–related structures, long tracts, and the reticular formation (Fig. 6-13B). Within the tegmentum are found the medial lemniscus and spinothalamic tract, both of which have shifted in orientation relative to medullary levels. The medial lemniscus stretches diagonally from a slightly dorsal position next to the midline to a more ventral position laterally (Fig. 6-13C). The medial lemniscus carries tactile, vibratory, and proprioceptive information from the contralateral legs, trunk, and arms. Lateral to the ventrolateral edge of the medial lemniscus, the spinothalamic tract carries pain and temperature information from the contralateral body toward the ipsilateral thalamus and thence to somatosensory cortex.

The cranial nerve nuclei present are a different group than those present in the medulla. Only one leftover is present: a vestige of the spinal trigeminal nucleus, its rostral pole. The facial nucleus, the cranial nerve nucleus related to the skeletomotor components of cranial nerve VII, sits ventrally in the second pie slice from the midline (see Chapter 5) because it contains motoneurons that innervate superficial facial muscles derived from branchial arches. During development, the facial motoneurons migrate dorsally toward the ventricle and then ventrally again, all the while dragging their axons behind them. This peculiar process results in a hairpin pathway for the axons of branchiomeric facial motoneurons. The facial colliculus, the bump in the floor of the fourth ventricle (see Fig. 6-3), marks the facial genu, where these axons curve around before traveling caudally and ventrolaterally to exit from the ventral surface of the brainstem at the pontomedullary junction. Only facial nerve axons of motoneurons innervating branchial arch–derived muscles—the superficial facial muscles and the stapedius—follow the circuitous route around the abducens nucleus. Somatosensory fibers from the ear, destined for the trigeminal nuclei, and taste input destined for the nucleus of the solitary tract enter the brainstem through the nervus intermedius.

The abducens nucleus is a compact spherical nucleus containing motoneurons that innervate the lateral rectus muscle, which, as you recall, abducts the eye. The abducens nucleus sits on the dorsal midline of the mid-pons, exactly the location expected for a somatomotor nucleus. The axons of abducens motoneurons travel ventrally to an exit point at the pontomedullary junction. In addition to causing

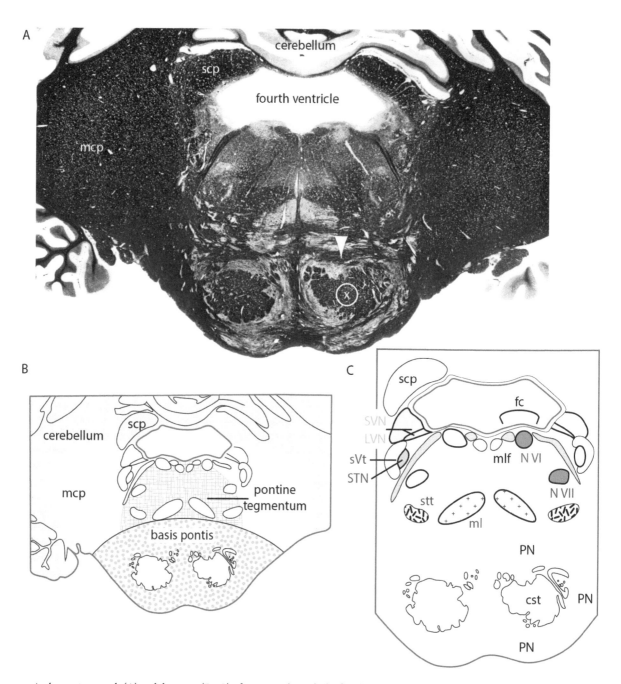

Figure 6-13 A photomicrograph (A) and diagrams (B–C) of a section through the facial colliculus. The most remarkable landmarks of the pons are the basis pontis, the middle cerebellar peduncle (*mcp*), the fourth ventricle, and the overlying cerebellum. Fibers descending from the cerebral cortex include corticospinal fibers, cut in cross-section (*circled x* in A) en route to the spinal cord, and corticopontine fibers that terminate in the pontine nuclei. Pontine nuclear neurons send axons across the midline, cut longitudinally in this transverse section (*arrowhead* in A), and into the middle cerebellar peduncle to reach their cerebellar targets as mossy fibers. B: The pons is divided into two divisions: the ventral basis pontis and the dorsal pontine tegmentum. C: A cut out from the region illustrated in A and B is shown. The basis pontis contains bundles of corticospinal tract fibers (*cst*) amid neurons of the pontine nuclei (*PN*). The remaining structures of interest are located in the pontine tegmentum and cerebellar peduncles. The spinothalamic tract (*stt*) travels lateral to the ventral edge of the medial lemniscus (*ml*), which is now diagonally oriented. Together, these two tracts carry all types of somatosensory information from the contralateral body. The facial nucleus (*N VII*) contains motoneurons that control muscles of facial expression. The axons of facial motoneurons travel dorsomedially toward the fourth ventricle and then bend back around the abducens nucleus (*N VI*) to form the facial genu underlying the facial colliculus (*fc*). After the facial genu, facial motoneuron axons travel ventrolaterally and caudally from the genu to exit laterally at the level of the pontomedullary junction. The vestibular nuclei present in mid-pons are the superior (*SVN*) and lateral vestibular (*LVN*) nuclei. The superior cerebellar peduncle (*scp*) contains the output of the cerebellum. At its rostral pole, the spinal trigeminal nucleus (*STN*) is small in size, whereas the spinal trigeminal tract (*sVt*), containing all the inputs destined for more caudal levels, is large. The medial longitudinal fasciculi (*mlf*) remain on either side of the dorsal midline. Photomicrograph reprinted and drawings modified with permission from deArmond S et al., *Structure of the human brain: A photographic atlas*. New York: Oxford University Press, 1989.

abduction of the ipsilateral eye, activation of the abducens nucleus can also produce adduction of the contralateral eye through the activation of a special class of interneurons (see Chapter 19). Thus, we can think of the abducens nucleus as a command center for horizontal gaze. The *paramedian pontine reticular formation*, often abbreviated as *PPRF*, abuts the abducens nucleus ventrolaterally. The PPRF contains neurons critical to controlling conjugate horizontal eye movements, and this region is often termed the *horizontal gaze center*.

It is the abducens nucleus that facial axons curve around at the facial genu. Thus, it is the abducens nucleus and the facial nucleus motoneurons that form the facial colliculus. The result of this close association is the potential for impairment of both ipsilateral facial expressions and lateral eye movements by small strokes in the region.

The cochlear nucleus is restricted to the rostral medulla and absent from the mid-pons. However, within the mid-pons, two vestibular nuclei are present. The two rostral vestibular nuclei nestle within the medial aspect of the middle cerebellar peduncle, just ventral to the superior cerebellar peduncle (Fig. 6-13). As this location suggests, the rostral vestibular nuclei are critically important in linking vestibular input with cerebellar control of eye movements, posture, and balance.

Anatomical structures that distinguish the pons are listed in Box 6-5.

THE FOURTH VENTRICLE GREATLY NARROWS IN ROSTRAL PONS

Within the rostral pons, the fourth ventricle narrows in anticipation of joining the mesencephalic cerebral aqueduct (Fig. 6-14). At this level, structures retained from more caudal levels include:

- Basis pontis containing bundles of corticospinal tract fibers and pontine nuclei
- Medial lemniscus
- Spinothalamic tract
- Medial longitudinal fasciculus
- Middle cerebellar peduncle
- Superior cerebellar peduncle

Although present more caudally, the superior cerebellar peduncle is particularly well-defined as it exits the

---

Landmarks related to major tracts:

Pyramidal fibers: Cut transversely, collect in bundles in the basis pontis

Medial lemniscus: Oriented diagonally from dorsomedial to ventrolateral

Spinothalamic tract: Travels lateral to the lateral edge of the medial lemniscus

Landmarks related to cranial nerves:

Facial nucleus: Branchial motor to muscles of facial expression (VII)

Spinal trigeminal nucleus: The rostral pole is present at mid-pontine levels

Vestibular nuclei: Occupy the medial and ventral portions of the middle cerebellar peduncle

Additional notable landmarks:

Pontine nuclei: Information from cerebral cortex destined for the cerebellum synapses here

Medial longitudinal fasciculus: Carries axons critical to coordination of eye and head movements

Reticular formation: Fills the core with neurons and axons important to horizontal gaze and postural control

Middle cerebellar peduncle: Carries cerebro-ponto-cerebellar input to the cerebellum

Superior cerebellar peduncle: Carries the output of the cerebellum to the midbrain and forebrain

---

cerebellum to form the eaves of the fourth ventricle rostrally (Fig. 6-14). Notice how much smaller the superior cerebellar peduncles are than the restiform bodies and middle cerebellar peduncles combined. The restiform bodies and middle cerebellar peduncles contain virtually all of the enormous quantity of input that enters the cerebellum, and the superior cerebellar peduncles carry most of the relatively small output. Through the peduncles, the cerebellum receives all possible data regarding movements that we want to make, as well as information on how movements are actually progressing. The cerebellum processes this information and then sends out, mostly via the superior cerebellar peduncles, either a message of "steady as she goes" or a course correction. The high input-to-output ratio of the cerebellum,

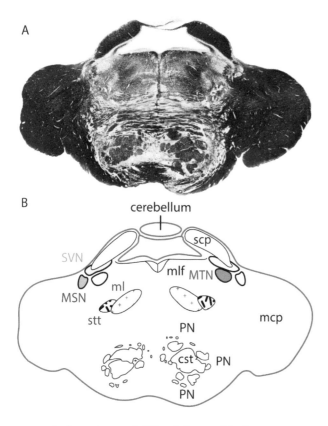

A

B

cerebellum

scp

SVN

mlf MTN

ml

MSN

stt

PN

mcp

cst

PN

PN

Figure 6-14 A photomicrograph (A) and diagram (B) of a section through the rostral pons. By now, familiar landmarks include the corticospinal tract bundles (*cst*) and pontine nuclei (*PN*) of the basis pontis, middle cerebellar peduncle (*mcp*), fourth ventricle (not labeled), spinothalamic tract (*stt*), medial lemniscus (*ml*), and medial longitudinal fasciculus (*mlf*). The motor trigeminal nucleus (*MTN*) contains motoneurons that innervate the branchiomeric muscles of mastication and tensor tympani of the middle ear. The main sensory nucleus (*MSN*) sits lateral to the motor trigeminal nucleus and processes mainly tactile input from the face. The superior cerebellar peduncle (*scp*) has left the cerebellum en route to the midbrain and forms the lateral walls of the fourth ventricle. The rostral pole of the superior vestibular nucleus (*SVN*) is nestled below the superior cerebellar peduncle. The roof of the fourth ventricle is formed by a thin layer of non-neural tissue called the superior medullary velum (not labeled). Above the roof of the fourth ventricle, a small region of tissue from the anterior cerebellum is present in this section. Fibers descending from the cerebral cortex include corticospinal fibers en route to the spinal cord and corticopontine fibers that terminate in the pontine nuclei. Pontine nuclear neurons send axons across the midline and into the middle cerebellar peduncle (*mcp*) to reach their cerebellar targets as mossy fibers. Photomicrograph reprinted and drawing modified with permission from deArmond S et al., *Structure of the human brain: A photographic atlas.* New York: Oxford University Press, 1989.

travel rostrally to the main sensory nucleus. Thus, roughly speaking, the main sensory nucleus is a trigeminal analog of a dorsal column nucleus because it is the first processing center for low-threshold somatosensory input from the face and oral cavity. The second trigeminal-related nucleus present in the rostral pons is the motor trigeminal nucleus (Fig. 6-14) that contains branchial motoneurons that innervate the muscles of mastication and the tensor tympani, a middle ear muscle.

The landmarks of the rostral pons are listed in Box 6-6.

Box 6-6 THE SUPERIOR CEREBELLAR PEDUNCLE AND NARROWING OF THE FOURTH VENTRICLE MARK THE ROSTRAL PONS

Landmarks related to major tracts:

Pyramidal fibers: Travel in bundles in the basis pontis

Medial lemniscus: Oriented diagonally from dorsomedial to ventrolateral

Spinothalamic tract: Travels lateral to the lateral edge of the medial lemniscus

Landmarks related to cranial nerves:

Main sensory nucleus: Receives somatosensory input, mainly low-threshold in nature, from the face and oral cavity

Motor trigeminal nucleus: Supplies branchiomotor innervations of the muscles of mastication and the tensor tympani of the middle ear

Vestibular nucleus: The most rostral portion of the vestibular nuclei is present just ventral to the superior cerebellar peduncle

Additional notable landmarks:

Pontine nuclei: Inputs from cerebral cortex destined for the cerebellum synapse here

Medial longitudinal fasciculus: Carries axons critical to coordination of eye and head movements

Reticular formation: Fills the core with neurons and axons important to sleep–wake control

Middle cerebellar peduncle: Carries cerebro-ponto-cerebellar input to the cerebellum

Superior cerebellar peduncle: Carries the output of the cerebellum to the midbrain and forebrain

about 40:1, reflects the powerful processing capacity of the cerebellum (discussed in much greater detail in Chapter 24).

Two nuclei related to the trigeminal nerve make their first appearances in the rostral pons. Taking the place, figuratively and literally, of the spinal trigeminal nucleus is the main or principal sensory nucleus (Fig. 6-14). Upon entering the pons, trigeminal afferents carrying low-threshold tactile and proprioceptive information turn to

THE CEREBRAL AQUEDUCT AND EMERGENCE OF THE TROCHLEAR NERVE ROOTS MARK THE PONTOMESENCEPHALIC JUNCTION

The emergence of the trochlear nerves from the dorsal side of the brainstem marks the pontomesencephalic junction (Fig. 6-15). The trochlear nerve innervates a

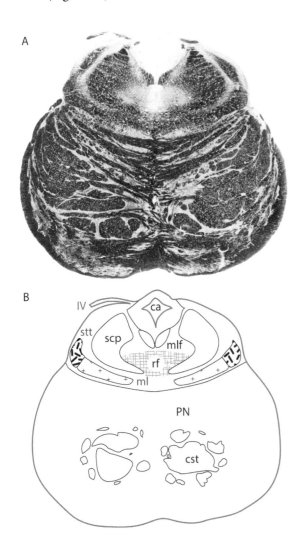

Figure 6-15 The exit of the trochlear nerve (*IV*) marks the pontomesencephalic junction in this photomicrograph (A) and diagram (B). The trochlear nerve, the only cranial nerve to exit from the dorsal surface of the brain, innervates the superior oblique muscle. The basis pontis containing the pontine nuclei (*PN*) and bundles of corticospinal tract fibers (*cst*) is still present. The medial lemniscus (*ml*), spinothalamic tract (*stt*), and medial longitudinal fasciculus (*mlf*) are in now familiar locations. The foremost landmark of a midbrain cross-section, the cerebral aqueduct (*ca*), appears. The superior cerebellar peduncles (*scp*) have dived into the brainstem and have begun to converge toward the midline. This convergence is the start of the decussation of the superior cerebellar peduncle, or decussation of the brachium conjunctivum, which occurs just rostral to this section (see Fig. 6-16). Reticular formation (*rf*) occupies the central core region of the dorsal tegmentum.   Photomicrograph reprinted and drawing modified with permission from deArmond S et al., *Structure of the human brain: A photographic atlas*. New York: Oxford University Press, 1989.

single extraocular muscle, the superior oblique muscle (see Chapter 5). The superior oblique, a somatic muscle—as are all the extraocular muscles—primarily depresses the eye.

The pontomesencephalic junction features the last vestige of the basis pontis, a pontine landmark, and the first appearance of the cerebral aqueduct, the quintessential sign of the midbrain (Fig. 6-15). The narrow cerebral aqueduct is the only section of the brain's ventricular system without any choroid plexus. This arrangement lessens the risk that the aqueduct will become occluded, a dangerous and potentially lethal situation. When a blockage of CSF flow through the cerebral aqueduct occurs, *hydrocephalus* is the result. Hydrocephalus elevates intracranial pressure by inflating the brain from the inside. It is a potentially lethal condition that luckily can be treated (see Chapter 8).

At the pontomesencephalic junction, axons from the cerebellum traveling in the superior cerebellar peduncles turn ventrally and medially en route to cross the midline a little more rostrally (Fig. 6-15). The medial lemniscus, carrying tactile information from the contralateral body, has shifted to an orientation that gently slopes dorsolaterally. Immediately lateral to the medial lemniscus is the spinothalamic tract. The mesencephalic reticular formation, occupying the central portion of the section, is important in locomotion, postural control, and arousal.

The anatomical structures that mark the pontomesencephalic junction are listed in Box 6-7.

Box 6-7 **THE TROCHLEAR NERVE EMERGES DORSALLY AT THE PONTOMESENCEPHALIC JUNCTION**

Landmarks related to major tracts:

Pyramidal fibers: Travel in bundles in the basis pontis

Medial lemniscus: Has shifted to a gentle arc from ventromedial to dorsolateral

Spinothalamic tract: Continues to travel lateral to the lateral edge of the medial lemniscus

Landmarks related to cranial nerves:

Trochlear roots: Somatic motoneurons that innervate the superior oblique muscle via cranial nerve IV

Additional notable landmarks:

Pontine nuclei: Neurons receive input from cerebral cortex and project into the cerebellum

Medial longitudinal fasciculus: Carries axons critical to coordination of eye and head movements

Superior cerebellar peduncle: Carries the output of the cerebellum to the midbrain and forebrain

The caudal midbrain is marked by the inferior colliculus and the decussation of the superior cerebellar peduncle, also known as the decussation of the brachium conjunctivum (Fig. 6-16). Fibers in the superior cerebellar peduncle cross the midline through the decussation of the superior cerebellar peduncle. Because of this decussation, cerebellar information about ipsilateral movements is carried across the midline to contralateral motor control centers in the forebrain. Thus, as mentioned earlier, movements on one side of the body are controlled by the contralateral motor cortex and smoothed by the ipsilateral cerebellum (see Fig. 6-4). Of great clinical importance, a lesion of this decussation is nearly equivalent to a lesion of the entire cerebellum. Because fibers from both sides of the cerebellum are present in the crossing of the decussation of the superior cerebellar peduncle, bilateral ataxia results.

Surrounding the aqueduct is an easily recognized donut-shaped area of gray matter termed the *periaqueductal gray*. The periaqueductal gray can be considered a caudal extension of the hypothalamus (see Chapter 7) and plays a critical role in coordinating homeostasis with motor behavior during mating, fighting, recuperation from injury, and so on.

Another landmark of the caudal midbrain is the trochlear nucleus, which nestles within the medial longitudinal fasciculus like an apple cupped in a hand (Fig. 6-16). The trochlear nucleus is small because it contains motoneurons innervating only one small muscle. The axons of trochlear motoneurons travel caudally and dorsally to exit. Upon exiting, the axons cross, so that the right trochlear nucleus innervates the left superior oblique and vice versa (see Chapter 19).

Corticospinal tract fibers from the basis pontis feed into the middle third of the cerebral peduncles, which mark the midbrain ventrum. Axons within the cerebral peduncles on either side of the corticospinal fibers are corticopontine fibers from either frontal or posterior regions of cerebral cortex. Corticobulbar fibers, headed for the motor trigeminal, facial, and hypoglossal nuclei, travel with the corticospinal fibers in the most medial portion of the middle third of the cerebral peduncle. The locations of the medial lemniscus and spinothalamic tract are slowly shifting dorsally as we move from pons and proceed rostrally through midbrain. In the caudal midbrain, the spinothalamic tract is just ventral to the inferior colliculus, and the medial lemniscus is ventromedial to the spinothalamic tract.

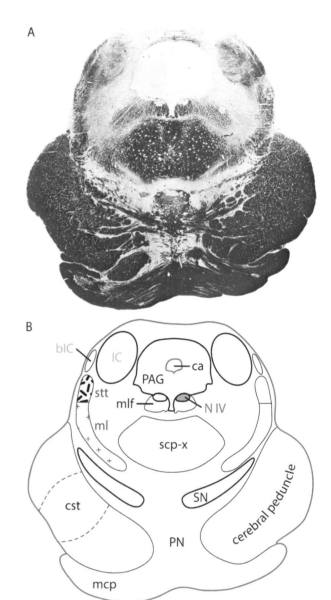

A

B

Figure 6-16 A photomicrograph (A) and diagram (B) of a section through the caudal midbrain. The basis pontis is largely gone, although small regions of pontine nuclei (*PN*) and mossy fibers destined for the middle cerebellar peduncle (*mcp*) remain. Taking the place of the basis pontis are the cerebral peduncles that mark the midbrain ventrum. The corticospinal tract (*cst*) travels in the middle third of the cerebral peduncle. The medial lemniscus (*ml*) and spinothalamic tract (*stt*) are in familiar locations. The cerebral aqueduct (*ca*) is present throughout the midbrain. Surrounding the aqueduct is the periaqueductal gray (*PAG*), a region that is important in coordinating homeostatic behaviors. The trochlear nucleus (*N IV*) is a small nucleus nestled within the medial longitudinal fasciculus (*mlf*) that, along with the inferior colliculus (*IC*) and decussation of the superior cerebellar peduncle (*scp-x*) distinguish the caudal midbrain. The output of the inferior colliculus carries bilateral auditory information through the brachium of the inferior colliculus (*bIC*) to the medial geniculate nucleus of the thalamus. Dorsal to the cerebral peduncle is the caudal pole of the substantia nigra (*SN*), an important component of basal ganglia circuits.   Photomicrograph reprinted and drawing modified with permission from deArmond S et al., *Structure of the human brain: A photographic atlas*. New York: Oxford University Press, 1989.

Dorsal to each cerebral peduncle stretches an arc of gray matter called the *substantia nigra*. The substantia nigra has two parts or pars, which have nothing in common beyond their neighboring locations. *Pars reticulata* is an output nucleus of the basal ganglia and functions similarly to the internal portion of the globus pallidus (see Chapter 25). As detailed in Chapter 25, substantia nigra pars reticulata sends out a continuous "don't move" signal, which is only interrupted when a movement becomes imperative. In the case of the major projection from pars reticulata to the superior colliculus, the continuous inhibitory signal prevents eye movements. When the inhibitory signal is briefly interrupted, the superior colliculus's plan for an orienting movement is released from suppression and thus is enacted.

The *substantia nigra pars compacta* consists of a group of dopaminergic cells that project heavily into the striatum of the basal ganglia. The roles of these dopaminergic cells are many, varied, and controversial. One clear role for nigral dopaminergic cells is to provide the "oil" necessary for movement. When pars compacta cells die, as occurs in Parkinson's disease, people initiate movements slowly and infrequently (see more in Chapter 25).

The structures that mark the caudal midbrain are listed in Box 6-8.

ROSTRAL MIDBRAIN IS MARKED BY THE OCULOMOTOR NUCLEUS, SUPERIOR COLLICULUS, AND RED NUCLEUS

Within the rostral midbrain, the cerebral peduncles containing the corticospinal and corticobulbar tracts are well developed (Fig. 6-17). Exiting from the medial edge of the cerebral peduncles are the roots of the oculomotor nerve. The oculomotor nucleus, a large sprawling nucleus, occupies the midline just ventral to the aqueduct. Recall that the oculomotor nucleus contains somatic motoneurons that innervate five different muscles:

- *Medial rectus*, an extraocular muscle that adducts eye

- *Inferior rectus*, an extraocular muscle that depresses the eye

- *Superior rectus*, an extraocular muscle that elevates the eye

- *Inferior oblique*, an extraocular muscle that elevates the eye

- *Levator palpebrae superioris*, a muscle involved in voluntarily elevating the eyelid

Also contributing to the oculomotor nerve is the Edinger-Westphal nucleus, which sits cradled within the

---

Box 6-8 **THE CAUDAL MIDBRAIN IS DISTINGUISHED BY THE INFERIOR COLLICULI AND THE DECUSSATION OF THE BRACHIUM CONJUNCTIVUM**

Landmarks related to major tracts:

Pyramidal fibers: Travel in the middle third of the cerebral peduncle contralateral to the muscles that they ultimately control

Medial lemniscus fibers: Continue to shift laterally

Spinothalamic tract: Travels dorsal to the medial lemniscus

Landmarks related to cranial nerves:

Trochlear nucleus: Somatic motoneurons that innervate the superior oblique muscle via the trochlear nerve

Additional notable landmarks:

Cerebral peduncle: Carries the corticospinal and corticobulbar tracts in the middle third and corticopontine fibers on either side

Medial longitudinal fasciculus: Carries axons critical to coordination of eye and head movements

Decussation of the superior cerebellar peduncle: Carries cerebellar output to the contralateral midbrain and thalamus

Caudal pole of the substantia nigra: A critical region for the timing and initiation of movements, caps the cerebral peduncles

---

oculomotor nucleus (Fig. 6-17C). The Edinger-Westphal nucleus contains visceromotor neurons that control pupillary constriction and lens shape via projections to the parasympathetic ciliary ganglion (see Chapter 5). Together, the oculomotor and Edinger-Westphal nuclei comprise the oculomotor complex. The medial longitudinal fasciculus is a highway dedicated to coordinating head and eye movements, and it is situated just lateral to the oculomotor complex. Neurons located adjacent to the medial longitudinal fasciculus at the level of the oculomotor complex *coordinate* vertical gaze and comprise the *vertical gaze center*.

The medial lemniscus and spinothalamic tract retain the same positions they occupied more caudally, although the surrounding landscape has changed. Instead of sitting near the edge of the brain, these somatosensory tracts now are positioned deep to the medial geniculate body, the thalamic nucleus critical to hearing. Because hearing from each ear is bilaterally represented in the brain above the medulla, even a lesion of the medial geniculate body does not noticeably alter hearing.

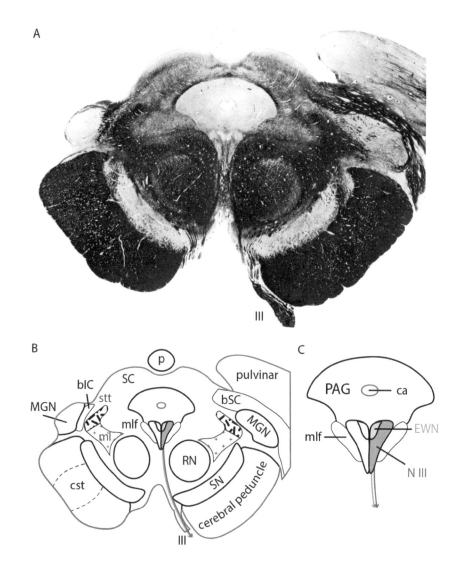

Figure 6-17 A photomicrograph (A) and diagrams (B–C) of a section through the superior colliculus (*SC*). B: At this level, the corticospinal tract (*cst*) travels in the middle third of the cerebral peduncle en route to the contralateral ventral horn. The medial lemniscus (*ml*) and spinothalamic tract (*stt*) continue to travel dorsal to the lateral edge of the cerebral peduncles. The red nucleus (*RN*), a motor control center, is evident as a large spherical nucleus. The substantia nigra (*SN*) is a clearly delineated gray matter region (unstained by myelin stains), which caps the cerebral peduncles. C: A magnified view of the central gray is illustrated. The oculomotor complex consists of the oculomotor nucleus (*N III*) and the Edinger-Westphal nucleus (*EWN*). Recall that the oculomotor nucleus contains somatic motoneurons that innervate four extraocular muscles and the levator palpebrae superioris, a muscle that raises the eyelid. The Edinger-Westphal nucleus contains autonomic motor neurons that innervate parasympathetic neurons in the ciliary ganglion, ultimately influencing pupillary diameter and lens shape. Axons from both oculomotor and Edinger-Westphal nuclei course ventrally and exit the midbrain just medial to the cerebral peduncles (*III* in A and B). The medial longitudinal fasciculus (*mlf*) is located just lateral to the oculomotor complex (B–C). The periaqueductal gray (*PAG*) continues to surround the cerebral aqueduct (*ca*) in the rostral midbrain. Although this section contains several structures of the rostral midbrain, it also contains a number of diencephalic structures including the medial geniculate nucleus (*MGN*), a thalamic nucleus that processes auditory information, and the pulvinar, a caudal thalamic nucleus involved in visual processing. The brachium of the inferior colliculus (*bIC*) carries input to the medial geniculate nucleus from the inferior colliculus. The brachium of the superior colliculus (*bSC*) carries visual information from the superior colliculus to the lateral geniculate nucleus (not present at this level) and to the pulvinar. Finally, nestled between the superior colliculi is the pineal gland (*P*), a non-neural gland that secretes melatonin.   Photomicrograph reprinted and drawing modified with permission from deArmond S et al., *Structure of the human brain: A photographic atlas*. New York: Oxford University Press, 1989.

Just as the inferior colliculi are landmarks of the caudal midbrain, the superior colliculi are a sure indication of the rostral midbrain. The superior colliculus is important in transforming multimodal sensory information—input from multiple senses—into a motor command for orienting movements. Thus, the superior colliculus is critical to shifting gaze toward unexpected stimuli. In lower animals without a well-developed cerebral cortex, the superior colliculus coordinates most visually driven behavior. In humans and other primates, the superior colliculi retain the capacity to drive orienting movements toward moving stimuli.

The substantia nigra is more fully developed in the rostral midbrain than in the caudal midbrain. In the rostral midbrain, the substantia nigra caps most of the width of the cerebral peduncles. Dorsal to the substantia nigra are large spherical nuclei that straddle the midline. These nuclei are the *red nuclei*, clear landmarks of the rostral midbrain. The red nuclei receive input from the cerebellum and from motor cortex and are the source of the *rubrospinal tract*, an important descending motor pathway. Hanging over the midbrain is a large thalamic nucleus, important to vision, called the *pulvinar*.

The landmarks of the rostral midbrain are reviewed in Box 6-9.

Box 6-9 **THE SUPERIOR COLLICULUS IS THE MAJOR EXTERNAL MARKER OF THE ROSTRAL MIDBRAIN**

Landmarks related to major tracts:

Pyramidal fibers: Travel in the middle third of the cerebral peduncle contralateral to the muscles that they ultimately control

Medial lemniscus fibers: Continue to shift laterally

Spinothalamic tract: Travels just deep to the medial geniculate nucleus and the brachium of the inferior colliculus

Landmarks related to cranial nerves:

Oculomotor nucleus: Somatic motoneurons that innervate four extraocular muscles and the levator palpebrae superioris

Edinger-Westphal nucleus: Visceromotor neurons that control pupillary constriction and lens accommodation via parasympathetic projections to the ciliary ganglion

Additional notable mesencephalic landmarks:

Cerebral peduncle: Carries the corticospinal and corticobulbar tracts in the middle third and corticopontine fibers on either side

Medial longitudinal fasciculus: Carries axons critical to coordination of eye and head movements

Substantia nigra: An important component of the basal ganglia and consists of two very different parts

Superior colliculus: Critical to visually guided movements and orienting movements to moving objects

Pineal gland: Non-neural tissue that secretes melatonin and is important in the coordination of circadian rhythms

---

THE POSTERIOR COMMISSURE MARKS THE MESODIENCEPHALIC JUNCTION

As the midbrain meets the diencephalon, the cerebral aqueduct elongates ventrally to form a slit; this is the opening of the third ventricle (Fig. 6-18). At this point, a transverse slice contains even more of a mixture of the two bordering regions than occurs at either the spinomedullary or pontomesencephalic junctions. This is simply because the brain does not develop in register with a grid, so that the actual demarcation between midbrain and diencephalon is an arc rather than a flat plane.

Clear signs of the midbrain at the mesodiencephalic junction include:

- *Red nucleus*: The source of the rubrospinal tract important in descending motor control

- *Superior colliculus*: A region important in coordinating orienting movements

- *Cerebral peduncles*: Containing corticospinal, corticobulbar, and corticopontine fibers

- *Substantia nigra*: Consisting of the pars reticulata, carrying the output of the basal ganglia to targets including the superior colliculus, and the pars compacta, the source of dopamine in the striatum

- *Posterior commissure*: Connects fibers on either side of the dorsal mid-brain important in coordinating a bilateral reaction to visual stimuli

The medial lemniscus and spinothalamic tracts remain in about the same relative location as more caudally as they near their targets in the posterior thalamus. Three thalamic nuclei are already visible:

- The *medial geniculate nucleus* processes auditory information from both ears and projects to the primary auditory cortex.

- The *lateral geniculate nucleus* processes visual information from the contralateral half of the visual field and projects to the primary visual cortex, also known as *striate cortex*.

- The *pulvinar* receives multimodal sensory inputs but serves as a primarily visual processing region in the posterior thalamus.

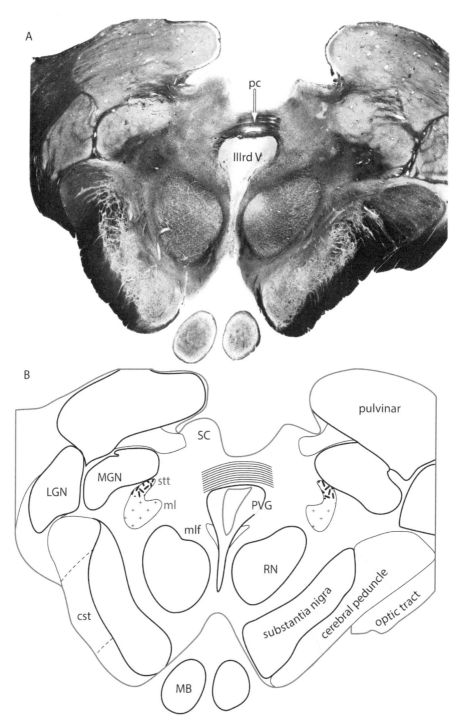

Figure 6-18 A photomicrograph (A) and diagram (B) of a section through the mesodiencephalic junction. In large part, midbrain features are concentrated centrally and diencephalic structures populate the edges. The cerebral aqueduct has elongated dorsoventrally as it transforms into the third ventricle (*IIIrd V* in A). The corticospinal tract (*cst*) continues to travel in the middle third of the cerebral peduncles. Although still present, the cerebral peduncles are oriented more dorsoventrally than is the case more caudally. Just anterior to this section, axons from the cerebral peduncles join the internal capsule of the forebrain. As they near their thalamic destination, the medial lemniscus (*ml*) and spinothalamic tract (*stt*) are poorly delineated. Consequently, damage in this region usually impairs the function of both pathways. Midbrain landmarks in this section include the red nucleus (*RN*), substantia nigra, and superior colliculus (*SC*). The rostral pole of the medial longitudinal fasciculus (*mlf*) is located just lateral to the periventricular gray (*PVG*), which surrounds the caudal third ventricle. The medial longitudinal fasciculus at this level serves to connect gaze control centers with more caudal areas containing extraocular and neck motoneurons. Capping the aqueduct is the posterior commissure (*pc* in A and lines in B), an easily visualized and therefore useful landmark in magnetic resonance images (MRIs). Diencephalic structures present include the medial geniculate nucleus (*MGN*) and its lateral neighbor, the lateral geniculate nucleus (*LGN*), a critical thalamic nucleus for vision. The pulvinar, another thalamic nucleus important in vision, appears as a pillow (*pulvinar* is Latin for cushion or pillow) atop the section. The optic tract (*ot*) carries visual information from the retina into the lateral geniculate nucleus, wrapping around the cerebral peduncles along the way. The neighboring positions of the optic and corticospinal tracts underlie the clinical syndrome of contralateral paralysis and hemianopia that follows damage in this region. Finally, the mammillary bodies (*MB*), important in memory formation, float below the midbrain, because they attach to the ventrum of the diencephalon more rostrally. Photomicrograph reprinted and drawing modified with permission from deArmond S et al., *Structure of the human brain: A photographic atlas*. New York: Oxford University Press, 1989.

Although not attached to the brain at this point, the mammillary bodies, an important part of the "limbic system" involved in memory, are seen floating below the section. The mammillary bodies participate in the Papez circuit, which is important in both memory and emotion (see Chapter 7). The mammillary bodies degenerate as a result of thiamine deficiency, giving rise to an amnesic syndrome called *Korsakoff syndrome*. Korsakoff syndrome, common in patients with advanced alcoholism, causes a deficit in explicit memory while leaving implicit memory relatively intact. An illustrative story involves the neurologist Éduoard Claparède, who placed a pin in his hand and then shook hands with a Korsakoff syndrome patient, causing the patient to experience a brief pricking pain. On the following day, despite having no recall of ever meeting Dr. Claparède, the patient refused to shake the physician's hand. Such subconscious memories that influence our actions without producing conscious awareness are termed *implicit memories*.

The mixture of mesencephalic and diencephalic structures present at the midbrain–diencephalon junction are listed in Box 6-10.

Box 6-10 **THE APPEARANCES OF DIENCEPHALIC NUCLEI, THE POSTERIOR COMMISSURE, AND THE THIRD VENTRICLE MARK THE MESODIENCEPHALIC JUNCTION**

Landmarks related to major tracts:

Pyramidal fibers: Travel in the middle third of the cerebral peduncle, which is about to merge with the internal capsule of the forebrain

Medial lemniscus fibers: Continue in the same relative position as they were more caudally

Spinothalamic tract fibers: Continue in the same relative position as they were more caudally

Landmarks related to cranial nerves:

None present at this level

Additional notable landmarks:

Cerebral peduncle: Shifts its orientation to transition into the internal capsule of the forebrain

Substantia nigra: An important component of the basal ganglia consisting of two very different parts

Superior colliculus: Critical to visually guided movements and orienting movements to moving objects

Posterior commissure: Joins the two sides of the tectum and provides a clear landmark for imaging studies

Optic tract: Refers to retinal fibers between the optic chiasm and the lateral geniculate nucleus

Medial geniculate nucleus: Receives auditory input from the inferior colliculus and projects to auditory cortex

Lateral geniculate nucleus: Receives retinal input and projects to visual cortex

Pulvinar: A caudal thalamic nucleus important in processing visual inputs

THE BRAINSTEM IS THE JACK-OF-ALL-TRADES OF THE NERVOUS SYSTEM

As diencephalic structures begin to overrun midbrain cross-sections, it is time to look back at our journey and to appreciate the "heavy-lifting" accomplished by the brainstem. The jack-of-all-trades character of the brainstem matches the array of functions served by specialized tissues of the head. The head has a mouth, ears, eyes, and an airway that supports breathing and speech. The brainstem *serves* the head, enabling the varied tissues of the head to look around, hear, speak, ingest solids and liquids, and sense head position with respect to gravity. The brainstem even contributes to the control of visceral function and postural control of the body. The functions of the spinal cord are less varied, being restricted to somatosensory, somatomotor, and autonomic motor functions. The concrete functions of the forebrain—smell, vision, hormone release—are also fewer than those of the brainstem. Because the brainstem is so integral to life as we know it, even a small lesion within the brainstem can be devastating, almost inevitably damaging multiple functions.

Hopefully, placing the brainstem in a larger perspective will help you realize the importance and worth of the material that you have taken the effort to learn in this chapter. Understanding and remembering the functions and structure of the brainstem takes effort and can feel overwhelming. Yet, millimeter for millimeter or milligram for milligram, the brainstem is worth it in terms of diagnostic power. Indeed, from the perspective of the brainstem, the forebrain is *easy*. So, onward to the easy part of the brain!

ADDITIONAL READING

Fins J. *Rights Come to Mind: Brain Injury, Ethics, and the Struggle for Consciousness.* Cambridge/New York: Cambridge University Press, 2015.

7.

FOREBRAIN

ACTION, PERCEPTION, EMOTION, AND THOUGHT

The deeply complex forebrain provides the substrate that infuses movements, stimuli, and situations with meaning. As hard as it is to identify any single forebrain feature that distinguishes us from other animals, it is clear that the collective properties of the forebrain are responsible for making us "human." The forebrain transforms movement into action, sensation into perception, and allows for the rich experiences of emotion and thought. Without the forebrain, we may be able to function physiologically, at least in forgiving conditions, but we could not do the things we do, be the individuals that we are, or live as communities. We could not build libraries, cook delicious meals, or whistle a happy tune. The forebrain leaves the hard work of keeping us alive to the brainstem and spinal cord while taking full credit and holding complete responsibility for all the lofty functions that we enjoy. In essence, "life" is possible, but certainly not as rich without the myriad contributions of the forebrain.

The forebrain presents an enormous challenge. On an anatomical level, as we saw in Chapter 3, the human telencephalon has taken twists and turns that render its three-dimensional visualization daunting. On a functional level, what the telencephalon "does" is more complex and nuanced than even the most skilled use of language can depict. Indeed, entire books and library sections are devoted to understanding each of the functions that are covered in this chapter. Linguistic limitations along with educational constraints force us to reduce brain areas, connections, pathways, and circuits into words, sentences, and paragraphs. Even so, the ultimate goal of providing future physicians with enough understanding of the brain to fuel their future careers is attainable. With that pep talk, let's dive in.

FUNCTIONAL GROUPINGS WITHIN THE FOREBRAIN

We start by dividing up the forebrain challenge into digestible bits. As you know, a fundamental embryological division

occurs between the diencephalon and telencephalon. The diencephalon contains two already familiar areas. The hypothalamus is critical to maintaining body homeostasis, responding to physiological challenges, and to expressing emotions. The hypothalamus also exerts control over the pituitary gland. The thalamus, or dorsal thalamus, includes about a dozen nuclei with functions primarily focused on sensory, motor, emotional, or executive processing. Nearly all inputs destined for the cerebral cortex have only indirect access to the cortex through a synapse in the thalamus. Thus, the thalamus translates the language of subcortical areas into language that is understandable by cerebral cortex.

Within the telencephalon, the cerebral cortex occupies the outer rind, or *mantle*. Cortical areas are modularly organized in that they have a primary function such as vision, hearing, or planning (Fig. 7-1). In this chapter, we discuss the following cortical areas:

- *Primary sensory cortices* are essential way-stations for somatosensory, visual, and auditory perception. The primary motor cortex is essential for volitional or voluntary movements.

- *Frontal cortex* contains a number of action-related areas, as well as the *prefrontal cortex* involved in executive function.

- *Parietal cortex* is critical to associating visual, somatosensory, and other sensory information for use in both perception and motor control.

- Circuits in *inferotemporal cortex* support recognition of the sensory world and translate sensory representations into meaning.

- The *hippocampus*, part of the *temporal cortex*, encodes new declarative, or factual, memories. Information arrives in the hippocampus, and memories are shipped out of the hippocampus to other regions of cerebral cortex for storage. The route out of the hippocampus passes through the *parahippocampal gyrus*.

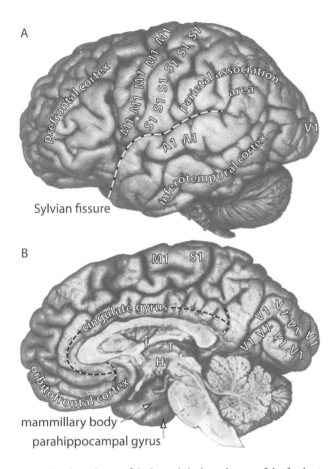

A

Sylvian fissure

B

mammillary body
parahippocampal gyrus

Figure 7-1 In a lateral view of the brain (A), the only part of the forebrain visible is the cerebral cortex. Primary motor (*M1*), somatosensory (*S1*), and auditory (*A1*) cortices, and a small bit of primary visual cortex (*V1*) are evident. The large Sylvian fissure or lateral sulcus (*dashed line*) divides the temporal cortex, housing auditory cortex, from parietal and frontal cortices, whereas the central sulcus (not labeled) separates the M1-containing frontal lobe from the S1-containing parietal lobe. Additional cortical areas visible are the prefrontal cortex, an area critical to organizing behavior; parietal association cortex where sensory inputs are integrated; and inferotemporal cortex where visual objects are identified and their meaning understood. Insular cortex, sometimes considered the fifth lobe, is deep within the Sylvian fissure and not visible from either the lateral or medial surfaces of the cerebral cortex (see Fig. 7-3). B: A mid-sagittal view of the brain reveals the thalamus (*T*), hypothalamus (*H*), and most of primary visual cortex. Small areas of primary motor and somatosensory cortices are also visible. The cingulate gyrus, posterior part of the orbitofrontal cortex, parahippocampal gyrus, and fornix (*f*) wrap around the diencephalon. Along with the hypothalamus, mammillary bodies, and amygdala (not visible here), these structures constitute the limbic system (Fig. 7-2). Photographs reprinted with permission from deArmond S et al., *Structure of the human brain: A photographic atlas.* New York: Oxford University Press, 1989.

- *Limbic structures* do not participate directly in either sensory or motor processing but rather contribute to emotional processing and to learning and memory.

The term *limbic* derives from the Latin word for "border," and, as originally defined by Pierre Paul Broca, refers to telencephalic structures that border the diencephalon (Fig. 7-2). Today, the term is used to refer to structures

that are central to emotional processing, learning, and memory but that do not participate directly in either sensory or motor processing. An influential formulation of the limbic system stems from a circuit originally proposed by American neuroanatomist James Papez in the early 20th century. This circuit, known as the *Papez circuit*, links the hippocampus to the mammillary bodies by way of the fornix, the mammillary bodies to the anterior nucleus of the thalamus, the anterior nucleus to the cingulate gyrus, and the cingulate gyrus to the parahippocampal gyrus, and then to the hippocampus. Additional regions now known to play critical roles in emotion, learning, and memory include the mediodorsal nucleus of the thalamus, amygdala, hypothalamus (beyond the mammillary bodies), and the orbitofrontal cortex.

Telencephalic structures deep to the outer rind of cortex are termed *subcortical* (Fig. 7-3). The two primary subcortical cell groupings are the striatum and pallidum of the basal ganglia and the amygdala. As you recall from Chapter 3, the striatum and pallidum develop from the ganglionic eminences of the ventral telencephalic vesicle. The striatum includes the caudate and putamen, functionally similar but separated anatomically by the internal capsule. Pallidum includes the internal and external globus pallidus, anatomical neighbors that serve related but different roles in basal ganglia function. The amygdala (Fig. 7-3C) is critical to processing emotional input and forming emotional memories.

Subcortical white matter tracts link the hemispheres with each other as well as with specific areas in the thalamus, brainstem, and spinal cord. As we already know, the corpus

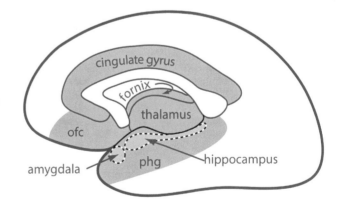

Figure 7-2 Limbic structures viewed on a cartoon of a mid-sagittal section through the brain. Pierre Paul Broca, a French neurologist who made numerous and varied contributions to our understanding of forebrain function, originally used the term "limbic" to refer to structures that border (*limbus* is the Latin word for "border") the diencephalon. These structures included the cingulate gyrus, hippocampus, orbitofrontal cortex (*ofc*), parahippocampal gyrus (*phg*), and fornix. Today, anterior thalamus, amygdala, and the hypothalamus including the mammillary bodies, are also considered to be limbic structures.

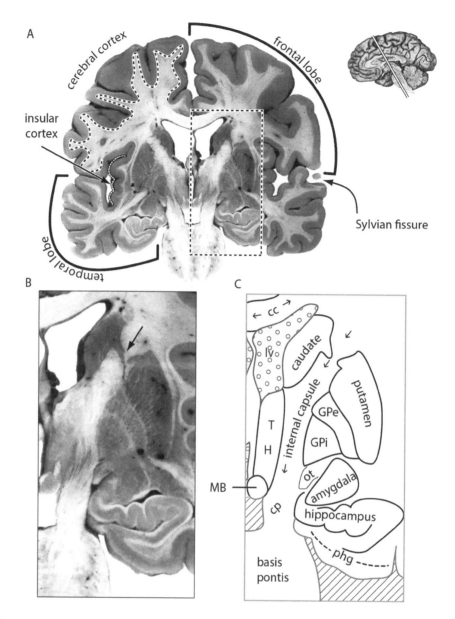

Figure 7-3 An unstained cross-section through the temporal and frontal lobes, at the level and angle illustrated in the inset. Since this section is unstained, regions containing neurons are gray in color and regions with myelinated axons are white in color. The region in the dashed box in A is shown at greater magnification in B and C. A: The gray matter mantle of the telencephalon is the cerebral cortex. The insular cortex is located deep within the Sylvian fissure. B–C: The hippocampus is a region of archicortex, or old cortex, that has only three laminae rather than the six layers that defines neocortex. Structures deep to the cortex (*dashed line* at top left of A) are termed *subcortical*. The major subcortical components of the telencephalon are the core components of the basal ganglia; namely, the caudate, putamen, external (*GPe*) and internal (*GPi*) globus pallidus. The caudate and putamen are split apart by fibers of the internal capsule during development. Nonetheless, occasional cellular bridges across the internal capsule between the caudate and putamen (*arrow* in B) remain in the adult brain. The striatum, consisting of the caudate and putamen, as well as the pallidum (external and internal globus pallidus) develop from the ganglionic eminences (see Chapter 3). The amygdala is the other major subcortical telencephalic structure. Additional structures labeled for orientation are the corpus callosum (*cc*), lateral ventricle (*lv*), thalamus (*T*), hypothalamus (*H*), optic tract (*ot*), mammillary bodies (*MB*), cerebral peduncles (*cp*), and parahippocampal gyrus (*phg*). In C, ventricular areas are filled with a pattern of circles on a pale background while regions outside of the brain are filled with diagonal lines.   Photomicrographs reprinted with permission from deArmond S et al., *Structure of the human brain: A photographic atlas*. New York: Oxford University Press, 1989.

callosum, the largest commissure, links cortical neurons in one hemisphere with cortical neurons in the corresponding region of the opposite hemisphere. The fornix (Fig. 7-4) carries traffic between the hippocampus of the temporal lobe and the medially located mammillary bodies, tracing a C shape as it follows the lateral ventricle.

Two white matter tracts, the *corona radiata* and internal capsule, make up the bulk of the white matter immediately underlying the cerebral cortex. These tracts provide the main access route to and from the cerebral cortex (Fig. 7-5A). The internal capsule contains axons that continue on from the corona radiata to reach midbrain,

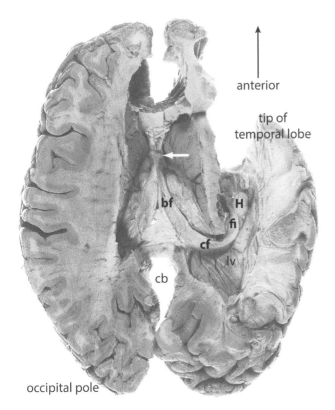

anterior

tip of
temporal lobe

occipital pole

bf

H

fi

cf

lv

cb

Figure 7-4 A horizontally oriented dissection through the cerebrum. The fornix is a large, easily recognizable tract that runs between the hippocampus and mammillary bodies. Most of the information carried in the fornix is traveling out of the hippocampal formation but some information comes into the hippocampal formation via the fornix. As fibers exit from the hippocampus (*H*), they initially form the fimbria (*fi*), which becomes the crus of the fornix (*cf*) as the axons leave the parahippocampal gyrus. Fibers of the fornix travel medially along the inside curve of the lateral ventricle. Upon reaching the midline, the fornix forms the body of the fornix (*bf*). At the white arrow, fibers of the fornix dive ventrally between the lateral ventricles as the columns of the fornix and ultimately reach the mammillary bodies. For orientation, the occipital pole, tip of the temporal pole, and lateral ventricle (*lv*) are labeled. Note that the brainstem has been removed; normally, the cerebellum (*cb*) would be visible caudally between the hemispheres. Photograph reprinted with permission from Bruni JE, Montemurro D. *Human neuroanatomy: A text, brain atlas, and laboratory dissection guide.* New York: Oxford University Press, 2009.

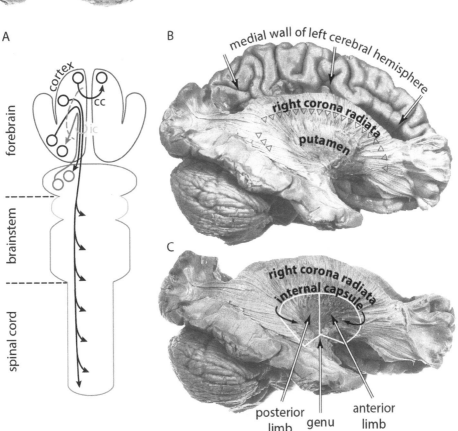

A

B

C

cortex

cc

ic

forebrain

brainstem

spinal cord

medial wall of left cerebral hemisphere

right corona radiata

putamen

right corona radiata

internal capsule

posterior
limb

genu

anterior
limb

Figure 7-5 A: The internal capsule (*ic*) connects the cerebral cortex with caudal regions of the neuraxis. All of the axons in the internal capsule are descending from the cerebral cortex en route to the diencephalon, brainstem, or spinal cord *except* axons that ascend from thalamus to reach cortex. Axons ascending from brainstem or spinal cord to thalamus do *not* travel in the internal capsule. Note that the corona radiata (*dashed brown line*) serves all axons leaving the cortex including those bound for the corpus callosum (*cc*) as well as the internal capsule. B: The corona radiata and internal capsule have been revealed by dissecting away the right cerebral cortex, leaving the right corona radiata evident and exposing the medial wall of the left hemisphere. The arrowheads point to where the corona radiata turns into the internal capsule; the latter is obscured by the putamen. C: Dissection of the putamen exposes the internal capsule carrying axons emanating from the cerebral cortex and ending in thalamus, brainstem, or spinal cord. The internal capsule consists of an anterior limb, genu, and posterior limb. Photograph reprinted with permission from Bruni JE, Montemurro D. *Human neuroanatomy: A text, brain atlas, and laboratory dissection guide.* New York: Oxford University Press, 2009.

hindbrain, or spinal cord. For example, axons of the corticospinal and corticobulbar tracts travel through the corona radiata and internal capsule before entering the cerebral peduncles. Extensive two-way traffic between the telencephalon and thalamus also travels in the internal capsule. Among the axons ascending to cortex from thalamus are the thalamocortical axons of the *somatosensory* and *optic radiations*.

In this chapter, we continue our journey up the neuraxis from caudal to rostral. We start by examining the functions of the hypothalamus. We then look at thalamic function, which necessarily involves an examination of the bidirectional interactions between the thalamus and cortex. Before exploring the function of several key cortical areas and of cortex as a whole, the amygdala and basal ganglia, two important subcortical structures are described. Circuits devoted to perception, action, emotion, and abstract thought are all unique products of the forebrain. However, we start with the hypothalamus, the forebrain region that most closely resembles the brainstem in terms of versatility and necessity.

THE HYPOTHALAMUS SERVES AS THE EXECUTIVE CENTER FOR REGULATING AND PROTECTING THE BODY'S PHYSIOLOGY

Nervous control of hormone secretion is the prime—or at least original—directive of the hypothalamus. Even invertebrates such as worms have cells that respond to sensory inputs (e.g., light) and control hormonal output. In people and other vertebrates, the hypothalamus controls the hormone-secreting pituitary gland. Thus, one could view the hypothalamus as an elaborate expansion of an evolutionarily ancient system that at its core serves to control hormones necessary for growth, reproduction, and circadian rhythms. Through its capacity to engage other brain regions (see later discussion) as well as to control hormones, the mammalian pituitary achieves a high level of flexibility and coordination for behaviors important to survival and reproduction.

The variety of processes with which the hypothalamus is concerned varies from critical but unexciting functions, such as electrolyte balance, to more lofty roles, such as facilitating pair-bonding with another individual. The hypothalamus projects to and employs the pituitary, or *hypophysis*,

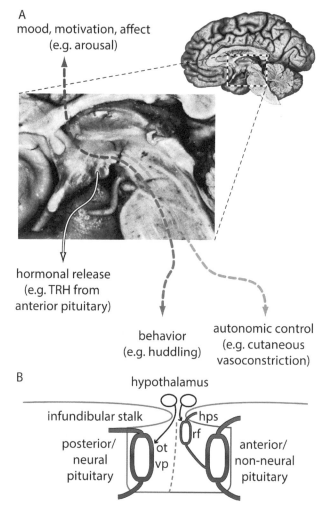

Figure 7-6 A: The hypothalamus is illustrated on a midsagittal section. The hypothalamus serves to maintain and protect the body's physiology by controlling hormonal release, motor behavior, autonomic function, mood, and motivation. As an example, when we walk outside on a very cold day, our hypothalamus coordinates a defense against the cold. The hypothalamus releases hormones, such as thyroid releasing hormone, which act on the pituitary to activate thyroid function and increase metabolism. The hypothalamus also sets into motion behavioral reactions, such as putting on a coat or huddling within a protected space. Autonomic reactions coordinated by the hypothalamus include cutaneous vasoconstriction, which restricts the exposure of warm blood to the cold elements. Finally, being challenged by a very cold environment causes arousal, preventing sleep and motivating action. To accomplish these diverse goals, the hypothalamus uses projections to the pituitary, brainstem, spinal cord, and cortex. B: The posterior part of the pituitary is the neural portion, also termed the *neurohypophysis*, and the anterior part is a non-neural gland often called the *adenohypophysis*. The hypothalamus controls the neural pituitary via direct release of hormones, oxytocin (*ot*) and vasopressin (*vp*), into the systemic circulation. In contrast, the hypothalamus controls release of several hormones from the anterior pituitary indirectly by releasing hormonal releasing factors (*rf*) into the hypophyseal portal system (*hps*). Endocrine cells in the anterior pituitary respond to releasing factors by releasing hormones into the general circulation. Photographs reprinted with permission from deArmond S et al., *Structure of the human brain: A photographic atlas*. New York: Oxford University Press, 1989.

as well as autonomic, somatomotor, and limbic pathways to effect coordinated changes in hormonal release, internal physiology, and skeletomotor actions, as well as emotion and motivation (Fig. 7-6). Some of the notable functions of the hypothalamus include:

- *Fluid and electrolyte balance*: Ensures adequate blood volume and keeps blood osmolarity and electrolyte concentrations within narrow ranges

- *Energy*: Ensures adequate energy intake through feeding and regulates energy expenditure to protect against starvation

- *Growth*: Regulates the release of growth hormone from the anterior pituitary, which in turn stimulates cell growth and division

- *Thermoregulation*: Maintains body temperature within a narrow temperature range appropriate to varying conditions

- *Mating and reproduction*: Regulates the drive to seek a sexual partner, as well as sexual motor acts themselves; directs the hormonal environment appropriate for pregnancy and lactation; initiates and contributes to puberty

- *Circadian rhythm*: Coordinates the daily rhythm of behavior, physiology, and hormone release

Although the hypothalamus is critical to maintaining the body within physiological limits, it only does so in partnership with the rest of the brain. The hypothalamus integrates information from multiple sensory modalities about the environment, both internal and external to the individual, with internal motivations, memories, and action plans. Because of the wide variety of information reaching the hypothalamus, our ability to react to challenges is highly flexible. For example, we may eat when we feel both chilly and hungry but move around if we feel chilly and not particularly hungry. As with all neural function, it is context that narrows down meaning from a wide range of possibilities ascribable to any one stimulus and which in turn dictates the hypothalamus's eventual interpretation.

Once the hypothalamus arrives at an interpretation of a situation, it directs appropriate reactions and coordinates responses of several types. For example, when a newborn suckles on the mother's breast, the neuropeptide oxytocin is released into the mother's hypothalamus and into the systemic circulation via the pituitary (see Chapter 27). Release of oxytocin, along with prolactin, into the circulation leads to milk letdown, whereas oxytocin released into the hypothalamus leads to a reduction in the emotional reaction to stressful events. In this way, mothers nurse while being biologically inclined to more easily absorb the stress of a dependent baby.

The hypothalamus is continuous caudally with the midbrain periaqueductal gray and together the two regions organize complex reactions to physiological challenges. The hypothalamus alone controls the pituitary and contributes to the regulation of mood and motivation. The hypothalamus and periaqueductal gray work together to coordinate skeletomotor and autonomic reactions to outside threats.

THE PITUITARY STALK SITS RIGHT BELOW THE OPTIC CHIASM

In humans and other mammals, the pituitary gland sits just below the base of the brain in a bony cavity called the *sella turcica*. The hypothalamus connects to the pituitary via the *infundibular stalk*, or *median eminence*, which penetrates through the dura just below the *optic chiasm*. Due to the high prevalence of pituitary tumors, the location of the optic chiasm atop the sella turcica is of great clinical importance.

Pituitary adenomas are common, perhaps present in 15% or more of the population, but typically are small and asymptomatic. Unfortunately, a small minority of pituitary adenomas grow and take up space. The bony sella turcica has no room to spare and prevents expansion in any direction but up and to the front. Therefore, space-occupying tumors that outgrow the sella turcica may impinge on neighboring structures. Pituitary adenomas can compress and consequently impair the function of the posterior pituitary, hypothalamus, or optic chiasm.

Since the optic chiasm is the most common site of compression, the most common presenting symptom associated with a pituitary tumor is blurred or restricted vision. As we shall see later in this chapter, the optic chiasm carries visual information from the temporal visual field to the contralateral lateral geniculate nucleus. Therefore, when a pituitary tumor presses on the optic chiasm, the temporal parts of the visual world become blurry or obscured altogether. The inability to see the temporal hemifield from either eye is termed *bitemporal hemianopia* and is a common symptom of space-occupying pituitary adenomas. A common treatment for pituitary adenomas is trans-sphenoidal surgery, which takes an approach through the nose. This procedure is usually successful. Radiation therapy is also used, often to treat recurrent tumors.

The pituitary consists of two parts, which the hypothalamus controls in different ways. The anterior portion is the non-neural pituitary or *adenohypophysis*. Hypothalamic cells control the adenohypophysis through an indirect pathway involving a private circulatory system—the hypophysial portal system, a set of capillary beds interconnected by veins (Fig. 7-6B). The posterior portion is the neural pituitary or posterior pituitary or neurohypophysis. Hypothalamic cells make and release hormones from axonal terminals in the neurohypophysis.

Within the posterior pituitary, hypothalamic cells release hormones directly into the systemic circulation so that, as is the case with motoneurons, hypothalamic cells directly alter peripheral function. *Oxytocin* and *vasopressin* (also known as *antidiuretic hormone*, commonly abbreviated as *ADH*) are hormones released from the posterior pituitary. Both are neuropeptides (see Chapter 12). Peripherally, oxytocin and vasopressin act to regulate fluid balance and also a number of reproductive functions.

As with other pituitary hormones, oxytocin and vasopressin are released centrally into the hypothalamus as well as peripherally. *The release of hormones into both the hypothalamus and the general circulation allows for coordinated hormonal regulation of skeletomotor, autonomic, emotional, and cognitive processes in service of complex goals such as hydration or maternal care.* For example, when an increase in plasma osmolarity is detected in the hypothalamus and afferents to the hypothalamus signal a decrease in blood pressure and a dry mouth, vasopressin is released into both the blood stream and the hypothalamus. Vasopressin acts on the kidneys to concentrate urine, reabsorb more water, and decrease urine output while acting on the brain to stimulate the search for and drinking of fluids. In this way, the coordinated actions of vasopressin on body and behavior rectify the original problem of dehydration, thus maintaining the body's physiology within acceptable limits.

The hypothalamus regulates the anterior pituitary only indirectly via the hypophysial portal system. Neurons in the hypothalamus release hormonal-releasing factors into the hypophysial portal system:

- *Corticotropin-releasing hormone* or CRH leads to the release of *adrenocorticotropic hormone* or ACTH, which has multiple effects on the brain and body, all of which are part of the reaction to stress.

- *Thyrotropin-releasing hormone* or TRH increases the release of *thyroid stimulating hormone*, also termed *thyrotropin* or TSH. Thyrotropin stimulates the thyroid gland to increase metabolism and energy expenditure.

- TRH release also increases, whereas dopamine decreases *prolactin* release, which in turn stimulates milk production and modulates sexual arousal.

- *Growth hormone-releasing hormone* or GHRH stimulates the release of growth hormone, also known as *somatotropin*. Somatostatin inhibits the release of growth hormone which, as the name suggests, increases bone and muscle growth.

- *Gonadotropin-releasing hormone* or GnRH stimulates the release of *luteinizing hormone*, or LH, which stimulates ovulation in women and testosterone production in men. GnRH also stimulates the release of *follicular-stimulating hormone*, or FSH, which is critical to reproductive function across the life cycle in both women and men. Puberty does not occur in individuals who lack hypothalamic GnRH cells, a condition known as Kallmann syndrome (see Chapter 5).

Secretory cells in the anterior pituitary respond to hypothalamic releasing factors by releasing hormones, which in turn act on glands and other tissues such as the gonads. Hormones released by the anterior pituitary exert effects on growth, metabolism, reproductive function, and the generalized stress reaction.

As an example of the hypothalamic influence on the adenohypophysis, consider the generalized stress reaction. In response to CRH released into the hypophysial portal system, the adenohypophysis releases ACTH. ACTH in turn acts on the adrenal gland to stimulate release of corticosteroids, principally *cortisol*, often referred to as the "stress hormone." The pathway from the hypothalamus to the anterior pituitary and then to the adrenal gland is termed the *hypothalamic-pituitary-adrenal axis*, typically abbreviated as the *HPA axis* (Fig. 7-7). Cortisol provides a hormonal jolt, mobilizing the body's resources for movement and action while shutting down immunological function. Cortisol also inhibits both ACTH release from the pituitary and CRH release from the hypothalamus, thus providing a termination signal and preventing cortisol release from accelerating out of control. It should be noted that stress reactions are necessary for normal physiological function. Although too much and too little cortisol are both problematic, too little is a far more serious and potentially fatal condition (see Chapter 27).

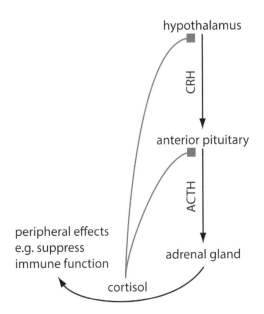

hypothalamus

CRH

anterior pituitary

ACTH

adrenal gland

peripheral effects
e.g. suppress
immune function

cortisol

Figure 7-7 The hypothalamic-pituitary-adrenal axis refers to the connection between the brain and adrenal gland. During stressful conditions, stress-activated neurons in the hypothalamus release corticotropin releasing hormone (*CRH*), which evokes the release of adrenocorticotropic hormone (*ACTH*) from the adenohypophysis or anterior pituitary. ACTH acts on the adrenal gland to release cortisol into the systemic circulation. Cortisol has diverse effects on the body, such as increasing gastric acid secretions and suppressing immune function. Cortisol exerts inhibitory feedback control (*red* ■ *symbols*) on both CRH release from the hypothalamus and ACTH release from the adenohypophysis.

SENSORY INFORMATION TRANSFERS WITHIN THE THALAMUS TO REACH THE CORTEX

Visual, auditory, somatosensory, and gustatory inputs all synapse in the thalamus en route to the cerebral cortex.

For example, the lemniscal pathway carrying touch and related information only reaches the somatosensory cortex after a synapse in a specific nucleus of the thalamus. The most important sensory nuclei of the thalamus are:

- The *lateral geniculate nucleus* contains neurons that receive visual input from the retina and provide input to primary visual cortex (see Table 7-1).

- The *medial geniculate nucleus* contains neurons that receive auditory input from the inferior colliculus and provide input to primary auditory cortex.

- Neurons in the *ventral posterolateral nucleus* (*VPL*) receive somatosensory input from the body, *from both the dorsal column-medial lemniscus and spinothalamic systems,* and provide input to primary somatosensory cortex.

- Neurons in the *ventral posteromedial nucleus* receive somatosensory input from the face and oral cavity via trigeminothalamic tracts. These thalamic neurons also receive gustatory input. Somatosensory information is sent to the appropriate region of primary somatosensory cortex, while gustatory information is sent to the gustatory cortex within the insula.

For most sensory information, the thalamus is a requisite way-station to get to cerebral cortex. The synapse within the thalamus is the penultimate step for the lemniscal and spinothalamic pathways that we have followed for several chapters now. Lemniscal (touch, vibration, and proprioception) and spinothalamic (pain and temperature) pathways from the body both synapse in the ventral posterolateral nucleus.

Table 7-1 **SENSORY PATHWAYS CONTAIN AT LEAST FOUR NEURONS**

| | | | SOMATOSENSATION | | |
	VISION	HEARING	DC-ML	STT	V
Sensory transduction cell	Retinal photoreceptor (rod or cone)	Cochlear hair cell	Dorsal root ganglion cell or sensory cell (e.g. Merkel cell)	Dorsal root ganglion cell	Trigeminal ganglion cell or sensory cell (e.g. Merkel cell)
Primary afferent Neuron	n.a.	Spiral ganglion	Dorsal root ganglion cell	Dorsal root ganglion cell	Trigeminal ganglion cell
Thalamic projection neuron	Retinal ganglion cell	Inferior colliculus neuron	Dorsal column nuclear cell	Spinothalamic tract cell	Main sensory/ Spinal trigeminal nuclear cells
Location of thalamic neuron	Lateral geniculate nucleus	Medial geniculate nucleus	Ventral posterolateral nucleus (VPL)		Ventral posteromedial nucleus (VPM)
Primary cortical target	Primary visual cortex	Primary auditory cortex	Primary somatosensory cortex		
Function	Visual perception	Auditory perception	Somatosensory perception from the body and face		

Trigeminal somatosensation and taste share the ventral posteromedial nucleus. Thalamic neurons then carry somatosensory information from all modalities and from both face and body to primary somatosensory cortex. Thus, the ventral posterior nuclei in the thalamus and the primary somatosensory cortex perform double duty, supporting more than one sensory pathway. The two thalamic nuclei serving somatosensation, the ventral posterolateral and posteromedial nuclei, are collectively termed the *ventrobasal complex*.

Damage to the ventrobasal complex or nearby posterior thalamic regions that interrupts the spinothalamic tract can cause a debilitating chronic pain condition called *central post-stroke pain*. This syndrome was previously known as *thalamic pain syndrome* or *Dejerine-Roussy disease* until it became clear that strokes outside of the thalamus could also produce a similar syndrome of central pain. Central post-stroke pain affects up to 10% of stroke victims and is associated with lesions to ascending pain pathways. Central post-stroke pain is a form of *neuropathic pain*, which means that no physical stimulus is present and responsible for the pain sensation (see more in Chapter 17). Instead, the pain results from errant signaling in the nervous system. Patients typically perceive a sensation of burning, searing pain in a contralateral distribution. Central post-stroke pain is typically treated with either tricyclic antidepressant or anticonvulsant drugs. These drugs are used at doses that would have little effect on depression or seizures and are thought to decrease pain by blocking burst firing in pain-signaling neurons. Narcotics are typically not used to treat central post-stroke pain because they are often ineffective.

Other sensory nuclei of the thalamus play similar roles to that of the ventral posterolateral nucleus. For example, damage to the lateral geniculate nucleus impairs contralateral visual perception, rendering the visual world contralateral to the lesion, termed the *contralateral visual hemifield* (see more later in this chapter), invisible to either eye. However, as described in Chapter 6, unilateral damage to the medial geniculate nucleus does not impact hearing.

SENSORY THALAMUS IS NOT JUST A RELAY STATION

Sensory thalamus is insinuated between the lowest and highest levels of central sensory processing. As a rule, sensory information reaches from the periphery to the cortex in a stereotyped manner:

> stimulus → primary sensory neuron → ≥1 secondary
> sensory neurons → thalamus → primary sensory cortex

For vision, the basic pathway is:

> light → retinal photoreceptor → → retinal ganglion
> cell → *lateral geniculate nucleus* → primary visual cortex

Despite there being two tracts carrying somatosensory input from the body, somatosensory pathways have a similar organization:

> touch, vibration, proprioception → primary somatosensory afferent → dorsal column nucleus → *ventral posterolateral nucleus* → primary somatosensory cortex
>
> pain and temperature → primary somatosensory afferent → spinal dorsal horn → → *ventral posterolateral nucleus* → primary somatosensory cortex

One way to view the synapse in thalamus is that it provides a "boost" or a "leg-up," a burst of metabolic and nutritive support for the long journey from here to there. Yet we know that many axons, including dorsal column axons and spinothalamic tract axons, can stretch a meter or more in some individuals. Therefore, it is unlikely that sensory pathways synapse in the thalamus because cortex is too far away for a direct, single axon projection. Rather, as this line of reasoning suggests, the thalamus serves as far more than a relay station. To appreciate the true contributions of the thalamus, consider vision. The input from retinal ganglion cells to lateral geniculate neurons comprises well under 5% of the entire input to these thalamic cells. Similarly, ventrobasal complex neurons receive only a small proportion of their input from the medial lemniscus or spinothalamic tract (Fig. 7-8).

Thalamic neurons that project to the cortex are called *thalamocortical projection cells*. As described earlier, only a minority of the synapses on thalamocortical projection cells arise from lemniscal pathways, which are those, such as the medial lemniscus, that carry sensory input. Instead, most synaptic input to thalamocortical projection cells in thalamic sensory nuclei arises from one of three sources:

- *Thalamic neurons*: Local neurons in the same thalamic nucleus as well as neurons in the surrounding *thalamic reticular nucleus* are sources of inhibitory input. Such inhibitory input can sharpen the distinction between stimulated areas and areas not stimulated, enhancing "edge" detection.

- *Brainstem nuclei*: Neurons in select brainstem nuclei release neuromodulators, such as *serotonin* and *norepinephrine*, which modulate the sensitivity of thalamic neurons to sensory inputs. The

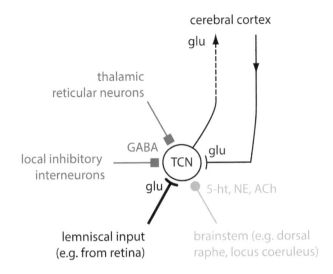

cerebral cortex

glu

thalamic
reticular neurons

GABA

local inhibitory
interneurons

TCN   glu

glu

glu   5-ht, NE, ACh

lemniscal input
(e.g. from retina)

brainstem (e.g. dorsal
raphe, locus coeruleus)

Figure 7-8 Thalamocortical projection neurons receive an enormous number of inputs, only a minority of which arises from lemniscal pathways. Thus, in terms of *number of synapses*, nonlemniscal inputs to thalamocortical projection neurons dominate over lemniscal inputs. Nonlemniscal inputs arise from a variety of brainstem nuclei, cortex, the thalamic reticular nucleus, and from local inhibitory interneurons. The corticothalamic input to thalamocortical projection neurons arises primarily from the same part of cortex to which the thalamic neurons project. Lemniscal inputs and feedback from cortex to thalamocortical projection neurons use the excitatory neurotransmitter glutamate (*black*). Inputs from local interneurons and the thalamic reticular nucleus utilize the inhibitory neurotransmitter γ-aminobutyric acid (*GABA*) (*red*). Because both local interneurons and thalamic reticular neurons receive excitatory inputs from lemniscal inputs and/or thalamocortical projection neurons, the GABAergic inputs onto thalamocortical projection neurons from these cells provide *inhibitory feedback*. Inputs from the brainstem arise from neurons in nuclei including the dorsal raphe and locus coeruleus, which use a monoamine neurotransmitter. Inputs from brainstem therefore release a variety of neurotransmitters (*blue*) including serotonin (*5-ht*), norepinephrine (*NE*), and acetylcholine (*ACh*). Although inputs from nonlemniscal sources dominate, lemniscal inputs onto thalamocortical neurons carry far more weight than do nonlemniscal inputs. As a consequence, the discharge of thalamocortical neurons most closely resembles firing in lemniscal pathways.

neuromodulatory substances released at any one moment depend on behavioral state. In this way, different complements of modulatory substances are released during wakefulness, non–rapid eye movement (REM) sleep, REM sleep, vigilance, and so on.

- *Cerebral cortex*: Cortical regions that receive thalamocortical input send corticothalamic projections back to thalamus. For example, primary visual cortex projects to the lateral geniculate nucleus. Such projections allow cortex to influence perceptions at an early point in sensory pathways.

Even though secondary sensory neurons provide only a small proportion of the input to sensory thalamic nuclei, this input has a stronger and more reliable influence than

the effect of any single synapse from the brainstem or cortex. To paraphrase George Orwell, some synapses "are more equal than others." Nonetheless, the picture that emerges is that *sensory input arising from the world is one component but certainly not the sum total of information that thalamus passes on to the cortex*. The large number of inputs to sensory thalamic neurons from areas of the brain other than pathways bringing in sensory input from the periphery reflects the fact that we *interpret* rather than faithfully record the sensory world (see Chapter 14).

SENSORY THALAMUS SERVES AS INTERPRETER, GATE-KEEPER, AND SPOTLIGHT OPERATOR

The requisite synapse in the thalamus allows sensory input to be translated into a message that is interpretable by the cortex. The thalamus can close the gate on sensory information, as occurs during sleep. The thalamus also plays a key role in setting attention to particular parts or features of the sensory world and to allowing expectation to either anticipate or color the perception of sensory events.

Key to the thalamus's role in interpreting and modulating sensory input to the cortex is a particular physiological characteristic of thalamocortical projection cells. Thalamocortical neurons are often termed "relay cells," but this is a misnomer. In fact, thalamocortical projection cells operate in one of two modes, only one of which is relay-like in nature:

- In *relay mode*, thalamic neurons faithfully pass on the message that they receive from secondary sensory neurons (Fig. 7-9A). The sequence of action potentials sent by the thalamic neuron matches nearly exactly the sequence of action potentials received by the thalamic neuron in a one-to-one fashion.

- In *burst mode*, thalamic neurons fire a batch of action potentials upon receipt of an action potential (Fig. 7-9B). By transforming one action potential into many action potentials, a thalamic neuron in burst mode can serve to "awaken" the cortex or to increase attention to a particular stimulus feature.

Thalamocortical projection cells operate in either relay or burst mode depending on inputs from brainstem nuclei that release neuromodulators (Fig. 7-8). The neuromodulators released within thalamus vary across behavioral states such as wake and sleep. Consequently, thalamic firing differs across behavioral states.

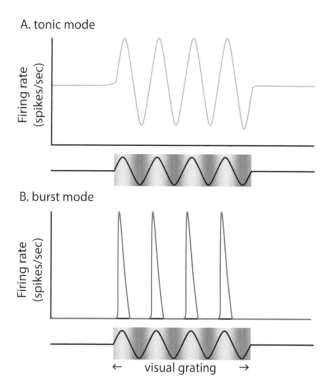

A. tonic mode

Firing rate (spikes/sec)

B. burst mode

Firing rate (spikes/sec)

← visual grating →

Figure 7-9 Thalamocortical projection neurons have two different modes of firing. In response to a sinusoidal grating of stripes (visual grating), lateral geniculate neurons respond differently when in tonic mode (A) or in burst mode (B). When in the tonic mode of firing, thalamic neurons faithfully represent the input that they receive. In contrast, when in burst mode, thalamocortical projection neurons burst in response to each stimulus cycle. In the absence of stimulation (flat lines on either side of the visual grating), neurons in tonic mode fire at a relatively steady rate of discharge whereas neurons in burst mode are hyperpolarized and do not fire. Modified from Sherman SM. Tonic and burst firing: dual modes of thalamocortical relay. *Trends Neurosci* 24:122–126, 2001, with permission of the publisher, Elsevier.

As an example of how the thalamus functions, consider the consequences of a tap on the shoulder during wake or sleep. During wakefulness, a tap will activate primary afferents that will ascend through the lemniscal pathway to eventually synapse in the ventral posterolateral nucleus of the thalamus. During wakefulness, neurons in the ventral posterolateral nucleus are in tonic mode (Fig. 7-9A). Therefore, virtually the same message that thalamic neurons receive from the dorsal column nucleus is sent to the somatosensory cortex. The result of this entire pathway is a faithful representation of the incident tap. Now, consider that the same tap occurs during non-REM sleep rather than during wakefulness. The tap still travels the same pathway to reach thalamus. However, during sleep, thalamic neurons are bathed in a complement of neuromodulators that puts them into burst mode (Fig. 7-9B). A light tap may elicit *no response at all* in a ventral posterolateral thalamic neuron. However, a stronger tap may elicit a burst of activity in thalamocortical projection neurons. When it does, the result is strong activation of the somatosensory cortex producing a perception *more notable for startle*

than for any of the sensory characteristics of the tap—location, duration, intensity. Thus, the sensory features of a stimulus are poorly represented in both thalamus and cortex when thalamic neurons are in burst mode. On the other hand, activation of thalamic neurons in burst mode increases detection of sensory stimuli and may radically shift the behavioral state toward greater arousal and vigilance.

It is interesting to note how that tap on the shoulder is processed during REM sleep. During REM sleep, the thalamus is bathed in a neuromodulator "soup" that resembles that during wakefulness, and, consequently, thalamic cells tend to be in relay mode. Thus, when the phone rings while a person is in REM sleep, information about the phone ringing reaches the cerebral cortex. However, during REM sleep, a state of *atonia*, a kind of reversible paralysis, precludes muscle contraction. Therefore, the person in REM sleep is very unlikely to pick up and answer a phone. Instead, that person may incorporate the ringing into a dream. By similar mechanisms, many of us incorporate actual events, such as a car alarm or a barking dog, into our dreams.

THE CEREBRAL CORTEX USES INPUT FROM THALAMUS TO MAP THE OUTSIDE WORLD

Thalamocortical projection neurons contact cortical neurons that are clustered together so that cortical neurons in *columns* stretching from the pia to the white matter share functional properties. Neurons in neighboring parts of thalamus project to neighboring parts of cortex. For example, somatosensory stimulation of adjacent parts of the cutaneous surface—the skin—excites neurons in adjacent parts of thalamus and, in turn, in adjacent bits of cortex. In this way, the external world is *mapped* within thalamus and then onto sensory regions of cortex. In the case of somatosensation, the topographic representation of the body across cortical columns is an example of *somatotopy*. In the case of vision, the systematic mapping of the visual field across primary visual cortex is termed *retinotopy*. Since maps in the visual field and in the retina are simply inverses of each other, the map present in the visual cortex is as representative of *visual field* topography as it is of *retinal* topography.

In sensory systems, some parts of the sensory world are more important than others and thus are represented by larger areas of neural tissue. For example, representation of the central 5 degrees of the visual field occupies more than half of primary visual cortex, whereas the peripheral 70 degrees on either side is represented in the remainder of the primary visual cortex. Similarly, in the somatosensory system, neurons receiving input regarding the fingertips and lips occupy far more territory than neurons that respond to stimulation anywhere on the trunk (Fig. 7-10). Clearly, the trunk contains far more surface area than do the fingertips, but, more importantly, it is far less sensitive to somatosensory stimulation than are the fingertips.

The somatosensory cortex maps tactile sensitivity rather than surface area. The common measure of tactile sensitivity is two-point discrimination. You can easily measure two-point discrimination with a consenting adult. First, ask your partner to look away. Then take two pencils or two stir sticks or two pointed objects of any type and place either one or both on the skin of your willing partner. Ask if your partner perceives one or two points. Stimulating two points in regions of low tactile sensitivity, for example the trunk, is typically perceived as only one point of contact. To detect that two separate points have been contacted, the two points have to be very far apart. In contrast, two points placed on regions of high tactile sensitivity, regions such as the lips or fingertips, are rarely interpreted as one point.

A similarly skewed representation of the periphery occurs in primary motor cortex, where the map of the body is termed a *homunculus*. Far more cortex is involved in controlling muscles capable of fine movements than in controlling muscles that are only capable of poorly controlled, ballistic movements. The brain overrepresents muscles of the hand, lips, and tongue, which produce the most articulated movements, and under-represents muscles of the trunk, arms, and legs, which produce far grosser movements. Similar but not identical topographic exaggerations mark somatosensory and motor cortices so that the sensory and motor homunculi are similar but different.

The overrepresentation of some information and under-representation of other information reflects the *interpretative nature of brain function*. As introduced in Chapter 1, the brain does not faithfully and objectively record the external world as does a camera, a tape recorder, or a gas chromatograph. Nor does the brain give equal weight to all outputs as does a wind-up toy. Instead, the brain infers what the outside world means for the brain's owner, ignoring inconsequential stimuli and accentuating salient features of the world. Then, the brain initiates the output reactions it deems most pressing in light of its interpretation of the most salient inputs.

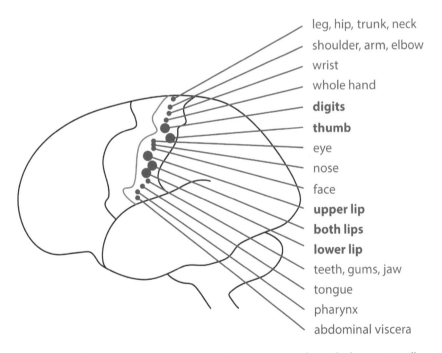

leg, hip, trunk, neck
shoulder, arm, elbow
wrist
whole hand
digits
thumb
eye
nose
face
upper lip
both lips
lower lip
teeth, gums, jaw
tongue
pharynx
abdominal viscera

Figure 7-10 The somatotopy in the portion of primary somatosensory cortex that is present on the cerebral convexity is illustrated. Starting from the saddle region and progressing rostrally, body parts are represented by neurons in progressively more lateral regions of cortex. Areas innervated by cranial nerves, such as the face, oral cavity, upper airway, and viscera, are represented most laterally with the top of the face represented most medially and the jaw and upper airway most laterally. Cortical maps are fractionated with jumps or discontinuities between regions of the body represented by neighboring cortical areas. Furthermore, maps contain multiple representations of some body parts. For example, the lips are represented individually, together, and as part of the face. The greatest neural territory of somatosensory cortex is devoted to regions with the highest tactile sensitivity. Therefore, small regions of the body, such as the lips and digits, are represented by large regions of cortex, whereas large body parts, such as the trunk, are represented by far smaller areas of cortex. Not shown are the representations of the genitalia, toes, and feet, all present on the medial surface of the hemisphere.

Neighboring cortical neurons receive and process information from thalamus in groups. Collections of cells that preferentially communicate with each other in patterned ways form functional circuits. The consequence of cortical circuits is cognition: perceptions, thoughts, emotions, and the initiation of actions. Because the cerebral cortex contributes to each component of cognition, one can view cognition as the total output of the cerebral cortex. Different regions of the brain give rise to different components of cognition. For example, activity in a particular circuit in somatosensory cortex may result in the perception of touch, whereas activity in motor cortex may result in an action and so on.

Cortical circuits show similar activity patterns "spontaneously" and in response to thalamic input. This is a remarkable finding because it means that circuits are primed to certain activity patterns, perhaps triggered by previous experiences, and that those patterns occur either in response to thalamic input or spontaneously without an obvious precipitating event. Taking this idea one step further, we conclude that *the perceptions, thoughts, emotions, or actions consequent to cortical circuit activity can occur with or without a precipitating stimulus.*

The existence of spontaneous firing patterns that resemble ones elicited by stimuli provides a framework by which to understand how dreams and hallucinations can be difficult to distinguish from reality. Consider a pattern of activity in a cortical circuit that results in the perception of your mother's face. If that pattern of activity occurs spontaneously in your brain, then you will perceive your mom's face even if she is nowhere near you. In this way, spontaneously occurring cortical circuit activity may produce *hallucinations.* Even in the absence of a frank hallucination, preset patterns of cortical activity may transform an actual input into an expected input. When you arrive at your job, you readily perceive a coworker's face, even if most of her face is hidden from you or is covered up by winter gear. However, if you see that same face outside of the *context* of your work, you have difficulty identifying the face. We can speculate that expectation is reflected in the spontaneous activity present in a cortical circuit. Although that activity may not be sufficient to elicit a hallucinatory perception, it may mean that less stimulus-driven activity is needed to reach the threshold for perception. Using this framework, we can imagine that, when at work, activity due to expectation and activity due to the actual stimulus summate to produce perception. However, in the absence of expectation, activity due to the stimulus alone, activity driven solely by thalamic input, is insufficient to trigger a perception. Just as expectation influences perception, it may also influence thoughts, actions, and emotions.

Recall from earlier that the cerebral cortex projects back to the part of thalamus from which it also receives input (Fig. 7-8). Through these corticothalamic projections, the output of cortical circuits reaches thalamus. In this way, information about expectation, attention, and the like can influence thalamic processing of secondary sensory input. *Thalamocortical firing, which is changed by cortical input, reaches cortex and is indistinguishable from thalamocortical firing that was not changed by cortical input*: both "feel" like the real deal, a true representation of the outside world. Such a scenario lends neural credibility to the idea of "seeing what you want to see." Imbuing perception with expectation is just one of many potential—and as of yet largely unexplored—ways in which cortical circuits may influence thalamic processing.

By now, you understand that specific thalamic nuclei translate sensory information into a form that is comprehensible

Table 7-2 **THE CONNECTIONS AND FUNCTIONS OF THREE THALAMIC NUCLEI THAT PROCESS INFORMATION RELATED TO MOTOR, LIMBIC, AND EXECUTIVE FUNCTION ARE LISTED**

THALAMIC NUCLEUS	CORTICAL AREA TARGETED BY THALAMIC NUCLEUS	INPUT TO THALAMIC NUCLEUS	FUNCTION
Anterior nucleus	Cingulate gyrus	Mammillary bodies, hippocampus	Learning and memory
Ventral anterior and ventral lateral nuclei	Primary motor cortex and prefrontal motor areas	Cerebellum and basal ganglia	Motor function and planning
Mediodorsal nucleus	Prefrontal cortex	Prefrontal cortex, cingulate gyrus	Executive function and emotion

by the cerebral cortex. Moreover, the cortex "talks back" to thalamus.

In addition to the thalamocortical circuits involved in perception listed in Table 7-1, the ventral anterior and ventral lateral nuclei translate motor information into a form used by motor areas of cortex (see Table 7-2). The ventral anterior and ventral lateral nuclei receive modulatory information related to movement, largely from the basal ganglia and the cerebellum, and send it on to motor areas of cortex. The anterior nucleus of the thalamus receives input from the hippocampus and mammillary bodies related to learning and memory and projects to cingulate cortex, part of the limbic system. The mediodorsal nucleus receives input from the cingulate gyrus and prefrontal cortex and projects back to the prefrontal cortex to support executive function. Although serving cognitive functions other than sensory perception, the way that these thalamic nuclei operate is thought to be analogous to the way that the sensory thalamic nuclei work.

In sum, thalamus appears to contribute a *method of processing* to the circuits that it participates in. It is as though the brain designed a clever computer chip, capable of transforming information in some particular way. The brain then uses this same chip to transform data of all types and from multiple sources for use by the cerebral cortex.

THE AMYGDALA IS CRITICAL TO EXPRESSING AND INTERPRETING FEAR AND FOR REMEMBERING EMOTIONAL EVENTS

The amygdala is a subcortical structure located just deep to the cerebral cortex at the anterior pole of the medial temporal lobe (Fig. 7-3C). Our initial understanding of amygdala function stems from lesion studies on macaque monkeys that suggested that the amygdala mediates most emotional reactions and that, in its absence, hypersexuality, hyperorality, and a release of social inhibition become evident (Box 7-1).

Recent experiments in animals, as well as the study of human patients who have bilateral damage to the amygdala (see Box 7-2, Fig. 7-11), have led to a modern, more nuanced, and still evolving view that the amygdala serves or contributes to several functions:

- Social distance from others both during normal conditions and in reaction to threats

Box 7-1 **BILATERAL TEMPORAL LOBECTOMIES**

In the late 1930s, Heinrich Klüver and Paul Bucy studied the effects of bilateral temporal lobectomies in monkeys. Lesioned monkeys consistently showed:

- *Social disinhibition*: Monkeys showed little fear and approached other monkeys readily.

- *Psychic blindness* and *hyperorality*: Monkeys handled all objects, including objects such as snakes that normally elicit an innate fear reaction, without any signs of fear. In fact, monkeys put every object into their mouths, a consistent behavior that was interpreted as evidence that the monkeys could not recognize objects using vision. We now think that the psychic blindness noted by Klüver and Bucy was in fact *visual agnosia* or the inability to recognize and interpret visual inputs, a deficit that resulted from a lesion of visual pathways within the temporal lobe.

- *Hypersexuality*: Monkeys showed greatly increased sexual interest in each other and in their own genitalia.

The Klüver-Bucy syndrome, comprising this set of symptoms, has profoundly influenced our thinking about temporal lobe function generally and amygdala function more specifically. Klüver and Bucy lesioned areas of the medial temporal lobe beyond the amygdala, but the symptoms that they observed were initially ascribed to impairment of the amygdala alone. This history played a large part in the still dominant notion that the amygdala is critical to expression of fear reactions and social inhibition.

More recently, selective and bilateral lesions of the amygdala in monkeys confirm a role for the amygdala in exhibiting and recognizing fear in social circumstances. Monkeys with amygdala lesions are hypersexual and friendlier with other monkeys, approaching the other monkeys and failing to respond to other monkeys' aggression. More remarkably, lesioned monkeys are viewed as *more approachable* by normal monkeys, evidence that the amygdala plays a role in both the expression and interpretation of social threat between individuals. In sum, Klüver and Bucy's experiments have greatly colored the modern view of the amygdala, supporting a strong emphasis on fear and other negative emotions reflective of threat or danger.

- Viewing, processing, and understanding the emotions in facial expressions, particularly fear

- Making emotional memories

- Evaluating the emotional valence of conditions or stimuli

Strokes cause bilateral damage to a single structure in the brain about as often lightning hits the same spot twice, which is to say, very rarely. For this reason, patients with bilateral damage to the amygdala are rare. Yet, there are two conditions that produce such damage with some frequency:

- *Limbic encephalitis* is a disease of varied etiology but usually involves a paraneoplastic (see Chapter 2) autoimmune attack on the medial temporal lobe bilaterally.

- *Urbach-Wiethe disease* is caused by a mutation in the gene for an extracellular matrix protein. Individuals with this inherited autosomal recessive disease have thickened tissues, most notably the skin and the larynx, resulting in numerous dermatological abnormalities, such as papules on the eyelids, and in hoarseness, respectively. Urbach-Wiethe disease is heterogeneous, arising from more than 40 different mutations. In roughly half of the patients, there is bilateral calcification of the blood vessels supplying the amygdala, and, as a result, the amygdala is effectively lesioned (Fig. 7-11).

Studies of patients with bilateral damage to the amygdala caused by either encephalitis or Urbach-Wiethe disease have reported several deficits. These patients appear behaviorally disinhibited. They make inappropriately sexual innuendoes to medical personnel. When looking at a person's face, they focus on the mouth instead of the eyes and, as a consequence, cannot recognize fearful expressions. Finally, these patients have poor memory for episodes from their own life. Since the patients have normal memory for autobiographical facts, the poor episodic memory has been interpreted as a deficit in emotional memory formation.

The amygdala's role in assessing the fear of a situation may not be entirely one of evaluation but may also involve how information is collected. When a patient with bilateral amygdala damage was asked to determine the emotion of a facial expression, she looked at the mouth rather than the eyes and consequently failed to detect a fearful expression (Fig. 7-12). When directly instructed to look at the eyes, the patient could correctly identify a fearful facial expression. It is interesting that the patient did not remember to look at people's eyes for long after the immediate instruction to do so and shortly lapsed back into looking only at people's mouths. This finding suggests that the amygdala may play a role in

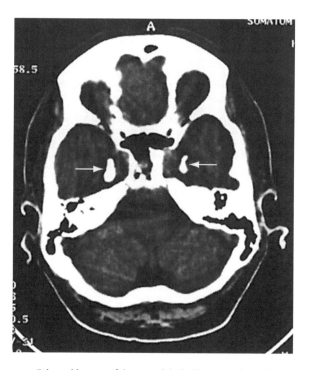

Figure 7-11 Bilateral lesions of the amygdala (*yellow arrows*) can be seen in this computed tomography (CT) scan of a patient with Urbach-Wiethe disease.   Modified from Siebert M, Markowitsch HJ, Bartel P. Amygdala, affect and cognition: evidence from 10 patients with Urbach-Wiethe disease. Brain 126(12): 2627–2637, 2003, with permission of the publisher, Oxford University Press.

emotional reinforcement of action patterns such as the eye movements used to scan a face. By changing gaze patterns, the visual data collected and used to evaluate emotion are also changed.

We make emotionally laden memories far more readily than emotionally flat ones. We remember the song playing on the radio when we had an accident but not the song that played during a routine commute. Thus, the assignment of an emotional value to a situation greatly facilitates memory formation. The amygdala is critical to forming emotional memories, subconscious memories of emotions associated with stimuli. Indeed, the amygdala has been implicated in the hypervigilance and easily triggered emotional memories associated with *post-traumatic stress disorder* (see Box 7-3).

One possible synthesis of the varied roles of the amygdala would hold that the amygdala is critical to evaluating the salience and threat level, or lack thereof, of objects and conditions, functioning as something akin to the body's own Department of Homeland Security. Just as Homeland Security constantly monitors data and updates the nation's threat level, the amygdala is likely to be important in updating the evaluation of objects and situations as they and the accompanying circumstances continually evolve.

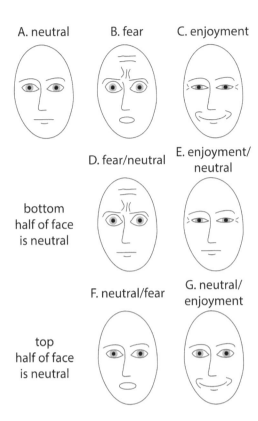

A. neutral   B. fear   C. enjoyment

D. fear/neutral   E. enjoyment/neutral

bottom half of face is neutral

F. neutral/fear   G. neutral/enjoyment

top half of face is neutral

Figure 7-12 Different parts of the face are key to the communication of different emotions. A fearful facial expression (B) depends primarily on features in the upper half of the face, whereas a smile of enjoyment (C) depends largely on the position of the mouth. When the upper half of a fearful expression and the lower half of a neutral face (A) are combined (D), the expression conveys fear. However, when the lower half of a fearful expression is combined with an upper face that is neutral (F), the expression does not convey fear. The converse is true for a smile of enjoyment. Combining the lower half of an expression of enjoyment with an upper face that is neutral (G) shows happy more than does the reverse (E).

THE BASAL GANGLIA IS BIASED TOWARD SUPPRESSING MOVEMENT

The basal ganglia are critical to choosing which actions, perceptions, thoughts, and emotions will occur at any one moment (see much more in Chapter 25). At rest, the basal ganglia continually inhibit target structures and thereby act like a big wet blanket, suppressing all movement. When the output from the basal ganglia pauses, action—or perception or thought or emotion—is released from the blanket inhibition exerted by the basal ganglia and the action, perception, thought, or emotion occurs.

Using just a basic understanding of basal ganglia function, we can understand the fundamental framework used to categorize basal ganglia movement disorders into hyperkinetic and hypokinetic types. As introduced earlier, the basal ganglia actively inhibit movements under resting conditions. Then, when the drive to take an action reaches

Unfortunately, many of us experience trauma, whether at the hands of other humans or through natural disasters. Of those who suffer through traumatic experiences, particularly military combat, rape, and disasters such as hurricanes or the 9/11 attacks on New York City, a minority develop a persistent anxiety disorder called *post-traumatic stress disorder* (PTSD). Post-traumatic stress disorder, colloquially referred to as *shell shock* in cases related to combat trauma, is marked by spontaneous or triggered flashbacks to the traumatic event, a flattening of affect, elevated vigilance, and a lowered startle threshold.

PTSD resembles an extreme version of fear conditioning in which a stimulus that does not carry an affective meaning, the *conditioned stimulus*, triggers a fear reaction, the *unconditioned response*, after being paired with a negative stimulus or event, the *unconditioned stimulus*. Furthermore, whereas normally repetition of the conditioned stimulus without a subsequent unconditioned stimulus extinguishes fear conditioning, the unconditioned responses of individuals with PTSD appear impervious to extinction. To concretize this analogy, consider a soldier quietly reading in a tent. All of a sudden, the light in the tent goes out and, moments later, shrapnel rips through the tent, resulting in the death of several comrades and the soldier's own severe injury. We can view the light going out as the conditioned stimulus and the shrapnel as the unconditioned stimulus. The pain and suffering of the soldier is the unconditioned response. For the individual who develops PTSD, the conditioning does not extinguish. Any version of the conditioned stimulus, even the nonthreatening occurrence of a light bulb burning out, triggers the unconditioned response. Such triggering continues to occur when the soldier returns home from the war zone. Many believe that fear conditioning without extinction serves as a good analogy for PTSD, although all would acknowledge that PTSD also involves additional more complex processes.

The amygdala may be critical to the development of PTSD. Attention was focused on the amygdala early, given the evidence that this structure is critical to fear conditioning, to the formation of emotional memories, and to the experience and expression of fear. The amygdala is not thought to work alone in establishing PTSD. The similarities between fear conditioning and PTSD point us in the direction of prefrontal cortex as a source of extinction. An inhibitory signal from medial prefrontal cortex to amygdala is thought to be necessary for the extinction of fear conditioning. This suggests that prefrontal cortex may fail to inhibit the amygdala and thus fail to extinguish fear and panic in PTSD patients.

It remains unclear why some individuals develop PTSD and others do not. If identification of the individuals most vulnerable to developing PTSD were possible, early and effective interventions may be able to prevent this potentially debilitating condition.

sufficient urgency, the basal ganglia release that action from inhibition. Although simplistic, this basic framework allows us to understand the clinical classification of basal ganglia–mediated movement disorders:

- *Hypokinetic disorders* result in a poverty of movement.
- *Hyperkinetic disorders* involve an excess of movements.

Hypokinetic disorders occur when the default output from the basal ganglia continues and does not shut off and therefore does not allow movements to occur. The archetypical hypokinetic disorder is Parkinson's disease, in which patients fail to initiate movements (*akinesia*) or move very slowly (*bradykinesia*).

Because hypokinetic disorders result from too much basal ganglia output, you should not be surprised that hyperkinetic disorders result from too little basal ganglia output. *Hemiballismus, Huntington's chorea,* and *dystonia* are hyperkinetic disorders that differ in pathophysiology and in the speed of the excess movements. In hemiballismus, ballistic flailing movements occur, whereas choreiform disorders like Huntington's chorea involve slower jerks and dance-like movements. Dystonia is a hyperkinetic disorder of posture in which patients adopt a fixed or slowly twisting position of their body, arm, head, or other body part.

THERE IS MORE INPUT TO THAN OUTPUT FROM THE BASAL GANGLIA

Strictly speaking, the term *basal ganglia* refers to the gray matter that arises from the medial and lateral ganglionic eminences (see Chapter 3). Yet, in modern parlance, we use the term to refer to a group of nuclei linked by conceptual function rather than developmental origin or anatomical location. The common usage of the term basal ganglia refers to the following seven structures (Fig. 7-13):

- Caudate
- Putamen
- External globus pallidus
- Internal globus pallidus
- Substantia nigra pars reticulata
- Subthalamic nucleus
- Substantia nigra pars compacta

Recall that the basal ganglia are key to choosing which action should occur at any one moment in time. Information about far more candidate actions, perceptions, thoughts, or emotions enter the basal ganglia than can occur at one time. The greater input to than output from the basal ganglia reflects a greater preponderance of anatomical projections into rather than out of the basal ganglia. In this regard, the basal ganglia resemble another region important in modifying cerebral cortical output—the cerebellum.

The caudate and putamen function together although they are anatomically distinct. *They are collectively termed the striatum and are the major input port for the basal ganglia.* These two structures arise together during development, before fibers that eventually become the internal capsule split them apart. At the rostral end of the striatum, the internal capsule is no longer present, and the putamen meets the front end, or head, of the caudate. The ventral portion of this rostral striatal tissue is the *nucleus accumbens*, an important area for signaling the rewarding aspects of stimuli and often included as part of the limbic system. Neurons throughout the striatum, including those in the accumbens, use *γ-aminobutyric acid* (*GABA*) as a neurotransmitter and are inhibitory.

Like the caudate and putamen, the internal globus pallidus and substantia nigra pars reticulata arise together before being divided by fibers, in this case by axons continuing on from the internal capsule into the cerebral peduncles (Fig. 7-13). Although there is no collective term for the internal globus pallidus and substantia nigra pars reticulata, these two areas are the two output nuclei of the basal ganglia. Targets of basal ganglia output include thalamus and brainstem regions such as the superior colliculus. The external globus pallidus contains GABAergic inhibitory interneurons, and the subthalamic nucleus contains excitatory interneurons. The role of these interneuronal populations will be explored in Chapter 25.

Dopaminergic, or dopamine-containing, cells populate the substantia nigra pars compacta and project to the striatum. The name of the substantia nigra arises from the Latin for "black substance." Indeed the *nigra*, as it is often called, is dark colored in unstained tissue due to large deposits of *neuromelanin* in the compacta cells that also contain the neurotransmitter dopamine (Fig. 7-13). The nigrostriatal pathway, formed by dopaminergic nigra cells that send their axons to the striatum, provides dopamine to the striatum. This pathway is absolutely critical to movement. In the same way that a motor cannot move without oil, we cannot move to pursue our goals without

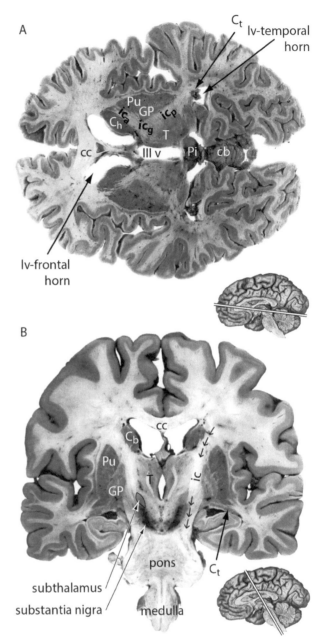

Figure 7-13 Sections in the horizontal (A) and coronal (B) planes illustrate the anatomy of the caudate, putamen, and pallidum. The caudate stretches the length of the lateral ventricle (*lv*) so that the head of the caudate (*C$_h$* in A) abuts the lateral ventricle in the frontal lobe, the body of the caudate (*C$_b$* in B) abuts the lateral ventricle in the parietal lobe, and the tail of the caudate (*C$_t$* in A and B) abuts the lateral ventricle in the temporal lobe. No other gray matter structure abuts the lateral ventricle: *the caudate is the only gray matter area next to the lateral ventricle*. Deep to the caudate, the internal capsule (*ic*) runs, carrying fibers from the cerebral cortex to targets in the thalamus, brainstem, and spinal cord along with fibers from thalamus to cortex. The three portions of the internal capsule—the anterior limb (*ic$_a$* in A), genu (*ic$_g$* in A), and posterior limb (*ic$_p$* in A)—can be seen in a horizontal section. *Genu* means "knee" in Latin. Corticospinal fibers travel in the posterior limb of the internal capsule, whereas corticobulbar fibers travel through the genu. Deep to the internal capsule sit the putamen (*Pu* in A and B) and the globus pallidus (*GP* in A and B). Together, the putamen and globus pallidus look like a lens and consequently are sometimes called the *lentiform nucleus*. The other components of the basal ganglia are the subthalamus, a lens-shaped nucleus, and the substantia nigra, both of which are visible in the section in B. Of note, in unstained sections of brain, neuromelanin contained in the neurons of substantia nigra pars compacta renders the nucleus black in appearance. For orientation, the pineal gland (*Pi*), cerebellum (*cb*), corpus callosum (*cc*), thalamus (*T*), pons, medulla, and ventricles (*lv, III v*) are labeled. Photomicrographs reprinted with permission from deArmond S et al., *Structure of the human brain: A photographic atlas.* New York: Oxford University Press, 1989.

striatal dopamine. Therefore, when dopaminergic nigra cells die, poverty of movement results, as exemplified by Parkinson's disease.

THE CEREBRAL CORTEX HOUSES NEURONS RESPONSIBLE FOR THE COMPLEXITY OF THE HUMAN MIND

Serving mundane and sublime functions alike, the cerebral cortex is flexible and variable enough to support the range of mammalian cognition. Due to our own human version of a cerebral cortex, we see colors, discuss what to have for dinner, make art, love passionately, aspire to explain the natural world, and build worldwide communication systems. In addition, our cerebral cortex supports a multitude of cognitive functions that we share with our mammalian relatives, functions as varied as recognizing our relatives, caring for offspring, finding palatable food, voiding only at appropriate times and places, and remembering the way home.

The function of different cortical areas follows *loosely* from the area's distances from primary sensory and motor cortices. In other words, cortical function across the vast cerebral mantle follows a logic that loosely connects to the functions and locations of primary cortical areas. An overview of cortical function from this perspective is explored next.

PRIMARY SENSORY CORTICES SUPPLY A FUNDAMENTAL PROCESSING STEP BUT NOT A COMPLETE COGNITIVE PERCEPT

Primary sensory cortices are necessary bottlenecks for sensory processing bound for perception. Visual information must pass through primary visual cortex, somatosensory information through primary somatosensory cortex, and so on in order for conscious perception to occur. Yet, on their own, primary sensory cortices do not support normal perception. Rather, they process the fundamental building blocks necessary for perception and pass this information on to other cortical areas. Furthermore, nonperceptual reactions, often termed *unconscious reactions*, to stimulation may occur through pathways that do not include primary sensory cortices.

The best example of the distinct pathways that support perception and nonperceptual reactions comes from a condition known as *blindsight*. People with blindsight may follow moving objects with their eyes but they do not consciously perceive any visual objects. Blindsight arises from a complete and bilateral lesion of primary visual cortex. This causes *cortical blindness*. In this condition, the retina and thalamus are fully operational, as is the superior colliculus. However, without the primary visual cortex as a gateway to higher visual processing cortical areas, no visual perception occurs. Thus, although primary sensory cortices are necessary for normal perception, they are not sufficient.

The rudimentary form of sensory processing in primary sensory cortices is well exemplified by the percepts that result from activity in the primary visual cortex arising during an epileptic seizure or a migraine aura. This activity is not a response to a stimulus but rather represents activity originating within, and restricted to, a local region. Therefore, the effects of seizure or aura-related activity tell us about the local information processing. Aberrant activity in the primary visual cortex makes people perceive flashing lights, rotating black-and-white patterns, or blind spots, termed *scotomas*. These percepts reflect the basic nature of sensory information in primary sensory areas.

Curiously, cortical blindness is often accompanied by *anosognosia* (i.e., a lack of awareness of the impairment). Patients with *Anton syndrome*, the term for cortical blindness with anosognosia, are blind. They do not blink in response to a threat, such as a rapidly approaching hand. Yet, they vehemently deny that they cannot see.

DIFFERENT VISUAL FIELD DEFICITS ARE ACCOMPANIED BY PREDICTABLE DEFICITS IN FOREBRAIN FUNCTIONS

We followed the three long pathways responsible for somatosensation and voluntary movement through the spinal cord and brainstem because knowledge of these pathways' anatomy allows us to deduce the location of most lesions located in the spinal cord or brainstem. Put another way, virtually all spinal and most brainstem lesions will cause a deficit in functions supported by at least one of the three long pathways introduced in Chapter 4. Upon reaching the forebrain, the diagnostic power of the three long pathways declines as all three pathways travel in the internal capsule and corona radiata to sensorimotor cortex. Since great swatches of the forebrain contain no part of the three long pathways, we need an alternate strategy to deduce the location of forebrain lesions. The most useful function to test in this regard is vision because the pathway from the retina to the primary visual cortex traverses regions of forebrain not visited by the three long pathways.

To understand the visual pathways, it is critical to first understand the concept of visual fields. Consider looking straight ahead. The point where you are looking is termed the *point of fixation*. This is the direction of your gaze. As you look straight ahead, the area to the right of your point of fixation is the right half of the visual field, and the area to the left of your point of fixation is the left half of your visual field (Fig. 7-14). Even if you turn your head to the right, the area to the left of your point of fixation remains your left visual hemifield, even if it is located on the right side of your body. In other words, the visual fields are named for their position *relative to your fixation point and not relative to your head or body*.

Each retina receives light from an entire monocular visual field, but each primary visual cortex receives input from only the contralateral hemifield, or half of a visual field. Therefore, information from each retinal nasal hemifield must cross to reach the visual cortex on the other side. The optic chiasm is where the crossing is made that provides contralateral, and only contralateral, visual field input to the cortex. Since the optic chiasm is interposed between the retina and the lateral geniculate nucleus, both visual cortex and thalamus process input from the contralateral hemifield exclusively. Remembering a minimal amount of information will allow us to logically deduce the basic visual pathway:

- Information from the ipsilateral hemifield (the nasal retina) crosses at the level of the optic chiasm to reach the contralateral lateral geniculate nucleus.

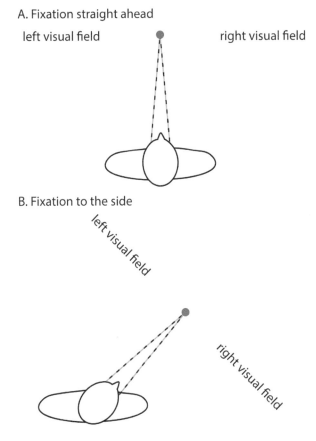

A. Fixation straight ahead

left visual field   right visual field

B. Fixation to the side

left visual field

right visual field

Figure 7-14 A: Everything to the right of the fixation point (*red dot*) is in the right visual field, and everything to the left is in the left visual field. The visual fields are always relative to the point of fixation rather than to the body axis. B: Thus, when a person fixates to the right, both the left and right visual fields are to the right of the body.

• Information from the contralateral hemifield (the temporal retina) bypasses the optic chiasm and heads directly for the lateral geniculate nucleus on the same side.

To understand the visual pathways, we consider the effect of lesions at every point in the path from the eye to the contralateral visual cortex, step by step (Fig. 7-15):

Lesions proximal to the chiasm (i.e., on the eye side of the optic chiasm) produce deficits restricted to input from the ipsilateral eye:

• *Retina*: Each retina sees light from both the ipsilateral and contralateral halves of the visual fields, with the nasal retina receiving ipsilateral and the temporal retina receiving contralateral visual field input. For example, the left eye's nasal retina receives input from the left, or ipsilateral, hemifield, and the left temporal retina receives input from the right, or contralateral, hemifield. Due to the chiasmal split of input from the two hemifields, the visual cortex will receive inputs from the ipsilateral temporal retina and the contralateral nasal retina.

• *Optic nerve*: The situation here is no different from that of the retina. Axons arising from the nasal retina carry input from the ipsilateral hemifield, and axons arising from temporal retina carry input from the contralateral hemifield. As above, optic nerve fibers from the nasal retina are ultimately destined for visual cortex on the opposite side, and optic nerve fibers from the temporal retina are destined for the ipsilateral visual cortex.

• *Optic chiasm*: The optic chiasm sits just over the pituitary, and damage to the chiasm most often results from a pituitary adenoma. Axons arising from each nasal retina cross in the optic chiasm and join the axons arising from the contralateral temporal retina to form the optic tract.

Lesions that are retrochiasmal (i.e., behind or caudal to the optic chiasm) produce homonymous, or corresponding, deficits restricted to the contralateral hemifield:

• *Optic tract*: The optic tract starts at the chiasm and ends at the lateral geniculate nucleus. En route from the chiasm to the lateral geniculate, the optic tract skirts around the cerebral peduncles, which, as you recall, carry the corticospinal and corticobulbar tracts. This means that lesions that disrupt the optic tract—resulting in a contralateral hemianopia—may also produce a contralateral motor deficit. Since the optic tract is past the crossing provided by the optic chiasm, all of its axons, whether originating from the ipsilateral or contralateral eye, carry input related to the contralateral hemifield.

• *Lateral geniculate nucleus*: The situation here is no different from that of the optic tract. Neurons in the lateral geniculate only respond to stimulation of the contralateral hemifield.

• *Optic radiation*: The optic radiation carries the axons of lateral geniculate neurons, which project to the primary visual cortex. As with the optic tract and lateral geniculate, the optic radiation carries inputs arising from both eyes that carry information about the contralateral hemifield exclusively. There is one additional wrinkle in the optic radiation's pathway:
  ◦ The optic radiation splits, so that the lower part of the visual field is represented by fibers that travel along a fairly straight path from the lateral geniculate nucleus to the primary visual cortex.
  ◦ Fibers carrying input from the upper part of the visual field make a fairly large detour, passing anterior to the temporal

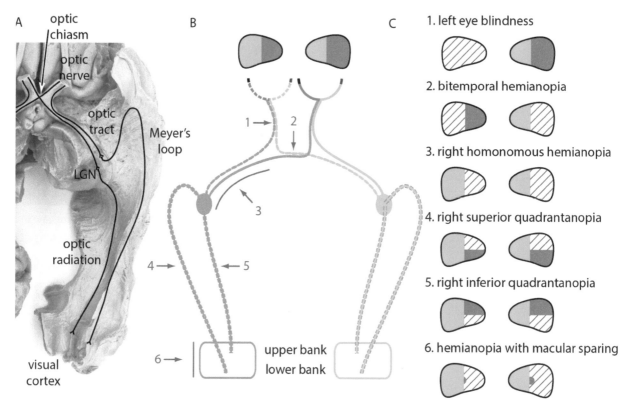

Figure 7-15 A: Visual pathways traverse the length of the telencephalon. Retinal ganglion cells carry preliminarily processed visual information from the retina to the lateral geniculate nucleus. The axons of retinal ganglion cells travel through three structures en route to the lateral geniculate: the optic nerve, optic chiasm, and optic tract. Only axons from the nasal retina cross in the optic chiasm with temporal fibers passing directly into the optic tract. Caudal to the chiasm, visual pathways carry *homonymous* visual field information. The optic tract travels laterally, past the cerebral peduncles, and ends in the lateral geniculate nucleus. After a synapse in the lateral geniculate nucleus, geniculate neurons project to primary visual cortex via the optic radiation. Axons carrying visual input from the contralateral upper quadrant of the visual field detour in front of the temporal horn of the lateral ventricle, a path known as Meyer's loop, before ending on the ventral bank of the calcarine fissure. B: A schematic of the visual pathways shows the left visual field in blue and the right visual field in gray. Anterior to the chiasm, in the retina and the optic nerve, both visual hemifields are represented. Caudal to the optic chiasm, all structures carry input exclusively from the contralateral visual field. C: The effects of the most common visual pathway lesions are shown. Damage to the retina or optic nerve (*1* in B) causes ipsilateral blindness. Damage to the optic chiasm (*2* in B), as occurs with a large pituitary adenoma, causes a bitemporal hemianopia. Lesions anywhere along the optic tract or in the lateral geniculate nucleus (*3* in B) cause a contralateral homonymous hemianopia. Damage to Meyer's loop (*4* in B) causes a contralateral superior quadrantanopia, whereas damage to the optic radiation within the parietal lobe (*5* in B) causes a contralateral inferior quadrantanopia. Damage to the occipital pole typically causes contralateral hemianopia with the central 5 degrees of the visual field spared (*macular sparing*).   Photograph in A reprinted with permission from Bruni JE, Montemurro D. *Human neuroanatomy: A text, brain atlas, and laboratory dissection guide*. New York: Oxford University Press, 2009.

horn of the lateral ventricle before traveling caudally to the occipital cortex, along a path known as *Meyer's loop*. Because of the split between fibers carrying inputs from the upper and lower portions of the contralateral hemifield, lesions in the optic radiation produce homonymous contralateral quadrantanopias (i.e., loss of a quarter of the entire visual field) rather than hemianopias.

- *Primary visual cortex*: Primary visual cortex is located along the calcarine fissure, a deep sulcus on the medial wall of the occipital lobe (Fig. 7-16). The gyrus dorsal to the fissure represents the lower visual field, and the gyrus ventral to the fissure represents the upper visual field. Along the caudal to rostral axis of the calcarine fissure, the visual field is represented retinotopically from the

center of the visual field, caudally, to the periphery of the visual field rostrally. As noted earlier, cortical retinotopy is marked by the disproportionate representation of the central visual field. In fact, the region representing central vision occupies more territory than is occupied by representations of all the rest of the visual field.

The visual pathways are logical. The cortex represents the contralateral visual hemifield, whereas each eye receives input from the entire binocular portion of the visual field. The necessary crossing of information from the nasal retina, receiving input from the ipsilateral visual field, occurs at the optic chiasm. The only other critical piece of information to memorize is that Meyer's loop contains fibers from the upper half of the contralateral hemifield.

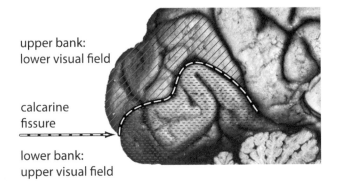

upper bank:
lower visual field

calcarine
fissure

lower bank:
upper visual field

Figure 7-16 The medial surface of the occipital lobe. Most of primary visual cortex is located along the *banks* of the calcarine fissure on the medial wall of the occipital lobe. The upper bank represents the lower visual field, whereas the upper visual field is mapped onto the lower bank. Central parts of the visual field are represented most caudally, and progressively more eccentric or peripheral locations in the visual field are represented at progressively more anterior locations. The representation of the central 5 degrees of the visual field occupies more territory (*red*) than does the representation of the remaining portions of the visual field (*black*). Photomicrograph reprinted with permission from deArmond S et al., *Structure of the human brain: A photographic atlas.* New York: Oxford University Press, 1989.

Finally, consider how we can use visual field deficits to narrow down the location of an anatomical lesion. First, every visual field deficit can be immediately narrowed down to a lesion located before or after the chiasm based on whether the same hemifield is affected in both eyes (see Box 7-4). Second,

---

Box 7-4 **LESIONS IN THE VISUAL PATHWAY LEAD TO PREDICTABLE VISUAL FIELD DEFICITS**

Because we have two eyes and a mostly binocular field of view, damage to the pathway from one eye only is often not even noticed. Even a small hole in the visual fields of both eyes is often compensated for by cortical mechanisms and therefore not noticed. However, careful visual field testing, mapping the visual field for each eye using small points of light, is extremely helpful in mapping the location of a lesion and can compete with modern imaging techniques in accurately locating a lesion.

Visual fields are always tested one eye at a time. The right eye's visual field is measured in a person with the left eye occluded and the left eye's visual field in a person with the right eye occluded. Recall that features to the right of the fixation point are in the right visual field of both the left and right eyes. Thus, the right visual field includes the temporal hemifield of the right eye (containing input from the nasal retina of the right eye) and the nasal hemifield of the left eye. The suffix *-anopia* or *-anopsia* is used to denote a loss of sight. With this terminology, we are now ready to name some of the common visual field deficits, all of which are illustrated in Figure 7-15.

A lesion at the midline of the optic chiasm, most frequently the result of a pituitary tumor, will cause a bitemporal hemianopia, which means that the patient cannot see the temporal hemifield of either eye. Since visual pathways beyond the chiasm carry only contralateral field information, retrochiasmal lesions produce homonymous, or consistent, visual field deficits in both eyes. For example, a complete lesion of the optic tract or lateral geniculate nucleus results in a contralateral *homonymous hemianopia*, meaning that the affected individual will be blind to the contralateral visual field. For example, a lesion of the left optic tract will impair vision of the right hemifield in both the right and left eyes.

Upon exiting the lateral geniculate nucleus, the optic radiation splits into two parts so that information from the upper and lower contralateral quadrants of the visual field travel separately. Lesions in the optic radiation typically knock out only one part of the radiation and, consequently, only a quarter of the visual field at most. For example, lesions that impinge on Meyer's loop impair vision of the upper half of the contralateral hemifield in both eyes, a condition termed *homonymous superior quadrantanopia*. Lesions at the back of the head, either due to blunt trauma or to ischemia in the territory of the posterior cerebral artery (see Chapter 8), can cause complete blindness if they are bilateral or a hemianopia if restricted to one side. Yet, in many occipital cortex stroke cases, central vision or some portion of it is spared. Such *macular sparing* likely results from a redundancy in the blood supply to visual cortex.

Very few lay people are familiar with either the term or the concept of visual fields. Therefore, a person's complaint of a problem with vision in one eye should simply serve as the impetus for visual field testing. The individual may be correct or more commonly, has misinterpreted a problem with a hemifield as a problem with the eye on that side.

Detailed visual field assessments are available using a computerized test of a patient's ability to detect spots of light randomly distributed throughout the visual field of each eye. Yet a crude version of visual field testing can be done by simply asking a patient to fixate straight ahead and report when she detects the appearance of an object such as the point of a pencil as the tester brings that object in from the periphery of each quadrant (nasal, nasal-superior, superior, temporal-superior, and so on). If all is well, the patient reports detecting peripheral objects throughout the visual field. If not, you have a crude estimate of the margins of the patient's visual impairment. Finally, in patients with compromised communication skills, testing whether a patient blinks to "*threat,*" a rapid movement of your hand toward the patient's face, can crudely map out the margins of a visual impairment. Normally, a person blinks if he or she can see the approach of the hand. However, an individual with, for example, bitemporal hemianopia will not blink when an object approaches rapidly from the temporal edge but will blink to a threat approaching from straight ahead.

the divergence of the optic radiation into tracts carrying input from the upper and lower quarter fields means that a lesion of the optic radiation will produce a deficit restricted to one or the other contralateral quarter fields. In contrast, a lesion in the optic tract or lateral geniculate nucleus typically produces a deficit that includes parts of both upper and lower quarter fields. Finally, since the visual pathway wends its way from the front to the back of the brain, a lesion caused by a stroke or a tumor will rarely affect visual pathways in isolation. Instead, accompanying symptoms, such as contralateral paralysis or a hormonal disturbance, greatly aid us in localizing lesions that cause visual field deficits.

VISUAL INPUT IS TRANSFORMED INTO INFORMATION NEEDED TO GUIDE MOVEMENT AND INFORM PERCEPTION

The occipital pole houses primary visual cortex. Cortical regions downstream from primary visual cortex provide an increasingly complex synthesis of the visual world, integrating visual building blocks—spots, edges, and the like—into complete scenes and recognizable objects. Two streams or pathways employed for different purposes emanate from visual cortex. The dorsal visual stream bound for the parietal cortex concerns the location and speed of visual objects (Fig. 7-17). This stream is used to identify the location of moving objects, visually guide movements, and understand the observed movements of others. Ultimately, information carried in the dorsal visual stream is sent toward motor and premotor areas, where it is invaluable to adjusting movements based on sensory input. Without such information, we might throw off target, break an egg by holding it with too much force, or injure ourselves by grabbing a thistle.

The ventral visual stream bound for the temporal cortex concerns the appearance of visual objects and is used to identify what we are seeing, so that we can understand the meaning of the visual world (Fig. 7-17). Somatosensory and auditory information joins with visual information in the inferotemporal lobe, where recognition and attachment of meaning to objects occurs.

The target of the ventral visual stream is critical to imbuing perceptions with meaning. The ventral visual stream carries information to the inferior temporal lobe where that information is used to not only build percepts of observed objects but also to connect those percepts to their meaning. The inability to connect a percept to its meaning, even when there is no impairment in sensory perception, is termed *agnosia*. There are many types of agnosia. For instance, the inability to recognize faces is termed *prosopagnosia*. An example of *form* agnosia, the inability to recognize a whole form despite accurately perceiving the form's components was described in Chapter 1. As the example of Dr. P. illustrates, seeing a green tube with red oblong petals does not a rose make. Since somatosensory, auditory, and olfactory as well as visual information reach the inferior temporal lobe, individuals with lesions that disconnect one sensory modality from the inferior temporal lobe may use a different sensory modality to identify an object. This was the case for Dr. P., who readily identified a rose by smell although he was unable to do so by sight.

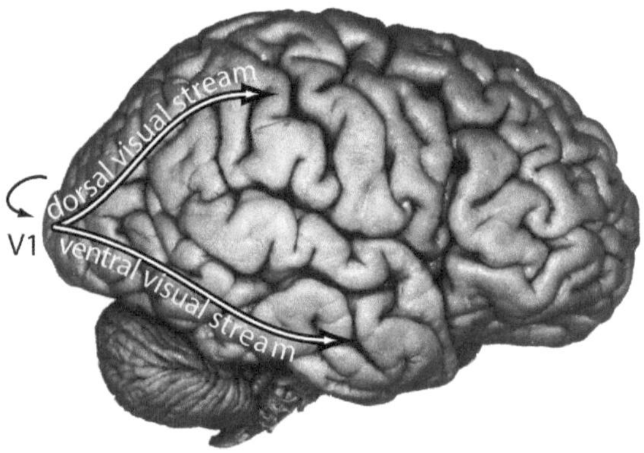

THE SENSORIMOTOR CORTEX IS CRITICAL TO VOLITIONAL ACTIONS

The primary motor cortex and neighboring regions, most notably the primary somatosensory cortex and regions anterior to primary motor cortex, give rise to the corticobulbar and corticospinal tracts. Instructions for voluntary actions reach motoneurons in the brainstem and spinal cord only by way of the descending tracts. Therefore, the sources of descending motor tracts from cortex, collectively termed the *sensorimotor cortex* (Fig. 7-18), form a bottleneck for voluntary movement. The impetus to act and the plan for a movement may arise elsewhere, but the most basic building blocks, the component movements, necessary for fully realized *voluntary actions* pass through primary motor cortex to the corticobulbar and corticospinal tracts.

Figure 7-17 From primary visual cortex (*V*1), information flows in two principal directions. The dorsal visual stream carries information about the location and movement of visual objects toward parietal cortex. The ventral visual stream, carrying information about the form, appearance, and, ultimately, meaning of visual objects, heads toward the lateral part of the inferior temporal lobe. Photomicrograph reprinted with permission from deArmond S et al., *Structure of the human brain: A photographic atlas.* New York: Oxford University Press, 1989.

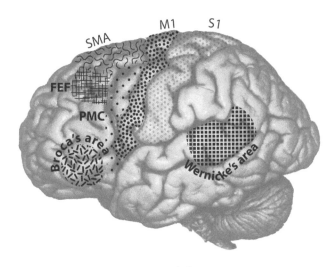

Figure 7-18 The sensorimotor cortex includes primary motor cortex (*M1*), supplementary motor area (*SMA*), premotor cortex (*PMC*), and primary somatosensory cortex (*S1*), all of which contribute to the corticobulbar and corticospinal tracts. Supplementary motor area and premotor cortex are located just rostral to primary motor cortex and are needed to plan any but the simplest one-muscle, one-joint movement. The primary somatosensory cortex receives somatosensory and vestibular information that provides critical information about where our body is, the state of our muscles and joints, the force needed to carry loads of different weights, and the consistency and texture of the objects that we manipulate. Broca's area and the frontal eye fields (*FEF*) are cortical areas needed for specialized movements: speech and eye movements, respectively. Wernicke's area is located in the superior temporal gyrus of the dominant hemisphere and is responsible for understanding language. Broca's area is located in the inferior frontal gyrus, anterior to representations of the tongue and larynx in primary motor cortex. Broca's area, present in the dominant hemisphere, is responsible for producing language. Photomicrograph reprinted with permission from deArmond S et al., *Structure of the human brain: A photographic atlas.* New York: Oxford University Press, 1989.

Reciprocal connections between motor cortex and the "motor" nuclei of the thalamus—ventral anterior and ventral lateral thalamus—allow the cerebellum and basal ganglia to modulate the final motor command arising from cortex and traveling in the corticospinal and corticobulbar tracts. Axons of the corticospinal and corticobulbar tracts course through the corona radiata before becoming part of the internal capsule. As you recall, corticospinal tract axons then travel through the cerebral peduncles, the basis pontis, and the medullary pyramids before entering either the ventral or dorsolateral funiculus of the spinal cord.

FRONTAL CORTEX TRANSFORMS MOTIVATION INTO A STRATEGY FOR ACTION AND THEN INTO COMMANDS FOR MOVEMENT

Anterior to the primary motor cortex are the premotor cortex and supplementary motor area, regions critical to movement planning. These areas chain together simple movements into more complex ones. For example, as we learn to play a new tune on the piano or how to flip an omelet, or even as we simply mentally rehearse these movements, we use our supplementary motor area. Two regions specialized for particular types of movements are found in the frontal cortex rostral to the primary motor cortex and premotor cortex. *Broca's area* is necessary for speech production (see later discussion), and the frontal eye fields are necessary for voluntary eye movements (Fig. 7-18). Collectively, primary motor cortex, premotor cortex, supplementary motor area, Broca's area, and the frontal eye fields constitute sensorimotor cortex.

The insula and limbic regions of frontal cortex are critical to the appreciation of tastes and odors and to the processing of the internal physiological state, inputs that have a particularly direct influence on our emotions and drive to act. A bad odor compels us to get away, just as a tasty odor motivates us to seek out its source, and sickness drains us of the motivation to do anything. From this perspective, we can view the frontal cortex as being bracketed by regions critical to motivation and regions critical to movement.

The intervening parts of frontal cortex are termed the *prefrontal cortex*. Prefrontal cortex organizes behavior by using working memory to translate personal and social motivations into a plan for movement. In essence, prefrontal cortex addresses the questions "Why move? Why do anything?" and answers either query by initiating an action or refraining from action. Therefore, prefrontal cortex organizes and prioritizes behavior to connect motivational areas to motor areas of cortex. In the absence of prefrontal function, little or no behavior is initiated.

The ability, or lack thereof, to play well with others, the capacity to stay on task or to divert one's attention, and myriad other high-level choices are worked out by anterior regions of prefrontal cortex. Progressively more caudal portions of frontal cortex then transform choices and strategy into an actual sequence of movements. Whereas damage to any part of motor cortex impairs some aspect of movement per se, individuals with damage to the prefrontal cortex often have problems in supervising or sequencing behavior, particularly when interruptions to the task at hand occur; these individuals therefore benefit from highly structured and consistent expectations, as well as a predictable environment. Taken as a whole, the prefrontal cortex is the center for prioritizing between various possible actions. The action strategies considered and the one adopted by an individual speak to that person's temperament and life experiences and are fundamental expressions of that person's self.

THE EFFECTS
OF PREFRONTAL DAMAGE

For several decades, neuroscientists have told the story of Phineas Gage in order to illustrate the function of the prefrontal cortex. Phineas Gage was a 19th-century railroad-building foreman who suffered a penetrating head wound and was said to never be the same. In the oft-told story, Gage was "no longer Gage" after the accident. Although popular prior to the accident, it was said that Gage became socially inappropriate and behaviorally disinhibited. Recent evidence raises strong doubts about the accuracy of the Gage story as commonly told. Specifically, the changes in Gage's behavior from before the accident to after his initial recovery are unclear, suggesting that the Gage story is at least partially apocryphal.

Despite the dubious nature of the Gage story, the effects of prefrontal damage are known. Unfortunately, this knowledge arrives through the painful lens of countless individuals who underwent a *frontal lobotomy*, the first widely used form of psychosurgery. Egas Moniz, a Portuguese neurologist, invented a surgical procedure that he called frontal *leucotomy* in 1935. Moniz was motivated by the desire to cure patients with mental illnesses such as depression, schizophrenia, and panic disorder, patients for whom only drastic treatments such as insulin shock therapy were available at the time. Moniz designed the leukotome, an instrument with a loop at the end, to sever the connections between the frontal lobes and the thalamus in an effort to deprive diseased parts of the brain an avenue of expression. He reported that most patients benefited and none was harmed by frontal leucotomy. After Moniz's pioneering work, many physicians began performing leukotomies, or variations thereupon, around the world. It is interesting to note that Moniz also invented cerebral angiography, a method for visualizing cerebral blood vessels in standard use today. Yet Moniz was awarded the 1949 Nobel Prize for Physiology and Medicine for the leucotomy, which has fallen into disrepute (see later discussion) and not for cerebral angiography.

The most active psychosurgeon in America was Walter Freeman, a neurologist who followed Moniz's work and performed frontal lobotomies, as he called them, in America from 1936 until 1967. To make the lobotomy accessible to the myriads of individuals he felt could benefit from it, Freeman simplified the procedure. Freeman lobotomized thousands by entering the brain through the eye with an ice-pick and then twirling the ice-pick around to cut the intervening brain tissue. Across the United States, Freeman performed this simple transorbital lobotomy in his office or in makeshift surgical arenas, including his own traveling bus.

Freeman took an evangelical view of the lobotomy, earning him infamy in the history of medical science. The fascinating story of Freeman and of psychosurgery more generally are detailed in *The Lobotomist* by Jack El-Hai and in *Great and Desperate Cures: The Rise and Decline of Psychosurgery and Other Radical Treatments for Mental Illness* by Elliot S. Valenstein. An emotionally wrenching account of a man who underwent a transorbital lobotomy in Freeman's office at the age of 12 is given in *My Lobotomy* by Howard Dully and Charles Fleming (2007).

The development of psychotropic drugs, notably the antipsychotic Thorazine, initiated the decline of the lobotomy. When first introduced, Thorazine was viewed as a chemical lobotomy. Currently, psychosurgery has made something of a comeback, but with important differences from the lobotomies performed by Freeman and others. First, the procedures are given to desperately ill patients, and informed consent is rigorously required. Second, the procedures are targeted at lesioning or stimulating specific parts of the brain, such as the cingulate gyrus or subthalamic nucleus and are performed using sterile surgical methods.

Moving beyond the history, what effect did lobotomies have on behavior? The general consensus is that destruction of frontal lobe white matter made individuals more docile and easier to manage. Yet the operations widely varied, as is to be expected from the twirling of an ice pick. Consequently, the effects of lobotomies widely varied. The stereotypical picture of lobotomized people is of individuals who seldom initiate behavior or conversation, an image that fits well with our conception that the frontal lobes are critical to turning motivation into planning and planning into action.

LANGUAGE AND
HANDEDNESS HEAD THE LIST
OF LATERALIZED FUNCTIONS

Throughout most of the spinal cord, brainstem, and forebrain, structures on the left and right side of the brain perform the same function for different body parts or regions of space. The left ventrolateral quadrant of the spinal cord carries pain and temperature information from the right body, and the right ventrolateral quadrant carries pain and temperature information from the left; left visual cortex codes for the right visual field, and right visual cortex codes for left visual field and so on. However, there are notable exceptions to this rule. One exception is that we, or at least the vast majority of us, have a dominant hand, a hand that we prefer to use over the other.

In most people, left- and right-handed alike, the left cerebral hemisphere is dominant, meaning that it is responsible for language. Understanding and producing speech primarily depends on Wernicke's and Broca's areas, respectively, *in the dominant hemisphere* (Fig. 7-18). Damage to either language area or to several nearby and related areas impairs language communication, causing some type of *aphasia*, or difficulty in language communication. Aphasia is a deficit in language *not* speech. For example, damage to Broca's area impairs sign language production in native signers just as it impairs speech in hearing individuals. Damage to the nondominant hemisphere can produce problems with understanding and producing *prosody*, the communicative tone that accompanies speech. A person who speaks without prosody sounds monotonic, and a person deaf to the prosody of speech has great difficulty understanding a speaker's intended meaning and emphasis. These topics are covered fully in Chapter 16.

THE HIPPOCAMPUS TURNS EXPERIENCES INTO MEMORIES AND THEN SENDS THE MEMORIES OUT FOR LONG-TERM STORAGE

In 1953, a young man named Henry Gustav Molaison, known as patient HM until his death in 2008, sought neurosurgical treatment for debilitating epileptic seizures. *Epileptic foci* are areas of the brain, typically in the cerebral cortex, where seizure activity begins. With time and with each seizure that begins at a focus, the threshold to elicit a seizure decreases, rendering the region increasingly epileptogenic. By the time that he sought neurosurgical treatment, HM's life choices were severely constrained by his seizures.

HM had bilateral epileptic foci, one in each temporal lobe. Consequently, William Scoville, a Connecticut neurosurgeon, removed both of HM's medial temporal lobes. The surgery had the intended effect of reducing the number of seizures that HM experienced. Unfortunately, the surgery also had an unintended consequence because HM, 27 years old at the time of the surgery, became profoundly amnesic, losing the ability to make new declarative memories for the remaining 55 years of his life.

There are several forms of memory. *Working memory* is a transient form of memory that is available only so long as it is held consciously. Thus, a working memory can be held continuously but never retrieved after a break. For example, when we are told a telephone number, we repeat it over and over until we can write it down or dial it. The contents of working memory either make it into long-term memory or are forgotten.

In contrast to working memory, *declarative memory* is the explicit and long-term memory of facts. It has two components: *semantic* and *episodic*. Semantic memory is essentially vocabulary: knowing the word for an apple or a flash drive, the name of your teacher or friend, and the name of a street and so on. Recalling the facts of events experienced utilizes episodic memory. So, for instance, in recollecting the trip to pick up a new puppy, the mode of transportation, destination, identities of traveling companions are all episodic memories. On the other hand, the smile on your face every time you pass the place where you picked up your now beloved dog is an implicit, emotional memory.

Testing for declarative memory is simple. First, a person is asked to remember a few words or numbers. To ensure that the person heard the list, he should immediately repeat the items. After a short interval, 5 minutes or so, the person is asked to recall the list. During the interval, the person must be distracted and engaged on another task to prevent continuous rehearsal of the list using working memory. When the interval is over, the person is asked to recall the words or numbers he was asked to remember. People with normal memories have total recall, whereas an individual like HM with *dense* (i.e., severe) amnesia will not even recall being asked to recall anything.

With an understanding of declarative memory in hand, we return to HM's story. Once Scoville realized that HM had a severe impairment of memory, he took HM to the Montreal Neurologic Institute. A neuropsychologist named Brenda Milner began to work with HM. Milner and her student Suzanne Corkin studied and performed rigorous psychological testing on HM over the course of six decades. Tests confirmed that HM had dense amnesia. Scoville and Milner published this fundamental result in 1957, and, consequently, no other patient has had the medial temporal lobes removed bilaterally. Additionally, Milner's and others' studies of HM and other patients with medial temporal lobe damage opened the door to our modern neurobiological view of memory, which includes the following essential ideas:

- The hippocampus is required for the formation of new, long-term declarative memories.

- Several forms of memory, including working, motor, procedural, and implicit memory, do not depend on the hippocampus. For example, HM learned to trace figures viewed through a mirror at a rate that did not differ from that of individuals without declarative memory problems.

- The long-term storage of declarative memories does not depend on the hippocampus. The import of this is that individuals with hippocampal damage, including HM, retain old memories made prior to the hippocampal damage. For example, in the early 1980s, HM was asked who was president, as part of a standard mental status exam. He was uncertain. When told that it was Ronald Reagan, HM responded with surprise and an embarrassed laugh saying, politely, "Well, he was a good actor." At each subsequent exam over several months, he responded in exactly the same manner. The examiner in each case had never heard HM laugh before.

Even without the ability to make new memories, HM remained the same affable person that he was before his operation. His good-natured personality shone through his disability, and, consequently, he was loved by those who worked with him. Although he was not survived by any family, HM left behind devoted friends among the scientists who tested him over the course of six decades, as well as myriads of grateful admirers who feel a deep indebtedness for all that he taught us.

The amnesia that results from bilateral hippocampal damage, as well as from a number of other conditions such as Alzheimer disease, differs from what many call "Hollywood amnesia," the version of amnesia seen in most movies. Alfred Hitchcock's *Spellbound* is a classic example of Hollywood amnesia. The character played by Gregory Peck has no idea of who he is and cannot recall any past events, but makes new memories completely normally. In stark contrast, amnesia is anterograde, meaning that new memories cannot be formed while old memories remain.

Anterograde amnesia is often accompanied by graded retrograde amnesia, meaning a failure to remember past events that is most severe for the immediate past and least severe for the long ago past. Retrograde amnesia rarely occurs unaccompanied by at least some period of anterograde amnesia, whereas states of anterograde amnesia are often accompanied by graded retrograde amnesia. For example, a person with graded retrograde amnesia may fail to remember the minutes or hours prior to a car accident while retaining normal recall of life prior to the accident. The same person also shows anterograde amnesia in failing to remember the immediate aftermath of the accident.

Long-term memories are not written in stone. Memories are retrieved when needed and then reconsolidated by the hippocampus. After each retrieval of a long-term memory, that memory is reformed or reconsolidated by the hippocampus before once again being shipped out to an area of neocortex. This idea allows us to understand several features of memory. First, memories degrade over time. Recall of an evening out is filled with far more details on the following day than when remembered a year later. Second, memory is facilitated by frequent recall and therefore frequent reconsolidation. A story that is told daily is more easily recalled than a story told once or infrequently. Third, memories can change. For example, eyewitnesses often recall one set of events immediately after a crime and a slightly different set of events years later.

We can use reconsolidation to understand graded retrograde amnesia. Consider two memories of equally strong emotional impact—one formed by HM at age 15, 12 years before his operation, and one formed by HM in the month before his operation. In the former case, HM presumably retrieved and consolidated the memory thousands of times. In contrast, in the case of a memory formed just a month before losing all hippocampal function, HM would have had time to retrieve the memory far fewer times. This perspective suggests that older memories are stronger and persist longer than more recently formed memories, as is indeed the case. In sum, reconsolidation may underlie the common finding that retrograde amnesia is graded, so that memories are lost in the reverse chronological order from which they are formed.

Although neurosurgeons no longer take out the temporal lobes bilaterally, bilateral hippocampal damage still occurs. Some of this is due to neurodegenerative diseases such as Alzheimer's disease or frontotemporal dementia. Another source of damage to the hippocampus is a lack of oxygen. As it turns out, the hippocampus is particularly sensitive to low levels of oxygen. Therefore, a fair number of individuals suffer bilateral hippocampal damage as a result of hypoxia, or low levels of oxygen. Hypoxia may occur for a number of reasons, including cardiac arrest. Since the brain region most sensitive to hypoxic damage is the hippocampus, the hippocampi of individuals who lack sufficient oxygen for a stretch of time, regardless of the cause, are often damaged bilaterally. These patients suffer bilateral medial temporal lobe damage "naturally."

THE PARAHIPPOCAMPAL GYRUS AND FORNIX PROVIDE PORTALS INTO AND OUT OF THE HIPPOCAMPUS

Since we form memories of all types of events, it should not be surprising that the hippocampus receives input from regions throughout the cortical mantle. Most of this input funnels into the hippocampus via the neighboring entorhinal cortex. Most of the output from the hippocampus also exits via a hippocampal neighbor, the subiculum.

The subiculum, entorhinal cortex, and hippocampus are all housed within the parahippocampal gyrus (Figs. 7-1, 7-3). Since most of the input to and output from the hippocampus courses through the parahippocampal gyrus, lesions there produce an amnesia very similar to that produced by lesions of the hippocampus proper.

The fornix is a prominent forebrain tract that serves hippocampal connections both into and out of forebrain areas more distant than the parahippocampal gyrus (Fig. 7-4). Axons leaving the hippocampus curve around the lateral ventricle as part of the fornix to end in the anterior thalamus and in the mammillary bodies. Medial diencephalic lesions, particularly those of the mammillary bodies, impair declarative memory.

CORTICAL ANATOMY IS THE SUBSTRATE FOR INTELLECTUAL ABILITY

In the past, psychologists have defined *g* as a factor that quantifies a measure of general intelligence. Under this construct, an individual's ability at each type of cognitive task is the product of *g* and a factor related to specific cognitive abilities. The concept of *g* has not been widely accepted in neuroscience. In contrast to the prediction that all types of intellectual aptitude are correlated, it is clear that normal individuals can have widely disparate abilities. Moreover, individuals with intellectual disability, a heterogeneous group of conditions previously termed "mental retardation," have gross deficits in some cognitive functions and no measurable differences from normal individuals in other cognitive functions. In fact, individuals with *savant syndrome* are characterized by an *exceptional* aptitude in one area— such as musical ability, visual memory, or calculations— and either normal or below-normal intellectual abilities in other areas.

One popular idea has been that, within a species, brain size is related to an individual's intelligence. This idea is supported by the prevalence of small brains (termed *microencephalic*) and brains with minimal gyrification (termed *lissencephalic*) among intellectually disabled individuals. Yet, *macrocephaly*, or a significantly larger than normal brain, can accompany either normal intelligence or intellectual impairment, as occurs in many conditions including autism and fragile X syndrome.

An evolving view holds that *intelligences* are emergent properties of the cerebral cortex. Different cortical areas support different cognitive abilities. Widespread anatomical changes, such as those found in individuals with Down syndrome, are likely to impair numerous cognitive functions. Moreover, cortical function may be delicately tuned, so that numerous types of changes— fewer neurons, more neurons, misdirected dendrites, extra synapses, loss of a signaling molecule, and so on—may all lead to cortical circuit dysfunction and therefore cognitive impairment. When these changes are restricted, the result may be tone deafness or poor language skills, and when the changes are widespread, the condition that we term intellectual disability may be the result.

Intellectual disability affects 1–3% of the population. It is a type of developmental disability in which children have a low intelligence quotient (IQ) and show impairment in additional cognitive functions. Intellectually disabled individuals typically fail to develop normal skills such as language, washing and dressing themselves, and socializing with others. Hundreds of causes result in intellectual disability, with the most common genetic defects being Down syndrome, phenylketonuria (PKU), and fragile X syndrome. Nongenetic causes of intellectual disability include maternal alcoholism, which gives rise to fetal alcohol syndrome; certain maternal or neonatal infections; hypoxia during delivery; and severe malnutrition. The latter is, tragically, a leading cause of intellectual disability in developing countries. Recently, microcephaly due to gestational infection by the Zika virus has become epidemic in some regions of the world.

Regardless of the cause, the anatomical substrate for below-average intellectual development appears to be distributed differentially across the cerebral—and in many cases cerebellar—cortex. In the case of Down syndrome, both the cerebral and cerebellar cortices are smaller, with fewer neurons and synapses than in individuals of normal intelligence. Cortical regions involved in language, motor control, and working memory are particularly impaired, as are the functions themselves. No treatment exists that either slows or reverses the deteriorating course of intellectual disability in most patients, including those with Down syndrome. In such cases, education, behavioral therapy, and management are employed to reduce stressors and optimize predictability in the patient's environment.

There is one notable exception to the lack of available treatments for patients with an intellectual disability-causing disease. If individuals with PKU adhere to a diet that lacks phenylalanine starting immediately after birth, a harmful buildup of phenylalanine can be avoided and normal intellectual development can occur. To enable the prompt identification of babies with PKU, typically caused by a mutation in the phenylalanine hydroxylase gene (see Chapter 12), all babies born in hospitals in industrialized countries are tested for PKU at birth. For the phenylalanine-free or "PKU diet" to be effective, it must be a life-long diet and must be followed with particular care during the developmental years.

ADDITIONAL READING

Albin RL, Young AB, Penney JB. The functional anatomy of basal ganglia disorders. *Trends Neurosci*. 12: 366–375, 1989.

Baxter MG, Murray EA. The amygdala and reward. *Nat Rev Neurosci*. 3: 562–573, 2002.

Corkin S. *Permanent Present Tense: The Unforgettable Life of the Amnesic Patient, H. M.* New York: Basic Books, 2013.

Dierssen M, Herault Y, Estivill X. Aneuploidy: From a physiological mechanism of variance to Down syndrome. *Physiol Rev*. 89: 887–920, 2009.

Emery NJ, Capitanio JP, Mason WA, Machado CJ, Mendoza SP, Amaral DG. The effects of bilateral lesions of the amygdala on dyadic social interactions in rhesus monkeys (*Macaca mulatta*). *Behav Neurosci*. 115: 515–544, 2001.

Gold JJ, Squire LR. The anatomy of amnesia: Neurohistological analysis of three new cases. *Learning Memory*. 13: 699–710, 2006.

Kay LM, Sherman SM. An argument for an olfactory thalamus. *Trends Neurosci*. 30: 47–53, 2007.

Klit H, Finnerup NB, Jensen TS. Central post-stroke pain: Clinical characteristics, pathophysiology, and management. *Lancet Neurol*. 8: 857–868, 2009.

Klüver H, Bucy PC. Preliminary analysis of functions of the temporal lobes in monkeys. Originally published in *Arch Neurol Psychiatry*. 42: 979–1000, 1939 and reprinted in *J Neuropsychiatry Clin Neurosci*. 9: 606–620, 1997.

Koenigs M, Grafman J. Post-traumatic stress disorder: The role of medial prefrontal cortex and amygdala. *Neuroscientist*. 15: 540–548, 2009.

Lonstein JS. Regulation of anxiety during the postpartum period. *Frontiers Neuroendocrinol*. 28: 115–141, 2007.

Macmillan M. Phineas Gage—unraveling the myth. *Psychologist*. 21: 828–831, 2008.

Penfield W, Rasmussen T. *The Cerebral Cortex of Man. A Clinical Study of Localization of Function*. New York: The Macmillan Company, 1950.

Rauschecker JP. Cortical control of the thalamus: Top–down processing and plasticity. *Nat Neuroscience*. 1: 179–180, 1998.

Rempel-Clower NL, Zola SM, Squire LR, Amaral DG. Three cases of enduring memory impairment after bilateral damage limited to the hippocampal formation. *J Neurosci*. 16: 5233–5255, 1996.

Ringach DL. Spontaneous and driven cortical activity: Implications for computation. *Curr Opin Neurobiol*. 19: 438–444, 2009.

Shallice T. The fractionation of supervisory control. In: Gazzaniga M, ed. *The Cognitive Neurosciences III*. 3rd ed. Oxford: Oxford University Press; 2004: 943–956.

Sherman SM. Tonic and burst firing: Dual modes of thalamocortical relay. *Trends Neurosci*. 24: 122–126, 2001.

Sherman SM. The thalamus is more than just a relay. *Curr Opin Neurobiol*. 17: 417–422, 2007.

Shin LM, Rauch SL, Pitman RK. Amygdala, medial prefrontal cortex and hippocampal function in PTSD. *Ann NY Acad Sci*. 1071: 67–79, 2006.

Siebert M, Markowitsch HJ, Bartel P. Amygdala, affect and cognition: Evidence from 10 patients with Urbach–Wiethe disease. *Brain*. 126: 2627–2637, 2003.

Slattery DA, Neumann ID. No stress please! Mechanisms of stress hyporesponsiveness of the maternal brain. *J Physiol*. 586: 377–385, 2008.

Squire LR. Memory and brain systems: 1969–2009. *J Neurosci*. 29: 12711–12716, 2009.

Wiest G, Lehner-Baumgartner E, Baumgartner C. Panic attacks in an individual with bilateral selective lesions of the amygdala. *Arch Neurol*. 63: 1798–1801, 2006.

Wrobel BB, Leopold DA. Clinical assessment of patients with smell and taste disorders. *Otolaryngol Clin N Am*. 30: 47–53, 2004.

8.

FOLLOWING THE NUTRIENTS

BLOOD SUPPLY, BLOOD–BRAIN BARRIER, AND VENTRICLES

ike all other organs, the brain requires oxygen and nutrients to function and waste disposal to prevent potentially toxic consequences. Yet the brain differs from most body tissues in important ways. First, the brain has the greatest oxygen requirement of any organ in the body. Second, the central nervous system (CNS) does not receive nutrients directly from capillary blood. Instead, a blood–brain barrier formed by specialized epithelial cells filters blood into a watery, clear fluid that lacks hemoglobin. Third, the brain is suspended within a sack of *cerebrospinal fluid* (*CSF*) that fits snugly within the bony cranium. As we shall see, the unyielding bony nature of the cranial cavity complicates the otherwise simple pressure relationship between arterial and venous blood flow.

To follow oxygen and nutrients from arrival in the cranium to disposal, we look at:

- The arterial blood supply to the brain and spinal cord

- The blood–brain barrier

- The collection and drainage of venous blood from the brain

As nutrients travel from arterial blood to brain and waste products from brain to venous blood, the paths critically involve the meninges that surround the brain and spinal cord. Therefore, we describe the anatomy of the meninges in some detail.

Within the brain, sufficient arterial blood flowing in and venous blood draining out depend on pressure relationships between the contents of the cranium:

- Arterial blood

- Venous blood

- CSF

- Brain tissue or *parenchyma*

Changes in the pressure relationships among these components can result in serious and relatively common brain failures. At the same time, our ability to intervene and remedy, or at least ameliorate, conditions such as stroke, traumatic brain injury (TBI), hemorrhage, encephalitis, and syncope (fainting) all depend on using an understanding of intracranial pressure (ICP) to advantage.

Stroke occurs when the brain's blood supply is interrupted through either vessel occlusion or vessel rupture and consequent hemorrhage within the cranium. Strokes can produce severe disability or even death. Moreover, strokes are extraordinarily common, striking nearly 800,000 in the United States each year. Strokes are the number one neurological cause for hospitalization and death in the United States; in fact, stroke causes 1 out every 20 deaths. We examine strokes in some detail.

THE BRAIN REQUIRES A STEADY AND CONSIDERABLE SUPPLY OF OXYGEN

The mammalian brain requires a disproportionately large proportion of the body's oxygen, about 25%, despite accounting for less than 3% of the body's mass. The delivery of oxygen to the brain is critical to brain function, so critical in fact that neurons show damage after seconds without oxygen and begin to die within minutes. *The brain suffers irreparable damage after only a few—less than 5—minutes without oxygen.* The heart, a runner-up to the brain in its oxygen requirement, continues to function for roughly 30 minutes without oxygen.

Altitude sickness provides a dramatic illustration of the brain's strong dependence on oxygen. On top of Tanzania's Mount Kilimanjaro, at an elevation of 5,900 meters (or 19,000 feet), the number of oxygen molecules per volume is lower than at sea level. This follows from the "thin air," a decrease in molecular density, at the low atmospheric pressures of higher altitudes. In other words, although air has 20% oxygen at both sea level and on high mountain peaks, there are far fewer molecules in a breath of thin air at high altitudes than in a breath of air at sea level. A single breath takes in about twice as much oxygen in San Francisco (at sea level) as on Mount Kilimanjaro. On top of Mount Everest, at an elevation that is roughly equivalent to the cruising altitude of passenger jets, oxygen molecules are still rarer.

Oxygen levels also fall to dangerous levels upon exposure to just a fraction of a percent of carbon monoxide (CO), resulting in death after only a few breaths at CO concentrations of more than 1%. Regardless of the cause, the clinical effects of a paucity of oxygen include headache, lightheadedness, confusion, and eventually loss of consciousness and possibly death, all consequences of brain dysfunction.

Arterial blood flow to the brain, about 15–20% of the heart's output, delivers oxygen to the threshold of the brain parenchyma, or tissue matter. Arteries dive into the brain, narrowing to arterioles and ultimately to capillaries. Oxygen diffuses out of cerebral blood vessels. Nutrients are ferried by transporters from the capillaries, across the blood–brain barrier, and into the parenchyma. Thus, *cerebral blood flow (CBF), the flow of blood through cerebral arterioles and capillaries, is critical to the healthy operation of the brain.* Cerebral blood flow in turn depends on *cerebral perfusion pressure (CPP)*, the pressure that drives blood through the cerebrum.

PRESSURE INSIDE THE RIGID CRANIUM LIMITS CPP

To provide the brain with oxygen, adequate perfusion by oxygenated blood of the brain is required. Normally, the perfusion pressure in an organ is simply the arterial pressure that flows into the organ less the venous pressure that drains blood from the organ. Since an average mean arterial pressure (MAP) is 80–100 mm Hg and venous pressure is about 5–10 mm Hg, organ perfusion pressure would be 70–95 mm Hg, sufficient to adequately drive physiological function. Yet, in the case of the brain, there is an additional and critical factor: *intracranial pressure*. The contents of the cranium—blood, CSF, and parenchyma—exist at a pressure that is normally about 15 mm Hg. Thus, ICP is greater than venous pressure. Consequently, ICP rather than venous pressure is subtracted from MAP to calculate CPP, the pressure that drives CBF through the brain:

$$CPP = MAP - ICP$$

For adequate CBF and oxygen delivery, CPP must be at least 60–80 mm Hg. A decrease in MAP or an increase in ICP, potentially due to a tumor, swelling, or subdural hemorrhage, can produce a dangerous reduction in CPP and thereby CBF (Fig. 8-1).

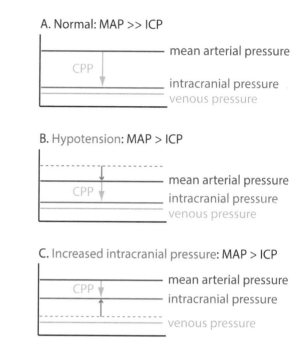

A. Normal: MAP >> ICP

B. Hypotension: MAP > ICP

C. Increased intracranial pressure: MAP > ICP

Figure 8-1 Cerebral perfusion pressure (*CPP*) depends on the difference between mean arterial pressure (*MAP*) and intracranial pressure (*ICP*). Normally, arterial pressure is much greater than intracranial pressure (A) so that cerebral perfusion pressure (*blue arrow*) is adequate, >60 mm Hg. However when systemic arterial pressure plummets (*red arrow*), as in hypotension, the difference between arterial pressure and intracranial pressure decreases, so that cerebral perfusion pressure becomes inadequate (B). Similarly, when intracranial pressure is elevated (*red arrow*), for any of a variety of reasons, the difference pressure decreases and cerebral perfusion pressure is inadequate (C).

CEREBRAL BLOOD FLOW IS HIGHLY REGULATED TO STAY WITHIN PHYSIOLOGICAL RANGE

Safeguards exist to ensure adequate, but not excessive, CBF even as CPP varies. *Autoregulation* refers to a physiological mechanism by which the blood flow to an organ is protected from changes in systemic arterial pressure within a given range. Because of autoregulation, an organ's perfusion pressure stays constant, or at least within a working range, even as systemic blood pressure changes. The range of arterial pressures tolerated and the mechanisms of autoregulation differ from organ to organ. In the case of cerebral autoregulation, *cerebral blood flow* is maintained at a steady level when the MAP is between 60 and about 140–150 mm Hg. Thus, cerebral autoregulation ensures that the brain is supplied with sufficient oxygen and nutrients across a fairly large range of circumstances (Fig. 8-2). Cerebral autoregulation is achieved through two principal mechanisms:

- *Myogenic:* The smooth muscles surrounding arterioles dilate in response to decreases in pressure and constrict in response to increases in pressure.

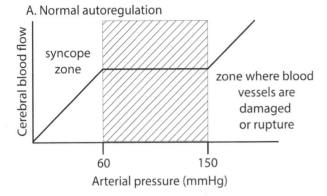

A. Normal autoregulation

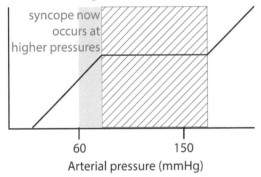

B. Shifted autoregulation

Figure 8-2 A: Normally, autoregulation keeps cerebral blood flow within physiological limits even as arterial pressure varies between about 60 and 150 mm Hg. If cerebral blood flow falls too low, syncope results, and if it rises too high, blood vessels, particularly small ones, are damaged and may even rupture. B: During periods of sustained elevations in blood pressure, as occurs during exercise or chronic hypertension, the range of autoregulation shifts to the right. This allows tolerance of higher pressures but it also puts an individual at increased risk of syncope because cerebral blood flow will be inadequate at pressures that are normally tolerated (*shaded area*).

- *Metabolic*: Increases in carbon dioxide (CO_2) and decreases in oxygen (O_2) result in the dilation of arterioles; decreases in CO_2 result in the constriction of arterioles.

Consider the effect of each mechanism on CBF. When blood pressure decreases, cerebral arterioles dilate, which serves to decrease resistance and thereby increase flow. When blood pressure increases, cerebral arterioles constrict, increasing vessel resistance and decreasing flow. *The myogenic contribution to cerebral autoregulation is the primary mechanism that keeps global CBF within physiological limits.*

Metabolic changes result from a number of factors, including neuronal activity. Active neurons generate CO_2 and utilize available O_2, leading to changes in local gas pressures. The increase in CO_2 and decrease in O_2 consequent to neuronal activity results in cerebral vessel dilation and, hence, an increase in local blood flow. This is the principle upon which modern imaging methods such

as functional magnetic resonance imaging (fMRI) are based. Conversely, vasoconstriction and a decrease in local blood flow follow a decrease in CO_2. The ultimate result of these metabolic autoregulatory reactions is that *CBF is diverted from less active brain areas to more active brain areas*. In this way, metabolic influences on CBF promote dynamic adjustments to local metabolic needs. The consequent change in the blood flow to different brain localities also means that local blood flow can deviate from the level defended by myogenic autoregulation in order to serve high levels of neuronal activity.

Myogenic and metabolic influences on CBF maintain adequate rates of flow globally and locally in the face of both changes in neuronal activity and cardiovascular function. In addition to these autoregulatory mechanisms, the brain influences CBF through additional pathways. For example, during exercise or during the clichéd conditions of "fight or flight," activation of sympathetic outflow results in a shift of the range of autoregulation to higher pressure values (Fig. 8-2B). This shift allows tolerance of a higher range of systemic blood pressure. Chronic hypertension also shifts the range of cerebral autoregulation to higher pressures much as sympathetic activation does. Although a rightward shift allows the brain to tolerate high blood pressures, it also increases the blood pressure threshold for insufficient CBF. As a result, insufficient CBF occurs when systemic pressure reaches values that are easily tolerated in normal healthy individuals at rest (Fig. 8-2B).

As the reader may imagine, there are circumstances when CBF falls outside of the autoregulation range. When CBF falls below the lower limit of autoregulation, about 60 mm Hg in healthy individuals, arterial perfusion of the cerebrum starts to decline with systemic blood pressure. Below about 30 mm Hg, CBF stops. If CBF falls too far and compensatory mechanisms such as increasing the rate of oxygen extraction fail, *syncope* occurs. Syncope refers to a loss of consciousness accompanied by a loss of postural tone, colloquially referred to as fainting. Note that a loss of consciousness can occur alone without falling, as it does during certain types of seizures, and a loss of postural tone without a loss of consciousness can also occur as in the case of *drop attacks*. It is the loss of both consciousness and postural integrity that constitutes syncope.

Syncope is a fairly common occurrence affecting about 10% of the population at one time or another. Cardiac problems such as hypotension or arrhythmia cause the majority of syncope cases, with only a minority initiated by a neural event such as a seizure. Regardless of the cause or trigger,

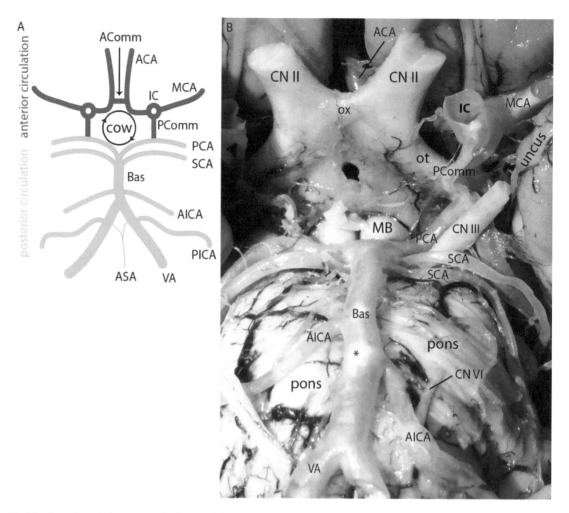

Figure 8-3 A: The blood supply to the brain is supplied primarily by the internal carotid (*IC*) and vertebral (*VA*) arteries. The main branches of the posterior or basilar circulation (*blue*) include the vertebral arteries, the anterior spinal artery (*ASA*), the basilar artery (*Bas*), and four sets of secondary arteries. The basilar artery is formed by the convergence of the two vertebral arteries. The posterior inferior cerebellar arteries (*PICA*) arise from the vertebral arteries, whereas the anterior inferior cerebellar arteries (*AICA*) and superior cerebellar arteries (*SCA*) come off the basilar artery. At the mesodiencephalic transition, the basilar artery splits into the two posterior cerebral arteries (*PCA*), the most anterior components of the posterior circulation. The main branches of the anterior circulation (*maroon*) include three communicating arteries and two pairs of cerebral arteries. The internal carotid, the major source of blood to the anterior circulation, splits into the middle and anterior (*ACA*) cerebral arteries. The two anterior cerebral arteries are connected by a single anterior communicating artery (*AComm*), which bridges the midline. The two posterior communicating arteries (*PComm*) link the middle cerebral arteries (*MCA*) to the posterior cerebral arteries of the posterior circulation. The circle formed by the cerebral and communicating arteries, termed the Circle of Willis (circle labeled *cow*), allows for compensatory blood supply in the case of occlusion to one artery. B: The blood supply has a stereotypical relationship to the underlying brain and cranial nerves as the following examples illustrate. The caudal end of the basilar artery occurs at the pontomedullary junction, where the abducens nerve (*CN VI*) emerges at a site caudal to where the anterior inferior cerebellar artery comes off the basilar artery. The optic chiasm (*ox*) sits in close proximity to the anterior cerebral and internal carotid arteries (*ACA, IC*). The oculomotor nerve (*CN III*) is sandwiched between the superior cerebellar and posterior cerebral arteries. Note that this individual has duplicate superior cerebellar arteries, a common finding present in roughly a quarter of the population. Additional structures labeled for orientation include the mammillary body (*MB*), optic chiasm (*ox*), optic nerve (*CN II*), pons, and uncus. The asterisk shows the location of an atherosclerotic plaque on the basilar.

syncope takes the form it does because of a global failure of cerebral function consequent to inadequate CBF.

At the opposite end from syncope, elevations in CBF are also dangerous. When CBF exceeds the upper limit of autoregulation, which happens at arterial pressures of about 140 or 150 mm Hg in nonexercising individuals, blood vessels can no longer maintain their resting tone and become passively dilated, resulting in damage to the vessel wall and potentially vessel rupture.

THE CIRCLE OF WILLIS CONNECTS BLOOD FROM ANTERIOR AND POSTERIOR CIRCULATIONS

Arteries that supply blood to the brain enter through specific holes in the skull and circumnavigate the base of the brain in a characteristic pattern. The brain receives blood from two major sources (Fig. 8-3):

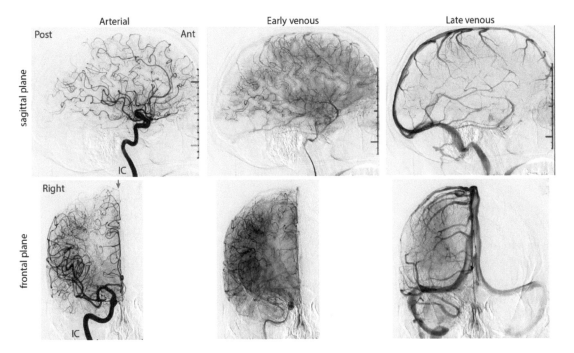

Figure 8-4 A time series of angiograms illustrate the reach of the anterior circulation in the sagittal (*top row*) and coronal (*bottom row*) planes. Injection of contrast agent into the internal carotid (*IC*) initially fills the arterial circulation. The extent of the territory served by the internal carotid through the middle and anterior cerebral arteries is evident. Contrast subsequently moves into the small arterioles and then venules of the *early venous* system. Blood from the venules collects into veins before entering the sinuses (*late venous system*). Note that contrast stays ipsilateral to the site of injection until a modest movement across the midline (*red arrow* in bottom left panel) within the superior sagittal and transverse sinuses during the late venous stage. In all sagittal views, posterior (*Post*) is to the left and anterior (*Ant*) to the right. In the frontal plane angiograms, right is on the left by convention.   Photographs kindly provided by Seon-Kyu Lee, MD, PhD, University of Chicago.

- The *posterior* or *basilar circulation* arises primarily from the *vertebral arteries* with a contribution from the anterior spinal artery. All three of the arteries supplying the posterior circulation enter the skull through the foramen magnum.

- The *anterior* or *carotid circulation* arises from the *internal carotid arteries*, which enter through the paired carotid foramina at the base of the skull.

The internal carotid arteries bring in about 70% of the circulatory input to the brain, with most of the remaining blood arriving via the vertebral arteries.

The anatomy of the arteries supplying the brain provides a major safeguard against inadequate cerebral perfusion. A continuous ring of arteries called the *Circle of Willis* connects the posterior and anterior circulations (Fig. 8-3A). Because the anterior and posterior circulations are connected, redundant blood supplies feed the brain. This redundancy reduces the chance that the

failure of one arterial source will render the brain *ischemic* (without blood supply) and therefore either *anoxic* (without oxygen) or *hypoxic* (with insufficient oxygen). For example, if one internal carotid artery becomes *occluded*, or blocked, the internal carotid on the other side can supply blood and thereby oxygen. Despite the potential for compensatory blood supply, one internal carotid provides blood to just one hemisphere under normal circumstances (Fig. 8-4). In fact, the territory normally supplied by the internal carotid only extends into the parietal cortex. The occipital and ventral temporal lobes of the cerebrum receive blood primarily or exclusively from the posterior circulation.

It is interesting to note that in most vertebrates, including most mammals, blood flows *caudally* in the *basilar artery* (formed by the convergence of the vertebral arteries within the posterior circulation), so that it is the anterior circulation that supplies blood to the hindbrain. Only in mammals with large cerebral hemispheres does the telencephalic need for blood exhaust the capacity of the anterior circulation, leaving nothing to share with the brainstem. A solution to this issue has evolved in humans and other primates. Blood flows from caudal to rostral in the basilar artery, rendering the posterior circulation a potential support, albeit a limited one, to ensuring sufficient blood supply in the forebrain.

THE POSTERIOR CIRCULATION SUPPLIES BLOOD TO THE BRAINSTEM

In the human, the vertebral arteries join to form the basilar artery at the junction between the pons and the medulla. Four important sets of bilateral arteries belong to the posterior circulation, one pair arising from the vertebral arteries and the remainder from the basilar (Fig. 8-3):

- *Posterior inferior cerebellar arteries (PICA)* come off the vertebral arteries.

- *Anterior inferior cerebellar arteries (AICA)* come off the caudal end of the basilar artery.

- *Superior cerebellar arteries (SCA)* come off the rostral end of the basilar artery.

- Rostrally, the basilar artery splits into two *posterior cerebral arteries (PCA)*.

Knowing the territories supplied by the major cerebral blood vessels is critical to understanding the symptoms that arise from a brainstem stroke. Most caudally, the posterior inferior cerebellar arteries emanate from the vertebral arteries to supply blood to the dorsolateral part of the caudal medulla and, as the artery's name suggests, to the posterior inferior part of the cerebellum (Fig. 8-5A). More anteriorly, the anterior inferior cerebellar arteries emanate from the basilar artery to supply blood to the dorsal part of the pons and the anterior inferior part of the cerebellum (Fig. 8-5B). At the pontomesencephalic junction, the superior cerebellar arteries emanate from the basilar artery to supply blood to the dorsal part of the midbrain and most of the convexity of the cerebellum (Fig. 8-5C). The basilar artery itself and the paramedian penetrators that come off the basilar artery supply blood to the ventral and midline parts of the pons and midbrain. At its rostral pole, the basilar artery splits into two posterior cerebral arteries, and thereby forms the back end of the Circle of Willis.

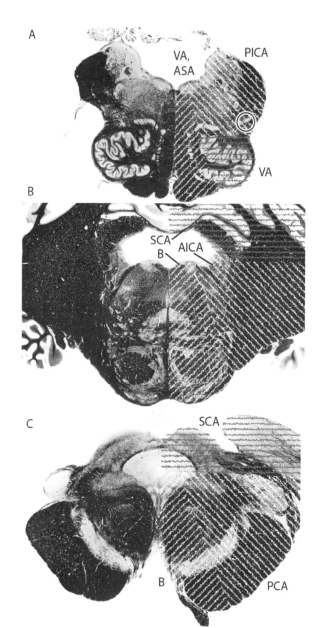

Figure 8-5 The blood supply to the brainstem is supplied by a mixture of at least six prominent arteries. In the medulla (A), the most medial regions receive blood from small offshoots called paramedian penetrators, which come off the anterior spinal (*ASA*) and vertebral (*VA*) arteries. Ventrolaterally, the inferior olive receives blood from the vertebral artery, and the dorsolateral medulla receives blood from the posterior inferior cerebellar artery (*PICA*). The location of the sympathoexcitatory tract from hypothalamus to thoracic sympathetic neurons is marked by a circle on the right, within the territory of the posterior inferior cerebellar artery. Interruption of the tract traveling in the encircled area, as occurs in lateral medullary strokes, produces an ipsilateral Horner syndrome. The most medial portions of both the pons (B) and midbrain (C) receive blood from paramedian penetrators arising from the basilar artery (*B*). B: Lateral parts of pons receive blood from the anterior inferior cerebellar artery (*AICA*). Note that the superior cerebellar peduncle, along with most of the convexity of the cerebellum (not shown), receives blood from the superior cerebellar artery (*SCA*). C: Ventrolateral midbrain receives blood from the posterior cerebral artery (*PCA*), whereas dorsal midbrain and caudal parts of thalamus receive blood from the superior cerebellar artery. Photomicrographs reprinted with permission from deArmond S et al., *Structure of the human brain: A photographic atlas.* New York: Oxford University Press, 1989.

THE ANTERIOR CIRCULATION SUPPLIES BLOOD TO THE TELENCEPHALON

The anterior circulation receives oxygenated blood from the internal carotid arteries, which supply 70–80% of the blood volume in the Circle of Willis. Along with the posterior cerebral arteries from the posterior circulation, two additional pairs of cerebral arteries and three communicating arteries comprise the arteries that complete the Circle of Willis:

- A pair of *anterior cerebral arteries (ACA)*

- A pair of *middle cerebral arteries (MCA)*

- One *anterior communicating artery (AComm)*

- A pair of *posterior communicating arteries (PComm)*

The Circle of Willis consists of the ring formed by the three communicating arteries and the proximal sections of the six cerebral arteries (Fig. 8-3A). *A large degree of congenital variability in the Circle of Willis exists across individuals, with up to 75% of the population possessing some variation on the standard circle.*

Each internal carotid splits into anterior and middle cerebral arteries. The two anterior cerebral arteries travel forward and supply the medial face of each cerebral hemisphere (Fig. 8-6). Between the two anterior cerebral arteries, there is the small—actually tiny—anterior communicating artery. The middle cerebral artery dives through the Sylvian fissure to provide blood to most of the convexity of the brain (Fig. 8-6). On the way laterally, it gives off *lenticulostriate arteries* that supply the caudate, putamen, globus pallidus, and posterior limb of the internal capsule. Since the corticospinal tract travels in the posterior limb of the internal capsule, it is useful to remember that the source of blood and oxygen for this structure is the stem of the middle cerebral artery. Upon reaching the Sylvian fissure, the middle cerebral artery splits into inferior and superior divisions supplying the temporal lobe and parietal lobe convexity, respectively. The posterior cerebral arteries provide

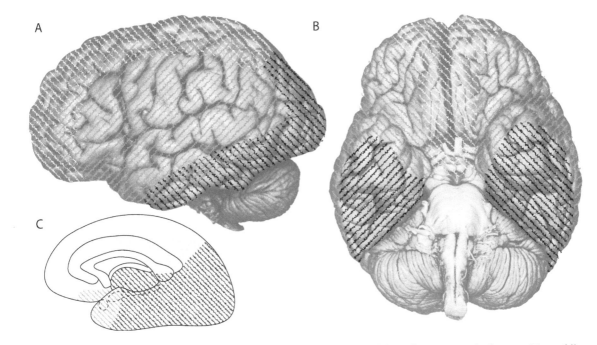

Figure 8-6 A–C: The blood supply to the forebrain derives principally from the anterior, middle, and posterior cerebral arteries. The middle cerebral artery (*blue lines*) supplies the largest territory, including most of the cerebral convexity (A). The anterior cerebral artery (*yellow lines*) supplies blood to most of the medial surface of the brain, all except the most posterior regions (C). The posterior cerebral artery (*black lines*) supplies blood to the caudal portions of the brain and to the ventrum of the temporal lobe (B). Watershed zones occur where the blood supplies from two cerebral arteries overlap, as occurs extensively on the cerebral convexity (A). In the event of hypotension, a sensory and motor loss in the trunk and proximal limbs results from lack of perfusion in the watershed zone between the anterior and middle cerebral arteries. This causes the so-called "man in the barrel" syndrome. Loss of perfusion in the watershed zone between the middle and posterior cerebral arteries produces a deficit in the contralateral visual field. As it travels laterally, the middle cerebral artery gives off small tributaries, the lenticulostriate arteries, which supply blood to the striatum and posterior limb of the internal capsule. This is important because the posterior limb of the internal capsule carries the corticospinal tract, with arms represented most anteriorly and legs most posteriorly. Upon reaching the Sylvian fissure, the middle cerebral artery splits into two divisions. The inferior division supplies the temporal lobe, whereas the superior division supplies the parietal and frontal convexities.   Photographs in A and B reprinted by permission of deArmond S et al., *Structure of the human brain: A photographic atlas.* New York: Oxford University Press, 1989.

blood to the ventral temporal lobe and the occipital lobe, including visual cortex (Fig. 8-6).

Anastomoses are interconnections between capillaries arising from different parent arteries. Networks of anastomoses exist on the convexity of the brain at the junctions of the anterior and middle cerebral arteries and of the middle and posterior cerebral arteries (Fig. 8-6). The region of brain supplied with blood by an anastomosis is termed a *watershed zone*. Since watershed zones receive blood from two major arterial systems, one can compensate for the other in cases of blockage.

In sensorimotor cortex, the representations of proximal leg, trunk, and proximal arm muscles fall within the watershed zone between the middle and anterior cerebral arteries. This is advantageous in that if one artery is occluded, motor cortex serving the proximal and trunk musculature is spared from harm because it can derive sufficient blood supply from the other (unaffected) artery. Yet watershed zones have a downside as well. Because anastomoses occur at the terminal ends of arteriolar domains, watershed zones are highly vulnerable to hypoxia consequent to low CBF when blood pressure is low. Thus, during episodes of pronounced hypotension, trunk and proximal limb weakness can occur, producing the *man-in-the-barrel* syndrome.

Small penetrating vessels that arise from major vessels of both the anterior and posterior circulations and do not communicate with any other blood vessels are the opposite of anastomoses. The brain regions supplied by such terminal vessels are referred to as *end zones*. Lenticulostriate arteries are examples of terminal vessels. Since each lenticulostriate end artery supplies only a small region of deep cerebral tissue, the damage that results from a stroke in one such artery occupies only a small area. Such restricted damage is termed *lacunar* (lacunae is the plural).

In *vascular dementia*, the second most common form of dementia among the elderly (Alzheimer's disease is the most common), lacunar strokes accumulate. With each stroke, small though it may be, cognition can degrade. This produces a characteristic step-wise decline in cognition including executive function, memory and recall, psychomotor speed, affective control, and so on. Vascular dementia is most common in older individuals with long-standing hypertension. There is no effective treatment for vascular dementia, and the prognosis is poor.

STROKES ARE THE MOST COMMON NEUROLOGICAL EMERGENCY

The failure of a vessel to deliver blood to the brain is termed a *cerebrovascular accident* or *stroke*. Strokes are very common. They are in fact the most common neurological emergency and the number one neurological cause of death. Most strokes, about 85%, are *ischemic*, meaning that blood flow to a region of brain is interrupted due to the occlusion of a vessel, causing an infarction. The remaining strokes occur when a vessel ruptures, resulting in a *hemorrhage* (i.e., leakage of blood into either the parenchyma or the space surrounding the brain). Regardless of the type, strokes can produce a sudden loss of brain function. It should be noted that not all strokes are symptomatic. *Silent strokes* are infarctions that are discovered through imaging or postmortem study but which are (or were) not associated with symptoms. It appears that silent strokes are quite common, far more frequent than symptomatic strokes. However, definitive information on prevalence and incidence do not exist currently.

Brain tissue left without normal blood flow, either because of vessel occlusion or vessel rupture, dies. In addition, the area around an ischemic stroke, the *penumbra*, is *in danger of dying*. Stroke is a medical emergency, and treatment is aimed at recovering function of as much of the penumbral area as possible. Although stroke results in significant mortality, the good news is that patients who survive show significant improvement over time. It is not unusual, for example, for a person who becomes aphasic and paralyzed on the right side of the body to be able to talk and move, albeit with some subtle deficits, weeks to months later.

A common cause of ischemic strokes is an *embolus*, which is any matter that occludes a blood vessel. The composition of emboli (the plural of embolus) varies. A *thromboembolus* is composed of clotted blood that detaches from a vessel wall where it forms. An embolus may also be composed of material thrown off from an *atheroma* or arthrosclerotic plaque, a pathological collection of cholesterol, cells, and calcium that sticks to the walls of arteries. One of the risks associated with certain broken bones is that fat from the bone marrow may enter the circulation as an embolus and clog small vessels in the brain.

Stroke can also result when an atheroma grows large enough to severely limit or even completely block flow through a cerebral artery. A final common cause of ischemic stroke is the occlusion of small vessels either from very small atheromata (plural form), termed *microatheromata*, or from a process known as *lipohyalinosis*. In lipohyalinosis, the smooth muscle of an arteriole degenerates and is replaced by collagen, which narrows the opening of the arteriole, ultimately leading to thrombosis and occlusion. Whatever the cause of the small-vessel blockage, the result is lacunar damage.

Ultimately, it is a failure of the circulatory system that causes strokes. Hypertension, smoking, diabetes, alcohol abuse, and a lack of exercise all adversely affect cardiovascular health and thereby greatly increase the risk of stroke. Although these risk factors can be ameliorated, additional risk factors, such as atrial fibrillation, are more difficult to address. In any case, odds are that an overweight smoker with diabetes and hypertension who experiences a sudden loss of the use of a limb, slurred speech, the ability to understand and use language, or the like has had a stroke.

Congenital *arteriovenous malformations* or AVMs are abnormal blood vessels where arteries connect directly to veins without intervening capillaries. Often there is a tangled "nest" of arteries and veins. Within AVMs, veins receive flow straight from arteries and therefore are under abnormally high pressures that are beyond their capacity. The vessels in a cerebral AVM become thin-walled and brittle over time and may rupture, producing a hemorrhagic stroke. Alternatively, an AVM may never rupture even in a person who lives into their 9th or 10th decade.

Chronic hypertension also places cerebral blood vessels at risk for rupture. At branch points, where cerebral arteries divide or join together, blood flow is particularly turbulent. The vessel wall may be especially thin in some individuals due to either a genetic predisposition or to trauma. Where the arterial wall thins, typically at branch points, outpouchings called *aneurysms* frequently develop. The most common aneurysm in the brain is a *berry*, or *saccular*, aneurysm. Berry aneurysms are so named because they are a round sack attached to the artery by a thin stem. Aneurysms are typically asymptomatic and most (~90%) are discovered incidentally during imaging for an unrelated symptom. However, if an aneurysm grows large enough, it can compress neighboring structures. Also problematic is that aneurysms can rupture. The resulting gush of blood produces an explosive headache and an often-fatal increase in ICP. Under the best of circumstances, an aneurysm stays small and causes no problem, whereas under the worst of circumstances, an aneurysm ruptures, leading to an intracranial hemorrhage and either death or severe disability.

Many aneurysms, once identified, can be treated with either an endovascular coil placed within the sac of the aneurysm or a clip placed on the outside, at the base of the aneurysm. Nowadays, endovascular coiling is the most common treatment because introducing an endovascular coil can be done through a vascular catheter and is therefore a minimally invasive procedure (Fig. 8-7). Placing a coil inside the aneurysm neck promotes clotting in the stem and prevents blood from entering the weak sacular portion of the aneurysm. Without the pressure provided by blood entering the aneurysm, there is no opportunity for rupture. However, the size and shape of some aneurysms do not lend themselves to being coiled. In these cases, the only possible intervention is the old-fashioned approach of intracranial surgery, during which a clip is placed on the outside of the aneurysm stem, thereby closing it off.

Neither clipping nor coiling an aneurysm is without risks. The decision to undergo intracranial surgery is a particularly difficult one to make. Of course, a nontrivial proportion (a few percent) of patients die during the invasive surgical procedure needed to clip an aneurysm. Avoiding this risk is attractive since, for many aneurysms, there is only

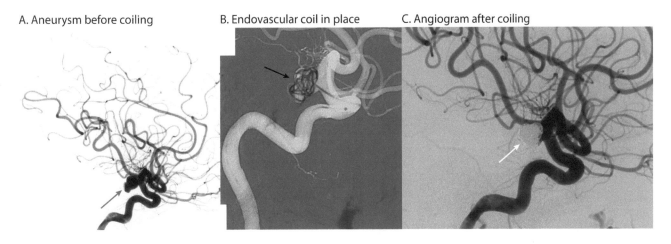

A. Aneurysm before coiling   B. Endovascular coil in place   C. Angiogram after coiling

Figure 8-7 An endovascular coil fills up a berry aneurysm, greatly reducing the risk of rupture. A: An angiogram taken prior to the coiling procedure shows an aneurysm (*red arrow*) in the left posterior communicating artery. B–C: After a coil (*black arrow* in B) is threaded into the aneurysm sac, arterial blood (and contrast) no longer has access to the weak walled aneurysm (*white arrow* in C). Even with the high image sensitivity used in the angiogram in C (compared to A), only the faintest outline of the empty aneurysm is apparent. Regions with patient-identifying material have been removed. Anterior is to the right and dorsal is at top.   Photographs kindly provided by Seon-Kyu Lee, MD, PhD, University of Chicago.

a minute chance (<1%) of rupture each year. (Note that the risk of rupture increases with increasing aneurysm size and reaches an annual rate of more than 50% for the largest aneurysms.) If an aneurysm does rupture, the chances of survival are about even with the chance of death within the first month; those who survive an aneurysm bleed are typically moderately to severely disabled. To add even more complexity to a patient's decision regarding surgery, consider the distress of living with a potentially ticking time bomb within one's head. For a riveting account of the physician's role in guiding patients to make the right decisions for themselves, as well as the operating room tension inherent in an aneurysm-clipping procedure, see *Do No Harm* by Henry Marsh, a British neurosurgeon.

The treatment of a stroke patient is two-pronged because, although the cause of stroke is a cardiovascular concern, the consequences are entirely neurological. Treatment aimed at the cardiovascular system requires an understanding of the cause of a stroke. Unfortunately, there is no fast or nontechnological way to assess the cause of a stroke; the only definitive way to determine whether a stroke is ischemic or hemorrhagic is to obtain an image such as a computed tomography (CT) scan. Knowing the type of stroke is important because, for example, drugs such as tissue plasminogen activator, which breaks down blood clots, may restore blood flow in the case of certain types of ischemic stroke but obviously are ill-advised in the treatment of hemorrhagic stroke. Rehabilitative treatment for the neurological consequences of a stroke is tailored to the particular deficits experienced by each individual.

Because stroke is the number one neurological cause of death, hospitalization, and serious illness, it is critical to understand both the cardiovascular and neurological contributions to this devastating and pervasive problem. Many if not most readers probably already know a friend or loved one who has experienced a stroke. Unfortunately, the chance of going through life without knowing someone—patient, friend, family member, or coworker—who has suffered a stroke is close to nil.

BRAINSTEM STROKES PRODUCE STEREOTYPICAL SYNDROMES

Understanding the neurological symptoms that will result from damage in different regions of the CNS is an excellent review of neuroanatomy. The reader who is able to predict the deficits that occur after damage to a defined area is one who successfully grasps the essentials of neuroanatomy.

The most common brainstem strokes, *Wallenberg syndrome* and *medial pontine strokes*, are in fact relatively rare, with each accounting for less than 10% of all strokes. In Wallenberg syndrome, also known as *lateral medullary syndrome*, the most common symptoms result from damage to the most superficially placed structures in the lateral medulla. Before reading on, try to use your knowledge of brainstem anatomy to predict the symptoms and signs that will result. In the medulla, what tracts are present most laterally? What nuclei are present laterally? What symptoms would you predict from damage to these structures? If you need hints, look back at Chapter 6.

Now, here are the answers. The structures most commonly damaged and the symptoms produced by that damage are:

- *Nucleus ambiguus*, leading to dysphagia, dysarthria, and hoarseness

- The *restiform body* or *spinocerebellar tracts* en route to the restiform body, leading to cerebellar symptoms such as ipsilateral ataxia, dysdiadochokinesia, and dysmetria (see Chapter 24)

- The caudal portion of the *spinal trigeminal tract and nucleus*, leading to headache, loss of pain and temperature sensation in the ipsilateral face, and abnormal sensations (paresthesia, dysesthesia, and allodynia)

- The *vestibular nuclei*, leading to vertigo, nausea, and abnormal posture

- The *spinothalamic tract*, leading to loss of pain and temperature sensation in the contralateral body along with abnormal sensations.

A lateral medullary stroke usually also produces ipsilateral ptosis and miosis due to Horner syndrome (see Chapter 4). In this instance, Horner syndrome results not from an interruption of the peripheral pathway from the thoracic cord to the eye but from damage of the excitatory pathway from hypothalamus to preganglionic sympathetic neurons in the thoracic cord (see Fig. 4-7). This excitatory pathway travels in the lateral medulla very near to the spinothalamic tract (Fig. 8-5).

Dysphagia, dysarthria, ataxia, facial and contralateral body analgesia and thermo-anesthesia, along with headache, are the immediate symptoms of the lateral medullary syndrome. Months later, the symptoms may be quite different. Despite a great deal of recovery, several symptoms including severe central pain and allodynia may persist and even worsen for months and years afterward. In this regard, the description of his own experience with a Wallenberg stroke provided by Japanese neurosurgeon Shuji Kamano is invaluable. It serves as a powerful reminder that the ramifications of injury and disease persist and change over time. Furthermore, patients are not as knowledgeable as a neurosurgeon. They may not connect post-stroke symptoms to the stroke event, as Dr. Kamano was able to do, and therefore may not seek help. Persistent follow-up on the part of a physician can stand between resigned acceptance of suffering and receiving help for a symptom that may be treatable.

Medial pontine strokes, typically lacunar in nature, damage the basis pontis, usually on one side. Consequently, the most common symptoms are hemiplegia affecting the control of muscles of the body and lower face contralateral to the site of damage. As a result, people are unable to willfully move their arms or legs, to make purposeful facial expressions, and often have dysarthria. All of these symptoms result from interruptions of the descending corticospinal and corticobulbar tracts. Large pontine strokes that produce locked-in syndrome, described in Chapter 1, are, thankfully, rare.

CEREBRAL STROKES PRODUCE STEREOTYPICAL SYNDROMES

Although strokes affecting the anterior circulation are highly varied, the most common strokes produce classic sets of symptoms. The location of more unusual strokes can be logically deduced from the observed symptoms.

Strokes in the anterior circulation most often occur in the middle cerebral artery or one of its tributaries. A stroke in the middle cerebral artery stem (i.e., before the artery has branched) has numerous severe consequences. Recall that the middle cerebral artery provides blood to most of the brain's convexity. As a result, the following structures can be damaged:

- Primary motor cortex
- Primary sensory cortex
- Optic radiation
- Frontal eye fields

Damage to these four regions produces contralateral hemiplegia, loss of contralateral sensation and sometimes contralateral dysesthesia (typically after a delay), contralateral homonymous hemianopia, and a loss of the ability to willfully look to the contralateral side. In addition, if the stroke occurs in the dominant hemisphere, the left one in most people (see Chapter 16), aphasia will result. A complete stroke of the middle cerebral artery in the nondominant hemisphere may impair prosody (see Chapter 16) and produce contralateral hemispatial neglect (see Chapter 15). Strokes in tributaries of the middle cerebral artery will produce some subset of this damage and respective symptoms. For example, one of the most common strokes involves sudden onset of aphasia and right face and arm paralysis, a constellation of symptoms that is pathognomonic for a stroke in the superior division of the left middle cerebral artery. Lacunar strokes often plague the lenticulostriate arteries, causing contralateral weakness due to interruption of the blood supply to the posterior limb of the internal capsule where corticospinal tract fibers travel.

Strokes in the posterior or anterior cerebral arteries cause more restricted damage because the brain territories supplied are smaller. Often, the only deficit resulting from a posterior cerebral artery stroke is contralateral homonymous hemianopia, an inability to see the contralateral visual field using either eye. Smaller strokes within the posterior cerebral artery territory cause smaller, but always homonymous, visual field deficits. With larger strokes that reach the diencephalic territory supplied by the posterior cerebral artery, pathways to and from the primary somatosensory and motor cortices may be interrupted, impairing contralateral somatosensation and voluntary movement.

Recall that the anterior cerebral artery supplies blood to the medial wall of the frontal and parietal lobes and extends, over the wall, to supply blood to the very dorsal part of the cerebral convexity (Fig. 8-6). Since the legs are represented medially in both somatosensory and motor cortex, a stroke in the anterior cerebral artery causes paralysis of and a loss of sensation from the contralateral feet and legs. Additionally, as large regions of prefrontal cortex receive blood from the anterior cerebral artery, impaired social competence, incontinence, and other behavioral symptoms may also occur.

THE BRAIN IS DIVIDED INTO THREE COMPARTMENTS BY FOLDS OF DURA

The dura and arachnoid, the two outer meninges (or membranes), serve to protect the brain from mechanical trauma by encasing the brain in a fluid-filled sack. The outermost membrane, the dura, is the toughest (dura is Latin for "hard") meningeal membrane (Fig. 8-8). The arachnoid, the middle membrane, adheres tightly to the inside of the cranial dura. Both the dura and arachnoid follow the curvature of the skull rather than the sulci and

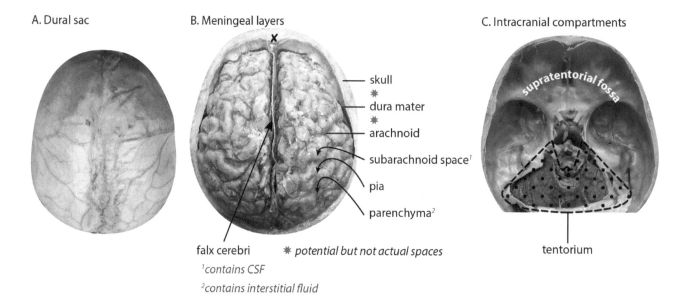

A. Dural sac **B. Meningeal layers** **C. Intracranial compartments**

skull
*
dura mater
*
arachnoid
subarachnoid space¹
pia
parenchyma²

falx cerebri   * *potential but not actual spaces*

¹*contains CSF*

²*contains interstitial fluid*

supratentorial fossa

tentorium

Figure 8-8 Three meningeal layers protect the brain from traumatic injury. A: The dura forms a complete sac around the central nervous system. B: The dura adheres to the skull (although it has detached, postmortem, at the site marked *x*) On its inner surface, the dura adheres to the translucent arachnoid. *Potential* but not *actual* spaces, which only contain fluid under pathological conditions, exist between each of these adhering pairs. The space between the arachnoid and the pia is an actual space, the subarachnoid space, and is filled with cerebrospinal fluid (CSF). The arachnoid includes trabeculae, thin filaments, that link the arachnoid membrane superficially to the pia below. These spidery filaments are the root of the name arachnoid, which derives from the Latin word for "cobweb." The pia adheres to the brain parenchyma. The falx cerebri is a fold of dura that separates the two hemispheres above the corpus callosum. C: With the telencephalon removed, the base of the dural sac is revealed. The area above the tentorium, another fold of dura, is termed the supratentorial fossa. The tentorium and falx form the barriers between the three compartments of the brain: infratentorial fossa, and left and right hemisphere. Both the falx and tentorium are made from folds in the inner layer of the dura; the outer layer of the dura affixes to the inside of the skull bone throughout the cranium.

gyri of the brain. Thus, the overall shape of the outer two meninges essentially forms an endocast of the brain cavity. Between the arachnoid and the brain, the subarachnoid space is filled with CSF (Fig. 8-8A). The arachnoid connects to the pia via gossamer-like trabeculae, or filaments. The pia, the innermost meningeal membrane, borders brain parenchyma.

Beyond providing mechanical protection, the meninges also provide a chemical barrier that prevents large molecules from entering the CNS. The chemical barrier is formed deep to the arachnoid in the innermost meningeal layer, the pia mater. Pia follows every sulcus and gyrus and every bump and crevice in the cerebral surface. Thus, pia is covered by the CSF-filled subarachnoid space and, in turn, pia blankets the brain surface situated deep to it.

The *falx cerebri* and the *tentorium cerebelli*, commonly referred to as simply the falx and the tentorium, serve as intracranial bulkheads that divide the brain into three compartments. The falx forms a divider separating the right and left cerebral hemispheres dorsal to the corpus callosum (Fig. 8-8B). The tentorium, interposed between the occipital cortex and the cerebellum, partitions the cranium into a supratentorial fossa and an infratentorial fossa (Fig. 8-8C). The forebrain is wholly supratentorial, whereas the hindbrain

is infratentorial. The three partitions formed by the falx and tentorium lend some protection to one compartment if pressure builds in a different compartment, akin to the protection formed by bulkheads in a ship's hull. Thus, the tentorium and falx restrict the damage inflicted by a localized mass, trauma, or swelling. Of course, the separation promoted by the falx cerebri and tentorium is insufficient in the face of a large enough mass or a large enough elevation in ICP, either of which can cause a shift in brain tissue through mass effect (Fig. 8-9).

When the falx and tentorium fail to keep ICP from spreading between compartments, *herniation* occurs. Herniation represents a failure of intracranial partitioning due to mass effect. In this context, "mass" refers to any space-occupying entity in the brain: a tumor, blood from a hemorrhage, or simply parenchymal swelling of unknown etiology. If the pressure at one location builds up to such a point that the gross shape of the brain changes, this is termed *mass effect*. The most subtle mass effect is *effacement*, meaning simply a smoothing of the outer cortical surface as the gyri fill in the spaces of the sulci. Far more dramatic examples of mass effect are when brain tissue no longer stays in its proper compartment. In such situations, a piece of the brain herniates or slips into a different compartment.

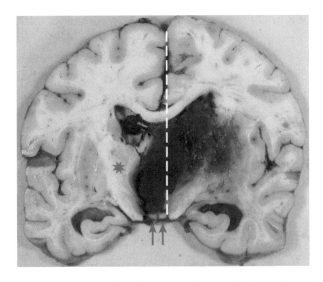

Figure 8-9 A sufficient buildup of intracranial pressure leads to substantial deformation of the brain through mass effect. In this patient, a hemorrhagic stroke led to a shift of subcortical structures deep to the corpus callosum. Some areas even moved across the midline (*dashed white line*). The mammillary bodies, which normally straddle the midline, are both present on the less affected side. The thalamus (*red star*), normally located adjacent to the midline, has moved laterally to a site where the pallidum would ordinarily be situated. The falx, which separates the two hemispheres, effectively prevented a major shift of tissue in the dorsal telencephalon. Photograph kindly provided by Peter Pytel, MD, University of Chicago.

Elevated pressure in the anterior fossa is likely to give rise to confusion and possibly loss of consciousness. Such an elevated pressure may also lead to *uncal herniation* in which the uncus (see Fig. 8-3), the anterior part of the parahippocampus gyrus, slips under the tentorium. Depending on the degree of herniation, the midbrain, third cranial nerve, posterior cerebral artery, and superior cerebellar artery may be compressed. A common sign of uncal herniation is a "blown pupil" (i.e., a pupil that is both dilated and unresponsive to light). This results from the herniated uncus compressing the third nerve as it exits the ventrum of the midbrain. Uncal herniation that is accompanied by a blown pupil is a medical emergency with a poor prognosis.

Additional types of brain herniation may occur on their own or in combination with other types. *Central herniation*, a form of transtentorial herniation like uncal herniation, is marked by parts of forebrain slipping under the tentorium at a site close to the midline. *Tonsillar herniation* is typically caused by increased pressure in the posterior fossa due to a tumor or hematoma. The tonsils of the cerebellum herniate down through the foramen magnum and press against the medulla and spinal cord. This is extremely dangerous because the pressure can interrupt connections critical to breathing and

other critical functions. Finally, the most common form of herniation is subfalcine, in which some portion of the cingulate gyrus slips under the falx. Although not always harmful or even symptomatic when occurring alone, a subfalcine herniation may be a harbinger of more consequential damage.

INTRACRANIAL BLEEDS ARE POTENTIALLY LETHAL

As we traverse from the outside to the inside of the head, we encounter the skull, dura, arachnoid, subarachnoid space filled with CSF, pia, and, finally, brain parenchyma (Fig. 8-10A). Ideally, the only fluid-filled space between skull and parenchyma should be the subarachnoid space interposed between pia and arachnoid, and the only fluid in this space should be CSF. No other spaces between bone and parenchyma *should* exist. All other spaces are *potential spaces*, meaning that they can be, but definitely should *not* be, filled with fluid. *In other words, potential spaces are actual*

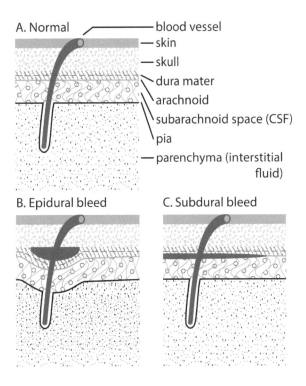

Figure 8-10 The actual and potential spaces in the meninges surrounding the brain. The subarachnoid space is an actual space between the arachnoid and the pia and is filled with cerebrospinal fluid (*CSF*). Blood vessels traverse the meninges and can rupture into the potential spaces either epidurally or subdurally. Epidural bleeds occupy the potential space between the unyielding skull and the dura (B). Subdural bleeds occupy the potential space between the dura and arachnoid (C). These potential spaces should not contain fluid and only do so under pathological conditions.

fluid-filled spaces only under pathological conditions. The two potential spaces are:

- The *epidural space*, sometimes called extradural, is the potential space between the outer layer of the dura and the skull (Fig. 8-10B).

- The *subdural space* is the potential space between the inner layer of the dura and arachnoid (Fig. 8-10C).

Cutting across from bone to pia are blood vessels, arterial and venal, that import oxygen and nutrients to the brain and remove waste products from the brain, respectively (Fig. 8-10A). Arterial vessels arrive from the periphery and penetrate the arachnoid and pia to provide oxygen and nutrients to the parenchyma. Venous blood is collected into sinuses formed by folds of dura and then emptied into the jugular veins that lead back to the heart. As blood travels in and out through the meninges, ripe opportunity exists for blood to accidently leak into one of the potential or actual spaces. Blood leaking out from cerebral vessels, due to trauma or other reasons, is a potentially life-threatening occurrence. When blood hemorrhages within the cranium, it fills any of four spaces:

- *Epidural*: A potential space between the dura and the skull that *should not contain fluid*

- *Subdural*: A potential space between the dura and arachnoid that *should not contain fluid*

- *Subarachnoid*: An actual space, between the arachnoid and pia, that should contain CSF and *not blood*

- *Parenchymal*: Brain tissue that should contain interstitial fluid, a fluid that is not different from CSF, and should definitely *not* contain blood

Hemorrhages, or bleeds, often occur after nonpenetrating traumatic injuries such as a blow to the head. Bleeds can also occur without any obvious precipitating trauma, as when an aneurysm or an AVM bursts or because of medical conditions such as hypertension. The amassed blood or *hematoma* usually causes sudden symptoms, with the patient complaining of a severe headache that arose explosively. The characteristics of bleeds in each of the four spaces listed above are discussed in turn.

An *epidural hematoma* involves blood amassed between the dura and the skull, usually due to a blow to the head (Fig. 8-10B). An epidural hematoma is a serious medical emergency because it typically results in death if not treated by shunting the blood, thereby relieving the elevated ICP.

The onset of symptoms, such as a loss of consciousness, may coincide with the onset of the epidural bleed or may follow a *lucid interval*, a period without symptoms during which blood presumably amasses to a dangerous and symptomatic level.

A *subdural hematoma* is blood amassed between the dura and the arachnoid (Fig. 8-10C). It often follows a traumatic injury but can also occur spontaneously in elderly people. Some small subdural hematomas shrink over time and are not life-threatening. A rupture of bridging veins is thought to be the most common cause of a chronic subdural hematoma. Bridging veins shuttle venous blood from the parenchyma to the dural sinuses. They travel straight out from the brain, like spokes on a wheel, to the dura where the veins are anchored firmly (Fig. 8-11). However, the bridging veins are not well anchored on the brain side. Therefore, when the brain moves within its dural sack, the bridging veins are stretched.

When the brain moves side to side, the falx limits the excursion traveled by the brain and therefore the potential of tearing the bridging veins. However, when the brain moves forward and backward, such as occurs during a whiplash or when a baby is shaken, the bridging veins are in particular danger of breaking. When bridging veins rupture, they usually do so at their thinnest spot, which is between the dura and the arachnoid, producing a subdural hematoma. Babies who are shaken, as occurs in abusive and criminal anger, are

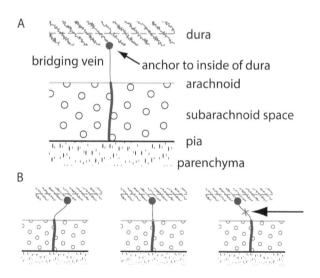

Figure 8-11 A: Bridging veins exit from the parenchyma at a right angle, traverse the arachnoid, and attach firmly (*circle*) to the dura. B: During vigorous shaking, particularly in the anterior-posterior axis, the brain moves within the dural sack. The bridging veins stretch and often break at their thinnest point, between the arachnoid and the dura. Rupture of bridging veins is believed to be the most common cause of subdural hematomas. Note that the space between the dura and arachnoid is microscopic and has been *greatly* exaggerated for illustrative purposes.

at risk of developing acute subdural hematoma, which is an often-fatal medical emergency.

A subdural hematoma caused by rupture of bridging veins often bleeds slowly—remember that venous pressure is low—and may take weeks to become symptomatic. In fact, some proportion of individuals with a subdural hematoma never seeks medical attention either because the hematoma is resorbed or because it never grows large enough to cause symptoms. As we age, our brain shrinks and this stretches the bridging veins, which also become more brittle with age. Consequently, the elderly are at a heightened risk of developing chronic subdural hematomata.

Rupture of an aneurysm or of an AVM and trauma are the most common causes of *subarachnoid hemorrhage*. Blood is released into the subarachnoid space between the arachnoid and pia, a space that should only contain CSF. *Algesic* (pain-evoking) components of blood, such as serotonin, strongly stimulate trigeminal afferents that innervate the vasculature itself, producing a particularly severe and sudden headache that is usually described as the worst ever or the worst imaginable. Typical accompaniments to the headache are neck stiffness and nausea. With time, a subarachnoid hemorrhage compromises an individual's mental status, creating mental confusion, a loss of consciousness, and sometimes death. Thus, subarachnoid hemorrhage is a medical emergency and must be treated immediately. Treatments are directed at preventing more bleeding by, for example, clipping an aneurysm and also at preventing *vasospasm*. Vasospasm refers to a pathological constriction of cerebral vessels that occurs after the vessels have been exposed to blood. It is important to prevent the development of vasospasm in order to avert the ischemia that results from pathologically constricted blood vessels. Even when treatment is attempted, the prognosis for individuals with subarachnoid hemorrhage is often poor.

A *parenchymal hemorrhage* is a bleed into brain tissue that results from trauma or from strokes associated with conditions such as hypertension, a brain tumor, or an AVM. *Intracerebral hemorrhages* are harmful because they kill and injure neurons as well as increasing ICP. The immediate neurological consequences of a cerebral hemorrhage are largely dependent on the location of the bleed and the functions supported by the affected neurons. As with most other intracranial bleeds that increase ICP, a cerebral hemorrhage is a medical emergency. Pharmaceutical treatments are aimed at reducing bleeding and swelling, whereas surgical procedures relieve ICP.

Hopefully, the reader understands the important takehome message: any severe headache or compromise to mental status with a sudden onset should be taken very seriously and treated as a medical emergency until proved otherwise.

EXTERNAL FORCES CAN OVERWHELM DURAL PROTECTION AND HARM THE BRAIN

As you know, the brain floats within a fluid-filled sack formed by the dura, arachnoid, and CSF-filled subarachnoid space. Under ideal circumstances, this arrangement protects the brain from damage caused by external forces. However, strong enough accelerating forces acting on the head overwhelm this protection and cause TBI. Medical imaging cannot be used to gauge the severity of a TBI. Except in the case of injuries that lead to intracranial bleeds, the injured brain does not look different from a normal healthy brain. Instead, assessment of TBI depends on a neurological exam and patient-reported symptoms.

TBI can cause symptoms that range from mild and transient to severe and permanent and, ultimately, in many cases to death. Singular TBIs with immediate and severe consequences—death or permanent impairment—are typically due to a percussive blow or penetrating wound. At the other end of the spectrum, nonpenetrating TBI may cause an impairment of cognitive function that ranges from mild to severe. TBI frequently results in headache, diplopia, nausea, difficulty with balance, mental confusion (such as not knowing one's location), unconsciousness, amnesia, and so on. Over time, additional symptoms such as heightened emotionality, attention deficits, slow recall, and sleep disturbances occur in addition to continued symptoms of headaches, nausea, and dizziness.

The colloquial term for a brain injury is *concussion*, and this term is even used by many in the medical community. The common definition of concussion includes two key elements: (1) caused by a blow to the head and (2) transient symptoms that resolve. Unfortunately, neither of these elements accurately describes TBI. As Sharp and Jenkins argue in a recent review, the term concussion has "no clear definition and no pathological meaning." The term may in fact function as a comforting euphemism that allows people to distance themselves from the realities that they or a loved one has in fact suffered a brain injury.

Direct blows to the head are one major cause of TBI. However, the brain can also be injured, even severely, from blows to the body as well as the head. The force of a blow to the body is communicated via the neck to the head. As the head rapidly accelerates back and forth *without hitting any external object*, the brain moves within its dural sac and can knock into the skull at both ends of its excursion. For example, a whiplash injury suffered from a hit from behind may result in damage to both the frontal and occipital poles of the brain. Traumatic impacts with rotational force tend to produce more severe brain injuries than do linear forces because they typically shear long-distance axonal connections.

The long-term consequences of TBI can be serious. TBIs, even ones that appear mild or are asymptomatic initially, may wreak severe damage after a delay. Repeated incidents of TBI greatly increase the chance of developing *chronic traumatic encephalopathy* or *CTE*, a devastating neurodegenerative tauopathy marked by neurofibrillary tangles (see Chapter 2). CTE is synonymous with the older term *dementia pugilistica*, which was named for its prevalence among former boxers. CTE is more descriptive than the older term and is the only term used today.

Although CTE is not the eventual fate of all who experience head trauma, head trauma is a prerequisite for CTE. And repeated head trauma greatly increases the odds. Accordingly, the prevalence of CTE in former professional players of American football, a "collision sport," may run as high as 95%. Even among high school football players, the prevalence is estimated at about 25%. Among football players, the likelihood of developing CTE appears more related to the number of hits to the head experienced rather than the number of immediately symptomatic TBI events. In other words, the thousands of hits incurred during practice that do not noticeably impair a player are the factor most highly associated with the development of CTE.

Head trauma happens not only during the collision sport of American football, but all the time and to multitudes of people. The causes are varied: a fall, violent assault, cycling accident, head-to-head collision incurred in the course of playing sports such as American soccer, body slamming in ice hockey, and so on. As a consequence, a physician is sure to encounter questions regarding TBI. Most notably, patients and their families want to know the best course of action after an incident of TBI. Current recommendations are based on the immediate consequences of head trauma and not on patients' health in either the medium- (months) or long- (years, decades) term, which remain unknown. It is particularly unclear how head trauma affects the brain of a child or teenager.

To best guide patients after a TBI, we need to know the answers to several open questions. Why do some individuals develop CTE and others do not, despite comparable histories of TBI? What accounts for the variable interval between TBI events and CTE symptoms? When is it safe

for an individual to return to normal activities, such as school or work, following a TBI? When, if ever, is it safe for an individual to return to contact or even collision sports following a TBI? As long as these questions remain unanswered, TBI will present a challenge for physicians who want to provide honest, truthful, and useful information to their patients.

THE BLOOD–BRAIN BARRIER ENSURES A SPECIFIC CHEMICAL ENVIRONMENT FOR THE CNS

The CNS exists in a molecular environment distinct from that of the rest of the body. This distinct environment is maintained by the *blood–brain barrier* (*BBB*), between blood and parenchyma and a *blood–CSF barrier* between blood and the CSF within the ventricles (Fig. 8-12). Arterial blood filtered through the BBB forms the *interstitial fluid* that bathes the brain parenchyma, whereas blood filtered through the choroid plexus becomes CSF. The composition of both interstitial fluid and CSF are different from that of blood and from extracellular fluid in the body. On the other hand, interstitial fluid within the CNS exchanges freely with and *is not different* in composition from the CSF that fills the ventricles and surrounds the brain and spinal cord (Fig. 8-12A). Consequently, *the two barriers—in parenchymal capillaries and in the choroid plexus—are collectively called the blood–brain barrier as I do here.*

Brain endothelial cells line capillaries to form the BBB, which keeps extracellular molecules of certain sizes and characteristics out of the brain. The capillaries where the BBB is actualized are densely distributed throughout the brain so that *virtually every cell has its own private access to a capillary*. It has been estimated that there are 400 miles of capillary in the brain of a mouse!

The lining of peripheral blood vessels is imperfect and leaky, allowing free exchange of blood between vessel and tissue. In contrast, capillaries in the brain and spinal cord are surrounded by unfenestrated endothelial cells that are connected to each other via tight junctions. Unfenestrated simply means that the capillary wall is effectively continuous (without "windows"); no gaps exist between the endothelial cells lining the capillary. Cerebral blood vessels allow free diffusion of gases including oxygen and some small amphiphilic substances access the brain by crossing directly through membranes. However, bacteria, parasites, fungi, white blood cells, red blood cells, platelets, and the like cannot enter the brain. Moreover, molecules beyond about 50 kD in size, including antibodies and many potentially

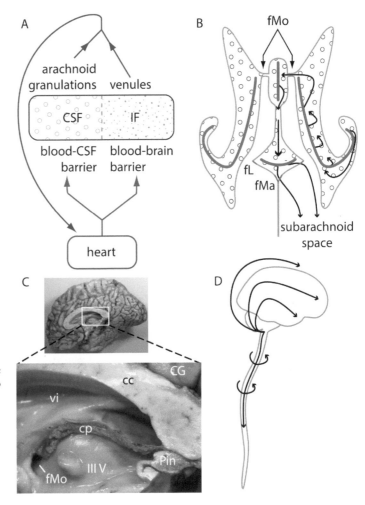

Figure 8-12 Arterial blood from the heart enters the brain parenchyma only after traversing the blood–brain barrier (BBB). Within the parenchyma, blood that has been filtered through unfenestrated endothelial cells becomes the interstitial fluid (*IF*) of the brain. Blood also enters the brain through capillaries in the choroid plexus. The choroid plexus forms a blood–cerebrospinal (*CSF*) barrier. Yet, there is no separation between CSF and brain interstitial fluid and the two barriers are typically referred to as simply the blood–brain barrier. Venules receive the fluid waste of the brain parenchyma, whereas arachnoid villi and granulations transport CSF into dural sinuses. Venous blood then returns to the general circulation. B: Choroid plexus (*red lines*) lines the lateral, third, and fourth ventricles and secretes CSF into the ventricles. CSF then flows (*black arrows*) through the ventricular system. CSF made within the lateral ventricles traverses the foramen of Monro (*fMo*) to reach the third ventricle. CSF leaves the ventricular system through three holes in the fourth ventricle: the bilateral foramina of Luschka (*fL*, only one side is labeled) and the midline foramen of Magendie (*fMa*). Note that this diagram is the same as that in Figure 3-7C, where the parts of the ventricular system are labeled. C: A midsagittal view of the brain shows the third ventricle (*III V*) and the foramen of Monro (*fM V*) that connects it to the lateral ventricle on each side. Also visible are the pineal gland (*Pin*), cingulate gyrus (*CG*), corpus callosum (*cc*), choroid plexus (*cp*), and velum interpositum (*vi*) located above the roof of the third ventricle. The massa intermedia that bridges the two thalami across the third ventricle is visible but not labeled. D: CSF escaping from the back of the fourth ventricle bathes the subarachnoid space surrounding both the brain and spinal cord.

therapeutic drugs, are unable to move from brain capillaries into the parenchyma. *Therefore, central and peripheral chemical environments are largely distinct.*

There are exceptions to the rule that large molecules do not enter the CNS. A small number of molecular transporters carry specific classes of molecules across the vessel wall and into brain. Of particular importance are transporters that bring glucose and various amino acids into the brain. Specific channels allow critical ions access to the CNS. The upshot is that *peripheral blood is filtered into a clear, watery fluid with no cells, very little protein, about 65% of the glucose present in blood, and nearly the same concentrations of ions as blood.* This composition is true of both interstitial fluid and CSF. Yet only CSF is accessible to the physician and therefore our knowledge of the chemical composition inside the CNS during health and disease is entirely based on CSF.

Upon a background of no (or few) cells and little protein, the presence in CSF of white blood cells and protein, including antibodies, indicative of an infection of the brain or meninges, stands out. *Meningitis* is an infection of the meninges, and *encephalitis* is an infection of brain parenchyma. In either case, the CSF of an affected individual will have an abnormal increase in white blood cells. A lumbar puncture is typically used to diagnose meningitis. Whether caused by a bacterium or a virus, meningitis causes a headache, heightened sensitivity to sounds and light, fever, and a characteristically painful and stiff neck.

As the CSF of patients with meningitis and encephalitis proves, cells and antibodies *can* enter the brain. Antibodies also reach the brain in autoimmune encephalitis diseases, stiff-person syndrome, and multiple sclerosis. As discussed in Chapter 2, immune cells including antibody-producing cells enter the brain through the process of *diapedesis*, which essentially means passing through (from Greek: *dia*, "through" and *pedēsis*, "leaping") an endothelial cell barrier. Crossing into the brain is accomplished either by passing between (*paracellular* dipedesis) or through (*transcellular* dipedesis) cells. Tight junctions between epithelial cells that line brain capillaries greatly deter paracellular dipedesis. Therefore, diapedesis in the brain occurs predominantly via the transcellular route.

Under pathological conditions, white blood cells stick to adhesion molecules expressed by endothelial cells and penetrate the endothelial lining. Transcellular diapedesis is upregulated, resulting in far more immune cells accessing the brain and retina. Inflammation resulting from stroke, TBI, or a neurodegenerative disease stretches the spaces between epithelial cells and increases the frequency of paracellular diapedesis. In sum, many brain pathologies are marked by a BBB through which immune cells penetrate. The cause-and-effect relationship between disease and BBB dysfunction is not well established. Thus, it may be that a failure in BBB function is a causal factor in disease. Alternatively, disease progression may cause BBB failure and then in turn be accelerated by the same.

The BBB works both for us and against us. The barrier helps us by keeping out toxins, bacteria, and antibodies against endogenous antigens. Yet, the BBB also keeps out many potentially helpful, therapeutic compounds. Furthermore, a breakdown in the BBB may initiate, accelerate, or contribute to the pathology of a number of neurological disorders including Alzheimer's disease, Parkinson's disease, and multiple sclerosis.

CSF FLOWS THROUGH AND AROUND THE BRAIN AND SPINAL CORD

Cerebrospinal fluid is made at a rate of roughly half of a liter, or 2 cups, per day. Yet only a fraction of the CSF produced is present at any one time. CSF flows through the ventricles and out into the subarachnoid space in a stereotyped fashion before being resorbed (Fig. 8-12). Before following the route of CSF flow, recall that choroid plexus is present in five specific places:

• Roof of the lateral ventricle, bilaterally

• Roof of the third ventricle

• Posterior-lateral region of the fourth ventricle, bilaterally

The cerebral aqueduct has no choroid plexus, and thankfully so because the aqueduct's opening is small and would be certainly be occluded if choroid plexus were present.

Although choroid plexus is found throughout the ventricular system, the bulk of the CSF is made in the lateral ventricles. Consequently, CSF flows out from the lateral ventricles, through the foramina of Monro, to fill the third ventricle (Fig. 8-12B, C). Cerebrospinal fluid

from the lateral ventricles, along with CSF made by choroid plexus in the roof of the third ventricle, then flows caudally through the narrow, Sylvian aqueduct present in the midbrain. As midbrain gives way to hindbrain, CSF flows into the large rhomboid-shaped fourth ventricle. More CSF is made by choroid plexus in the caudal roof of the fourth ventricle. From the fourth ventricle, CSF leaks out to the subarachnoid space surrounding the brain's convexities through three holes—the midline foramen of Magendie and the two laterally located foramina of Luschka. CSF that exits the fourth ventricle flows up and around the convexity of the brain and also flows caudally to surround the spinal cord and spinal roots (Fig. 8-12D). Recall from Chapter 4 that a pool of CSF termed the *lumbar cistern* surrounds the cauda equina and that we can sample CSF through a lumbar puncture at this level of the spinal column.

Hydrocephalus, colloquially referred to as "water on the brain," is any impairment of CSF flow as it moves through the ventricles, into the subarachnoid space, and then out of the cranium. In most cases, an obstruction to CSF flow results in an increase in ventricular CSF and then in ventricular pressure, leading to enlarged ventricles and, ultimately, to an increase in ICP. *Pediatric hydrocephalus*, a relatively common problem, occurs for a number of reasons, such as birth defects that block CSF flow. For example, *Chiari malformations* are a heterogenous group of structural abnormalities that can occlude the flow of CSF out of the fourth ventricle and into the subarachnoid space. Cerebrospinal fluid builds up and, if untreated, affected babies will develop an unusually large head. When hydrocephalus occurs early enough in development, a baby's fontanelles, the soft junctions between cranial bones, may fail to close and bulge out due to the excess ICP. Babies with hydrocephalus fail to thrive, showing lethargy, poor appetite, and vomiting along with a characteristic enlarged head.

Neurosurgeons treat hydrocephalus by inserting a shunt that provides a route for CSF to follow from the ventricles to either the atrium of the heart or the peritoneal cavity. Shunts typically have a valve that permits CSF flow out of the brain when a pressure threshold is exceeded. Patients with many forms of hydrocephalus require life-long shunting. Unfortunately, a shunt can malfunction, become infected, or simply fail, and, when it does, there will be a renewal of the symptoms of hydrocephalus. The frequency of shunt failure is revealed by the fact that only a minority of shunt operations for hydrocephalus represent the first such operation for the patient.

In other words, patients undergo repeated shunt "fix-ups" through their lifetimes.

A single neurosurgical operation is fiscally and logistically difficult to arrange, and circumstances make multiple operations extremely unlikely, particularly in developing countries. Therefore, a preferred approach to hydrocephalus is to perform an endoscopic third ventriculostomy, which means creating a hole between the third ventricle and the subarachnoid space of the interpeduncular cistern, a pool of CSF located between the cerebral peduncles. This procedure has the advantage that no route for foreign material to access the brain and create an infection is introduced.

CIRCUMVENTRICULAR ORGANS ALLOW THE BRAIN ACCESS TO CERTAIN SYSTEMIC SUBSTANCES

In five special CNS regions, capillaries are *fenestrated*, which means that there is an incomplete BBB at these sites. Leaky areas include the posterior or neural pituitary (see Chapter 7) and five *circumventricular organs* (*CVO*):

- Subfornical organ
- Organum vasculosum of the lamina terminalis (OVLT)
- Subcommissural organ
- Median eminence
- Area postrema

Each circumventricular organ serves a particular function that requires access to and monitoring of blood contents. For instance, the subfornical organ monitors the blood levels of *angiotensin*, a liver hormone, in order to maintain homeostatic water balance. The area postrema monitors blood for certain emetic, or vomit-inducing, substances. In response to, for example, hypotonicity, activation of area postrema neurons leads to vomiting. The organum vasculosum of the lamina terminalis monitors blood for fever-producing substances, called *pyrogens*, and engages fever production when pyrogens are detected.

Circumventricular organs are isolated from the rest of the brain by *tanycytes*, ependymal cells that are connected by gap junctions. Thus, even the substances that reach circumventricular organs do not have free access to the brain's extracellular space and thence to the CSF circulation.

BLOOD AND CSF FEED INTO SINUSES EN ROUTE TO VENOUS DRAINAGE OUT OF THE CEREBRUM

Within the brain, interstitial fluid returns to venous blood through capillary venules. Veins collect venous blood from the venules and shuttle it into sinuses via bridging veins that cross the subarachnoid space and flow into the sinuses. The sinuses, pockets formed by folds in the dura, drain into the jugular veins that leave the brain. Within the falx, there are two sinuses: the *superior sagittal sinus* receives blood from the superficial cerebrum, and the *inferior sagittal sinus* captures blood from deeper parts of the cerebrum. For example, blood from the thalamus and basal ganglia drains into the great vein of Galen, which empties into the inferior sagittal sinus, which eventually becomes the straight sinus (Fig. 8-13). The straight sinus drains into the transverse sinus, which continues into the sigmoid sinus and then into the jugular vein. The spot where the superior sagittal, straight, and transverse sinuses come together is termed the *confluence of the sinuses*.

Cerebrospinal fluid is transported from the subarachnoid space directly into sinuses. Minute volumes of CSF are endocytosed by arachnoid prominences termed *villi* when small or *granulations* when larger. *Arachnoid granulations* absorb a vacuole of CSF, transport it across the cell, and release it into a sinus. Within the sinuses, resorbed CSF mixes with venous blood collected through venules. Some proportion of CSF may leak out from the dural sac along with exiting cranial and spinal nerves.

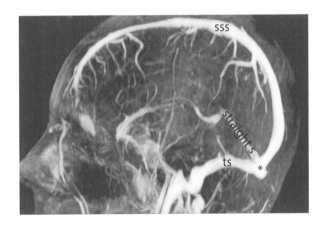

Figure 8-13 This angiogram shows the major sinuses and veins that drain venous blood and cerebrospinal fluid (CSF) from the brain. The asterisk marks the confluence of the sinuses. Abbreviations: straight sinus (*straight s*); superior sagittal sinus (*sss*); transverse sinus (*ts*). Photograph reprinted with permission from Bruni JE, Montemurro D. *Human neuroanatomy: A text, brain atlas, and laboratory dissection guide.* New York: Oxford University Press, 2009.

THE DURA OF THE SPINAL CORD DOES NOT ADHERE TO THE VERTEBRAL BONES

The meninges are somewhat differently arranged within the vertebral column compared to inside the cranium. Most notably, the outer layer of dura does not attach to the vertebral bones as it does to the cranium (Fig. 8-14). Instead, there is a layer of fat, termed *epidural fat*, interposed between dura and bone. This epidural space is of great clinical utility because drugs can be administered into the actual epidural space that exists in the spinal column, a delivery venue known as *epidural*. Since the epidural space only exists in the spinal column, all epidurals are spinal epidurals. Epidural drugs, used for pain relief during child birth and medical procedures, are given into the actual space between the vertebral column and the outside layer of the dura surrounding the spinal cord (Fig. 8-14). This space is not present in the cranium since cranial dura affixes directly to the skull periosteum.

Because it is not contained in a rigid casing, the spinal cord is not under pressure, as is the brain. Therefore, perfusion pressure is simple: arterial pressure less venous pressure. Spinal strokes can happen, but fortunately only rarely. The source of blood for the spinal cord arises from a hodgepodge of anastomoses involving the anterior spinal artery and segmental radicular arteries that circle the spinal cord.

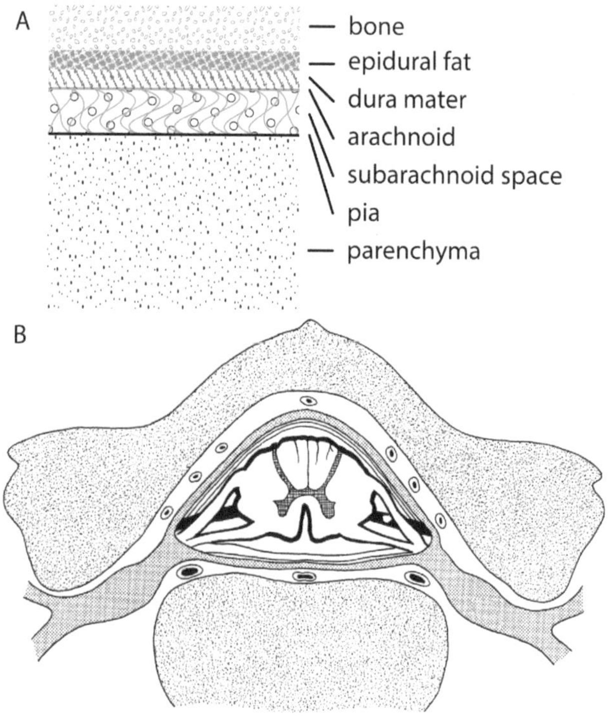

— bone
— epidural fat
— dura mater
— arachnoid
— subarachnoid space
— pia
— parenchyma

Figure 8-14 The meningeal covering of the spinal cord differs from that of the brain in one key way. The dura surrounding the spinal cord does not adhere to the bone of the vertebral column. Instead, a layer of epidural fat is interposed between bone and dura. As a result, the epidural space, which is a potential space in the cranium, is an *actual* space in the spinal cord.   Diagram in B reprinted with permission from Bruni JE, Montemurro D. *Human neuroanatomy: A text, brain atlas, and laboratory dissection guide.* New York: Oxford University Press, 2009.

ADDITIONAL READING

Carman CV. Mechanisms for transcellular diapedesis: Probing and pathfinding by 'invadosome-like protrusions.' *J Cell Sci.* 122: 3025–3035, 2009.

Franco AF. Cerebral autoregulation and syncope. *Prog Cardiovasc Dis.* 50: 49–80, 2007.

Fukuoka T, Takeda H, Dembo T, et al. Clinical review of 37 patients with medullary infarction. *J Stroke Cerebrovasc Dis.* 21: 594–599, 2012.

Greve MW, Zink BJ. Pathophysiology of traumatic brain injury. *Mt Sinai J Med.* 76: 97–104, 2009.

Kamano S. Author's experience of lateral medullary infarction--thermal perception and muscle allodynia. *Pain.* 104: 49–53, 2003.

Kataoka S, Hori A, Shirakawa T, Hirose G. Paramedian pontine infarction. Neurological/topographical correlation. *Stroke.* 28: 809–815, 1997.

Marsh H. *Do No Harm.* New York: Thomas Dunne Books, 2014.

Rekate HL. A contemporary definition and classification of hydrocephalus. *Semin Pediatr Neurol.* 16: 9–15, 2009.

Sharp DJ, Jenkins PO. Concussion is confusing us all. *Pract Neurol.* 15: 172–186, 2015.

UCAS Japan Investigators, Morita A, Kirino T, et al. The natural course of unruptured cerebral aneurysms in a Japanese cohort. *N Engl J Med.* 366: 2474–2482, 2012.

Warf BC. Hydrocephalus in Uganda: The predominance of infectious origin and primary management with endoscopic third ventriculostomy. *J Neurosurg.* 102: 1–15, 2005.

Yamashima T, Friede RL. Why do bridging veins rupture into the virtual subdural space? *J Neurol Neurosurg Psychiatry.* 47: 121–127, 1984.

Zlokovic BV. The blood–brain barrier in health and chronic neurodegenerative disorders. *Neuron* 57: 178–201, 2008.

SECTION 3

NEURAL COMMUNICATION

Perception, action, thoughts, and emotions all require active communication between neurons and either other neurons or peripheral organs. In this section, we examine the varied ways that neurons communicate using electrical and chemical signaling. First, we cover the electrical properties of a single neuron *at rest* that provide the electrochemical basis for all neuronal messages. We then consider how a single neuron integrates multiple messages to come up with one outgoing message that is communicated to a target cell. This communication typically occurs across long distances through the use of patterned sequences of action potentials. Action potentials are then turned into chemical messages through the release of packets of neurotransmitters released upon the arrival of the action potential trigger. This process enables one cell to send a *timed* chemical message to another cell. We also consider how the packets of neurotransmitters are formed and the mechanisms that terminate the actions of neurotransmitters so that every neural message has an end as well as a beginning. Finally, we consider how the binding of neurotransmitters to receptors on target cells is transformed into a received message. Our treatment of neuronal communication takes us full circle, from the integration of inputs to sending a message, and, finally, to receiving that message.

In the end, we stand in awe of the diverse electrochemical and molecular mechanisms that allow neurons to metaphorically whisper or shout, to cover their ears or turn up the volume on headphones.

9

THE NEURON AT REST

eurons communicate with other cells and also between their own near and distant parts by using electrochemical signaling. Here, we describe the electrical properties of the neuron under *resting* conditions. When a neuron is at rest (i.e., it is not firing an action potential), two features dominate the neuron's electrical landscape:

- The resting membrane potential

- Graded synaptic inputs

The resting membrane potential represents the default electrical potential (see Box 9-1 for review of electrical terms) of the neuron in the absence of any inputs. Neurons return again and again to this default, but critical, electrical potential. A failure of neurons to maintain an adequate resting membrane potential results in a complete disruption of function. The second influence on a neuron's membrane potential is synaptic input. In this chapter, we consider subthreshold synaptic inputs that cause graded responses but do not cause a neuron to fire an action potential.

Box 9-1 **MOST ELECTRICAL TERMS ARE EASILY CONCEPTUALIZED BY CONSIDERING PLUMBING ANALOGIES**

The meaning of most electrical terms can be visualized using a water analogy. For those needing a brief reminder of fundamental principles and terms of electricity, consider the following analogies:

- *Electrical potential or voltage*: Water at the top of a tall waterfall can fall a long way and thus has a large amount of potential energy. Water on top of a short waterfall has a lower potential. Water in a land-locked lake has no potential and thus represents zero potential or the *ground* state. Note that electrical potential, symbolized as E, and voltage, symbolized as V, are synonymous for our purposes.

- *Current*: The amount of water flowing past a point, in terms of volume per unit of time, represents the current.

- *Charge*: The integrated current over time is charge. In a water analogy, water volume is therefore analogous to charge.

- *Resistance or impedance*: Narrower channels or pipes offer greater resistance to water flow than do wider pipes. For this reason, firefighters use wide hoses rather than garden hoses to put out fires. Higher resistance wires allow less current flow. In neuronal processes, resistance is inversely proportional to the caliber (diameter) of a dendritic or axonal process.

- *Conductance*: The inverse of resistance, conductance is higher in wide, unimpeded channels, such as a firefighter's hose, than in narrow pipes.

- *Capacitance:* There is no good water analogy for capacitance, which relates to how voltage changes over time. As a very rough approximation, consider that water in one lake must fill a bucket before entering a stream. The water will reach the stream *more slowly* if a large intermediary bucket must be filled than if a small one needs to be filled. Thus, the large bucket transfer system has a higher capacitance than does the small bucket one. Capacitance impacts the rate of charge transfer—or water transfer in this case—but does not change the eventual outcome: given enough time, all the lake water will make its way into the stream, regardless of whether it is transferred by a small or large bucket. Although this analogy fails under scrutiny, the important point to remember is that *voltage changes slowly across a high-capacitance membrane and rapidly across a low-capacitance membrane.*

MEMBRANES PREVENT THE FREE DIFFUSION OF CHARGED MOLECULES

As the biological version of a wall, *membranes* are absolutely necessary for life and indeed serve the fundamental role of defining the limits of an organism. Within living beings, membranes separate *cells*, the structural units of life. Membranes that surround cells, including neurons, termed cellular or *plasma membranes*, separate the inside of a cell, the *intracellular compartment*, from the outside or *extracellular space*.

Glycerophospholipids are the main constituents of biological membranes. Glycerophospholipids possess one hydrophilic, or water-friendly, head and two hydrophobic, or water-repelling, tails (Fig. 9-1A). In biological membranes, two layers of lipids are arranged in a tail-to-tail fashion, termed a *bilayer*, with the hydrophobic tails intermingling (Fig. 9-1B). The hydrophilic heads of the lipids face either the extracellular space or the intracellular cytosol. The action of specific enzymes, including *flippases* and *scramblases*, can alter the composition of the inner and outer leaflets, or layers, so that different lipids predominate in the inner leaflet (the one bordering the cytosol) and the outer leaflet (bordering the extracellular space).

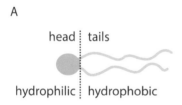

A

head ⋮ tails

hydrophilic ⋮ hydrophobic

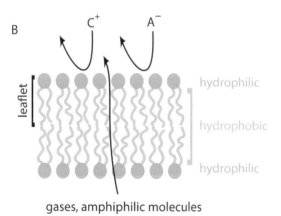

B

C^+ A^-

leaflet

hydrophilic

hydrophobic

hydrophilic

gases, amphiphilic molecules

Figure 9-1 A: The lipids that make up biological membranes, primarily glycerophospholipids, have a hydrophilic head and two hydrophobic tails. Two layers of tail-to-tail aligned lipids form a bilayer, so that a wide hydrophobic core is bounded on either side by shallow hydrophilic borders. B: Flipases and scramblases are membrane enzymes that move lipids between the two layers or leaflets of a biological membrane. As a result, the two leaflets of a plasma membrane typically contain somewhat different lipid compositions (not illustrated). Ultimately, membranes prevent the free diffusion of charged molecules, anions (A^-) and cations (C^+) while allowing gases and amphiphilic molecules, compounds that have both hydrophilic and hydrophobic regions, to freely move between the separated compartments.

The hydrophobic core of biological membranes, formed by lipid tails, repels charged molecules. As a result, charged molecules cannot penetrate the tail region of the lipid bilayer and thus cannot cross the membrane (Fig. 9-1B). *The plasma membrane's hydrophobicity prevents the free diffusion of both large and small charged molecules*; the latter are termed *ions*. In contrast, gases and small amphiphilic substances, such as fats, cholesterol, and—importantly—most *general anesthetics*, diffuse easily through biological membranes.

Although charged molecules cannot move across lipid bilayers, they do move across biological membranes through several specialized routes that extend into both the extracellular and intracellular compartments. The routes are formed by membrane proteins, proteins that are anchored within the membrane and span the bilayer. Typically, multiple protein subunits complex together and extend across the lipid bilayer to provide routes through which ions can cross a lipid bilayer or membrane. Broadly speaking, there are three types of transmembrane or membrane-spanning protein complexes that allow for the movement of ions and/or large molecules across the membrane:

- Ion channels

- Transporters

- Gap junctions

When appropriate conditions occur, ion channels switch from a *closed conformation* to an *open conformation*. The open conformation of an ion channel forms a pore through which ions pass (Fig. 9-2A). The pore is typically *selective*, so that only a particular ion or set of ions, distinguished by size and/or charge, passes through. The formation of the pore is termed *opening the channel*. Channel-opening is triggered or *gated* when the voltage difference across the membrane reaches a certain value (in the case of *voltage-gated channels*) or when a ligand, such as a neurotransmitter, binds to the channel (in the case of *ligand-gated channels*; see later discussion and discussion in Chapter 13). Ligand-gated channels are also called *ionotropic receptors*; the two terms are synonymous. If one thinks of a channel as a door, then *gating* refers to the mechanism that opens that door. Ligand-gated channels are analogous to doors that open with a key, whereas voltage-gated channels can be thought of as swing or pocket doors that open with force.

Unlike channels, transporters never form a pore that stretches from inside to outside the cell. Instead, transporters open to either the cytosol or to the extracellular space. Using a variety of mechanisms, transporters transfer molecules across the lipid bilayer membrane. Transporters exist in many varieties, including pumps and exchangers or carriers; they use energy from adenosine triphosphate (ATP) or from an existing electrochemical gradient to move molecules across the membrane without forming a pore (Fig. 9-2B).

Gap junctions are pores that extend between cells. In other words, a gap junction pore stretches from the cytosol of one cell to the cytosol of a closely adjacent cell. Molecules up to a certain size may pass through a gap junction *in either direction* (Fig. 9-2C). In the nervous system, ions, metabolites, and signaling molecules may all pass through gap junctions. The size and characteristics of gap junction channels can be modulated so that, under different circumstances, the same gap junction may pass nothing, only ions, or large signaling molecules as well as ions. Since gap junctions are physical connections, molecules cross from one cell to another virtually instantaneously.

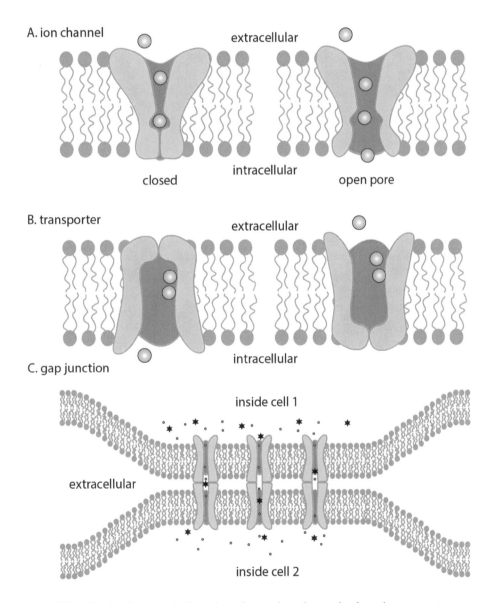

Figure 9-2 Charged molecules (*blue spheres*) only traverse biological membranes through specialized membrane-spanning proteins. An ion channel, a transporter, and a gap junction, three different types of membrane proteins, are shown in cross section. A: Ion channels can be either open or closed. In the closed configuration (*left*), ion channels do not allow ion movement across the membrane. In the open configuration (*right*), ion channels form a pore that allows ions to cross between the cytosol and the extracellular space. B: Transporters move ions and other small molecules across the membrane without ever forming a membrane-spanning pore. There are several different types of molecular transporters, only one of which is illustrated. C: Gap junctions form a conduit between the inside of two different cells (in this case, cell 1 and cell 2) through which a variety of ions (*small dots*) and large molecules (*larger black stars*) can move. At the site of a gap junction, the membranes of the two cells involved are closely juxtaposed, being separated by about 3 nm rather than the normal synaptic gap of 30 nm or so. Complementary membrane proteins, termed *connexins*, in the two cells join to form an actual pore.

All cells have a resting membrane potential that stems from an uneven distribution of charged molecules across the plasma membrane. As with the rest potential of glial, epithelial, muscle, blood, and other types of cells, the potential of a neuron at rest is negative with respect to the extracellular fluid. Yet the value of a neuron's resting membrane potential is of far less importance than are the mechanisms that maintain that potential. To understand why the mechanisms matter so much more than the actual membrane potential, consider a nightclub at two different times: just before opening and just after closing. The inside of the club boasts the same number of workers and the same lack of patrons at both times. However, just after closing, the workers are tired, the liquor depleted, and the line of people outside is gone, whereas at opening, the workers are fresh, supplies replenished, and a long line of energetic people are lined up outside. We could say that the nightclub is in the same empty state at both times but that would not accurately reflect the huge difference between the nightclub at the two times. At opening time, another tick of the clock will usher in a noisy, crowded, vibrant social scene, a scene that is an impossibility after closing time.

Just as the nightclub's circumstances are more important than the number of people in the nightclub, the mechanisms that support the resting membrane potential are more important than the particular millivolt value of the resting membrane potential. These mechanisms possess special significance because they determine *the degree to which a neuron defends its resting membrane potential even in the face of inputs that cause deviations.* The ease with which inputs can or cannot activate a cell is termed *excitability.* Cells that deviate easily from rest potential can reach the threshold for an action potential quickly and thus are highly excitable, whereas those that deviate briefly and rarely from rest, nearly always returning quickly to the resting membrane potential, are far less excitable. *Two neurons with the same rest potential, supported by different electrochemical mechanisms, may have very different levels of excitability.* For this reason, it is important to not only remember that the resting membrane potential of most neurons is −60 to −70 mV but also to understand the electrochemical forces contributing to that rest potential, our task in this chapter.

Only three species, or types, of ions move across the neuronal membrane at rest. These ions include two positively charged ions, or cations, potassium (K^+) and sodium (Na^+), and one small anion, chloride (Cl^-). Each of these ions is differentially distributed across the membrane of a neuron, with potassium ions more prevalent inside the cell and sodium and chloride ions more prevalent outside. When a cell is at rest, each ionic species exists in steady state, with the same number of ions leaving the cell as entering it. Before considering how all three ions arrive at steady state, we consider how just one ionic species, K^+, reaches electrochemical equilibrium.

Potassium ions exist at a much higher concentration inside the mammalian neuron (155 mM) than outside (5 mM) so that a chemical driving force pushes potassium ions outward (Fig. 9-3). However, since neurons are negative with respect to ground, electric forces attract potassium ions inward. Thus, chemical and electrical driving forces oppose one another, with the electrical driving force pushing potassium ions to the negative side, which is the intracellular side of the membrane, and chemical forces pushing

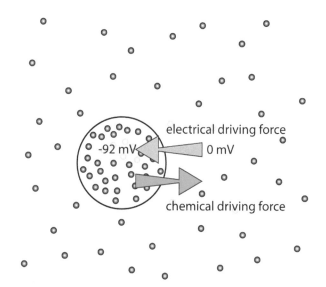

Figure 9-3 The steady-state potential, where there is no net flux of ions (*spheres*), occurs at the potential where the chemical (*outward arrow*) and electrical (*inward arrow*) forces exerted on any given ionic species are equal and opposite. In the case of potassium ions, the ionic concentration inside cells is roughly 30-fold higher than that in the extracellular fluid. Therefore, chemical forces push potassium ions out. Since cells are negative with respect to ground, electrical forces push the positively charged potassium ions in. If we consider potassium ions exclusively, the steady state potential predicted by the Nernst equation is about −92 mV.

potassium ions to the extracellular side where the potassium ion concentration is lower.

At steady state, the chemical and electrical driving forces exerted on potassium ions are equal but opposite (Fig. 9-3). The electrical potential (E), where the chemical and electrical forces on any given ionic species, X, are exactly opposing is given by the *Nernst equation*. By calculating the value of a term encompassing several constants at human body temperature, the Nernst equation can be simplified to:

$$E_X = 62 * z * \log \frac{[X]_0}{[X]_i}$$

where $[X]_0$ and $[X]_i$ are the extracellular and cytosolic concentrations of the ionic species in question. The term z refers to the valence of the ionic species. For potassium ions and other monovalent cations, the valence is $+1$, and, for monovalent anions such as the chloride ion, $z = -1$. This brings us to an expression of the Nernst equation for potassium ions:

$$E_K = 62 * (+1) * \log \frac{[K]_0}{[K]_i}$$

where $[K]_0$ and $[K]_i$ are the extracellular and intracellular concentrations of potassium ions. If we plug in physiological values for $[K]_0$ and $[K]_i$, 5 and 155 mM, respectively, we can solve the Nernst equation for potassium ions:

$$E_K = -92 \, \text{mV}$$

Thus, when the neuron is at a potential of -92 mV, the Nernst potential for potassium ions—the electrochemical gradient for potassium ions—is at steady state, with the same number of potassium ions leaving as entering the cell.

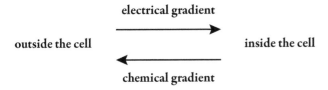

Furthermore, if an outside current perturbs the cell's membrane potential, taking it away from -92 mV, the cell will, in short order, return back to -92 mV. For example, if one injected negative current into a cell so that the membrane potential reached -100 mV, the excess electrical gradient, opposed by an unchanged chemical gradient, would now *drive* potassium ions into the cell:

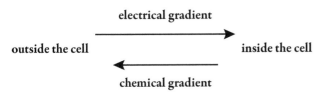

until the cell's membrane potential returned to the E_K value of -92 mV.

Let us now use our understanding of the rest potential to predict the consequences of an elevation in extracellular potassium ion concentration on neuronal membrane potential. An elevation of the potassium ion concentration in blood, termed *hyperkalemia*, produces a similar elevation in the extracellular fluid, including within the central nervous system (CNS). Kidney failure, certain congenital conditions, or a number of drugs can cause hyperkalemia. Elevation of the extracellular potassium ion concentration has one critical consequence. It decreases the chemical gradient. Note that the electrical gradient does not change. The decrease in the chemical gradient results in more potassium ions entering than leaving the cell:

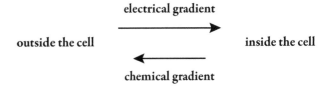

until a new steady state potential is reached. As earlier, more potassium ions would enter than leave the cell until the electrical and chemical gradients once again were exactly opposite.

A higher than normal extracellular potassium ion concentration, as occurs in hyperkalemia, changes the Nernst potential for potassium ions, E_K, in this case to a more positive value than -92 mV. For example, if $[K]_0$ were raised from a normal value of 5 mM (range of normal values is 3.5–5.0 mM) to 7 mM, the new Nernst potential for K^+ would be -83 mV. The dominant clinical concern in hyperkalemia is cardiac related, as will become clear in the next chapter.

FROM REST POTENTIAL TO EXCITABILITY

Recall that the mechanisms that produce a neuron's rest potential are more important than the actual value of that potential. To understand this, let's consider the effect of a perturbation in membrane potential, as would be caused by a synaptic input. For now, we remain concerned with a cell that is permeable only to potassium ions and therefore "sits" at E_K at rest. If synaptic input moves the membrane potential away from rest, what will the cell's electrochemical response be? Two concepts guide us:

• The *driving force* is proportional to the difference between the membrane potential (V_m) and the Nernst potential ($V_m - E_X$). In the case of potassium ions, the further away from E_K that the membrane potential deviates, the more driving force ($V_m - E_K$) exists to redistribute potassium ions until V_m returns to E_K.

- The *reversal potential* is the membrane potential, where the driving force equals zero. In our example, where we are only concerned with potassium ions, the reversal potential is E_K or −92 mV, the potential where $V_m - E_K = 0$. Above the reversal potential, potassium ions leave the cell, and below the reversal potential, the net flow of potassium ions reverses, so that potassium enters the cell. Thus, when the membrane potential is more polarized (from ground), or *hyperpolarized*, than −92 mV, potassium ions enter the cell; when the membrane potential is less polarized, or *depolarized*, than −92 mV, potassium ions leave the cell.

The driving force concept tells us that deviating from E_K by 5 mV will elicit a larger and faster response than will deviating by only half of a millivolt. Because of the reversal potential, potassium ions will move across the membrane in opposite directions depending on whether the membrane potential is perturbed above or below E_K. Using these two principles, we can predict the so-called passive responses of a cell, which are any responses that do not involve an action potential. However, there is a catch. The preceding only holds when potassium ions are the exclusive ionic species that crosses the membrane at rest, as is true of astrocytes and cardiac muscle cells. However, as we shall see in the next section, neurons at rest are permeable to sodium and chloride ions as well as to potassium ions. To understand the neuronal resting potential, we must take into account all three ionic species with permeability.

THREE IONIC SPECIES CONTRIBUTE TO THE NEURONAL RESTING MEMBRANE POTENTIAL

Ionic permeability occurs when at least a portion of the ion channels that pass a particular ionic species are open. The ion channels that concern us here are those that are gated by voltage. The probability that a voltage-gated ion channel is open depends on the membrane potential. Only ion channels that open at rest potentials contribute to the resting membrane potential. For example, ion channels that allow potassium ions to pass have a high probability of opening at the astrocytic resting membrane potential. In contrast, there is no chance that ion channels that allow sodium ions to pass

will open at the resting membrane potential of an astrocyte. Thus, potassium ions contribute to the resting membrane potential of an astrocyte, and sodium ions do not.

The situation is different in a typical neuron. In addition to channels permeable to potassium ions, channels permeable to sodium and chloride ions may also open at rest potential. Thus, the resting membrane potential, the default potential of a cell, depends on two factors:

- *The ionic species to which a neuronal membrane is permeable at rest*: Permeability depends not only on the presence of ion channels through which an ion can pass but also on the conformation of the ion channel. As an analogy, there may be many doors into a nightclub, but if they are all locked and thus impermeable, then no one gains entrance.

- *The concentrations of the permeant ions on the two sides of the membrane*: Obviously if it is 8 A.M. and no one is waiting to get into the nightclub, it does not matter whether the doors are locked or open.

As mentioned earlier, three ionic species—potassium, chloride, and sodium—permeate neuronal membranes at rest. We already know that $E_K = -92$ mV. Given the distribution of chloride and sodium ions, we can calculate E_{Cl} and E_{Na} as follows:

$$E_{Cl} = 62 * (-1) * \log \frac{[Cl]_0}{[Cl]_i} = -62 * \log \frac{100}{7} - 71 \, mV$$

and

$$E_{Na} = 62 * (+1) * \log \frac{[Na]_0}{[Na]_i} = 62 * \log \frac{145}{12} = 67 \, mV$$

Clearly, neuronal resting membrane potentials of −50 to −70 mV must be more influenced by the negatively valued E_K and E_{Cl} than by the positively valued E_{Na}. To quantify the relative contributions of each ionic species on steady-state membrane potential, we use the *Goldman-Hodgkin-Katz* (or *GHK*) *equation*. The GHK equation weights the contributions of each ion's equilibrium (Nernst) potential by the membrane's permeability for that ion. As with the Nernst equation, we simplify the GHK equation by calculating the constant terms at human body temperature:

$$V_m = 62 * \log \frac{(P_k * [K]_0 + P_{Na} * [Na]_0 + [P_{Cl}] * [Cl]_i)}{(P_k * [K]_i + P_{Na} * [Na]_i + [P_{Cl}] * [Cl]_0)}$$

where P_K, P_{Cl}, and P_{Na} are the relative permeabilities for each ionic species in a neuron at rest. Like astrocytes, neurons are most permeable to potassium ions at rest. We therefore set P_K to 1.0 and then express the permeabilities of sodium and chloride ions relative to P_K. The most definitively established resting permeability values come from experiments using a very large axon found in the squid. For the squid giant axon, the permeabilities of potassium, chloride, and sodium ions are:

$$P_K = 1.00$$
$$P_{Cl} = 0.45$$
$$P_{Na} = 0.04$$

Another way to view this is that potassium ions carry 60–70% of the current in a typical resting neuron, chloride ions carry 25–35%, and sodium ions carry only about 3–4% of the current. The influence of sodium ions on the resting potential is substantial despite the relatively low permeability of sodium ions at rest. This is because of the very large driving force that results from the positive Nernst potential for sodium ions (+67 mV).

If we use ion permeabilities from the squid giant axon along with ion concentrations observed in mammalian neurons, we can use the GHK equation to calculate the resting membrane potential as:

$$V_m = 62 * \log \frac{((1)*(5)+(0.04)*(145)+(0.45)*(7))}{((1)*(155)+(0.04)*(12)+(0.45)*(100))}$$
$$= 62 * \log \frac{(5+6+3)}{(155+0+45)}$$
$$= -72\,mV$$

The GHK equation quantifies the reality that *the equilibrium potential of any ionic species only influences a cell's membrane potential to the extent that the cell is permeable to that ionic species*. The number, selectivity, and conformational state of ion channels limit the movement of ions across the cell membrane just as the number, type, and state of doors limit access to a room. A cat door lets cats in and out but not large dogs or people; bats and birds can fly in through windows but cats cannot. Each ion channel is permeable to some ions and not to others. Potassium ions contribute the most to the resting membrane potential because of the high permeability to potassium ions at rest.

To appreciate how the membrane potential of a neuron, dependent on three ionic species, differs from that of a cell that is only permeable to one ionic species at rest, let us return to hyperkalemia. In astrocytes and cardiac muscle cells, potassium ions are the only game in town, so to speak. In such cells, raising $[K]_o$ from 5 to 7 mM results in a resting membrane potential that is depolarized by 9 mV. Now consider a neuron. In a neuron, potassium ions contribute hugely to the membrane potential, but they are not the only contribution. Therefore, we expect that the effect of hyperkalemia on neuronal resting membrane potentials will be tempered by the contributions of other ions. Indeed, the same change in $[K]_o$ that would be expected to depolarize a cardiac muscle cell (or astrocyte) by 9 mV will depolarize a neuron by less than 4 mV.

The relative permeabilities of chloride and sodium ions in mammalian neurons are likely to be close to these values. The relative ion permeabilities of potassium, sodium, and chloride ions—P_K greater than P_{Cl}, which in turn is far greater than P_{Na}—are the same in human neurons as in the well-studied squid axon. Yet, the absolute values of these permeabilities surely do not hold for every mammalian neuron. What consequence would different values in P_{Cl} or P_{Na} have for the rest potential?

- The calculated rest potential, −72 mV, is very close to our calculated E_{Cl} of −71 mV. Therefore, changing P_{Cl}, even by a large amount, will not shift the GHK equation-calculated rest potential by much, if at all. This holds as long as chloride ions are far more concentrated outside than inside the cell, a condition which is itself modified under certain circumstances (see later discussion).

- Even very small changes in the relative resting permeability to sodium ions can substantially alter the calculated rest potential. This conclusion follows from the large driving force, calculated as the difference between the positively valued E_{Na} and the negative rest potential.

In truth, the rest potential of mammalian neurons varies from about −70 mV, close to our calculated value, to about −50 mV. A rest potential substantially more depolarized than our GHK equation-calculated potential may result from a greater permeability to sodium ions, additional minor permeabilities such as one to calcium ions, or from changes in the chloride ion distribution across the membrane that in turn result in a more depolarized E_{Cl}.

The movement of only about 1/1000th of 1% of all the free ions in the cell is needed to maintain the resting membrane potential of a typical neuron. Yet, over extended time, if ions followed their electrochemical gradients, the intracellular concentration of potassium ions would decrease and the intracellular concentration of sodium ions would increase. To counteract these changes, the cell continuously and at considerable cost pumps out sodium ions while pumping in potassium ions. The Na$^+$/K$^+$ ATPase is a pump, a type of ion transporter that requires the hydrolysis of one ATP molecule in order to pump three sodium ions out and two potassium ions in. Because more sodium ions leave the cell than potassium ions enter, the Na$^+$/K$^+$ ATPase is *electrogenic* (i.e., it generates a current), in this case an outward current, or net positive movement to the extracellular side of the cell (Fig. 9-4). The outward current resulting from the Na$^+$/K$^+$ pump hyperpolarizes the resting membrane potential by roughly 5 mV in a typical neuron.

Blocking the ATPase pump is toxic, and, at sufficient doses, drugs that do so are lethal. Two such drugs are *ouabain* and *digitalis*, also called *digoxin*. The initial result of blocking Na$^+$/K$^+$ transport is a depolarization of cellular membrane potentials. As with hyperkalemia, ATPase failure depolarizes cardiac muscle cells and can lead to paralysis and *asystole*, or cardiac silence, and thus to death. Alternatively, when the dose is carefully titrated, digitalis can be used to regulate irregular heartbeats. The reasons that depolarization leads to paralysis and asystole will become evident later.

Chloride ions are also transported across the cell membrane by two types of chloride transporters:

- A sodium/potassium/chloride carrier, NKCC, transports chloride ions *into* the cell.

- A potassium/chloride carrier, KCC, transports chloride ions *out* of the cell.

The net result of NKCC and KCC activity is that there are far more chloride ions outside the cell than inside. However, neonates do not express KCC transporters and therefore have a greater internal concentration of chloride ions. The presence of more chloride ions internally produces a shallower chloride gradient and a more positive Nernst potential for chloride ions, E$_{Cl}$. Thus, in the neonate, the rest potential is more depolarized because E$_{Cl}$ is more depolarized.

The resting membrane potential is, of course, more a concept than a reality. Even the least active neurons do not maintain a flat-line membrane potential. Neurons in the CNS are constantly bombarded with synaptic inputs that alter their electrochemical gradients away from steady state. The electrical currents consequent to synaptic inputs are mediated by either the opening or closing of ion channels. By altering the conformation of ion channels, synaptic inputs generate synaptic currents. Synaptic inputs that result in the closing or opening of channels also alter the *input resistance*, or total resistance across the membrane, of a neuron. Thus, synaptic inputs may change the ionic current that flows across the membrane while also changing the membrane resistance.

Synaptic inputs that alter the ionic current or flux across a cell membrane will alter the membrane potential. Currents that lead to a more positive membrane potential are termed *inward currents* and those that hyperpolarize a cell are termed *outward currents* (Fig. 9-4). Neurons use two different mechanisms to achieve inward and outward currents. First, increasing or decreasing the *efflux* of potassium ions from a cell by opening or closing potassium channels

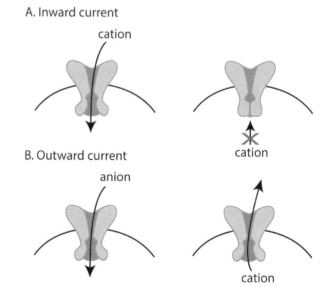

A. Inward current

cation

B. Outward current

anion

cation

cation

Figure 9-4 A: Inward currents make the inside of the cell more positive. Most typically, they arise from a net influx of cations, typically sodium and/or calcium ions or from a *reduction* (*red X*) in the ongoing efflux of cations, typically potassium ions. B: Most outward currents, which make the inside of the cell more negative, arise from the influx of anions, typically chloride ions, or an increase in the efflux of cations, typically potassium ions.

produces outward or inward currents, respectively. Second, an *influx* of anions or cations produces outward and inward currents, respectively. The anion that produces an outward current is a chloride ion. Inward currents can be carried by cations, such as sodium or calcium ions, entering the cell. Nonspecific cation channels, which allow sodium ions to pass into the cell and potassium ions to leave the cell, have a reversal potential of about 0 mV. Thus, opening a nonspecific cation channel produces an inward current.

Synaptic input affects a neuron's excitability through changes in the input resistance as well as through changes in membrane potential. To understand how changes in input resistance affect the excitability of a neuron, we recall Ohm's Law from basic physics:

$$V = I*R$$

where V is voltage, I is current, and R is resistance. In the case of a neuron responding to a synaptic input, the change in voltage (V) elicited by a synaptic input will equal the synaptic current (I) multiplied by the input resistance (R). Thus, a synaptic current is less effective in changing membrane potential when membrane resistance is low. Conversely, when membrane resistance is increased, as occurs when channels are closed, a synaptic current is more effective in changing membrane potential. As a consequence, one must know whether input resistance increases or decreases—as well as knowing whether the input elicits an inward or outward current—in order to predict the effect of a given synaptic input.

Consider the consequences of closing potassium channels open at rest:

- An inward current

- An increase in input resistance

The inward current results from a decrease in the outward flux of positively charged potassium ions, which will have the effect of accumulating positive charges inside the cell and thus depolarizing the cell. The increase in input resistance follows simply from the *closing* of the potassium channels. Together, the increase in input resistance and the inward current powerfully depolarize a cell and make it more excitable as well.

Broadly speaking, we can divide inputs from chemical synapses into two categories:

- Excitatory synaptic inputs make it more likely that a neuron will fire an action potential. These inputs typically elicit an inward current that depolarizes the

neuron. Although excitatory inputs that cause an inward current through an increase in cation influx necessarily decrease input resistance as a result of opening the cation channels, the excitatory effect of the inward current outweighs the inhibitory effect of the drop in resistance.

- Inhibitory synaptic inputs make it less likely that a neuron will fire an action potential. Inputs that elicit an outward current and/or decrease the cell's input resistance make a neuron less likely to fire an action potential.

The most prevalent type of excitatory synaptic input causes a large inward current through a nonspecific cation channel that takes the cell toward the action potential threshold. The most prevalent inhibitory synaptic input results in the opening of a chloride channel. Since E_{Cl} is often more hyperpolarized than the rest potential, chloride ions flow into the cell, causing an outward current (remember that currents are named in the direction of net positive charge movement, Fig. 9-4). In addition, the open chloride channels reduce the cell's input resistance. The outward current and decreased input resistance combine to keep the cell hyperpolarized, far from the threshold for an action potential, and in a "leaky" state or state of low resistance that makes it harder for any synaptic input to elicit a large response.

Box 9-2 **A LIGAND IS A MOLECULE THAT BINDS TO A RECEPTOR**

Ligands are molecules that bind to receptors just as keys fit into locks. A ligand that changes the activity of a receptor is called an *agonist*. In contrast, when *antagonists* bind to a receptor, they decrease either agonist binding or the effect of agonist binding without directly changing the receptor's activity. There are two major types of antagonists:

- *Competitive antagonists* bind to the same site as agonists do and thus directly compete for the binding site.

- *Noncompetitive antagonists* bind to a different site than do agonists and alter the conformation of the receptor to decrease either agonist binding or the effect of agonist binding.

Some ligands have intermediate or mixed effects. For example, a molecule that binds inefficiently to the agonist-binding site can weakly activate the receptor—as an agonist would—while also functioning as a competitive antagonist by denying other agonists access to the binding site.

Channels that open after binding directly to a neurotransmitter are *ionotropic receptors*. In other words, *an ionotropic receptor is both a receptor and a channel* (Fig. 9-5). In the next section, we consider how current through two such ligand-gated ion channels changes the membrane potential of a neuron initially at rest (see Box 9-2). Note that a *ligand-gated ion channel is the same thing as an ionotropic receptor*; the two terms are synonymous, simply different ways to refer to the same physical entity.

WHEN AGONISTS BIND TO LIGAND-GATED IONOTROPIC RECEPTORS, IONIC PERMEABILITIES CHANGE

In physical terms, ligand-gated channels are transmembrane protein complexes that contain a neurotransmitter-binding region linked by three-dimensional structure or conformation to a pore region that can open or close and through which ions flow when open (Fig. 9-5). Typically, the ligand-binding site sits on the outside of the transmembrane protein. The binding of a neurotransmitter causes the membrane protein to undergo a conformational shift that opens the pore running through the membrane. These pores are selective for ions, which will then travel down their electrochemical gradients.

We focus here on the two most common ligand-gated channels in the CNS: a glutamate receptor called the α-amino-3-hydroxyl-5-methyl-4-isoxazole propionic acid (AMPA) receptor (after a particularly selective receptor agonist) and a γ-aminobutyric acid ($GABA_A$) receptor:

- The AMPA receptor is an ionotropic receptor that binds glutamate. It is a nonselective cation channel that allows sodium ions to enter the cell and potassium ions to leave the cell. The net effect of opening an AMPA receptor is an inward current and, ultimately, membrane depolarization (Fig. 9-5B).

- The $GABA_A$ receptor is an ionotropic receptor that binds GABA, resulting in an open pore that selectively passes chloride ions. Thus, the $GABA_A$ receptor carries an outward current and ultimately produces membrane hyperpolarization.

To understand the effects of AMPA and $GABA_A$ receptor activation, we use the same concepts introduced earlier to understand the resting membrane potential. *The voltage achieved after transmitter binding depends on the selective permeabilities and consequent reversal potential of the ligand-gated channels opened and on the driving force.*

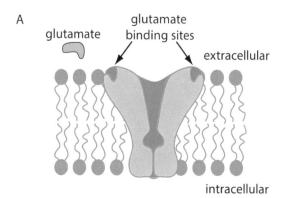

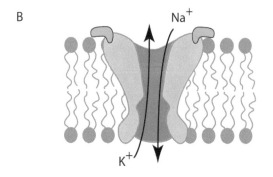

Figure 9-5 Ionotropic receptors, such as the glutamate receptor shown here, possess a pore region through which ions can travel. Ionotropic receptors are a class of ligand-gated channels in which a ligand, in this case glutamate, binds directly to the channel and *gates* a pore. In the absence of glutamate, the pore is shut (A). When two glutamate molecules bind to the two glutamate binding sites, the pore opens, allowing both potassium and sodium ions to pass (B).

WHEN GLUTAMATE BINDS THE AMPA RECEPTOR IN THE BRAIN, A PORE OPENS THAT ALLOWS BOTH SODIUM AND POTASSIUM IONS TO PASS

When open, the AMPA receptor is permeant to the two monovalent cations sodium and potassium, with the permeabilities of the two ions nearly equal so that the AMPA receptor's reversal potential is about zero. Thus, when glutamate binds the AMPA receptor, sodium ions enter the cell and potassium ions exit the cell through the pore region of the receptor (Fig. 9-5B). For a cell sitting near the rest potential, −50 to −70 mV, opening an AMPA receptor will cause a net inward current and a cell depolarization. This depolarization is called an *excitatory postsynaptic potential* (*EPSP*). Although a unitary AMPA receptor–mediated EPSP may be quite small, many such EPSPs can summate to reach threshold and trigger an action potential, thus *exciting* the cell. The summation of postsynaptic potentials, both excitatory and inhibitory, across time and space is described in the next chapter.

Glutamate opens the AMPA receptor only briefly. The glutamate concentration in the synaptic cleft is reduced rapidly by effective reuptake (much more on this in Chapter 12). In addition, the AMPA receptor, like most ionotropic receptors, desensitizes. This means that the AMPA receptor enters a desensitized state in which no ion flux occurs even though glutamate is still bound to the receptor. Consequently, the effect of glutamate on a postsynaptic cell with AMPA receptors is transient: a quick depolarization followed by a return to the resting membrane potential. Some degree of desensitization marks all ionotropic receptors; thus, postsynaptic potentials mediated by ionotropic receptors are fast, beginning and ending rapidly.

ACTIVATION OF GABA$_A$ RECEPTORS OPENS A CHLORIDE CHANNEL

Now, consider the consequences that follow GABA's binding to its ionotropic receptor, the GABA$_A$ receptor. The GABA$_A$ receptor is a chloride channel, meaning that it is permeable to chloride ions. Yet, because E$_{Cl}$, calculated earlier as −71 mV, is so close to the resting membrane potential that we calculated for a typical neuron, −72 mV, the actual driving force is negligible. As a consequence, the absolute magnitude of the synaptic current—and consequently the change in voltage—elicited by GABA$_A$ receptor activation can be small to nonexistent, particularly for neurons with membrane potentials near −70 mV. For neurons with a rest potential closer to −50 mV, GABA$_A$ receptor activation causes an outward current that results in a small hyperpolarization toward E$_{Cl}$.

Relative to the small outward current that flows through GABA$_A$ receptors in a neuron near the rest potential, the increased permeability to chloride ions and consequent decrease in input resistance often have a greater influence on the cell. The flux of chloride ions through open chloride channels (aka open GABA$_A$ receptors) reduces input resistance of the membrane (R). A reduction in input resistance (R) will result in a reduction in the membrane voltage change (V) evoked by a given synaptic current (I); remember that V = I * R. In a neuron with open GABA$_A$ receptors, coincidentally occurring EPSPs such as those caused by glutamate's binding to AMPA receptors will be smaller. In essence, *the high permeability to chloride ions through GABA$_A$ receptors serves to clamp a neuron at E$_{Cl}$, near the rest potential and render that cell difficult to depolarize.* For this reason, neurons receiving many active GABA$_A$ inputs are far less easily brought to action potential threshold than are neurons with few active GABA$_A$ inputs. Thus, the net effect of GABA$_A$ receptor–mediated inputs is inhibitory, and the resulting potential is termed an *inhibitory postsynaptic potential* (*IPSP*).

Since the GABA$_A$ receptor causes both an outward current and a decrease in membrane resistance, this receptor is very effective in lowering excitability:

- The outward current causes a hyperpolarization that takes a neuron farther from the threshold for an action potential so that the neuron requires more additional excitatory input to reach threshold than does a more depolarized cell.

- The decrease in input resistance decreases the voltage change evoked by any given synaptic current so that a neuron needs more EPSPs to reach threshold and is therefore less excitable.

Because of the strong inhibitory effect of the ubiquitous GABA$_A$ receptors, a number of important drugs—sedatives, sleep aids, and general anesthetics—act on the GABA$_A$ receptor to reduce the general excitability of the CNS. Drugs that act on GABA$_A$ receptors comprise a pharmaceutical treasure trove. In addition, GABA$_A$ receptors contain *allosteric sites*, sites other than the neurotransmitter-binding site, where a number of modern pharmaceuticals act to facilitate GABA$_A$ receptor-mediated transmission. One such allosteric site is the *benzodiazepine* site where anxiolytics (drugs that decrease anxiety) and hypnotics (drugs that promote sleep) bind and facilitate the opening of the GABA$_A$ receptor's chloride channel. A variety of general anesthetics and alcohol bind to other sites on the GABA$_A$ receptor and thereby facilitate chloride ion flux through the receptor's chloride channel.

Recall that the distribution of chloride ions is set up by the activity of chloride transporters NKCC and KCC. If KCC, which transports chloride ions out of the cell, is less active, the intracellular concentration of chloride ions increases. It does not take much intracellular accumulation of chloride ions to raise E$_{Cl}$ above the rest potential so that chloride ions leave the cell in response to GABA signaling. This greatly increases excitability because the brake normally supplied by GABA$_A$ receptor–mediated inhibition is disabled. In essence, the major inhibitory signal in the brain, GABA, now depolarizes rather than hyperpolarizes neurons. It should not be surprising then that a genetic defect in the KCC transporter is at the root of a rare form of temporal lobe epilepsy, a disorder marked by the abnormally high excitability of cortical neurons in the temporal lobe.

CHANGES IN MEMBRANE POTENTIAL ARE LARGELY DEPENDENT ON CHANGES IN CONDUCTANCES

Two principles are critical to understanding the membrane potential of a neuron. First, we need to identify the *conductances* that are present at any moment in time. Second, we need to know the distributions of permeant ions. Unlike the situation with the patrons of a nightclub, the distribution of potassium, sodium, and chloride ions does not change appreciably across the course of a minute, hour, or even day. Therefore, in healthy individuals, changes in conductance dictate most changes in membrane potential. At rest, conductance to potassium ions is highest, with smaller conductances to chloride and sodium ions also present. The membrane potential at rest is therefore close to E_K. When other channels, such as ligand-gated ion channels, open, the membrane potential changes in a way that is predicted by the conductances afforded by the newly opened channels. For example, when an AMPA channel opens, the conductance for sodium ions greatly increases, and the membrane potential briefly approaches E_{Na}. When GABA$_A$ receptors open, a chloride ion conductance dominates, and the membrane potential remains around E_{Cl}, which happens to be close to the rest potential. Using this same framework, we are now ready to understand the electrochemical basis of the action potential.

ADDITIONAL READING

Ben-Ari Y. Excitatory actions of GABA during development: The nature of the nurture. *Nat Rev Neurosci.* 3: 728–739, 2002.

Huberfeld G, Wittner L, Clemenceau S, et al. Perturbed chloride homeostasis and GABAergic signaling in human temporal lobe epilepsy. *J Neurosci.* 27: 9866–9873, 2007.

10.

ELECTRICAL COMMUNICATION WITHIN A NEURON

eurons continually receive information in the form of synaptic currents, and, with the arrival of each new input, the neuronal membrane potential may change. As discussed in the previous chapter, the voltage change resulting from each synaptic input is the product of the synaptic current and the membrane resistance. In this chapter, we examine how neurons integrate incoming synaptic inputs and communicate the resulting integral to the synaptic terminal. Although the mechanisms of postsynaptic potential (PSP) integration are common to all neurons, the mode of transferring that information to the synaptic terminal differs in different cell types. Some compact neurons and most neuroepithelial sensory cells (e.g., hair cells of the inner ear) lack an axon and do not use an action potential to transfer electrical signals within the cell. However, the majority of neurons project to distant enough targets that an axon is required to physically reach the destination. For these cells, action potentials provide the only means of communication that can travel the length of the axon to the synaptic terminal. This chapter focuses on three subjects:

- The integration of PSPs received across time and space

- The transformation of excitatory information sufficient to reach threshold and produce an action potential and a full consideration of threshold

- The conduction of action potentials along axons, both unmyelinated and myelinated

Upon reaching the threshold for an action potential, a membrane depolarization is greatly amplified, increasing by tens of millivolts in a millisecond or so (see "A Large Increase in Sodium Permeability Through Voltage-Gated Channels Produces the Rising Phase of the Action Potential"). Thus, the action potential is said to depend on *active* currents. In contrast, graded potentials are integrated without any amplification. Because of this key difference, physiological processes that do not depend on an action potential, such as the spatial and temporal integration of

synaptic potentials and the resting membrane potential, are termed *passive*.

THE PSP THAT RESULTS FROM AN INPUT DEPENDS ON THE RECEPTOR INVOLVED AND THE PAST HISTORY OF THE NEURON

In the previous chapter, we considered two common types of synaptic inputs:

- An excitatory PSP (EPSP) mediated by an α-amino-3-hydroxyl-5-methyl-4-isoxazole propionic acid (AMPA) receptor

- An inhibitory PSP (IPSP) mediated by a γ-aminobutyric acid (GABA$_A$) receptor

The AMPA receptor–mediated EPSP and the GABA$_A$ receptor–mediated IPSP are both fast potentials, deviating from and then returning to the rest potential all within milliseconds (Fig. 10-1A). Yet, PSPs come in nearly infinite variety as they differ in magnitude, latency to onset, time course of rise, and time course of decay. The variety in PSPs stems from two factors:

- *The large number of different receptor types*: Different receptor types open or close a different channel or set of channels, doing so either directly and thus rapidly in the case of ionotropic receptors or indirectly and therefore more slowly in the case of metabotropic receptors (Fig. 10-1B and see Chapter 13).

- *The past electrical history of a neuron*: The history of electrical inputs to a cell confers a unique state of excitability to the cell.

Since the voltage change (V) produced by a synaptic input is the product of synaptic current (I) and input resistance (R), recent or simultaneous synaptic inputs

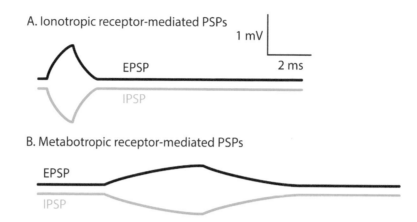

A. Ionotropic receptor-mediated PSPs

1 mV

2 ms

EPSP

IPSP

B. Metabotropic receptor-mediated PSPs

EPSP

IPSP

Figure 10-1 Postsynaptic potentials (PSPs) mediated by ionotropic receptors, such as the AMPA receptor for glutamate and the $GABA_A$ receptor for γ-aminobutyric acid (GABA), reach their peak potentials rapidly and also return to baseline rapidly (A). In contrast to these fast postsynaptic potentials, slow postsynaptic potentials mediated by metabotropic receptors, such as the $GABA_B$ receptor, have a delayed onset and can last for hundreds of milliseconds or even seconds or minutes (B). When a ligand binds to a metabotropic receptor, a series of intracellular steps may eventually result in the opening or closing of ion channels and consequently a change in membrane potential. The magnitude of postsynaptic potentials, mediated by either receptor type, varies widely and only representative examples are shown here. The time course of metabotropic receptor–mediated postsynaptic potentials also varies a great deal; relatively short metabotropic receptor–mediated postsynaptic potentials are illustrated here.

that change input resistance will also change the voltage response to simultaneous and subsequent synaptic inputs. The voltage resulting from a synaptic current will be larger if input resistance increases due to closed channels and smaller if input resistance decreases, as occurs when ion channels open. For example, any input received during a long-lasting, conductance-increasing IPSP will cause less of a voltage change than if it arrived during a period of rest. Thus, the influence of any single input on the membrane potential of a neuron is strongly dependent on recent and synchronous inputs.

Synaptic inputs to a neuron arrive at widespread sites on the neuronal membrane, and they arrive at different times. If we consider a single site within a neuron, the influence of distant inputs, as well as past potentials depends on how membrane potential changes across space and time, the topics considered in the following sections.

NEURONS SUMMATE PSPS ACROSS BOTH TIME AND SPACE

Most neurons in the human central nervous system (CNS) receive at least hundreds and typically thousands of synaptic inputs. At any one moment, dozens of the synapses impinging on a neuron may release neurotransmitter that elicits a PSP. Postsynaptic potentials occurring at the same time summate over the entire cell surface, a process known as *spatial summation*. Postsynaptic potentials also summate across time, a process known as *temporal summation*.

Neurons continually summate inputs across time and space, employing spatial and temporal summation concurrently.

A LONG LENGTH CONSTANT ALLOWS POTENTIALS FROM WIDESPREAD REGIONS OF A NEURON TO EFFECTIVELY SUMMATE

To understand spatial and temporal summation, we need to understand how voltage changes across space and time, respectively. The term *length constant*, symbolized by the Greek letter lambda (λ), quantifies how a potential change decays as it travels down a cellular process. Lambda is the length that a potential travels down a cylindrical structure, such as a dendrite or axon, before it is reduced to 37%, or $1/e$, of its initial magnitude. If an EPSP has an initial amplitude of 100 μV, then after one length constant down the neuronal process, that same EPSP will have a peak amplitude of 37 μV. The length constant is dependent on only two parameters:

$$\lambda = \sqrt{\frac{r_m}{r_a}}$$

where r_m is the *membrane resistance* and r_a is the *axial resistance*. Membrane resistance is a familiar concept by now. Whereas we symbolized "resistance" as R in referencing Ohm's law, now that we are considering multiple values of resistance, we will use r_m to represent *membrane* resistance.

Axial resistance (r_a) is simply the resistance encountered as current travels *within* the inside of a process, either an axon or a dendrite. Axial resistance is greatest in the thinnest of neuronal processes and lowest in fibers with the largest diameter. The formula for the length constant essentially tells us that PSPs spread further as the membrane resistance increases and/or as the axial resistance decreases. Therefore, the largest values of length constant, some number of millimeters, are found in wide-diameter processes with a large r_m (i.e., very few channels are open) and low r_a. The axial resistance in large-diameter processes is low by virtue of the process caliber, and this holds regardless of whether a process is a dendrite or an axon. The smallest length constant values, a fraction of a millimeter, are found in the thinnest dendrites and axons.

To understand how the neuronal length constant relates to the change in potential across space, we use the water analogy introduced previously. Consider injecting 1,000 mL of water at one point along a pipe. If the pipe walls are very leaky, the injected water will leak out and will not get very far so that, before too long, only 370 mL, or 37%, remain; this is an example of a short length constant. If the pipe diameter is thin, axial resistance will be very high and water will encounter so much resistance that it will not travel far; again, the length constant will be short. However, if the pipe diameter is wide with impermeable walls, injected water will travel a long distance, and the length constant will be long.

In sum, potentials travel the farthest with the least degradation in neurons with the greatest length constants. Therefore, *neurons with long length constants summate potentials arriving at widely dispersed sites. In contrast, neurons with short length constants only summate synaptic potentials from closely spaced inputs.*

THE TIME CONSTANT REFLECTS THE PERIOD OF TIME OVER WHICH NEURONS EFFECTIVELY SUMMATE POTENTIALS

Before considering the time constant, we consider the capacitance of a neuronal membrane and then work through the implications of a membrane's electrical properties on changes in cellular potential across time. First, think of a capacitor that you purchase from an electrical supply store. A store-bought capacitor consists of two charged *plates* separated by a nonconductive space, the *dielectric*. The arrangement of a nonconductive dielectric between the two plates sets up an electrical field between and around the plates. If we think of the capacitance as the "ability" to keep

charge separated, then we can understand that capacitance increases as the area (and charge) of the conductive plates increases and as the separation between the two conductive plates *decreases*.

In the case of a lipid bilayer, one conductive "plate" is the cytoplasm of the cell and the other is the interstitial fluid. The membrane serves as the nonconductive dielectric between the two plates. Because the thickness of biological membranes does not vary much, it is the size of the cell that is the primary influence on membrane capacitance. As a consequence, a large cell forms a large conductive "plate" and therefore has a higher *membrane capacitance* (c_m) than a small cell.

The bulk (i.e., free) solutions within the cytosol of a spherical cell and within the surrounding extracellular space are isopotential, with every charged molecule balanced by nearby charges that are equal and opposite. Thus, the entirety of the neuronal membrane potential falls across the width of the plasma membrane. The resting membrane potential of a neuron, −50 to −70 mV, may appear to be an inconsequential voltage because it is only a tiny fraction of what is readily available in the wall outlets ubiquitous to modern societies or even in the small batteries that run common household devices. However, this small voltage drop is maintained across 5–10 nm, the width of a lipid bilayer. Even for the smallest neurons, with the smallest sized "plates," maintaining a separation of 50–70 mv across a membrane is roughly equivalent to keeping a lightning bolt about 4 inches or 100 mm away. The powerful charge separation exhibited by neuronal membranes is accomplished by the very high membrane capacitance common to all neurons.

By now, it should be clear that every membrane has a resistance and a capacitance. In electrical terms, we would call this is a resistor-capacitor (RC) circuit. RC circuits transfer charge exponentially. It is this exponential rate of membrane potential change that is captured by the *time constant*, typically symbolized by the Greek letter tau (τ). The time constant is the time that it takes a potential to change by 63%, or by $1 - (1/e)$. Using the same example as previously of an EPSP that will peak at 100 µV, the membrane will reach 63 µV above the rest potential after one time constant has passed. Similarly, the membrane potential will decay to 37 (100 − 63) µV at a time point that is one time constant after the peak amplitude is reached.

As with the length constant, the time constant is dependent on r_m, but it is also dependent on membrane capacitance or c_m. Just as in an RC circuit, a biological membrane has a time constant that is the product of resistance and capacitance:

$$\tau = r_m * c_m$$

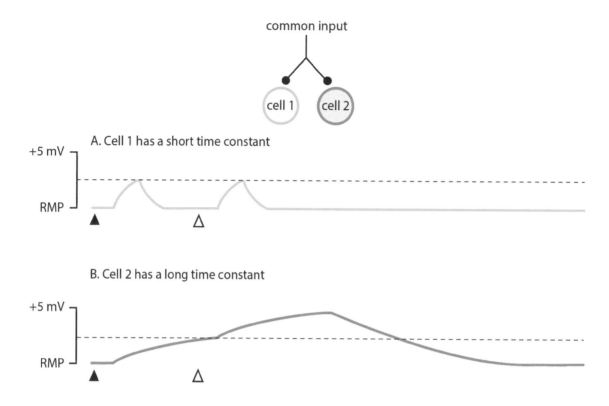

Figure 10-2 The time constant, τ, is the time needed for the membrane potential to change by 63%, en route to either the peak or nadir of a postsynaptic potential (PSP) or during the decay back to baseline. Consider two cells that differ only in their relative time constants. These cells receive the same synaptic input (inset at top) that elicits an excitatory postsynaptic potential (EPSP) after the same latency. Cell 1 has a short time constant, and its synaptic response reaches 63% of its maximal value (*dotted line*) after a shorter time (A) than does the synaptic response of cell 2 with a longer time constant (B). A second input (*hollow arrowhead*) that occurs shortly after a first input (*filled arrowhead*) elicits temporal summation in cell 2 but not in cell 1. Cell 1, which has a short time constant, has the same response to both inputs. Thus, cells with longer time constants summate inputs over a longer period of time.

The time constant increases as membrane resistance increases so that PSPs change more rapidly in neurons with low membrane resistance. Membrane capacitance also influences the time constant: as membrane capacitance increases, more time is needed to charge the membrane. The membranes of neurons with low capacitance charge up rapidly and, therefore, potential changes reach their peaks or troughs rapidly and then decay rapidly. In contrast, neurons with high-capacitance membranes charge up and decay slowly, thereby stretching out the effect of a given synaptic input over a longer time.

The time constant, taking into account both membrane resistance and capacitance, informs us of the time needed to change the potential in either the hyperpolarizing or depolarizing direction. Neuronal time constants typically range from a few milliseconds to tens of milliseconds. In neurons with a long time constant, the membrane potential responds to a synaptic input by slowly reaching the peak potential followed by a slow decay back to rest, resulting in a lengthy period during which

the arrival of another PSP will result in temporal summation. The memory of earlier events lasts for a longer time in neurons with a long time constant. *In sum, if a neuron receives two synaptic inputs separated by a few tens of milliseconds, a neuron with a lower time constant will not show any summation whereas one with a longer time constant will* (Fig. 10-2).

THE ACTION POTENTIAL IS AN ALL-OR-NONE UNIT OF EXCITATION

Incoming IPSPs and EPSPs sum, spatially and temporally, to alter a neuron's membrane potential. For a minority of neurons and sensory cells, the summation of PSPs alone determines the amount of transmitter released. In these cells, transmitter release is *graded*, with more transmitter released when the cell is depolarized and less when it is hyperpolarized. However, the vast majority of neurons employ an additional, very important mode of electrical

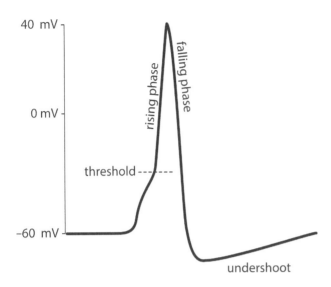

40 mV

0 mV

threshold

-60 mV

rising phase

falling phase

undershoot

Figure 10-3 During an action potential, the membrane potential shoots up from rest, anywhere from −70 mV to −50 mV, to a positive value before returning to rest. An undershoot or afterhyperpolarization occurs as the membrane potential initially repolarizes beyond the rest potential before eventually, and relatively slowly, returning to the rest potential. The entire action potential occurs in one to a few milliseconds, with the rising phase occurring in a millisecond or less.

signaling: the action potential (Fig. 10-3). In these cells, when the membrane reaches a certain depolarized threshold, an action potential, often termed a *spike*, results. Lord Edgar Adrian, who along with Sir Charles Sherrington received the Nobel Prize for Physiology or Medicine in 1932, likened this process to the operation of a gun trigger. Pressure can build and build on the trigger, but a bullet is fired only when pressure on the trigger passes a threshold. Just as a bullet's trajectory cannot be reversed once released, an action potential cannot be interrupted once it starts. We now turn to the action potential for the remainder of the chapter.

ACTION POTENTIAL ARE BITS AND SPIKE TRAINS SPELL INFORMATION BYTES

The action potential provides the boost needed to send information to synaptic terminals located hundreds of length constants from the soma. The action potential is key to triggering communication from one neuron to another through chemical synapses. In sum, the action potential serves two critical functions:

- It travels across long distances through action potential conduction.

- The depolarization associated with the action potential triggers neurotransmitter release from synaptic terminals (detailed in Chapter 11).

Here, we consider the action potential and its conduction along neuronal processes. In the next chapter, we examine how the action potential affects neurotransmitter release machinery upon reaching the synaptic terminal. As we learned in the previous chapter, neurons receiving one or a few depolarizing inputs quickly return to the resting membrane potential. However, if the depolarizing input is sufficient to reach threshold, then an action potential results. This action potential takes the cell's membrane potential from the rest potential to a positive potential and then back down to rest all within a few milliseconds (Fig. 10-3).

There are no half or partial action potentials. As an all-or-none signal, the action potential resembles the binary computer bit of information. A bit is either 0 or 1, never any fraction. As in computer language, information comes in the way that bits—in this case action potentials—are strung together (Fig. 10-4A). The number and frequency of action potentials fired by a neuron within a *spike train* (i.e., a sequence of spikes) code information just as strings of bits make up bytes and eventually kilobytes, megabytes, gigabytes, and terabytes of information. Understanding the exact nature of the neuronal code evidenced in a spike train remains an exciting challenge.

A LARGE INCREASE IN SODIUM PERMEABILITY THROUGH VOLTAGE-GATED CHANNELS PRODUCES THE RISING PHASE OF THE ACTION POTENTIAL

The action potential can be understood using the same framework used to understand the rest potential. In essence, the action potential depends on rapid changes in ionic conductances. At the start of the action potential, sodium ion permeability increases to a level that is at least 20 times greater than the potassium ion permeability at rest. Because of this high sodium ion permeability, the membrane potential is dominated by the Nernst potential for sodium ions, E_{Na}, which is positive with respect to ground due to the far greater abundance of sodium ions outside of the cell relative to inside.

Sodium ion conductance during the rise of the action potential is carried by a special class of ion channels.

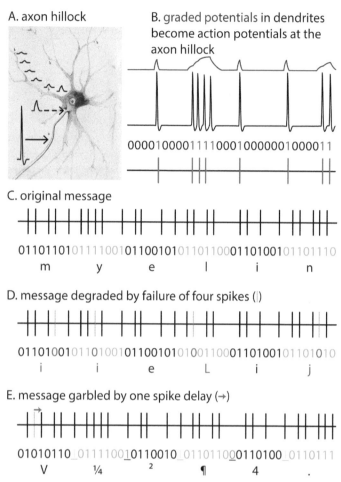

A. axon hillock

B. graded potentials in dendrites become action potentials at the axon hillock

0000100001111000100000010000011

C. original message

01101101 01111001 01100101 01101100 01101001 01101110
m   y   e   l   i   n

D. message degraded by failure of four spikes (|)

01101001 01110100 01100101 01001100 01101001 01101010
i   i   e   L   i   j

E. message garbled by one spike delay (→)

01010110 _0111100 _10110010 _01101100 _0110100 _0110111
V   ¼   2   ¶   4   .

Figure 10-4 A: The axon hillock is a specialized region where a high density of voltage-gated sodium channels (VGSCs) most easily transforms a graded potential into an action potential (*dashed arrow*). Graded potentials received by a neuron's dendrites and soma may elicit an action potential in that neuron's axon (*arrow*). B: The dendrites receive graded potentials (*top trace*), including sub-threshold excitatory potentials and inhibitory potentials (not shown). Excitatory potentials that pass the threshold lead to the generation of an action potential in the axon hillock. The action potential can then travel down the axon to distant targets. Action potentials are analogous to bits in computer language so that, at every moment in time, the axon's activity can be denoted as zero (no action potential) or one (action potential). C: A spike train can be translated into zeroes and ones and then read as bytes (sequential groups of 8 in black or blue) to spell "m-y-e-l-i-n" in ASCI code. D: Failure of only a few action potentials (*red*) leads the message in C to be degraded so that it spells "i-i-e-L-i-j". E: A single added delay in the spike train (*red arrow*) garbles the message completely, spelling "V-¼-²-¶-4-."   Image in A reprinted with permission from deFelipe J, *Cajal's Butterflies of the Soul*, New York: Oxford University Press, 2009.

Unlike the AMPA or GABA$_A$ receptors, which are gated by the binding of a ligand such as a neurotransmitter, *voltage* gates the sodium channels responsible for the rapid rise of the action potential. Since depolarization itself activates *voltage-gated sodium channels (VGSCs)*, and since sodium ion influx depolarizes the cell, the sodium ion conductance is regenerative (see Box 10-1). In other words, sodium ion conductance through VGSCs feeds upon itself. Once past threshold, VGSC opening does not stop until all available VGSCs have opened. In fact, the threshold is the point at which VGSC opening becomes regenerative. Put another way, the opening of available VGSCs cannot be stopped once the action potential threshold is surpassed.

Because the permeability for sodium ions is so high, the action potential, at its maximum, overshoots zero and becomes positive. The peak of the action potential does not reach E$_{Na}$ because the chloride and potassium channels that are open at rest remain open. At the positive potentials of the action potential, the driving force on chloride and potassium ions is greatly increased. Therefore, chloride ions enter the cell and potassium ions leave the cell, producing outward

Tetrodotoxin, often abbreviated as *TTX*, is a toxin produced by bacteria naturally present in a number of animals including pufferfish, newts, and sea stars. This powerful toxin derives its lethality from binding to the pore of VGSCs and thereby preventing the inward sodium current that generates action potentials. Tetrodotoxin has proved to be an invaluable tool in understanding VGSCs. Luckily, it presents only a minor medical threat; cases of tetrodotoxin poisoning in humans are rare and largely restricted to those who eat inadequately prepared sushi. In contrast, *saxitoxin* and *brevetoxin*, toxins that also target the VGSC pore, can present important health risks on occasion. Saxitoxin and brevetoxin are made by dinoflagellates, a type of plankton, but accumulate in shellfish, thereby posing a potential health risk to humans. Sporadically, the population of plankton explodes, causing *red tide* that ultimately leads to the illness and sometimes to the death of wildlife and humans that eat affected shellfish. The cause of death is respiratory failure due to paralysis for reasons that are described in the text.

currents that counteract the depolarization carried by VGSCs and keep the membrane potential from reaching E_{Na}.

Action potentials are generated at *trigger zones*, which in many neurons are located at the *axon hillock* that marks the start of the axon (Fig. 10-4A). Regardless of location, the trigger zone is a specialized region where VGSCs are at high density, 100 or more times greater than the density in somatodendritic membranes. This high density of VGSCs explains why a given depolarization is far more likely to elicit an action potential at the trigger zone than elsewhere. The same EPSP that opens three VGSCs in a patch of membrane at the soma would open 300 or more VGSCs in the same-sized patch of membrane located at the trigger zone. An action potential is far more likely to occur in the latter scenario than in the former one.

VOLTAGE-GATED POTASSIUM CHANNELS REPOLARIZE THE MEMBRANE POTENTIAL AFTER THE PEAK OF AN ACTION POTENTIAL

Depolarization opens voltage-gated potassium channels as well as VGSCs. The channel carrying the ensuing potassium ion conductance, referred to as the *delayed rectifier*, opens after a delay and does not contribute appreciably to the membrane potential until after the rising phase of the action potential is completed. Yet, soon after the action potential peak, voltage-gated potassium channels are maximally activated. The large potassium ion conductance carries potassium ions out of the cell, repolarizing the cell toward the rest potential. The potassium ion conductance develops slowly and lasts long enough to produce an undershoot or *afterhyperpolarization*, often abbreviated as AHP, which takes the membrane potential briefly toward E_K from rest (Fig. 10-3). Voltage-gated potassium channels are only triggered by depolarized potentials so that, once the membrane reaches potentials as hyperpolarized as the rest potential, the voltage-gated potassium ion conductance turns off. By repolarizing the membrane potential, the delayed rectifier is important for swiftly terminating the action potential.

INACTIVATION OF VOLTAGE-GATED SODIUM CHANNELS ALSO CONTRIBUTES TO ACTION POTENTIAL TERMINATION

Beyond the delayed rectifier, there is another contributor to termination of the action potential: VGSC *inactivation*.

Immediately after a brief opening, VGSCs inactivate (Fig. 10-5). Sodium ions cannot pass through the pore of an inactivated VGSC. More importantly, *an inactivated channel cannot open; it is not activatable*. To be activated again, a VGSC must return to a hyperpolarized voltage around the rest potential. Thus, even if there were no delayed rectifier conductance to repolarize the cell, the cell would slowly return to rest potential because the VGSCs would all inactivate and not reopen, whereas resting chloride and potassium ion conductances would repolarize the cell. The presence of voltage-gated potassium channels greatly accelerates the rate of membrane repolarization after an action potential.

THE THRESHOLD FOR AN ACTION POTENTIAL DEPENDS ON THE PROPORTION OF INACTIVATED VGSCS AND THEREFORE ON PRIOR ELECTRICAL HISTORY

Depolarization above rest activates VGSCs. The larger the depolarization, the greater the probability is that a closed VGSC will open. *The action potential threshold represents the tipping point at which one more sodium ion entering the cell will trigger a regenerative sodium ion conductance, and, alternatively, one more potassium ion leaving the cell would take the cell back to rest potential.* The direction in which this unstable situation tips depends in large part on how many VGSCs are *closed* versus inactivated. Remember that closed VGSCs are available for opening, but inactivated VGSCs are not (Fig. 10-5A).

Let us consider two different paths from rest to −40 mV, a journey that takes us from a potential where most VGSCs are closed to a potential that is clearly above the spike threshold under normal circumstances. If a large inward current takes the membrane potential from rest to −40 mV in the course of a couple of milliseconds, an action potential is highly likely to occur (Fig. 10-5B). However, if the membrane potential moves from rest to −40 mV over seconds to minutes, then an action potential is highly unlikely. Why? Because as the membrane potential drifts upward, the cumulative probability that a closed VGSC will open increases (Fig. 10-5C) far faster than the possibility that an inactivated VGSC will recover from inactivation. Remember that VGSC opening is favored at depolarized potentials, and recovery from inactivation is favored at hyperpolarized potentials. Thus, across a gradual depolarization, more and more VGSCs open and inactivate, thereby becoming unavailable for future opening. Moreover, in the absence of any strong hyperpolarizing influence, the inactivated

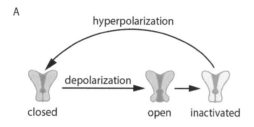

A

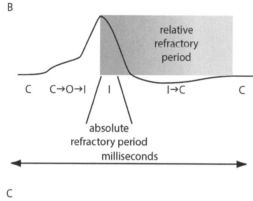

B

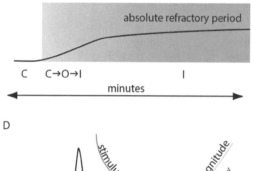

C

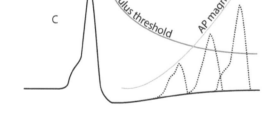

D

Figure 10-5 A: Voltage-gated sodium channels (VGSCs) change conformation from the closed (*C*) to the open (*O*) state when the membrane potential depolarizes above rest. *Immediately* after opening, VGSCs enter an inactivated (*I*) state. The transition from the open to the inactivated state is automatic and cannot be bypassed. To recover from inactivation and reenter the closed state, the membrane potential must hyperpolarize to near rest potential. B: The rapid opening of VGSCs (C→O) is responsible for the rising phase of the action potential. Yet, VGSCs enter the inactivated state immediately after opening (C→O→I), rendering the membrane unexcitable because the inactivated VGSCs cannot open. During the rising and initial decay phases of the action potential, most of the VGSCs are inactivated and there are not enough closed VGSCs to support an action potential; this period is the absolute refractory period. As the membrane potential approaches the rest potential, more and more VGSCs transition from inactivated to closed (I→C), a period that is termed the relative refractory period. C: If a cell depolarizes slowly, over seconds to minutes, VGSCs open and become inactivated, just as they do when a cell depolarizes quickly over a few milliseconds. However, in the case of a slow depolarization, no action potential can occur because not enough VGSCs are closed and available for opening once threshold is reached. Therefore, a slow depolarization leads to a persistent state of absolute refractoriness. D: When a cell repolarizes from an action potential to near the rest potential, the relative refractory period starts. During the relative refractory period, action potentials can occur. However, the depolarization needed to trigger an action potential (stimulus threshold) is greater than normal, and the action potential peak (AP magnitude) is lower. After more and more time at a hyperpolarized potential, more and more VGSCs recover from inactivation, and, consequently, the action potential returns to normal in terms of both threshold and magnitude.

VGSCs are extremely unlikely to recover from inactivation. If this process continues long enough, most of the VGSCs end up in the inactivated or unopenable state, at which point *no amount of depolarization or inward current can trigger an action potential.*

In sum, a fixed action potential threshold does not exist. Instead, the point at which an action potential is triggered depends not only on the potential reached but also on the state of the VGSCs, which in turn depends on the cell's electrical history.

The dependence of the action potential threshold on prior history has major implications for the hyperkalemic patient whom we initially considered in Chapter 9. As already discussed, this patient's neurons would have a rest potential more depolarized than normal by a few millivolts, perhaps resulting in some errant neural functioning. However, far more worrisome are the consequences of elevated potassium ion levels for cardiac function. Contraction of cardiac muscle is driven by action potentials in cardiac muscle cells. Although the action potential of cardiac muscle differs from that of a typical neuron, the rising phase is the same, carried by an influx of sodium ions through VGSCs. Thus, VGSCs are necessary for cardiac muscle action potentials that produce the cardiac muscle contractions necessary for life. How does hyperkalemia affect cardiac function? Remember that cardiac muscle cells have a rest potential dominated by potassium ion conductance and that this rest potential would increase by almost 10 mV in a hyperkalemic patient. Such a large increase in membrane potential greatly increases the likelihood of VGSC opening and consequent inactivation while decreasing the probability that channels will recover from inactivation. If enough VGSCs enter the inactivated state, action potentials can no longer be supported and cardiac muscle contractions cease. Therefore, if unrecognized and untreated, hyperkalemia is fatal.

Although rare, *hyperkalemic periodic paralysis*, an autosomal dominant disease, is dramatically illustrative of the importance of the VGSC cycle between closed, open, and inactivated channel states. Patients with hyperkalemic periodic paralysis have a mutation in a VGSC allele that is expressed in skeletal muscle cells, cells that fire action potentials that are quite similar to neuronal ones. The mutation in hyperkalemic periodic paralysis prevents mutated channels from inactivating when in the presence of an elevated potassium ion concentration. Thus, mutated channels that open *remain open* during and after exercise when the extracellular concentration of potassium ions is elevated in skeletal muscles. Mutant VGSCs open and stay open, keeping the membrane potential depolarized and preventing the normal VGSCs from ever closing. This renders the muscle unable to contract, and, consequently, patients with hyperkalemic periodic paralysis become weak, sometimes sufficiently so that they are unable to move (hence the name) immediately after exercise.

REFRACTORY PERIODS FOR ACTION POTENTIALS LIMIT THE RATE AT WHICH NEURONS CAN FIRE ACTION POTENTIALS

As should be clear by now, VGSCs in the inactivated state cannot open, even at depolarized potentials that would normally trigger an action potential. Therefore, immediately after a patch of membrane supports an action potential, that same area cannot support another action potential. The inability to fire an action potential for 500 microseconds—half a millisecond—or so after an initial action potential defines the *absolute refractory period* (Fig. 10-5C). *During the absolute refractory period, VGSCs are inactivated, unavailable to open, and therefore no amount of depolarizing current can trigger an action potential.* The absolute refractory period

ends when enough VGSCs leave the inactivated state upon repolarization of the membrane potential (Fig. 10-5D). Thus, VGSC inactivation is the root cause of the absolute refractory period.

After the membrane repolarizes from an action potential, increasing numbers of VGSCs transition from inactivation to a closed, but *activatable*, state. As VGSCs enter the closed state, they come back "online," available once again to contribute to the rising phase of another action potential. At the same time as the VGSCs emerge from inactivation, conductance through voltage-gated potassium channels is very high, causing a hyperpolarization beyond the normal rest potential. During this afterhyperpolarization, a much larger inward current than normal is needed to reach the threshold for an action potential because of both the decrease in input resistance and the hyperpolarized membrane potential. This period, which can last a few milliseconds, is termed the *relative refractory period* (Fig. 10-5D).

The length of the action potential, which varies across different sizes and types of axon (see "Unmyelinated Axons Conduct Action Potentials at Speeds Proportional to Their Diameter"), determines the length of the refractory period. The lengths of the absolute and relative refractory periods in turn limit the rate at which neurons can fire action potentials. Since action potential durations vary from <1 ms to 3–4 ms, the maximum rate of firing varies from about 50 to 1 kHz, or 1,000 Hz, or more.

THE REFRACTORY PERIOD SERVES TO POLARIZE ACTION POTENTIAL CONDUCTION

Beyond providing an upper limit on the rate of neuronal firing, the absolute refractory period also provides directionality to action potential conduction. To understand this, consider the axon below that connects the soma and dendrites on the left to the synaptic terminal on the right:

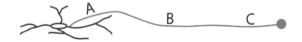

Now consider an artificial situation in which an action potential is initiated somewhere along the length of an axon, at point B in the case illustrated here. An action potential initiated at point B may travel to both points A and C because the axonal membrane between B and A, as well

as that between B and C, can support an action potential. However, once at A or C, the action potential cannot travel back to B since the membrane at B, as well as that between B and A or between B and C, is refractive. This example illustrates how *action potential conduction, rather than the axon itself, is polarized by the absolute refractory period*. Under physiological situations, an action potential starts in one place and travels in only one direction down neuronal processes, *away from where it has been*. In this way, the absolute refractory period is at the root of the polarization of axons.

LOCAL ANESTHETIC AND SOME ANTICONVULSANT DRUGS ACT THROUGH BLOCKING VGSC FUNCTION

Local anesthetic and select anticonvulsant drugs, along with several antidepressant and Class I antiarrhythmic drugs, all act on a common molecular target, the VGSC, but have distinctly different clinical effects. Here, we briefly examine the former two drug classes. Commonly used local anesthetics include lidocaine, known as Xylocaine, and procaine, typically used for dental procedures and known in the vernacular as novocaine. Anticonvulsant drugs that act on VGSCs include phenytoin, carbamazepine, and lamotrigine, which are known as Dilantin, Tegretol, and Lamictal, respectively, in the United States. There are additional types of anticonvulsant drugs, such as those acting on the $GABA_A$ receptor (see Chapter 13), that employ mechanisms of action unrelated to VGSCs.

All four types of drugs listed here act by reducing sodium ion flux through VGSCs. They have less affinity for the baseline, closed state of the VGSC than for either the open or inactivated state. Therefore, in the presence of these drugs, VGSCs are less likely to be in the baseline, closed state and consequently less likely to be available for opening. Because of their limited affinity for channels in the closed state, local anesthetic and anticonvulsant drugs have little to no effect on hyperpolarized and quiescent neurons. The dependence of drug efficacy on neuronal activity is a property known as use- or state-dependence. There is a key difference between the nature of the use-dependence exhibited by local anesthetic and anticonvulsant drugs. Local anesthetic drugs block action potentials that occur at moderate rates as well as *bursts* of action potentials, whereas the anticonvulsant drugs primarily block high-frequency discharge while leaving less frequent firing relatively unchanged.

In *epilepsy*, there are paroxysmal bursts of action potentials that "ride" on top of a depolarized plateau. During an epileptic burst, anticonvulsant drugs remain bound because the membrane potential remains depolarized between action potentials. In contrast, during normal activity, when a cell returns to the rest potential between action potentials, anticonvulsant drugs have the chance to dissociate from VGSCs. In this way, anticonvulsant drugs block epileptic activity that involves an underlying depolarization but do not interfere with normal spiking that does not involve a plateau potential.

Local anesthetic drugs have a slower off-rate from closed VGSCs than the anticonvulsant drugs just discussed. This means that it takes more time for a local anesthetic than an anticonvulsant to dissociate from a closed VGSC in a hyperpolarized membrane. As a result, local anesthetic drugs remain bound to VGSCs between action potentials that occur at moderate to high frequencies. More local anesthetic molecules remain bound with every subsequent action potential. Thus, local anesthetic drugs powerfully suppress rapidly firing neurons and have little effect on lower frequency discharge. Such a mode of action is commonly termed *use-dependent block*.

UNMYELINATED AXONS CONDUCT ACTION POTENTIALS AT SPEEDS PROPORTIONAL TO THEIR DIAMETER

An action potential travels along neuronal membranes because the inward sodium current at one spot depolarizes the adjacent membrane enough to start opening the VGSCs located there. Once the spike threshold is crossed, closed VGSCs open, and a regenerative action potential occurs. In this fashion, *by sequentially activating VGSCs in adjacent membrane regions, action potentials travel down unmyelinated axons*. Consider the process by which an action potential at site A results in an action potential at an adjacent site on the axon B:

1. The inward current at A travels down the interior of the axon, through *axoplasm*, to reach B.

2. The membrane at B depolarizes over time until it reaches the threshold for an action potential.

Thus, the speed with which an action potential propagates down an axon, typically termed the *conduction velocity*, depends on the inward current traveling down the inside of the axon. The speed at which current travels through axoplasm is inversely related to the product of the axial resistance of the axon, r_a, and the capacitance of the axonal membrane, c_m:

$$\text{conduction velocity} \propto \frac{1}{r_a c_m}$$

As we saw earlier, axial resistance is greater in smaller diameter fibers than in larger diameter fibers. What this means is that *action potentials propagate faster in large-diameter axons with low r_a values than in small-diameter axons with high r_a values.*

Now recall that as membrane capacitance increases, more time is needed to charge the membrane. Due to their high capacitance, unmyelinated axonal membranes require milliseconds to "charge up." Therefore, the action potential of unmyelinated axons is typically two or more milliseconds in duration. Both the slow conduction of current through small-diameter fibers and the extended time needed to charge up a bare neuronal membrane are responsible for the slow conduction velocity of unmyelinated axons. In humans and other vertebrates, the range of unmyelinated axonal diameters and therefore of conduction velocities is limited. The largest unmyelinated axons are 1–2 microns in diameter and conduct at maximal speeds of 1–2 meters/second. Smaller unmyelinated axons, a half-micron in diameter, conduct at speeds of about a half-meter/second.

MYELINATION GREATLY INCREASES THE SPEED OF ACTION POTENTIAL CONDUCTION

Action potential propagation is slower in smaller diameter fibers and faster in larger diameter fibers for two reasons. First, small-diameter fibers have greater axial resistance than do large-diameter axons. The second reason has to do with capacitance. Although the specific capacitance of neuronal membranes (the capacitance per given membrane surface area) is relatively uniform across neurons, membrane capacitance or c_m increases as the circumference (=2 * π * radius) of an axon increases. Thus, the capacitance of axonal membranes is greater in larger diameter fibers than in smaller diameter fibers. As membrane capacitance increases, the time needed for an action potential to depolarize and then repolarize increases. Overall, conduction

velocity increases in proportion to the radius of a fiber. This holds because:

- c_m is related to the circumference of an axon and thus increases in proportion to the radius.

- r_a is related to the cross-sectional area of an axon and thus decreases in proportion to the radius *squared*.

- conduction velocity is proportional to $(r_a * c_m)^{-1}$.

In sum, conduction velocity increases as axonal radius increases; action potentials conduct more quickly down larger diameter axons than smaller diameter axons. Although conduction velocity is considerably faster in all myelinated axons for reasons detailed next, the same relationship exists for myelinated as for unmyelinated axons, with larger myelinated fibers conducting action potentials more rapidly than their smaller myelinated counterparts and larger unmyelinated fibers conducting action potentials more rapidly than their smaller unmyelinated counterparts.

In invertebrates, only axons that are *hundreds of microns in diameter* achieve the high conduction velocities needed for fast escape reactions. If vertebrates, including humans, were to use the same mechanism for ensuring rapid action potential conduction, we would have to be enormous—meaning large dinosaur size—to accommodate the large number of fast-conducting axons that we possess. Instead, vertebrates evolved a different mechanism, rather than axonal diameter, to solve this problem. In vertebrates, *specialized glial cells make an insulating membrane, termed myelin, that wraps around axons and greatly speeds up conduction of action potentials.*

Axons wrapped by myelin are termed *myelinated axons*. Myelin is a membrane, containing mostly lipids (about 80% by weight) along with proteins. *Myelin, as well as the neuronal membrane that it covers, has few channels and thus has a high resistance, probably more than tenfold higher than that of a typical neuronal membrane.* Moreover, myelin-producing cells wrap around a myelinated axon 10–160 times, more for larger axons and less for smaller diameter axons (Fig. 10-6). Each wrap of myelin consists of two lipid bilayers and the intervening cytoplasm (Fig. 10-7A). The lipid bilayers between two wraps are joined by extracellular adherens junctions (see Box 10-2), interspersed with the occasional tight junction, all of which greatly increases the resistance of the myelin wrap. The cytoplasm within the myelin-producing cell is squeezed out, so that the intracellular space is narrower than even the thickness of a single lipid bilayer, which in turn greatly increases *axial resistance within the*

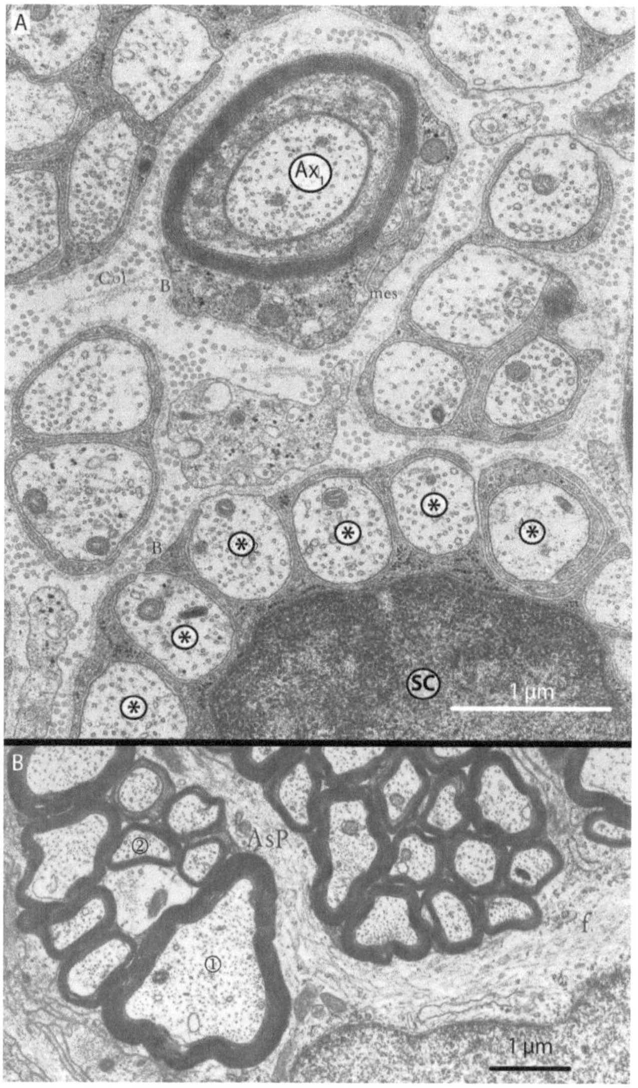

Adherens junctions are regions of cell-to-cell adhesion or, more accurately, membrane-to-membrane adhesion. Molecules such as cadherins and integrins span a membrane and bind to a like molecule on an adjacent membrane. In the case of myelin, membranes in the myelin wrap belonging to the same glial cell are brought in tight proximity by adherens junctions. *Tight junctions* are occluding junctions that prevent fluid from flowing between two cell membranes. Importantly, tight junctions may allow small organic ions, such as potassium ions, to pass. *Gap junctions*, introduced in the previous chapter, join two intracellular domains with a small conduit through which molecules may travel. Note that, in myelin, the cytoplasm that is joined by the gap junctions belongs to the same cell, either a Schwann cell or an oligodendrocyte (see Chapter 2). Mutations in the *GJB1* gene, which codes for gap junction protein connexin32, are one of the most common causes of Charcot-Marie-Tooth disease. It is the impairment of gap junction function that leads to demyelination in this X-linked form of Charcot-Marie-Tooth disease.

Figure 10-6 A: An electron micrograph through the sciatic nerve of a rat shows one myelinated axon (Ax_1) with the myelin provided by a Schwann cell. Another Schwann cell (*SC*) embeds a group of unmyelinated axons (*encircled asterisks*). Although Schwann cells surround unmyelinated axons, they do not wrap these axons in myelin. B: An electron micrograph through the rat optic nerve reveals a pure population of myelinated axons. The width of the myelin sheath is thicker for axons of larger diameters (e.g., *1*) than for axons of smaller diameters (e.g., *2*). Photomicrographs are reprinted from Peters A, Palay SL, Webster H deF. *The fine structure of the nervous system: Neurons and their supporting cells*, 3rd edition. New York: Oxford University Press, 1991.

myelin sheath. The result of myelin's high membrane resistance, as well as the glial cell's high axial resistance, is that *no easy path exists along which current can escape*; current cannot easily travel across the myelin wraps nor can it spiral down the center of the myelin-producing cell. In electrical circuit terms, each membrane within each myelin wrap has a resistance, and each membrane is in series with every other membrane in the myelin sheath. Since resistances placed in series are additive, the resistance between the inside of an axon and the outside of the myelin is huge, as much as hundreds of times greater than that of a bare axon. The bottom line is that *the path of least resistance for the current due to an action potential is straight down the axon.*

Now, let's look at the capacitance of a myelinated axon. The capacitance of a myelinated axon plummets because the conductive *plates* are now separated by the axonal membrane and myelin wraps. In essence, the axoplasm inside the axon is separated from the interstitial fluid by far more than the 4–5 nm of a single membrane. This wide separation of the two plates gives a myelinated axon a very low capacitance. The low capacitance of myelinated axon means that the membrane charges up really quickly wherever myelin exists.

Myelin does not cover the entire axon. Instead, myelin covers evenly spaced stretches, *internodes*, separated by patches of bare axon called *nodes of Ranvier* or simply nodes (Fig. 10-7). As a result of the infinitesimal capacitance of the membrane in the internode, action potentials travel lightning fast down axons covered in myelin. However, when the action potential reaches the bare node, a normally timed action potential results. As a result, action potentials

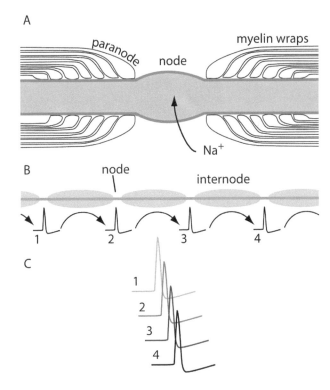

Figure 10-7 A: At axonal nodes, no myelin is present and voltage gated sodium channels (VGSCs) that are packed at high density support sodium ion (*Na+*) influx during action potentials. In the paranode, the myelin wraps begin. The myelin wrapping around myelinated axons is restricted to the internodes. B: Action potentials move along a myelinated axon by saltatory conduction, meaning that the action potential is conducted so rapidly through the internodes that it appears to jump from one node to the next. In this example, the action potential is moving from left (*1*) to right (*4*). C: At any one moment, action potentials occur in multiple nodes (four are illustrated) as the rising phase of an action potential in one node leads to the depolarization of the next node, which then fires an action potential, which in turn depolarizes the subsequent node and so on. Action potentials are numbered for the node from which they arise, as labeled in B.

appear to *jump* from one node to the next, a process termed *saltatory conduction* (Fig. 10-7B, C). Finally, it is important to remember that VGSCs are packed into the nodal membrane at densities of more than a thousand channels per square micron, ten times even the density of VGSCs at the trigger zone. The high density of VGSCs at nodes works to prevent action potential conduction failure.

In general, axons greater than about 1 or 2 microns in diameter are myelinated. The amount of myelin wrapped around an axon increases as the diameter of the axon increases, up to a maximal axon diameter of 20 microns or so in vertebrates, including humans. An axon with a diameter of 10 microns will be wrapped by about 7 microns of myelin. This axon will conduct action potentials at about

60 meters/second. The conduction velocities of myelinated fibers vary from about 5 to as much as 120 meters/second.

DEMYELINATING DISEASES DISRUPT THE MYELIN WRAP AROUND AXONS

Peripheral and central myelin differ in several ways. As you recall from Chapter 2, peripheral myelin is produced by Schwann cells and central myelin by oligodendrocytes. In the periphery, the myelin wrap of each internode is produced by a single Schwann cell. In contrast, one oligodendrocyte provides myelination for the internodes of up to 40 central axons. Despite some shared components, such as *myelin basic protein*, many of the molecules in central and peripheral myelin are distinct. This is of great clinical importance because *demyelinating diseases affect either central or peripheral myelin, but not both*. An example of a central demyelinating disease is *multiple sclerosis*, and examples of peripheral demyelinating disease include the acute inflammatory *Guillain Barré syndrome* and a heterogenous group of progressive, hereditary neuropathies termed *Charcot-Marie-Tooth disease* or *hereditary sensorymotor neuropathy*.

Demyelination does not interfere with neuronal function or synaptic transmission. Instead, demyelination prevents action potentials from being faithfully and rapidly conducted down an axon. Demyelination essentially ruins the game of "telephone" from the soma of a neuron to its synaptic terminals. Demyelination may be of varying severity from a loosening of the myelin wrap to an outright loss of myelin, resulting in anything from a slowing to a complete failure of conducting action potentials. Altering the pattern of action potentials in turn changes information content (Fig. 10-4C–E). We can picture the effects of demyelination on neuronal communication by using the analogy to the bits and bytes of computer language introduced earlier. Let's say that, at every moment in time, the value of a bit is either one (action potential) or zero (no action potential) and that a sequence of 8 bits makes up a byte. As shown in Fig. 10-4, the loss of just a small number of spikes will substantially change meaning, and a single frame-shift will irreparably garble the message. This analogy is not perfect because it is too harsh in some respects and overly forgiving in others. Nonetheless, the exercise shows the sensitivity of neuronal communication to axonal myelination.

A. Pes cavus, hammer toes, wasting

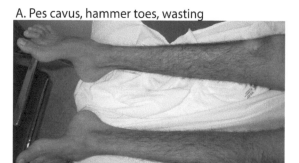

B. Hammer toes

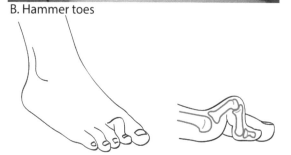

The effects of peripheral demyelination most commonly include weakness and loss of touch sensation, reflecting the contributions of well-myelinated peripheral axons to movement, proprioception, and touch sensation. In Charcot-Marie-Tooth disease, motor weakness and the lack of proprioceptive feedback lead to skeletomotor abnormalities including hammer toes, pes cavus (a very high arch), muscle atrophy, and even scoliosis (Fig. 10-8). Along with the diversity of symptoms caused by demyelinating diseases, the pathophysiology varies across and even within a disease such as Charcot-Marie-Tooth disease. For example, some forms of the disease result from a defect in the axon and other forms from a defect in Schwann cells. Regardless of whether the initial defect affects the axonal membrane or the myelinating glial cell, the end result is a loss of myelination and the consequent disruption to neuronal communication.

Figure 10-8 A: Charcot-Marie-Tooth is a demyelinating disease that produces musculoskeletal abnormalities. A: A patient shows pes cavus (high arches due to plantar flexion), hammer toes, and muscle wasting (in calves), all symptoms that are common in patients with Charcot-Marie-Tooth disease. B: A loss of strength and proprioceptive feedback due to impaired action potential conduction in the axons of well-myelinated motoneurons and sensory afferents can produce abnormal positioning of the toe joints that results in hammer toes. Panel A is reprinted with permission from The Hereditary Neuropathies by S Herskovitz in Peripheral Neuropathies in Clinical Practice (S Herskovitz, S Scelsa, H Schaumburg, eds.) New York: Oxford University Press, 2008. Panel B is reprinted with permission from Musculoskeletal problems by Simon C et al. in Oxford Handbook of General Practice (4 ed.; C Simon, H Everitt, F van Dorp, M Burkes, eds.) New York: Oxford University Press, 2014.

Multiple sclerosis is the consequence of an autoimmune attack on central myelin. Unfortunately, the antigen targeted for immune attack in multiple sclerosis remains unclear, although many features of this disease are mimicked in *experimental autoimmune encephalomyelitis*, which is elicited by an immune response to myelin basic protein in experimental animals. The particular symptoms associated with central demyelination depend on the identity of the axons affected. The most common symptoms are related to the functions of the most heavily myelinated axons in the CNS, those involved in voluntary movement, motor coordination, somatosensation, vision, eye movement, balance, and equilibrium. The good news in multiple sclerosis is that *remyelination* is possible although, unfortunately, not assured. Because demyelination in multiple sclerosis is associated with oligodendrocyte death, remyelination appears to stem from the proliferation and terminal differentiation of precursor cells into new oligodendrocytes that, in turn, can remyelinate bare axons.

ACTION POTENTIALS ARE TRANSLATED BACK INTO GRADED POTENTIALS AT THE SYNAPTIC TERMINAL

In this chapter, we examined how a neuron integrates inputs. We saw that information is supported by graded potentials in the dendrites and soma and by action potentials in axons. For neural communication to occur, the ultimate target of intracellular signaling is the synaptic terminal. As will be explored in the next chapter, information is once again carried by graded potentials in the synaptic terminal. Cells that lack an axon, such as retinal neurons and non-neuronal sensory hair cells of the inner ear employ graded potentials exclusively. However, for cells with an axon, the all-or-none language of spike trains is translated back into a graded potential within the synaptic terminal. The graded potential of the synaptic terminal in turn drives neurotransmitter release, the central topic explored in the next chapter.

ADDITIONAL READING

Cummins TR, Zhou J, Sigworth FJ, et al. Functional consequences of a Na+ channel mutation causing hyperkalemic periodic paralysis. *Neuron.* 10: 667–678, 1993.

Dyer CA. The structure and function of myelin: From inert membrane to perfusion pump. *Neurochem Res.* 27: 1279–1292, 2002.

El Waly B, Macchi M, Cayre M, Durbec P. Oligodendrogenesis in the normal and pathological central nervous system. *Front Neurosci.* 8: 145, 2014.

Kleopa KA. The role of gap junctions in Charcot-Marie-Tooth disease. *J Neurosci.* 31: 17753–17760, 2011.

Lipkind GM, Fozzard HA. Molecular model of anticonvulsant drug binding to the voltage-gated sodium channel inner pore. *Mol Pharmacol.* 78: 631–638, 2010.

Scherer SS, Arroyo EJ. Recent progress on the molecular organization of myelinated axons. *J Periph Nerv Syst.* 7: 1–12, 2002.

Strichartz GR, Wang G-K. State-dependent inhibition of sodium channels by local anesthetics: A 40-year evolution. *Biochem (Mosc) Suppl Ser A Membr Cell Biol.* 6: 120–127, 2012.

11.

NEUROTRANSMITTER RELEASE

nce a neuron sums up and integrates all incoming information into a coherent message, the neuron *sends* that message on to other cells via synapses. The crux of the challenge here is to ensure a tight correspondence between neuronal activity and the synchronous release of neurotransmitter. Ideally, whenever excited, a cell sends a loud and clear message. In the moments between being activated, a cell may "mutter" but not loudly enough that nearby neurons mistake the utterances for an intentional communication. By tying neural communication to neuronal activity, messages are meaningful and easily distinguished from background noise.

In this chapter, we examine the biochemical processes by which neurons send a chemical message to a postsynaptic cell. As explored in the next chapter, the chemical used in neural communication is a *neurotransmitter*. Neurotransmitters are packed by the thousands within *synaptic vesicles*, small (30–100 nm in diameter) spherical organelles that are present in synaptic terminals. Synaptic vesicles are released from the *active zone*, a stretch of synaptic membrane that faces a postsynaptic cell across the divide of the *synaptic cleft*. A minority of synaptic vesicles are *docked* at the active zone and then *primed* for release by protein complexes that bring them into extreme proximity to the plasma membrane. Release results when the membrane of a synaptic vesicle fuses with the plasma membrane so that neurotransmitter from the inside of the synaptic vesicle is now in the synaptic cleft. Molecules of neurotransmitter then passively *diffuse* across the synaptic cleft to reach a postsynaptic cell where they have effects as described in Chapter 13. Finally, the nervous system is anything but wasteful. Because of the fusion of synaptic vesicle membranes into the plasma membrane, the active zone membrane of working synapses is rich in valuable membrane proteins. This active zone membrane is endocytosed, and synaptic vesicle proteins are then reassembled into recycled synaptic vesicles, allowing for more rounds of neurotransmitter release.

SYNAPTIC VESICLE FUSION IS TIGHTLY CONTROLLED

At the core of neurotransmitter release is membrane fusion between a synaptic vesicle and the plasma membrane. Yet membrane fusion is a ubiquitous process required for all living cells—from yeast to plant to human—to survive. Constitutive membrane fusion serves basic cell biological functions such as the synthesis and trafficking of proteins through the endoplasmic reticulum and Golgi apparatus, the insertion of proteins into the plasma membrane, the construction of internal organelles, and cell division. Because membrane fusion events occur constitutively throughout all cells, it is not surprising that few, if any, inherited or autoimmune diseases involve a primary defect in membrane fusion machinery. It is equally unsurprising that bacteria and predatory animals have evolved the ability to synthesize, accumulate, and use toxins and venoms that specifically disable membrane fusion associated with neurotransmitter release. These toxins and venoms are used to temporarily immobilize or kill bacterial hosts and prey and can prove lethal to humans as well (see more "Clostridial Toxins Block Synaptic Transmission by Cleaving One of the SNAREpin Proteins").

Unlike constitutive membrane fusion, *membrane fusion associated with the release of neurotransmitters must be tightly controlled so that it occurs synchronously when triggered by neuronal activity*. Thus, the challenge to neurons is not membrane fusion per se but rather gaining complete control over the timing of membrane fusion. Neurons must yoke membrane fusion between synaptic vesicle and plasma membranes to an intended neural message. Thus, control over neurotransmitter release requires two fundamental functions:

• Minimizing spontaneous release

• Tying synchronous release to neuronal activity

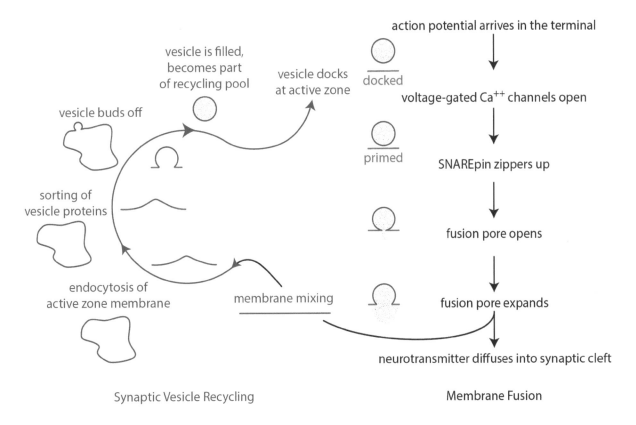

action potential arrives in the terminal

voltage-gated Ca⁺⁺ channels open

SNAREpin zippers up

fusion pore opens

fusion pore expands

neurotransmitter diffuses into synaptic cleft

vesicle is filled, becomes part of recycling pool

vesicle docks at active zone

docked

primed

vesicle buds off

sorting of vesicle proteins

endocytosis of active zone membrane

membrane mixing

Synaptic Vesicle Recycling

Membrane Fusion

Figure 11-1 Neurotransmitter release involves the coordination of neuronal activity leading to membrane fusion (*black on right*) with synaptic vesicle recycling (*blue on left*). Synaptic vesicles dock at the active zone, are primed, and, when triggered by a sharp increase in local calcium ion concentration, fuse to the membrane (*red insets*). When an action potential arrives in the synaptic terminal, calcium ion influx is triggered, and a high concentration of calcium ions is reached at the active zone. The high concentration of calcium ions at the site of docked synaptic vesicles zippers up the SNAREpin so that docked vesicles are primed for release. When the SNAREpin is completely zippered up, synaptic vesicles merge with the plasma membrane and a fusion pore forms. Neurotransmitter may leak out through the fusion pore, but free diffusion of neurotransmitter into the synaptic cleft requires an expanded pore. The insets show cartoons of docked and primed vesicles along with the initial fusion pore and the expanded "omega" fusion pore. Membrane from the active zone is endocytosed, and recycled vesicles are formed anew from the functional vesicle proteins. Synaptic vesicle recycling can occur either through endocytosis of just enough membrane to form a single synaptic vesicle (cartoons inside of circle) or through bulk endocytosis followed by budding off of single vesicles (cartoons outside of circle). In both cases, vesicle proteins (*blue*) must be sorted from plasma membrane proteins (*red*) and nonfunctional proteins (not shown), which are degraded. After a recycled vesicle is formed, it is filled with neurotransmitter and becomes part of the recycling pool.

Suppressing spontaneous release prevents neurons from "crying wolf," releasing gobs of neurotransmitter in the absence of an intended message. More accurately, spontaneous release is not prevented but rather minimized, sufficient to avert a multitude of neuronal "whispers," born of spontaneous and asynchronous release, from accumulating into a crescendo that a postsynaptic cell mistakenly interprets as an intentional message. Tying synchronous release to neuronal activity is the essence of neural communication. Neurons have optimized the connection between message and neurotransmitter release by using a sharp rise in the concentration of calcium ions at the active zone as the requisite trigger for the vast majority of synaptic release. Spontaneous vesicle fusion occurs but only sporadically and at low frequency.

In sum, substantial neurotransmitter release should reliably accompany every neuronal message and should not occur in the absence of a neuronal message. This ideal one-to-one relationship between neuronal activity and synchronous neurotransmitter release is accomplished by an exquisite dance of biochemical interactions between a large number of proteins. Before examining the details of the *neurotransmitter release dance* step by step, we consider an overview of what is currently understood about the release process. It should be noted that work in this field is intense, and, although our understanding is evolving rapidly, complete agreement on all steps currently evades us. With those caveats, the process of neurotransmitter involves the following elements (Fig. 11-1):

- A small number of synaptic vesicles are docked at the active zone by a protein complex called the *SNAREpin*.

- Synaptic vesicles are primed for triggered release by conformational changes in the SNAREpin and simultaneously prevented from spontaneous release through interactions between *complexin* and the SNAREpin.

- Depolarization of the synaptic terminal triggers calcium ion influx through *voltage-gated calcium channels* located near primed synaptic vesicles at the active zones.

- A high calcium ion concentration in the immediate vicinity of the active zone is sensed by *synaptotagmin*, which interacts with the SNAREpin of primed vesicles.

- A further conformational change of the SNAREpin, termed *zippering up*, results in a *fusion pore* that runs from the inside of the synaptic vesicle, through the plasma membrane, to the synaptic cleft.

- The fusion pore expands as the synaptic vesicle forms an omega shape (Ω) and then flattens out, allowing neurotransmitter contained within the vesicles to freely diffuse into the synaptic cleft.

- The protein and lipid constituents of the membrane from the emptied synaptic vesicle mix with the protein and lipid of the plasma membrane.

- Plasma membrane near the active zone, which is rich in synaptic vesicle proteins, is endocytosed into the synaptic terminal.

- Synaptic vesicles are regenerated, refilled with neurotransmitter, and returned to a *recycling pool* of vesicles available for future docking, priming, and eventual release.

Although we are most interested in neurotransmitter release per se, the actual release of neurotransmitter is relatively trivial—transmitter simply diffuses from a vesicle into the synaptic cleft through an opening or pore—compared to the complex process of *membrane fusion triggered by neuronal activity*. Consequently, this chapter focuses on the process of triggered membrane fusion.

There are two fundamentally different types of synaptic vesicles and, consequently, two processes of neurotransmitter release. In this chapter, we focus on the more common process, the release of small, low-molecular-weight neurotransmitters (see Chapter 12) such as glutamate or γ -aminobutyric acid (GABA) from small, clear synaptic vesicles. There are relatively few species, or types, of low-molecular-weight transmitters. Yet, these transmitters are ubiquitous, present in all, or nearly all, synaptic terminals in the nervous system (Fig. 11-2). The release of low-molecular-weight neurotransmitters from small synaptic vesicles is tightly regulated so that release accompanies neuronal activity, whereas release from inactive neurons is rare.

In the final section of this chapter, we consider the release of a different class of neurotransmitter, the *neuropeptides*, from large, dense-core vesicles. The type of neuronal activity that triggers release from large vesicles, as well as the molecular details of this release, differs substantially from the process of release from small synaptic vesicles.

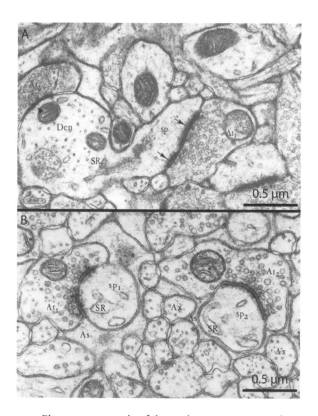

Figure 11-2 Electron micrographs of chemical synapses in rat visual cortex (*A*) and macaque cerebellum (*B*). The illustrated synapses are characterized by a large number of clear synaptic vesicles in the synaptic terminals (*At₁, At₂*) and by the electron-dense (therefore dark in an electron micrograph) membranes of both the active zone and the postsynaptic density. The presynaptic density marking the active zone is crowded with calcium channels, and the postsynaptic density is crowded with receptors. A: One presynaptic terminal (*At₁*) contains concentrations of synaptic vesicles at each of two active zones (*arrows*). The terminal is synapsing onto a spinehead (*sp*) that emerges from a dendrite (*Den*). That same dendrite also receives a synapse from an additional terminal (*At₂*) at the upper left. B: As in A, one presynaptic terminal (*At₁*) has two active zones, whereas a second presynaptic terminal (*At₂*) has a single active zone. Both terminals are synapsing onto Purkinje cell spines (*sp₁, sp₂*) in the cerebellum. Additional abbreviations: Ax: axon; As: astrocytic process; SR: smooth endoplasmic reticulum.   Photomicrographs are reprinted from Peters A, Palay SL, Webster H deF. *The fine structure of the nervous system: Neurons and their supporting cells*, 3rd edition. New York: Oxford University Press, 1991.

CALCIUM ION INFLUX IS NEEDED FOR NEUROTRANSMITTER RELEASE

Calcium ions are more concentrated, by at least a thousand-fold, outside of neurons (2–5 mM) than in the cytosol (10–100 nM). Thus, the calculated Nernst potential for calcium ions is a potential of hundreds of millivolts, far more positive than even the peak of the action potential. The enormously steep gradient in free calcium ions dictates that when calcium-permeable channels on the plasma membrane are open, *calcium ions will always enter the cell* and will do so with a great deal of driving force.

Unlike other ions, most calcium ions within a cell are sequestered in intracellular stores or deposits rather than existing freely within the cytosol. For example, the calcium ion concentration is 100–500 μM in the endoplasmic reticulum and reaches millimolar levels in mitochondria. Within the cytosol, calcium ions act as critical second-messengers that can modify enzyme activity and change ion channel properties (see Chapter 13). Calcium ions, present in nearly every intracellular organelle, can reach the cytosol through two types of calcium channels: inositol-1,4,5-trisphosphate (IP_3) and ryanodine receptors. However, for our purposes of understanding the role of calcium ions in triggering synaptic vesicle release, we now focus our attention solely on voltage-gated calcium channels in the plasma membrane at the active zone.

A depolarization from rest to about −20 mV activates calcium channels that, as is the case with voltage-gated sodium channels (VGSCs), are gated by a depolarized voltage. However, unlike sodium channels, *calcium channels do not rapidly inactivate but instead remain open for as long as the membrane is sufficiently depolarized.* Consequently, the total amount of calcium ion influx increases as the time that a synaptic terminal is sufficiently depolarized increases. Since the waveform of the all-or-none action potential can vary, the calcium ion influx accompanying action potentials varies as well. Remember that the time course of an action potential can vary with differences in membrane capacitance so that unmyelinated axons fire slower action potentials than do myelinated axons. The longer that an action potential lasts, the more calcium ion influx occurs. Thus, depending on its particular waveform or time course, an action potential causes more or less calcium ion entry into the synaptic terminal (Fig. 11-3). The amount of calcium ion influx in turn determines the amount of transmitter released, so that as more calcium ions enter the cell, more neurotransmitter is released. Consequently, the end result of the action potential—the amount of neurotransmitter released—varies between action potentials with different

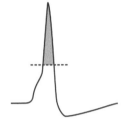

A. Brief action potential permits little Ca^{++} influx

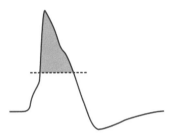

B. Prolonged action potential enables greater Ca^{++} influx

Figure 11-3 Short-duration action potentials (A) spend less time above the voltage threshold (*dashed line*) for voltage-gated calcium channels (*gray*) than do longer-duration action potentials (B). As a result, fewer calcium channels open, fewer calcium ions enter the cell, and less neurotransmitter release results.

time courses. Finally, it is important to remember that the depolarization needed to open calcium channels can arise from an action potential invading the synaptic terminal, as is the case for most neurons, or from a graded depolarization in the case of nonspiking neurons and sensory cells.

Calcium channels are located at the active zone immediately adjacent to sites where docked synaptic vesicles are primed and where membrane fusion occurs. Because of this architecture, calcium ions achieve a very high concentration at the active zone. This high concentration of calcium ions triggers fusion of the plasma and synaptic membranes (Fig. 11-4C). It should be noted that calcium ion–triggered vesicle fusion occurs even when the calcium ion concentration within the total cytosol of the neuron remains unchanged. Thus, *neurotransmitter release is triggered by a very high but very localized concentration of calcium ions.*

The importance of calcium channels to release is exemplified by *Lambert-Eaton syndrome*, a rare (<5 cases per million) autoimmune disease in which antibodies are directed against a subset of voltage-gated calcium channels. As mentioned in Chapter 2, paraneoplastic Lambert-Eaton syndrome arises from antibodies made in response to a malignancy, typically a small-cell lung carcinoma. In up to half of the patients with Lambert-Eaton syndrome, there is no malignancy and the disease is not paraneoplastic.

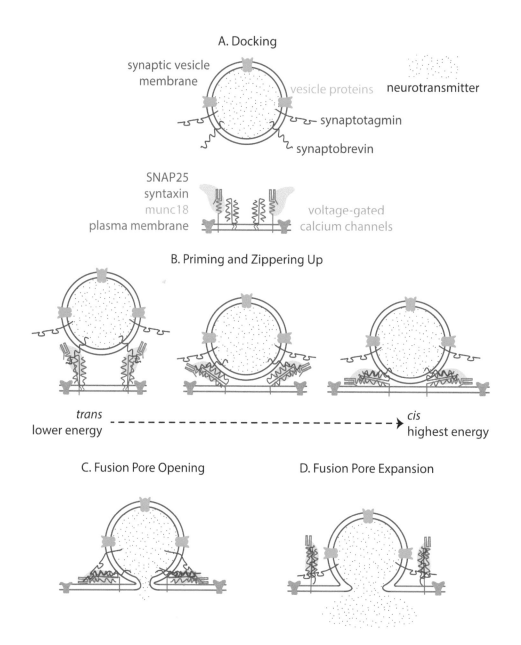

A. Docking

synaptic vesicle
membrane

vesicle proteins   neurotransmitter

synaptotagmin

synaptobrevin

SNAP25
syntaxin
munc18   voltage-gated
plasma membrane   calcium channels

B. Priming and Zippering Up

trans   *cis*
lower energy   highest energy

C. Fusion Pore Opening   D. Fusion Pore Expansion

Figure 11-4 Clear synaptic vesicles are docked (A), primed (B), and ultimately fuse to the plasma membrane (C–D), releasing their contents into the synaptic cleft. A: When a synaptic vesicle moves close to the plasma membrane, it is docked to the plasma membrane by RIM and associated proteins (not illustrated). B: Synaptic vesicles are brought progressively closer to the plasma membrane when the SNAREpin forms and zippers up, moving from a *trans* to a *cis* configuration and climbing an energetic mountain. C: When a high concentration of calcium ions (not illustrated) is reached in the immediate vicinity of the docked vesicle, synaptotagmin interacts with the SNAREpin to complete the latter's change in configuration. As a consequence, the vesicular and plasma membranes fuse, opening a small pore through which neurotransmitter may leak out. D: Using energy provided by NSF and other ATPases, membrane mixing is facilitated and the fusion pore expands, allowing neurotransmitter to freely diffuse into the synaptic cleft.

Regardless of etiology, Lambert-Eaton syndrome causes a loss of voltage-gated calcium channels critical to triggering synaptic release of neurotransmitter. This loss greatly impairs the synchronous release of neurotransmitter triggered by neuronal activity.

The antibodies involved in Lambert-Eaton syndrome do not cross the blood–brain barrier and therefore only affect peripheral terminals, primarily the neuromuscular junction between a motoneuron and skeletal muscle. Due to a decrease in the number of functional voltage-gated calcium channels within motoneuronal synaptic terminals, patients typically present with motor weakness as their chief complaint. With fewer calcium channels, each action potential results in less neurotransmitter release and therefore less muscle contraction. Diagnostic of Lambert-Eaton syndrome is an increasing or incremental response to repeated stimulation. The increasing response occurs because calcium ions, entering through the remaining voltage-gated calcium channels, progressively build up in the motoneuron terminal, eventually reaching levels that are sufficient for vesicle fusion with the plasma membrane. Thus, repeated stimulation circumvents the primary defect in Lambert-Eaton syndrome. Treating patients with *diaminopyridine*, a potassium channel blocker, is an effective therapeutic because it increases calcium ion influx by blocking repolarization of the action potential and thereby prolonging spike duration.

SPECIALIZED PROTEINS TETHER SYNAPTIC VESICLES AND CALCIUM CHANNELS TO THE ACTIVE ZONE

The active zone is a highly specialized cellular region where synaptic vesicles, the plasma membrane, and voltage-gated calcium channels exist in close proximity to one another (Fig. 11-2). Ensuring the proximity of these key active zone elements requires a number of proteins. Three *SNARE* (a catchy acronym for *s*oluble *NSF* *a*ttachment *r*eceptor proteins) *proteins* form the core of the SNAREpin. Two of the three SNARE proteins, SNAP-25 and syntaxin, are anchored within the plasma membrane while the third, synaptobrevin, is anchored within the synaptic vesicle membrane. The SNAREpin holds a docked synaptic vesicle near the plasma membrane of the active zone. When a high calcium ion concentration leads to a change in SNAREpin conformation, synaptic vesicles are brought so close to the plasma membrane that fusion is inevitable and unstoppable (more on this later).

SNARE proteins cannot work without a number of partners. Chief among these partners are *SM* (a not-so-catchy acronym for Sec1/Munc18-like) *proteins*, exemplified by Munc18. Munc18 associates with the SNAREpin, and, in the absence of Munc18, there is no neurotransmitter release. Finally, a close association between synaptic vesicles and the plasma membrane is insufficient for triggered release. Voltage-gated calcium channels must also be in close proximity to the other two active zone elements. A set of proteins, including *RIM* (Rab3-interacting molecule) *proteins* and their binding partners, tether voltage-gated calcium channels contained in the plasma membrane to docked and primed synaptic vesicles.

Within relatively inactive synaptic terminals that release only one or a few vesicles rarely, the number of docked vesicles is far less than the number in highly active synaptic terminals. Accordingly, the structure of the active zone varies to accommodate the docking of anywhere from a few to many vesicles. In a number of specialized sensory cells with high rates of neurotransmitter release, a proteinaceous "ribbon" extends into the cytosol, with synaptic vesicles docked on all sides of the ribbon. Ribbon-containing synapses are present in sound- and light-sensing cells, as well as in vestibular sensory cells that respond to accelerating forces.

A CHANGE IN SNAREPIN CONFORMATION BRINGS ABOUT MEMBRANE FUSION

Docked vesicles are held close to the plasma membrane by SNAREpins, the macro-molecular bundles of three SNARE proteins. Recall that two of the SNARE proteins (syntaxin, SNAP-25) are anchored in the plasma membrane while the third (synaptobrevin) is anchored in the vesicle membrane. Because of their molecularly distant attachments, these proteins only overlap at their untethered ends. Thus, the association is loose initially and the complexed proteins are in the *trans-* conformation. Thus, when a vesicle is simply docked at the active zone, the SNAREpin holds the vesicle at some distance from the plasma membrane (Fig. 11-4B). The process of priming a synaptic vesicle involves bringing the vesicle membrane closer to the plasma membrane, a feat that is accomplished as the SNARE proteins form a more tightly coiled bundle. The coiling process is referred to as "zippering up" the SNAREpin. As the SNAREpin becomes progressively more zippered up, the attached vesicles are moved closer and closer to the plasma membrane, progressively readying them for fusion.

When primed, vesicles are so close to the plasma membrane that membrane integrity is destabilized (Fig. 11-4B). Vesicle and plasma membranes would fuse if it were not for two interacting molecules, complexin and synaptotagmin. Recall that synaptotagmin is the calcium ion sensor that links release to calcium ion influx. In the absence of a high calcium ion concentration, complexin and synaptotagmin act together to prevent fusion of primed vesicles, thereby "clamping" down on spontaneous synaptic release.

When zippering up is complete, even complexin and syntagmin cannot keep the membranes from fusing. In other words, a zipped-up SNAREpin brings the membrane of a synaptic vesicle so close to the active zone membrane that a fusion pore is inevitable and resistance futile. At this point, the SNAREpin is in the *cis-* conformation. The vesicle and plasma membranes fuse, and a pore connects the inside of the synaptic vesicle to the extracellular space of the synaptic cleft (Fig. 11-4C). SM proteins facilitate lipid mixing between the now continuous membranes of the vesicle and cell, leading to expansion of the fusion pore. Pore expansion initially results in the synaptic vesicle adopting an omega shape (Ω) before eventually flattening out. Unlike the narrow fusion pore, the expanded pore allows neurotransmitter contained within the vesicles to freely diffuse into the synaptic cleft (see Fig. 11-4D).

Complexin lives up to its name because it is required for activity-triggered vesicle release as well as for clamping down on spontaneous vesicle release. Different parts of the complexin molecule partner with synaptotagmin to clamp down on spontaneous release or, alternatively, to tie triggered release to calcium ion influx. Once the calcium ion trigger for fusion arrives, synaptotagmin activates the SNAREpin and SM protein complex so that the SNAREpin finishes "zippering up."

Synaptic vesicles climb an energetic mountain as they move from the cytosol of a synaptic terminal to the active zone and ultimately fuse with the plasma membrane to open a pore. At the peak of the energetic mountain, the synaptic vesicle is docked and primed, held close to but remaining distinct from the plasma membrane. The energy needed to climb the mountain is provided by the energy-releasing conformational change of SNAREpins from *trans* to *cis* along with a number of specialized ATPases, such as NSF.

The synaptic delay, the time between a presynaptic action potential and a postsynaptic response, is less than a millisecond. The vast majority of the synaptic delay involves the time needed within the presynaptic terminal, time for an incoming signal to trigger calcium ion influx and then membrane fusion. Diffusion of neurotransmitter across the synaptic cleft and activation of postsynaptic receptors require far less time. Variations across neurons in the number and isoform of synaptotagmin molecules, as well as in the number of SNAREpins per vesicle, contribute to variations in the timing of neurotransmitter release across neurons. For example, the synaptotagmin isoform present in sound-localizing neurons is extremely fast, whereas the isoform in limbic neurons is slow. This difference matches the need for *microsecond* timing in localizing high-frequency (up to 15–20 kHz) sounds and the adequacy of more lackadaisical timing in limbic areas that support thoughts and emotions.

CLOSTRIDIAL TOXINS BLOCK SYNAPTIC TRANSMISSION BY CLEAVING ONE OF THE SNAREPIN PROTEINS

Clostridial toxins include *tetanus toxin* and several varieties of *botulinum toxin* made by bacteria of the *Clostridium* genus. Clostridial bacteria can only survive in an anaerobic environment and are killed by exposure to oxygen. Tetanus and botulinum toxins cleave a SNARE protein, causing irreparable harm that prevents neurotransmitter release until new SNARE proteins are synthesized. Fundamentally, the two clostridial toxins work very similarly, but they arrive at their destinations through different routes.

Botulinum toxin, produced by *C. botulinum*, causes *botulism* (from *botulus*, the Latin word for "sausage"), a condition originally described by Justinus Kerner in early 19th-century Germany when poor kitchen hygiene led to the production of rotten meat which in turn caused a rise in deaths from "sausage poison." Botulinum toxin is endocytosed by peripheral neuronal terminals, preferentially those that release acetylcholine, which includes motoneurons, preganglionic autonomic neurons, postganglionic parasympathetic neurons, and sympathetic ganglion cells that innervate sweat glands (see Chapter 13). Once inside the cell, botulinum toxin cleaves one of the molecules in the SNAREpin. Three strains of the toxin, including the one most widely used for therapeutic purposes, cleave SNAP-25; four strains cleave synaptobrevin; and one cleaves syntaxin. Cleavage of any part of the SNARE complex prevents neurons from releasing neurotransmitter. Since it is preferentially taken up by motoneurons that utilize acetylcholine as their transmitter, *botulinum toxin kills people by preventing the acetylcholine release necessary for breathing*. There is no treatment save for placing patients on a ventilator and waiting the weeks or months—depending on the strain involved—that it takes to break down and clear the toxin.

Kerner predicted that botulinum toxin could be used as a therapeutic and even experimented on himself to that end. Kerner was right. Despite its powerful lethality, botulinum toxin is now used at very low doses and with highly localized application as a treatment for a variety of medical conditions including *strabismus* or crossed eyes, *blepharospasm* or excessive blinking, *laryngeal dystonia* or spasm of the vocal cords, and even for certain types of incontinence.

Even more widespread than modified botulinum's therapeutic uses are its cosmetic uses, chiefly for the erasure of facial wrinkles. This latter use works because wrinkles are sustained by motoneuron-produced muscle contractions. Therefore, injection of modified botulinum into and near wrinkles blocks release of acetylcholine from motoneurons and therefore blocks activation of the facial muscles involved. The pharmaceutical relaxation of wrinkles lasts for months, as long as it takes to clear the injected toxin, typically strain A. The "safety" of injecting one of the most threatening agents of biological warfare into healthy people requires the usage of extremely low doses in restricted

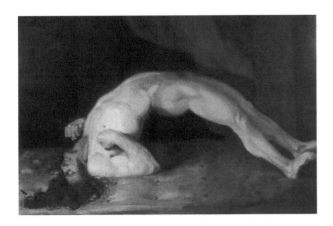

Figure 11-5 This painting, titled *Opisthotonos*, by Charles Bell, shows an individual suffering from tetanus. Physiological extensor muscles (see Section 5) are most affected, resulting in hyperextension. "Opisthotonos" is the term applied to a posture balanced on the heels of the feet and the crown of the head. This posture is a classic sign of severe tetanus. Photograph kindly provided by the Royal College of Scottish Surgeons of Edinburgh.

locales. Even so, reports of patients leaving a physician's office after receiving an injection of botulinum toxin for forehead wrinkles with an entirely frozen face are not uncommon.

C. tetani is the clostridial species that produces tetanus toxin. Like botulinum toxin, tetanus toxin cleaves a molecule in the SNARE complex, in this case synaptobrevin. Unlike botulinum toxin, tetanus toxin does not act on the synaptic terminals into which it is originally endocytosed. Instead, it is transported retrogradely (i.e., against the normal direction of action potential conduction) from the terminal to the soma of a motoneuron. The toxin is then further transported, again retrogradely but now trans-synaptically. This means that the toxin leaves the dendrites and soma of a motoneuron and travels "backward" *across the synaptic cleft* to presynaptic terminals. Another curious feature of tetanus toxin is that it invades only a subset of the motoneuron's presynaptic terminals, only those belonging to inhibitory neurons. Thus, tetanus toxin ends up in the synaptic terminals of inhibitory interneurons that contact motoneurons, and it is here that tetanus toxin exerts its pathogenic effects. The mechanisms targeting tetanus toxin specifically to the presynaptic terminals of inhibitory interneurons are not known.

Within the inhibitory interneuron terminals, tetanus toxin prevents neurotransmitter release. This in turn releases postsynaptic motoneurons from inhibitory control. The result is continuous motoneuron discharge and consequently unremitting muscle contractions causing lockjaw and *opisthotonos*, a characteristic arching of the back, memorialized in a powerfully emotive painting by the Scottish painter, Charles Bell (Fig. 11-5). Muscle contractions due

to tetanus are sufficiently severe that they cause severe pain and can even break bones. Luckily, tetanus vaccine is effective and widespread, rendering tetanus a disease largely of the past.

SYNCHRONOUS RELEASE DOMINATES BUT SPONTANEOUS RELEASE HAPPENS AND IS IMPORTANT

The synaptic terminal machinery is well-suited to tying neuronal activity to rapid and synchronous neurotransmitter release. Synchrony is critical for presynaptic cells to speak in a loud and coherent "voice." Yet the whispers continue as, occasionally, neurons spontaneously release vesicles of neurotransmitter. On average, each presynaptic terminal may spontaneously release a vesicle about once every couple of minutes. Yet, under certain conditions, for example in the presence of certain modulators, the rate of spontaneous release can increase to as much as every other second. Since typical neurons receive thousands of synapses, one or more vesicles may be released onto a neuron during any given millisecond. While this low level of spontaneous release is unlikely to elicit an action potential, it may change the membrane potential or alter excitability. In essence, untriggered, spontaneous vesicle fusion can produce a significant background hum in the neuronal conversations of the brain.

The molecules, membrane region, and mechanisms of spontaneous release appear to partially, but not fully, overlap with those of triggered synchronous release. As with synchronous release, spontaneous release depends on membrane fusion. Yet there are also differences between spontaneous and triggered release. For example, spontaneous release is not dependent on a high concentration of calcium ions throughout the active zone, as is required for activity-triggered release. Thus, at rest, single vesicles of neurotransmitter are released intermittently, perhaps in association with stochastic openings of single calcium channels. Then, when an action potential triggers sufficient calcium ion influx, fusion pores are formed at multiple terminals and neurotransmitter spills simultaneously into multiple synaptic clefts. Now, consider the consequences of losing voltage-gated calcium channels, as occurs in Lambert-Eaton syndrome. As we have already observed, triggered release from motoneurons is decreased. More action potentials are required for a triggering concentration of calcium ions to enter through fewer voltage-gated calcium channels. What about spontaneous release? Well, spontaneous release does not depend on a high calcium ion concentration throughout the active zone and therefore it is normal in Lambert-Eaton syndrome.

Exciting recent findings suggest that spontaneous release is critical to formation and stabilization of synapses during development. In adults, spontaneous release appears to be an important signal that is used in maintaining synapses at a roughly constant strength across time, a homeostatic process called *synaptic scaling*. For example, if spontaneous release from a presynaptic terminal plummets, perhaps due to injury or disease, a compensatory boost in synaptic efficacy will result. One mechanism by which synaptic efficacy can be increased is by the insertion of additional postsynaptic receptors.

VESICLES ARE THE SYNAPTIC UNIT OF INFORMATION

The vesicle is the smallest unit of information used by the chemical synapse, essentially the synaptic byte. Upon sufficient depolarization, some small number of vesicles fuses with the plasma membrane and dumps neurotransmitter into the synaptic cleft. The average number of vesicles released per action potential varies from hundreds at the neuromuscular junction to one at many central synapses. A difference in the number of active zones per synapse largely explains this variation. Many central synapses, such as those in the hippocampus, contain a single active zone, whereas the neuromuscular junction contains hundreds of active zones.

When a single action potential arrives at an active zone, either a vesicle is released or no vesicle is released. Put into probabilistic terms, the probability of release can vary between zero—release never happens—and one—release happens in response to every action potential. Release probability at hippocampal synapses is roughly 0.5, whereas at other, more reliable synapses, such as the neuromuscular junction, release probability may approach 0.8 or so.

The lower number of active zones and thus vesicles released at central synapses enables one postsynaptic cell to receive and sum up information from multiple inputs. A low number of active zones per synapse, and thus a low number of vesicles released per action potential, prevents a ceiling effect for each synaptic input (i.e., the cell is not maximally affected by input at any one synaptic contact). Because one input cannot saturate or even come close to saturating the postsynaptic response, inputs from an increasing number of excitatory inputs produce an increasingly large response. In practice, most central neurons integrate thousands of inputs without reaching a maximal or saturated response level. This wide dynamic range, the range of inputs over which a response varies, is critical in sensation, allowing us to, for example, hear a whisper as a quiet sound and a jet's takeoff as a loud sound. A wide dynamic range also enables us to issue a motor command to produce a force that varies between very low—sufficiently gentle to stroke a baby's cheek—to very high—strong enough to open a tightly sealed jar. Beyond these examples, all neurons operate within a dynamic range that is sufficient to allow for graded responses to graded inputs.

Integration of numerous inputs is not needed at the neuromuscular junction where only one motoneuron axon makes a single contact with each postsynaptic muscle fiber (see Chapter 21). Yet a motoneuron endplate contains many active zones. Since one vesicle is released at each active zone and there are hundreds of active zones, hundreds of vesicles are released per action potential in the presynaptic axon. This arrangement prevents a *floor effect*, meaning that when an action potential arrives in the motoneuron, the sole source of input to a muscle fiber, the effect will be large enough to ensure that the muscle responds. Thus, an action potential in the motoneuron innervating a skeletal muscle reliably causes a muscle fiber twitch.

SYNAPTIC VESICLES ARE RECYCLED

As synaptic vesicles fuse with the plasma membrane, the presynaptic membrane expands in area. If unchecked, this expansion would result in a ballooning presynaptic membrane that is out of register with a static postsynaptic membrane. As it turns out, the plasma membrane at the active zone is endocytosed in the terminals of active neurons. The endocytosed membrane contains contributions from the fused vesicle along with lipids and proteins native to the plasma membrane. The membrane components are sorted, and functional synaptic vesicle proteins are used to make new synaptic vesicles, whereas synaptic vesicle proteins that are no longer good are transported to the cell body for degradation. There are two major routes for recycling vesicles:

- Enough clathrin-coated membrane to form an individual vesicle is endocytosed and forms a new vesicle in a matter of seconds.

- Membrane from numerous vesicles is bulk endocytosed and numerous synaptic vesicles bud off from the internalized membrane, a process that requires tens of minutes.

At slow rates of neurotransmitter release, the amount of active zone membrane that is endocytosed is about the same as the amount of membrane contained within a synaptic vesicle. Under these circumstances, clathrin, a protein that self-assembles into basket-like structures, coats just enough plasma membrane at the active zone to form a single vesicle. Recycled vesicles are then refilled with neurotransmitter through processes described in Chapter 12. At faster rates of release, a larger area of membrane, including membrane from many vesicles, is taken up through bulk endocytosis into endosomal structures. From these endosomes, a small area of membrane becomes coated with clathrin and then buds off as a single synaptic vesicle.

THE POOL OF READILY RELEASABLE SYNAPTIC VESICLES IS REPLENISHED AFTER SYNAPTIC ACTIVITY

The synaptic vesicles abutting the membrane at the active zone are the ones released upon depolarization and calcium ion entry; these synaptic vesicles form the terminal's *readily releasable pool* (Fig. 11-6). The proportion of vesicles that is readily releasable is low, generally less than 2% of the synaptic vesicle population. Because of its small size, the readily releasable pool could, in theory, be depleted by fewer than two dozen action potentials occurring at high frequency (i.e., in rapid succession). Depletion does not occur because vesicle recycling *replenishes* the readily releasable pool.

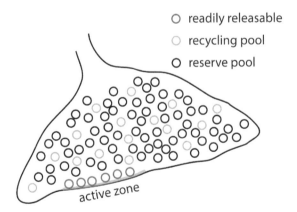

○ readily releasable
○ recycling pool
○ reserve pool

active zone

Figure 11-6 Synaptic vesicles that are docked and primed for release form the readily releasable pool. After fusing to the plasma membrane, the membrane from synaptic vesicles of the readily releasable pool is endocytosed. The endocytosed vesicles form the recycling pool, which is scattered throughout the synaptic terminal and which ultimately replaces the depleted readily releasable pool. The majority of synaptic vesicles in the synaptic terminal belong to the reserve pool. Reserve vesicles are tethered to the internal cytoskeleton and only move to the active zone under extremely active conditions.

Recycled vesicles comprise a *recycling pool,* consisting of 10–20% of the total number of synaptic vesicles in the synaptic terminal. Note that the recycling pool denotes a functional distinction, vesicles that were recently released and then endocytosed and recycled, but not a spatial one because the recycling vesicles are found interspersed with vesicles of a final group of synaptic vesicles, the *reserve pool* (see later discussion and Fig. 11-6). The recycling pool of vesicles not only arises from vesicles recycled from the readily releasable pool but also feeds the readily releasable pool. Thus, the readily releasable pool receives a constant influx of vesicles from the recycling pool, thereby ensuring the availability of enough vesicles for fusion upon a subsequent depolarization and preventing depletion of releasable synaptic vesicles from the synaptic terminal.

To summarize, under normal circumstances, an action potential arriving in the synaptic terminal sets in motion the recycling cycle:

- An action potential arrives, and a readily releasable vesicle fuses to the plasma membrane.

- Recycled vesicles join the recycling pool.

- A vesicle from the recycling pool moves toward the active zone and is docked, thereby joining the readily releasable pool of vesicles.

In this way, vesicle movement from the recycling pool to the readily releasable pool replenishes the pool of readily releasable synaptic vesicles docked at the active zone when needed.

A LARGE RESERVE POOL OF SYNAPTIC VESICLES SUPPLIES VESICLES WHEN HIGH-FREQUENCY RELEASE DEPLETES THE RECYCLING POOL

The vast majority of synaptic vesicles, 80–90% of the total, belong to the reserve pool. The reserve pool is intermingled with vesicles of the recycling pool. Under circumstances of unusually high activity, the recycling pool becomes depleted, and vesicles from the reserve pool are recruited to the active zone for release. At rest, molecules called *synapsins* tether reserve pool synaptic vesicles to the cytoskeleton. Upon strong stimulation, calcium ions accumulate in the synaptic terminal's free cytosol, not only in the region just inside the active zone membrane. A high cytosolic calcium ion concentration in the terminal triggers the phosphorylation of synapsin. When phosphorylated, synapsin releases the reserve pool's synaptic vesicles from their tether to the cytoskeleton so they can then move to the active zone, dock, and become primed for release.

LARGE DENSE-CORE VESICLES ARE RELEASED USING DISTINCT MECHANISMS

Small vesicles containing low-molecular-weight neurotransmitters make up the readily releasable pool of synaptic vesicles packed around the active zone, as well as the recyclable and reserve pools. As discussed earlier, a highly localized concentration of calcium ions confined to the active zone is sufficient for the fusion of small vesicles and consequent release of low-molecular-weight neurotransmitters. Remember that calcium channels crowd the active zone. Therefore, a local elevation of calcium ion concentration at the active zone can be achieved by the invasion of *a single action potential*.

No readily releasable pool of large, dense-core vesicles exists. Rather, large vesicles are scattered throughout the synaptic terminal, typically in locations relatively far from the active zone (Fig. 11-7). The fusion of large vesicles is only triggered when the concentration of calcium ions rises at the locations of the vesicles dispersed throughout the cytosol of the synaptic terminal. Although the calcium ion concentration required for large-vesicle fusion is quite a bit lower than that needed for small-vesicle release, that concentration must be achieved globally within the cytosol of the terminal. Therefore, release from large vesicles typically requires a high-frequency train of action potential firing to achieve the needed calcium ion concentration throughout the synaptic terminal. In sum, *single action potentials preferentially release small vesicles containing low-molecular-weight neurotransmitters, whereas it often takes a train of action potentials to release large vesicles containing a mixture of peptides and low-molecular-weight neurotransmitters.*

WIDESPREAD SYNAPTIC DISRUPTION MAY BE AT THE CORE OF SEVERAL DISEASES

Babies with *Rett syndrome*, a severe developmental disorder that causes intellectual disability, repetitive behaviors, and seizures in girls, begin to diverge from a normal developmental course at about 18 months. Similarly, babies with autism develop normally before regressing at some point after the first year of life. Thus, in both of these developmental

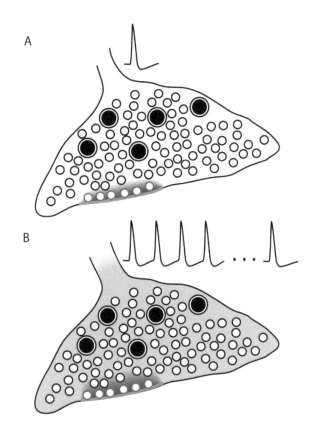

Figure 11-7 Some synaptic terminals contain both small, clear vesicles and large, dense-core vesicles. As illustrated here, the number of small vesicles is usually much greater than the number of large vesicles. A: Readily releasable small vesicles (*red circles*) can fuse to the plasma membrane when the calcium ion concentration increases locally (*dark blue cloud*). A single action potential is capable of increasing the local calcium ion concentration and thus of triggering fusion of a small synaptic vesicle. B: In contrast, large, dense-core vesicles only fuse when the calcium ion concentration increases throughout the synaptic terminal (*light blue*). The calcium ion concentration needed to trigger dense-core vesicle fusion is far lower (B) than is needed for fusion of clear vesicles (A). Yet a train of high-frequency action potentials is typically needed to produce this increase in calcium ion concentration *globally* throughout the terminal. Even as a train of action potentials produces a small increase globally, it also greatly increases calcium ion concentration locally at the active zone.

disorders, *affected individuals show symptoms postnatally after a period of normal development.* At the time point when symptoms arise, the brain has already formed and neurons (with the exception of many neurons in the cerebellum) have been born. Synaptic connections have even formed. The timing of disease onset is suggestive that these developmental disorders are disorders that alter the operations of synaptic connections. In 2003, Huda Zoghbi proposed the idea that Rett syndrome and autism are *synaptopathies*, diseases of synaptic function. Since that time, genetic evidence has accumulated to suggest that at least some forms of neurodegenerative disorders (Parkinson's disease, Alzheimer's disease, age-related hearing loss) and neurospsychiatric diseases (e.g., schizophrenia) are also synaptopathies.

The implication of synaptic proteins in complex diseases brings home the fundamental importance of understanding how the array of molecules involved in synaptic function produce diverse modes of neuronal communication that vary in time and space, appropriately operating under different circumstances and across widespread brain areas.

ADDITIONAL READING

Erbguth FJ, Naumann M. Historical aspects of botulinum toxin: Justinus Kerner (1786-1862) and the "sausage poison." *Neurology.* 53: 1850–1853, 1999.

Kaeser PS, Regehr WG. Molecular mechanisms for synchronous, asynchronous, and spontaneous neurotransmitter release. *Annu Rev Physiol.* 76: 333–363, 2014.

Kavalali ET. The mechanisms and functions of spontaneous neurotransmitter release. *Nat Rev Neurosci.* 16: 5–16, 2015.

Kononenko NL, Haucke V. Molecular mechanisms of presynaptic membrane retrieval and synaptic vesicle reformation. *Neuron.* 85: 484–496, 2015.

Neher E, Sakaba TC. Multiple roles of calcium ions in the regulation of neurotransmitter release. *Neuron.* 59: 861–872, 2008.

Rizzoli SO, Betz WJ. Synaptic vesicle pools. *Nat Rev Neurosci.* 6: 57–69, 2005.

Südhof TC, Rothman JE. Membrane fusion: Grappling with SNARE and SM proteins. *Science.* 323: 474–477, 2009.

Südhof TC. A molecular machine for neurotransmitter release: Synaptotagmin and beyond. *Nat Med.* 19: 1227–1231, 2013.

Südhof TC. Neurotransmitter release: The last millisecond in the life of a synaptic vesicle. *Neuron.* 80: 675–690, 2013.

Zhai RG, Bellen HJ. The architecture of the active zone in the presynaptic terminal. *Physiology.* 19: 262–270, 2004.

Zoghbi HY. Postnatal neurodevelopmental disorders: meeting at the synapse? *Science.* 302: 826–830, 2003.

12.

SYNTHESIS, PACKAGING, AND TERMINATION OF NEUROTRANSMITTERS

eurotransmitters carry messages from one neuron to another. By most estimates, there are more than a hundred different neurotransmitters. Neurotransmitters comprise a set of molecules that are heterogeneous in chemical structure, stability, and mode of action. Some neurotransmitters, such as glutamate and adenosine triphosphate (ATP), are present in all cells of the nervous system and body. Numerous other neurotransmitters, such as serotonin and the peptide neurotransmitters, are far more concentrated in non-nervous tissue than in neurons and glia. Thus, *neurotransmitters are not a special set of biological molecules dedicated to neural communication but rather a diverse group of molecules serving multiple duties in various tissues of the body, including the nervous system.*

Neurotransmitters within the nervous system are extremely heterogeneous in their distribution, ubiquity, physiological effect, and ultimate function. Some neurotransmitters participate in a myriad of functions and others in only a few. Examples of the ubiquitous type are γ-aminobutyric acid (GABA) and glutamate, each of which participates in arguably every circuit within the central nervous system (CNS). Glutamate is a critical player in cellular learning regardless of whether the neurons participate in learning to ride a bike, speak a new language, recognize a new acquaintance, or solve a quadratic equation. Although a shared function for GABA is less clear, GABA appears to be important in accentuating differences, such as the edge of a visual object or the pause between spoken words. At the other extreme, some neurotransmitters participate in a relatively small number of functions. Histamine, a major signaling molecule in the immune system that is released from mast cells, is present in neurons of a *single* brain nucleus that coordinates brain function with sleep–wake status. Another example is the peptide growth hormone releasing hormone or GHRH, which is also synthesized by only one small group of hypothalamic neurons and, critically, stimulates growth hormone release from the pituitary.

Most neurotransmitters occupy a middle ground between the extremes of GABA and glutamate on one hand and histamine and GHRH on the other. For example, the neuropeptide substance P serves several functions. Substance P provides an important signal in the transmission of noxious information that can result in a perception of pain. It is also contained in afferents from the stomach that trigger vomiting, or emesis. Substance P's actions in the brainstem, striatum, substantia nigra, amygdala, and a number of other regions are varied. And, yet, there are circuits, such as those supporting sound localization, where Substance P is not present and, thus, plays no functional role.

NEUROTRANSMITTERS COME IN THREE BASIC VARIETIES

All neurotransmitters must be synthesized, released, and then effect a response in the targeted cell. The modes of synthesis and release, the manner in which a neurotransmitter causes a response, and the fashion in which a neurotransmitter's effect comes to an end differ widely across the more than 100 neurotransmitters. Within this extreme heterogeneity, there are groups of neurotransmitters that operate similarly. Thus, we can think of neurotransmitters as belonging to one of three classes, each possessing a different feature set with respect to synthesis, packaging, and action:

1. A dozen or so *low-molecular-weight molecules* are enzymatically synthesized in the synaptic terminal and packaged in small clear vesicles; these comprise the so-called classical neurotransmitters.

2. There are *more than a hundred* small *peptides* that are made through transcription in the cell body and transported to the synaptic terminal within large dense-core vesicles.

3. At least two gas neurotransmitters are employed for neural communication.

There is a fundamental difference between low-molecular-weight and peptide neurotransmitters on one hand and gas neurotransmitters on the other. Low-molecular-weight and peptide neurotransmitters support orthodromic (*right-running*) communication, from a synaptic terminal to the dendrites and somata of other cells. Gas neurotransmitters are fundamentally different in that they are typically made in and released from dendrites, thereby supporting antidromic (*against-running*) communication from dendrites back onto synaptic terminals. In this chapter, we delve into low-molecular-weight and peptide neurotransmitters in some depth, leaving a cursory discussion of gas neurotransmitters for the end.

NEUROTRANSMITTERS SHARE A RESTRICTED NUMBER OF MECHANISMS FOR SYNTHESIS, PACKAGING, AND TERMINATION OF EFFECT

Although no physical property distinguishes the set of molecules that serves neural communication and any given molecule may serve multiple roles in the body, *only hormones and neurotransmitters are packaged into vesicles*. Neurotransmitters fill vesicles at far higher concentrations, as much as one molar, than are present in either the surrounding cytosol or other parts of the body. The manner in which neurotransmitters are packaged into vesicles differs between low-molecular-weight and peptide neurotransmitters. The former are packed into vesicles using *vesicular transporters* that shuttle synthesized neurotransmitter from the cytosol into the vesicle. Packaging of low-molecular-weight neurotransmitters occurs within the synaptic terminal. In contrast, peptides are packed into synaptic vesicles within the cell body where they are synthesized as the product of translation and transcription. Synaptic vesicles containing peptide neurotransmitters reach the terminal through axonal transport from the cell body to the terminal (see Chapter 2).

As described in Chapter 11, the start of neurotransmitter release is highly regulated so that it starts synchronously upon the influx of calcium ions. In order for the message of synchronous neurotransmitter release to be meaningful, neurotransmitter must be transiently present, lending an end as well as a beginning to the message. An interminable message, like an interminable lecture, loses meaning. The end of a neurotransmitter's message is regulated in several ways that are understood and in some ways that warrant further investigation.

A major contributor to both the onset and termination of a neurotransmitter's action is *diffusion*. Neurotransmitter diffuses from the site of release to the sites of the receptors to which the neurotransmitter binds. At a typical synapse in the CNS, the synaptic cleft across which a neurotransmitter diffuses to reach the postsynaptic cell is narrow, about 30 nanometers across, whereas at the neuromuscular junction, the synaptic cleft is 100 nanometers wide. At other synapses, no classic synaptic cleft exists, and the location of the receptors may be some distance from the site of release. In still other cases, perhaps the majority of central synapses, neurotransmitter acts on receptors located both near and far from the site of release. As a result of diffusion, neurotransmitter concentration and thus the probability of a neurotransmitter's binding to a receptor decrease rapidly with distance from the site of release. In this way, *diffusion contributes enormously to terminating the message of every neurotransmitter*.

A set of transporters present in cellular membranes takes neurotransmitter from the extracellular space to the inside of a neuron or glial cell. This recycling process is termed *uptake* and effectively ends the action of many neurotransmitters, including most of the low-molecular-weight neurotransmitters. Transporters involved in uptake sit in the plasma membrane and comprise a distinct group, with distinct affinities from the vesicular transporters present in the membrane of synaptic vesicles. For example, a single vesicular transporter can move serotonin, dopamine, and norepinephrine across a vesicle membrane whereas three different uptake transporters preferentially move serotonin, dopamine, or norepinephrine across the plasma membrane. *Degradation* also plays a primary role in terminating the message of some neurotransmitters. For example, extracellularly located enzymes break down excess acetylcholine, thereby ending the synaptic message. As another example, peptides are degraded by extracellular peptidases.

Uptake and degradation are processes upon which many drugs act. Widely used psychotropic therapeutics, as well as abused drugs such as cocaine, act on transporters responsible for neurotransmitter uptake. Other therapeutics, as well as toxins including pesticides and biological weapons, disable enzymes that degrade neurotransmitters. In addition, a number of mutations in uptake transporters are associated with personality traits such as impulsiveness or aggression.

The modes of synthesis, packaging, and release and the activated receptors and mechanisms of termination of neurotransmitter action for low-molecular-weight and peptide neurotransmitters are summarized in Table 12-1.

Table 12-1 FUNDAMENTAL PROPERTIES OF LOW-MOLECULAR WEIGHT AND PEPTIDE NEUROTRANSMITTERS

	LOW-MOLECULAR-WEIGHT MOLECULES	PEPTIDES
Synthesis	Mostly in the terminal	In the soma
Packaging	In either small clear vesicles or large dense-core vesicles	In large dense-core vesicles only
Release trigger, location	Ca^{2+}-dependent, single action potentials, from active zones	Ca^{2+}-dependent, trains of action potentials, from peri-synaptic regions outside the active zone
Effect	Activates ionotropic and metabotropic receptors, located both synaptically and peri-synaptically	Activates metabotropic receptors located peri-synaptically
Termination of action	Diffusion, uptake, and/or enzymatic degradation	Diffusion and proteolysis (enzymatic degradation)

As the reader is aware, most neurons use chemical transmission, and, at most chemical synapses, at least one low-molecular-weight neurotransmitter is released. Four low-molecular-weight neurotransmitters—glutamate, GABA, acetylcholine, and norepinephrine—are particularly abundant, with one of these four used as a neurotransmitter in virtually all peripheral and central neurons. In contrast, any one peptide may be employed by only a small number of neurons.

A common feature of low-molecular-weight neurotransmitters is that their production is tied to neuronal activity. How can this be? As you recall from basic chemistry, enzymatic activity depends on the concentrations of substrate and product (termed the *law of mass action*). The dependence of enzyme activity on the concentrations of substrate and product is critical to understanding neurotransmitter synthesis in the nervous system. When neurotransmitter—the product—is abundant, the rate of neurotransmitter synthesis decreases, whereas when neurotransmitter supply is depleted, the rate of synthesis increases. Therefore, an important modulator of the activity of many neurotransmitter-synthesizing enzymes is neural activity.

When neural activity changes for a sustained period of time, adaptive changes may occur. Persistent increases in neural activity can lead to increased production of neurotransmitter by any number of modifications, such as increasing the activity of the synthesizing enzymes or the affinity of the enzymes for a co-factor or by decreasing the affinity of an enzyme for an inhibitor. Regardless of the mechanism, short- and long-term mechanisms that link the rate of neurotransmitter synthesis to neurotransmitter release ensure that the supply of neurotransmitter remains in line with demand.

After synthesis, low-molecular-weight neurotransmitters are transported into vesicles. The membranes of all synaptic vesicle membranes house an ATPase, an ATP-fueled pump, that uses cytosolic ATP to transport protons from the cytosol to the inside of the vesicle. As a result, *all synaptic vesicles have a high proton concentration. This proton gradient—low in the cytosol to high in the vesicle—is then used by the vesicular transporters to "load" neurotransmitter into the vesicle.* ATP is also present in high concentrations within most vesicles, including vesicles containing non-nucleotide neurotransmitters.

As mentioned earlier, we divide low-molecular-weight neurotransmitters into five categories based on the synaptic vesicle transporters. The correspondence between the five types of vesicular transporters and the five classes of low-molecular-weight neurotransmitters is shown in Table 12-2.

Acetylcholine is the neurotransmitter released by all somatic motoneurons as well as by all preganglionic autonomic motor neurons. In addition, acetylcholine is found in neurons in a restricted number of brain regions such as the basal forebrain. The small number of cholinergic, or acetylcholine-containing, neurons have widespread axonal projections that reach throughout the brain and spinal cord, playing a key role in facilitating learning and attention. Similarly, a relatively small number of monoaminergic neurons, neurons containing a monoamine transmitter, project extensively throughout the CNS and have important functions. For example, histaminergic (histamine-containing) neurons are only found in the tuberomammillary nucleus of the hypothalamus but reach all parts of the brain and spinal cord through widely projecting axons. Histaminergic signaling in the CNS promotes wakefulness, and histamine receptor antagonists cause drowsiness. In the same vein, dopamine, norepinephrine, and serotonin are monoamines that critically modulate virtually every function of the CNS from thermoregulation to muscle tone and posture to sleep–wake cycling, motivation, and affect. Epinephrine, an important hormone released by the adrenal medulla, is found in restricted sites within the CNS mostly having to do with homeostatic regulation of blood pressure, salt balance, and the like.

NEUROTRANSMITTER CLASS	VESICLE TRANSPORTER	LOW-MOLECULAR-WEIGHT NEUROTRANSMITTERS
Acetylcholine	Acetylcholine transporter VAChT; <u>v</u>esicular <u>a</u>cetyl<u>ch</u>oline <u>t</u>ransporter	Acetylcholine
Monoamine	Monoamine transporter VMAT; <u>v</u>esicular <u>m</u>ono<u>a</u>mine <u>t</u>ransporter	Dopamine, norepinephrine, epinephrine (catecholamines) Serotonin Histamine
Excitatory amino acid	Glutamate transporter VGLUT; <u>v</u>esicular <u>g</u>lutamate <u>t</u>ransporter	Glutamate Aspartate
Inhibitory amino acid	GABA and glycine transporter VIAAT; <u>v</u>esicular <u>i</u>nhibitory <u>a</u>mino <u>a</u>cid <u>t</u>ransporter	GABA Glycine
Nucleotide	ATP transporter VNUT; <u>v</u>esicular <u>n</u>ucleotide <u>t</u>ransporter	ATP Adenosine

Central acetylcholine and monoamines operate primarily through *modulation*. A common misconception is that *modulation* is a code word for an unimportant contribution with only minor consequences. However, modulation is key to nervous functions that range from motor reflexes, thermoregulation, and walking to attention, learning, and cognition. Dysfunctions of modulatory pathways can lead to severe neurological diseases such as dementia (Box 12-1) or schizophrenia.

Glutamate is the most prevalent excitatory neurotransmitter in the brain. Aspartate, another amino acid, acts as an excitatory neurotransmitter in relatively few select regions of the brain. γ-Aminobutyric acid and glycine are amino acids that serve as inhibitory neurotransmitters, with GABA employed throughout the brain and spinal cord and glycine used primarily in the spinal cord and a few select areas in the brainstem. As mentioned earlier, ATP is contained in all synaptic vesicles and thus is released from most, if not all, neurons. Yet ATP is a particularly important signaling molecule at select synapses. Notably, ATP excites primary afferent synapses to signal sharp pain as well as a full bladder. Adenosine, a purinergic nucleoside present in all cells, acts as an inhibitory neurotransmitter and may be important in promoting sleep. As most readers are personally aware, the adenosine receptor antagonist caffeine promotes wakefulness.

Space does not permit us to cover every neurotransmitter. Therefore, in the following sections, the synthetic pathway, vesicular packaging, and mode of termination of action for acetylcholine, three monoamines (serotonin, dopamine, norepinephrine), glutamate, and GABA are described. We then consider peptide neurotransmitters as a group.

Box 12-1 DIMINUTION OF CHOLINERGIC TRANSMISSION IN THE FOREBRAIN CONTRIBUTES TO THE DEVELOPMENT OF DEMENTIA

During normal aging, cholinergic neurons die, and this may contribute to the mild memory problems and other cognitive compromises that are common among the elderly. In contrast, individuals with Alzheimer's disease have a gross loss of cholinergic neurons, including those in the basal forebrain that innervate the cerebral cortex. Loss of cholinergic function contributes to the cognitive decline in Alzheimer's disease. *Anticholinesterase* drugs slow the breakdown of acetylcholine. Anticholinesterase drugs are used to treat patients with Alzheimer's disease because they prolong the action of acetylcholine released from the remaining cholinergic neurons. These drugs do not address the underlying pathophysiology of Alzheimer's disease nor do they miraculously improve cognitive function. However, they may delay symptoms in some people and improve function in fewer people. Thus, treatment with anticholinesterases represents one of the only hopes, modest though it may be, available to Alzheimer's disease patients and their families.

ACETYLCHOLINE IS SYNTHESIZED IN THE NEURONAL TERMINAL AND RAPIDLY DEGRADED IN THE SYNAPTIC CLEFT

Acetylcholine is very important in the peripheral nervous system. Recall that it is the neurotransmitter used by all somatic motoneurons, preganglionic autonomic neurons, and postganglionic parasympathetic neurons. Acetylcholine's critical role in movement and autonomic function and the easy access to the neuromuscular junction have facilitated detailed studies of acetylcholine synthesis, packaging, and degradation. As evidence of acetylcholine's critical role in movement and autonomic function, a number of naturally occurring diseases and toxins, as well as synthetic agents such as pesticides, target acetylcholine neurotransmission. In the brain, acetylcholine plays a critical role in cognitive health through modulating attention, memory, arousal state, and the like (see Box 12-1).

Choline acetyltransferase, an enzyme present in the cytosol of synaptic terminals, transfers the acetyl moiety from acetyl coenzyme A to choline, thereby resulting in acetylcholine (Fig. 12-1). Under normal circumstances, dietary intake is the source of choline, the substrate for choline acetyltransferase. Foods rich in choline include egg yolks, soybeans, and liver. The choline transporter within the plasma membrane of cholinergic terminals transports

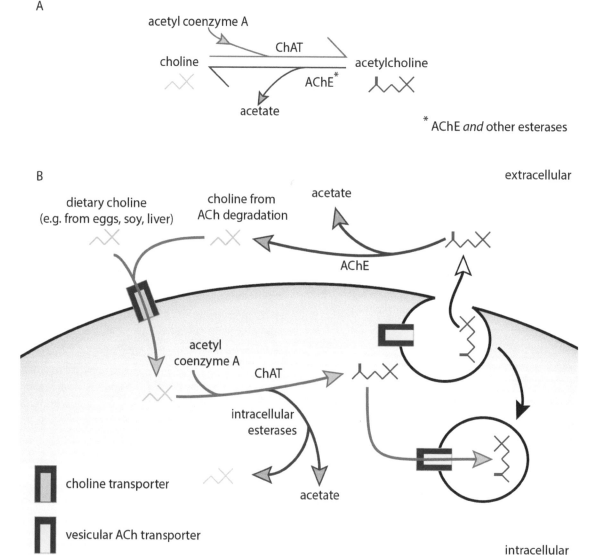

Figure 12-1 A: Acetylcholine (*ACh*) is synthesized from choline and acetyl coenzyme A by choline acetyltransferase (*ChAT*). Acetylcholinesterase (*AChE*) and several other esterases break acetylcholine down into choline and acetate. B: The synthesis, packaging, release, breakdown, and uptake mechanisms involved in cholinergic transmission are illustrated in situ. Choline (*light blue symbol as in A*) from dietary sources and from the extracellular breakdown of released ACh (*dark blue symbol as in A*) is taken up into cells by the choline transporter. Within cholinergic terminals, ChAT catalyzes the synthesis of ACh from choline and acetyl coenzyme A. The vesicular ACh transporter shuttles ACh from the cytoplasm into synaptic vesicles. Upon release, ACh is rapidly degraded by AChE. Within the terminal, esterases, including but not limited to AChE, break down ACh.

choline from the extracellular space and into the synaptic terminal. The choline transporter has a high affinity for choline, meaning that it can act on choline that is present at very low concentrations.

The vesicular acetylcholine transporter sits within the membrane of synaptic vesicles present in cholinergic terminals and transports acetylcholine into the vesicles (Fig. 12-1). Production of acetylcholine follows the law of mass action, by which the rate of any reaction in dynamic equilibrium is proportional to the cytosolic concentrations of the substrate—choline in the case of the end-product acetylcholine. As acetylcholine is transported into recycling vesicles, free acetylcholine concentration decreases and production increases. Substrate availability also plays a role because a higher concentration of choline than of acetylcholine will favor acetylcholine production, whereas a higher concentration of acetylcholine than of choline favors acetylcholine degradation.

Numerous *esterases*, enzymes that break acetylcholine down into choline and acetate, are present in the cytosol of the synaptic terminal. These esterases complicate the situation with neuronal production of acetylcholine because two enzymatic reactions are involved: choline acetyltransferase that produces acetylcholine and esterases that break it down. Acetylcholine is a substrate for esterases as well as the end-product of choline acetyltransferase, whereas choline is the substrate for choline acetyltransferase as well as the end-product of esterases. When acetylcholine builds up, choline acetyltransferase activity decreases and esterase activity increases, leading to a net breakdown of acetylcholine. In contrast, when choline builds up, choline acetyltransferase activity increases and esterase activity decreases, leading to a net synthesis of acetylcholine. In this way, large deviations in the concentration of acetylcholine away from equilibrium are prevented.

After release into the synaptic cleft, acetylcholine is degraded *extremely rapidly* by a large pool of extracellular acetylcholinesterase (Fig. 12-1). Extracellular choline is taken up by a choline transporter in the synaptic terminal, providing substrate for further synthesis of acetylcholine. A large number of drugs and toxins ranging from efficacious therapeutics to insecticides to agents of biological warfare interfere with acetylcholinesterase function (see Box 12-2).

MONOAMINES SHARE A COMMON PACKAGING MECHANISM

There are five monoamines: histamine, serotonin, dopamine, norepinephrine, and epinephrine. Two catecholamines go

Box 12-2 ANTICHOLINESTERASES ARE IMPORTANT THERAPEUTICS AND ALSO LETHAL WEAPONS

Anticholinesterases, drugs that interfere with acetylcholinesterase activity, prolong the effect of acetylcholine. Prolonging cholinergic signaling is therapeutic in conditions such as myasthenia gravis, in which cholinergic signaling is reduced. *Myasthenic* patients are weak because of a reduction in the number or clustering of acetylcholine receptors present on skeletal muscles (see Chapter 13). *Edrophonium*, a very short-acting anticholinesterase, is used as a diagnostic tool: a patient with myasthenia gravis can sustain a stronger muscle contraction for a longer time after edrophonium. Longer acting but still reversible anticholinesterases such as *neostigmine* provide effective treatment for patients with myasthenia gravis. Insecticides such as *parathion* are irreversible anticholinesterases and, at sufficient doses, can kill humans as well as insects. Finally, agents designed to kill humans, such as *sarin*, are, like insecticides, irreversible anticholinesterases. Sarin is highly volatile and easily passes through the skin. Even minute amounts of sarin are lethal to humans.

by different names in America and Europe. Norepinephrine is synonymous with noradrenaline and epinephrine with adrenaline. Customarily, Americans use norepinephrine and epinephrine, as I do in this book, whereas Europeans employ noradrenaline and adrenaline. Note that neurons that contain norepinephrine are referred to as *noradrenergic* and those that contain epinephrine are referred to as *adrenergic* in America and Europe alike. Receptors that bind norepinephrine or epinephrine are universally referred to as *adrenergic receptors*.

The five different monoamines depend on different synthetic pathways, and their actions are terminated by different mechanisms. Yet, they all share a requirement for the vesicular monoamine transporter (VMAT) that transports histamine, serotonin, dopamine, and epinephrine, synthesized within the cytosol, into synaptic vesicles. An additional monoamine, norepinephrine, is synthesized within synaptic vesicles from dopamine transported into the vesicles by VMAT (Fig. 12-2). Because of their shared dependence on VMAT, the monoamines can be viewed as a single neurotransmitter class, albeit a highly heterogeneous one (Table 12-2).

A second similarity among monoamines is the paucity of classical synapses involving a presynaptic element and a postsynaptic element separated by a narrow synaptic cleft. Instead, monoamines appear to depend primarily on

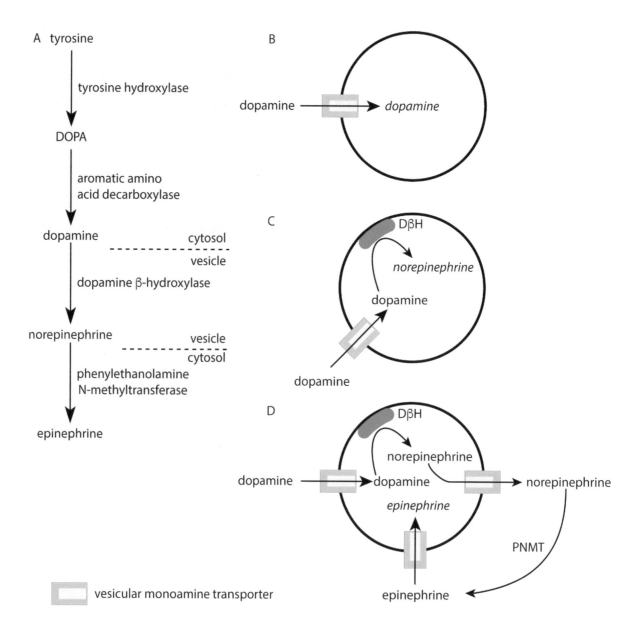

Figure 12-2 A: Tyrosine hydroxylase, the rate-limiting step in catecholamine synthesis, converts tyrosine into 3,4-dihydroxyphenylalanine (*DOPA*). Aromatic amino acid decarboxylase converts DOPA into dopamine, and dopamine β-hydroxylase (*DβH*) converts dopamine into norepinephrine. Finally, phenylethanolamine N-methyltransferase (*PNMT*) converts norepinephrine into epinephrine. All of these reactions *except* the conversion of dopamine into norepinephrine take place in the cytoplasm, and this exceptional reaction takes place within the synaptic vesicle. B: In dopaminergic, or dopamine-containing, terminals, the vesicular monoamine transporter transports dopamine, made in the cytoplasm, into synaptic vesicles. Neither DβH nor PNMT are found in dopaminergic terminals. C: In noradrenergic, or norepinephrine-containing, terminals, the vesicular monoamine transporter transports dopamine, made in the cytoplasm, into synaptic vesicles and DβH, present in the vesicle, then converts dopamine into norepinephrine within the synaptic vesicle. PNMT is not present in noradrenergic terminals D: The adrenergic terminal builds upon the noradrenergic terminal by *reverse* transporting norepinephrine out of the synaptic vesicle and into the cytoplasm. PNMT then converts norepinephrine into epinephrine within the cytoplasm. Cytosolic epinephrine is transported back into the synaptic vesicle by the vesicular monoamine transporter. Note that adrenergic, or epinephrine-containing, terminals contain all of the catecholaminergic enzymes. B–D: The dominant neurotransmitter in the synaptic vesicle is shown in italics. In dopaminergic terminals (B), only dopamine is synthesized and transported into vesicles. However, in noradrenergic terminals (C), norepinephrine predominates but lesser amounts of dopamine are present. Similarly, in adrenergic vesicles (D), some dopamine and norepinephrine are present along with mostly epinephrine.

volume, also termed *paracrine, transmission* meaning that monoamine neurotransmitters may act at some distance from the site where they are released. Thus, the presynaptic monoaminergic release site is often simply a varicosity at some distance from the postsynaptic receptors where a released monoamine binds. By current estimates, monoamines can travel up to 20 microns, a staggering distance, before decreasing to an ineffective concentration.

Considering that a typical synaptic cleft is on the order of 30 nanometers across, the extracellular distance potentially traveled by monoamines is almost 1,000 times greater than the distance traversed by a neurotransmitter at a classical synapse. *The upshot of volume transmission is that monoamines released from one site act on a large number and variety of cells located anywhere within a large radius from the site of release.*

MONOAMINES ARE CRITICAL TO MOOD AND AFFECT

Of the five monoamines used as neurotransmitters, we focus here on serotonin, dopamine, and norepinephrine. It is with some trepidation that we give short shrift to epinephrine. In cautioning against making light of the importance of central epinephrine, Arvid Carlsson, winner of the Nobel Prize in 2000 for studies on dopamine and Parkinson's disease, said "we have to take into account the fact that the brain is not a democracy," adding, "that is perhaps the reason why it works so well most of the time" (Fuller, 1982). Epinephrine-containing neurons are contained in both the brainstem and hypothalamus and appear to be important for cardiovascular regulation as well as for other homeostatic functions. Although brain epinephrine systems are not as well studied as dopaminergic and noradrenergic ones, they may nonetheless play as of yet unheralded and critical roles.

Serotonin, dopamine, and norepinephrine modulate virtually every brain pathway. Because pharmacological manipulations of these transmitters consistently alter affect and mood, drugs that affect the synthesis and uptake of serotonin, dopamine, and norepinephrine are typically termed *psychotropic*. Psychotropic drugs affect our psychological functioning and are used to treat a number of disorders that are typically classified as psychiatric.

Although many think that a decrease in serotonergic transmission leads to depression, an excess of serotonin to aggression, and so on, precise alignments between particular monoamine deficits and particular psychiatric disorders have eluded investigators to date. One reason for this difficulty is that many psychotropic drugs, such as those used to treat depression, must be taken for weeks before providing any relief, presumably because long-term changes in transmitter metabolism and receptor responsiveness are necessary for clinical efficacy. Furthermore, although one monoamine *may* play a primary role in any given psychiatric disorder, serotonin, dopamine, and norepinephrine are all likely to contribute.

CATECHOLAMINES SHARE SYNTHETIC AND PACKAGING STEPS

A series of synthetic steps leads to the formation of the catecholamine neurotransmitters. Two steps convert tyrosine to dopamine, which is then the substrate from which norepinephrine is synthesized, which in turn can be converted to epinephrine (Fig. 12-2A). The first step in making any catecholamine is the conversion of tyrosine into L-3,4-dihydroxy-L-phenylalanine (DOPA) by tyrosine hydroxylase. Aromatic amino acid decarboxylase (AAAD) then converts DOPA, often called L-DOPA, into dopamine. The two-step process from tyrosine to dopamine occurs entirely in the cytosol of synaptic terminals. VMAT transports available dopamine into synaptic vesicles. For a neuron that releases dopamine (i.e., a dopaminergic neuron), the synthetic pathway is complete, and additional catecholaminergic enzymes are not present (Fig. 12-2B).

In noradrenergic neurons, those that synthesize and release norepinephrine, the enzyme dopamine β-hydroxylase (DBH) converts dopamine contained *within a vesicle* into norepinephrine. Norepinephrine synthesized in situ within the vesicles is released upon appropriate stimulation (Fig. 12-2C). It may seem strange that norepinephrine is made in the vesicle rather than the cytosol. However, this odd detour allows a noradrenergic cell to package norepinephrine *preferentially* over dopamine; if norepinephrine were made in the cytosol along with dopamine, VMAT would transport both monoamines into vesicles in comparable amounts. In fact, norepinephrine-containing vesicles also contain a small amount of dopamine.

The pathway to epinephrine synthesis requires a strange-but-true step wherein norepinephrine is transported by VMAT *back out of the vesicles and into the cytosol*! Once in the cytosol, phenylethanolamine N-methyltransferase (PNMT) methylates the amine group of norepinephrine to form epinephrine. Cytosolic epinephrine is then transported into synaptic vesicles by VMAT (Fig. 12-2D).

As evident from the preceding descriptions, the synthetic enzymes that are present within a terminal determine the type of catecholaminergic neurotransmitter produced in that terminal (Fig. 12-2A). Thus, neurons that contain tyrosine hydroxylase and AAAD but lack DBH and PNMT synthesize dopamine. In contrast, cells that contain tyrosine hydroxylase, AAAD, and DBH but not PNMT, make and release norepinephrine. Cells that contain all four enzymes are *adrenergic* (i.e., they make epinephrine).

The rate-limiting step in all catecholamine production is the very first enzymatic step converting tyrosine to DOPA. For this reason, providing DOPA to patients with

Parkinson's disease who have greatly reduced levels of dopamine bypasses the bottleneck in catecholamine synthesis, thereby boosting the synthesis of all catecholamines including dopamine.

As with acetylcholine, the law of mass action applies to catecholaminergic synthesis. The more catecholamine product present, the less is synthesized; the more substrate present, the more catecholamine is synthesized. Another similarity to acetylcholine is the presence of an enzyme, *monoamine oxidase (MAO)*, which degrades the neurotransmitter product within synaptic terminals. The relative activities of MAO on one hand and synthetic enzymes for monoamines on the other determine the presynaptic concentration of any catecholamine. When MAO is inhibited by any of a number of clinically used MAO inhibitors (MAOI), then the amount of catecholamine available for release increases. Until the advent of tricyclic antidepressants and subsequently selective serotonin reuptake inhibitors (SSRIs), MAOIs were often the first drug prescribed in cases of clinical depression. It is interesting to note that the discovery of MAOIs' efficacy in treating depression occurred serendipitously when an MAOI was used to treat tuberculosis. Clinicians noticed that treated patients appeared happier although their tuberculosis remained problematic.

Genetic variation in the gene for MAO is associated with abnormalities in aggressive behavior. A rare X chromosome mutation present in a Dutch family results in a complete absence of one of the two forms of MAO. Men in this family exhibit a pathological and explosive form of aggression and impulsive destructive behavior. More commonly, naturally occurring mutations in the promoter or coding regions of the gene for MAO alter the expression or activity of MAO but do not necessarily lead to pathological behavior. An area of active investigation concerns how mutations in the MAO genes, both located on the X chromosome, interact with life events to change the likelihood of extreme aggressive and criminal behavior.

PHENYLKETONURIA IS A METABOLIC DISORDER THAT CAN CAUSE SEVERE BRAIN DYSFUNCTION

In healthy individuals, tyrosine, the starting material for all catecholamine synthesis, is a nonessential amino acid. This is because, normally, phenylalanine hydroxylase converts phenylalanine, an essential amino acid, into tyrosine. However, deleterious mutations in both copies of the gene

for phenylalanine hydroxylase impairs tyrosine synthesis and thereby results in *phenylketonuria (PKU)*. Different mutations give rise to different degrees of phenylalanine hydroxylase dysfunction from less efficient catalysis to no activity in the case of null or missense mutations. For PKU-affected individuals, tyrosine becomes an essential amino acid that must be acquired through diet. Patients with PKU also accumulate phenylalanine, which causes intellectual disability and seizures among adverse neurological and nonneural consequences. Luckily, a genetic test applied via heel stick to babies born in hospitals serves as a screen for high serum levels of phenylalanine, which can be a sign of PKU. A positive heel stick will lead to genetic and metabolic testing for PKU.

The adverse consequences of PKU can be largely avoided by strict adherence to a specialized diet lacking phenylalanine throughout childhood and adolescence. Since virtually every natural source of protein, including eggs, meat, fish, eggs, cheese, nuts, flour, and soy contains phenylalanine and should be avoided, amino acid supplements are necessary. The PKU diet is bland in taste and challenging to obtain at low cost. Moreover, holding to the diet is socially awkward and potentially isolating. The goal of the diet is simple: to keep phenylalanine below levels that cause neurological damage. The challenge arises because any slip-up in following the diet during the formative years can have severely adverse effects on brain function that undo the protection achieved by years of strict adherence.

It remains unclear how detrimental high levels of phenylalanine are in adults. However, gestational exposure to high phenylalanine levels results in stunted brain growth and severe intellectual disability in babies that come to term. Therefore, it is critical that PKU-afflicted women who are interested in and able to have children maintain a strict PKU diet during their reproductive years. Furthermore, phenylalanine and other amino acids are actively transported across the placenta, resulting in far higher concentrations of phenylalanine in the fetal circulation than in maternal blood. As a result, the fetuses of mothers with mild PKU may be exposed to far more than mild elevations in phenylalanine.

Beyond diet, innovative approaches to managing PKU are on the horizon. Novel approaches include administration of large neutral amino acids in order to flood the blood–brain barrier (BBB) transporter of the same name, thus lessening the transport of excess phenylalanine. Use of a plant enzyme, phenylalanine ammonia lyase, to degrade phenylalanine within the digestive tract is under development. This approach would prevent phenylalanine from ever building up peripherally, much less centrally, and therefore would allow a PKU sufferer to eat a more normal diet than is currently advisable.

SEROTONIN IS FORMED FROM TRYPTOPHAN BY TRYPTOPHAN HYDROXYLASE

Serotonin synthesis requires the essential amino acid tryptophan. To reach the CNS, tryptophan must be carried across the BBB by a transporter of large neutral amino acids—valine, leucine, isoleucine, tyrosine, tryptophan— and related molecules such as DOPA. Tryptophan competes with other possible substrates for transport across the BBB by the large neutral amino acid carrier. Eating meals rich in carbohydrates and proteins increases serum tryptophan levels, which in turn increases brain tryptophan levels and may underlie a postprandial serotonin surge within the brain following a large meal of both carbohydrates and fish or meat.

Tryptophan hydroxylase is thought to have arisen by gene duplication of its close relative, tyrosine hydroxylase. Tryptophan hydroxylase converts tryptophan into 5-hydroxytryptophan (Fig. 12-3). The same AAAD that converts DOPA into dopamine also decarboxylates 5-hydroxytryptophan to give serotonin, which is 5-hydroxytryptamine (5-HT). Once synthesized, serotonin is transported into synaptic vesicles by the same VMAT that loads catecholamines and histamine into vesicles (Fig. 12-3).

As in the case of catecholamines, the first enzymatic reaction in the synthesis of serotonin is rate-limiting. In contrast to catecholamines, however, the supply of the initial amino acid substrate, in this case, tryptophan, is also a key determinant in how much serotonin is made. Dietary restriction of tryptophan intake impacts serotonin levels and alters brain function, whereas tryptophan loading increases serotonin synthesis, and, when excessive, can cause the *serotonin syndrome*. The serotonin syndrome involves symptoms secondary to massive autonomic activation such as sweating, hyperthermia, nausea and vomiting, and palpitations along with muscle contractions and cognitive symptoms such as confusion and agitation. The symptoms of the serotonin syndrome are a dramatic reminder that serotonin plays a modulatory role in virtually every function of the nervous system. The incidence of serotonin syndrome is increasing as the psychotropic use of serotonin-boosting drugs increases and the lack of widespread recognition of the serotonin syndrome fuels a dangerous level of underdiagnosis for this potentially lethal condition.

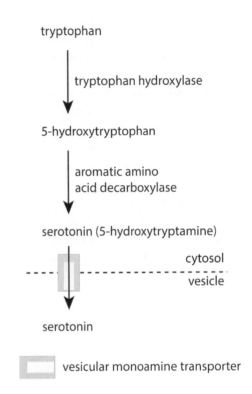

Figure 12-3 Tryptophan hydroxylase catalyzes the formation of 5-hydroxytryptophan from tryptophan and is the rate-limiting step in the synthesis of serotonin. Aromatic amino acid decarboxylase, the same enzyme that converts DOPA into dopamine, decarboxylates 5-hydroxytryptophan to form serotonin (5-hydroxytryptamine often abbreviated as 5-ht). Serotonin is transported into vesicles by the vesicular monoamine transporter, the same transporter that carries catecholamines into vesicles.

THE TERMINATION OF MONOAMINERGIC ACTION OCCURS LARGELY THROUGH REUPTAKE

The speedy termination of catecholamine and serotonin action occurs through reuptake back into the synaptic terminal via specific transporters. Dopamine, norepinephrine, and serotonin are taken up by dopamine (DAT), norepinephrine (NET), and serotonin (SERT) transporters, respectively. Thus, although all monoamines share a single vesicular transporter—VMAT—they are taken up through a set of more selective transporters present on the plasma membrane of the synaptic terminal. DAT, NET, and SERT are far more selective than the promiscuous vesicular transporter VMAT. Still, their names imply a specificity that does not reflect reality. Each reuptake transporter has modest affinity for at least one other monoamine beyond its eponymous neurotransmitter (Fig. 12-4). Thus, in addition to transporting the neurotransmitter for which it is named,

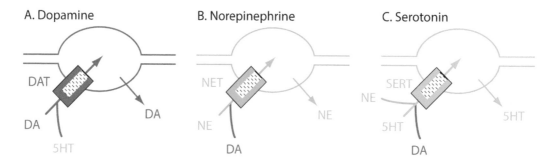

Figure 12-4 A: The plasma membrane of monoaminergic synaptic terminals, typically varicosities, that release dopamine (*A*), norepinephrine (*B*), or serotonin (*C*) possess transporters with high affinity for the transmitter released. Yet, each transporter has some affinity for other monoamines. The dopamine transporter (*DAT*) has low affinity for serotonin in addition to high affinity for dopamine. The norepinephrine transporter (*NET*) has nearly equivalent affinity for dopamine as for norepinephrine. Finally, the serotonin transporter (*SERT*) has low affinity for both dopamine and norepinephrine, as well as high affinity for serotonin.

NET transports dopamine, DAT transports serotonin, and SERT transports both norepinephrine and dopamine.

Transporters responsible for rapid monoamine reuptake are targeted by a number of important psychotropic therapeutics such as *tricyclic antidepressants* and SSRIs. Tricyclic antidepressants are minimally selective monoamine reuptake inhibitors that inhibit the transport of both norepinephrine and serotonin through actions at the respective reuptake transporters. Inhibiting norepinephrine and serotonin reuptake results in elevated extracellular concentrations of norepinephrine and serotonin. However, the efficacy of tricyclic antidepressants in relieving depression is due to longer term effects rather than to the acute increase in monoamine neurotransmitter levels. Tricyclic antidepressants were originally used to treat depression, but, since the advent of SSRIs, they are less often prescribed for depression. Now, this class of historically named antidepressants is often used to treat other conditions such as chronic pain. SSRIs, such as fluoxetine and sertraline, preferentially inhibit SERT and increase the amount of serotonin in the extracellular space. SSRIs are used to treat a variety of conditions including depression, anxiety, and obsessive-compulsive disorder.

Several important drugs of abuse, such as *cocaine* and *amphetamine*, produce psychotropic effects through inhibiting rapid monoamine reuptake. Cocaine is a nonselective monoamine reuptake inhibitor that inhibits the transport of dopamine, norepinephrine, and serotonin. The addictive nature of cocaine is thought to derive primarily from cocaine's effects on dopamine reuptake through DAT. With dopamine reuptake blocked, dopamine lingers at receptors for a longer than normal time. Amphetamine, another addicting substance, increases the concentration of dopamine in dopaminergic terminals through effects on VMAT as well as DAT. By acting on VMAT to reverse the

direction of dopamine transport, *amphetamine results in the transport of dopamine from synaptic vesicles to the cytosol.* The concentration of intracellular dopamine increases to such an extent that *DAT transports dopamine from the cytosol to the extracellular space.* Although both cocaine and amphetamine greatly increase the dopamine present extracellularly, the actual mechanism of addiction for both of these substances is likely to depend on changes in receptor properties as well as on increases in dopamine levels.

Genetic variations in monoamine transporters are associated with personality traits such as aggression, impulsivity, and susceptibility to depression. For example, within the serotonin transporter promoter region, there is a polymorphism known as the *serotonin transporter-linked polymorphism* (5HTTLPR). The short allele of 5HTTLPR decreases the amount of SERT made. Individuals with one or two copies of the short allele are more neurotic and less extroverted than are those with the long allele. Yet the story is not a simple one of genetic inheritance acting alone. An individual with the short allele is not fated to develop depression. Instead, there is an interplay between genes and environment that determines how particular genetic variations play out in a person's life. With respect to depression, short allele carriers who have experienced severe trauma are those most likely to develop depression.

Recall from our earlier discussion that monoamines participate in paracrine transmission, meaning that they may act on postsynaptic elements that are present within a relatively large volume of tissue. In fact, monoamines can reach high concentrations, in the millimolar range, at release sites and therefore can diffuse long distances measured in tens of microns. Consequently DAT, NET, and SERT, which are present only on the plasma membrane of monoaminergic terminals, are simply not present where monoamine concentrations remain substantial. Additional monoamine transporters such as the *organic cation transporter (OCT)* mop up monoamine molecules that escape from the reach of the reuptake transporters.

OCT is a poorly selective, low-affinity, and high-capacity transporter that is present on postsynaptic neurons and astrocytes. OCT has a far lower affinity for monoamines than do DAT, NET, and SERT and therefore can take up monoamines present at low concentrations. In essence, *OCT acts to mop up excess monoamine in the extracellular space of the brain but does so in a manner that is largely indiscriminate between the monoamines.* Now, consider that tricyclic antidepressants, SSRIs, amphetamines, and anxiolytics increase the concentration of extracellular monoamines by blocking (or reversing) high-affinity, rapid reuptake. By clearing excess extracellular monoamines, OCT and other low-affinity monoamine transporters may account for the resistance of some individuals to drugs that act on monoamine reuptake transporters.

Although the termination of monoaminergic neurotransmitter action is achieved most rapidly and completely by reuptake into the synaptic terminal, there is a contribution from *catechol-O-methyl transferase (COMT)*, which degrades catecholamines extracellularly. Although it would be natural to think that COMT inhibitors increase the time that catecholamines spend extracellularly, *reuptake (through DAT and NET) is so fast* that any effect of COMT inhibitors is minor. Thus, COMT inhibitors are not used therapeutically. Increasing COMT activity, on the other hand, can have effects on catecholaminergic transmission, but not therapeutic ones. One natural variation in the COMT gene involves a substitution—valine for methionine at codon 158—that results in greater enzymatic activity than normal. It is thought that a large increase in COMT activity decreases the extracellular concentration of catecholamines available to postsynaptic receptors. As we have seen repeatedly, genetics do not determine fate on their own, and the val158met variant of the COMT gene does not, on its own, lead to abnormalities. However, when coupled with adverse life events, people with this variant become more likely to show personality traits such as extreme risk-seeking behavior. The potential for a mutation in a single gene to influence high-order cognition speaks to the importance of catecholamines in psychological function.

NEURONS AND GLIA COOPERATE TO SYNTHESIZE GLUTAMATE

Glutamate, a nonessential amino acid, derives from diet or from one of at least two synthetic pathways. Neurons, like all cells, form glutamate when synthesizing either pyruvate or oxaloacetate from α-ketoglutarate, a key player in cellular metabolism (Fig. 12-5). Neurons also possess a neuron-specific synthetic pathway that utilizes mitochondrially located glutaminase to convert glutamine to glutamate. Once formed, glutamate is packaged into vesicles by the vesicular glutamate transporter (VGLUT).

After glutamate release, excitatory amino acid transporters located in both neuron terminals and in surrounding astrocytes take up free glutamate (Fig. 12-5) with the energy derived by co-transporting sodium and potassium ions down their respective electrochemical gradients. Although most released glutamate appears to end up in glial cells rather than in neuronal terminals, excitatory amino acid transporters are present on synaptic terminals as well.

The concentration of glutamine is higher, by at least ten times, than any other amino acid both peripherally in blood and centrally in cerebrospinal fluid (CSF). Yet, negligible amounts of glutamine enter the brain from the blood. Instead, astrocytes produce glutamine, converted from glutamate by glutamine synthetase, within the brain and thus are responsible for the high concentration of glutamine centrally. Because of the high concentration of glutamine (nearly 1 millimolar) in the extracellular fluid, neurons readily take up glutamine into synaptic terminals using glutamine-specific transporters. Within the synaptic terminals, glutamine is converted to glutamate, which is then packaged into synaptic vesicles, thus completing the glutamate–glutamine cycle of synthesis, packaging, and release of glutamate by the neuron and reuptake of glutamate and synthesis and release of glutamine by the astrocyte (Fig. 12-5).

Glutamate uptake is particularly crucial because prolonged exposure to glutamate is toxic. As discussed earlier, uptake of neurotransmitters or some other mode of terminating transmitter action is important in punctuating the message sent by neurotransmitter release. Rapid and efficient uptake of glutamate is particularly critical because prolonged exposure to glutamate causes *excitotoxicity* that ultimately results in death of neurons. When glutamate persists in the synaptic cleft, it sets in motion a series of events resulting in a large influx of calcium ions into the cell; this, in turn, triggers a number of deleterious events, including the activation of a variety of degradative enzymes. The excitotoxic effects of glutamate are most pronounced in neurons with the most calcium-permeable glutamate receptors (see Chapter 13) and with the weakest calcium-buffering capacity, features that mark hippocampal neurons. Thus, glutamate excitotoxicity preferentially damages neurons

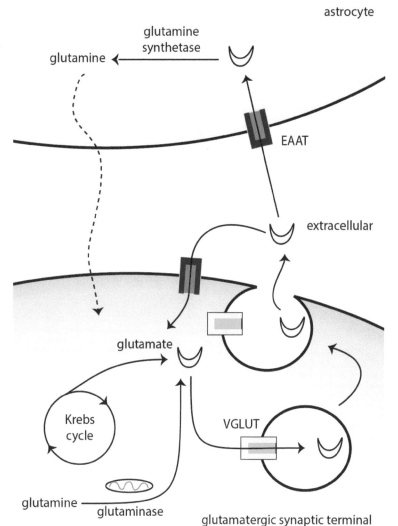

astrocyte

glutamine synthetase

glutamine ←

EAAT

extracellular

glutamate

Krebs cycle

VGLUT

glutamine ——— glutaminase

glutamatergic synaptic terminal

Figure 12-5 Astrocytes and neurons both participate in the synthesis, uptake, and degradation of glutamate (*yellow banana symbol*). Within synaptic terminals, glutamate is synthesized from glutamine by the mitochondrial enzyme, glutaminase. Glutamate is also a by-product of the Krebs cycle in all cells. Glutamate within synaptic terminals is transported into synaptic vesicles by the vesicular glutamate transporter (*VGLUT*) and, after release, is taken up by both astrocytes and synaptic terminals through the excitatory amino acid transporter (*EAAT*). Within astrocytes, glutamate is converted into glutamine by glutamine synthetase. The molecules involved in transporting glutamine out of astrocytes and into terminals are not yet identified molecularly. Yet glutamine does make it out of astrocytes and into neuronal terminals.

in the hippocampus, disrupting new memory formation at least temporarily. Excitotoxicity accompanies seizures, strokes, ischemic attacks, mechanical brain trauma, and neurodegenerative diseases such as Huntington's disease. Finding therapeutics that mitigate the excitotoxic effects of glutamate is an active area of investigation.

GLUTAMATE IS THE SUBSTRATE FOR GABA SYNTHESIS

In an odd twist of fate, glutamate, the most widely used excitatory neurotransmitter, is the substrate for synthesizing GABA, the most widely used inhibitory neurotransmitter. *Glutamic acid decarboxylase (GAD)*, converts glutamate into GABA (Fig. 12-6), which is then packed into synaptic

vesicles by the vesicular inhibitory amino acid transporter (VIAA). This packaged GABA can be released from the presynaptic terminal upon appropriate stimulation.

It is instructive to look at the consequences of impaired glutamic acid decarboxylase activity. *Stiff-person syndrome*, previously called stiff-man syndrome, is a rare disease associated in more than 80% of the cases with the presence of antibodies to GAD. By interfering with GABA synthesis, GABA synthesis is reduced, resulting in less GABA-mediated (GABAergic) inhibition, including less inhibition of motoneurons. Releasing motoneurons from inhibition is immediately apparent as an increase in muscle tone. The muscles of patients with stiff-person syndrome are both rock-hard and painful. Because stiff-person syndrome symptoms rarely progress to affect breathing, the disease is rarely fatal.

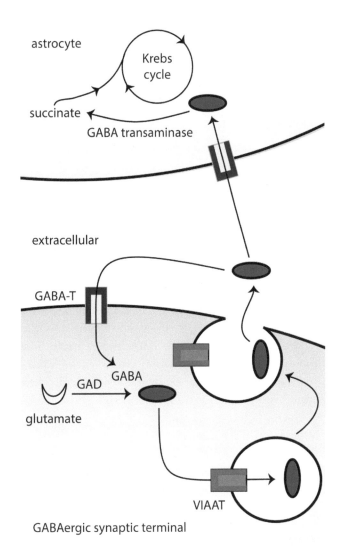

astrocyte

Krebs
cycle

succinate

GABA transaminase

extracellular

GABA-T

GAD

GABA

glutamate

VIAAT

GABAergic synaptic terminal

Figure 12-6 Astrocytes and neurons both participate in the synthesis, uptake, and degradation of γ-aminobutyric acid (*GABA*). GABA (*blue oval*) is formed from glutamate by glutamic acid decarboxylase (*GAD*) and then put into vesicles by the vesicular inhibitory amino acid transporter (*VIAAT*). After release, GABA is taken up by astrocytes and terminals by the GABA transporter (*GABA-T*). In synaptic terminals, GABA is recycled to fill synaptic vesicles anew, whereas in astrocytes GABA is converted to succinate by GABA transaminase. Succinate is used in the Krebs cycle.

Epilepsy and diabetes mellitus are symptoms in stiff-person syndrome that do not occur in individuals afflicted with tetanus, even though both conditions involve dysfunction of GABAergic neurons. The differences stem from two important dissimilarities in the pathophysiology. First, tetanus selectively affects a small subset of all GABAergic neurons, only those that directly synapse onto motoneurons, whereas all GABAergic neurons are impacted in stiff-person syndrome. Second, tetanus blocks all neurotransmitter release from GABAergic premotor neurons, whereas stiff-person syndrome is associated with the failure of the synthetic pathway for GABA. Since neurons may

release multiple neurotransmitters, a GABAergic neuron in a patient with stiff-person syndrome may continue to synthesize and release, for example, neuropeptides, a monoamine, or ATP.

The non-motor, and indeed non-neural, symptoms of stiff-person syndrome occur because of the variety of cells that use GAD to synthesize GABA. A high incidence of epilepsy is caused by a reduction in cortical inhibition by cortical inhibitory interneurons that release GABA. Reduced function in the GABAergic interneurons of startle circuits leads to nonhabituating reactions to unexpected stimuli such as a tap on the shoulder, hearing a honking horn, or viewing a bolt of lightning. A patient may freeze up and drop "like a log" to the ground upon the first and tenth iteration of a stimulus alike.

Diabetes mellitus (commonly known as type 1 diabetes) occurs because antibodies attack GAD that is contained within insulin-producing pancreatic β cells. Patients with stiff-person syndrome are typically treated by a combination of immunotherapy to suppress antibody formation and sedating benzodiazepines, which facilitate transmission via the GABA$_A$ receptor (see Chapter 13).

Extracellular GABA is taken up by GABA transporters present in the plasma membrane of both astrocytes and synaptic terminals. Within astrocytes, GABA is metabolized by GABA transaminase and ultimately returned to the Krebs cycle as succinate (Fig. 12-6). It should now be evident that the synthetic pathways of glutamate and GABA are highly interdependent.

PEPTIDES ARE DERIVED FROM LARGE PRECURSORS

Around 100 genes code for proteins that are processed into more than 100 peptide neurotransmitters. Peptides are short proteins, 3–80 amino acids in length, that are translated by ribosomes as larger pro-peptides and enzymatically processed to a mature, or released, peptide in the endoplasmic reticulum, Golgi apparatus, and vesicles. Once neuropeptide-containing vesicles—the large vesicle types—are transported to the synaptic terminal, the neuropeptides can be released by appropriate depolarization.

Neuropeptides are released from the synaptic terminal, far from the site of their synthesis and processing, in the cell body. Furthermore, neuropeptides are not recycled or taken up as are low-molecular-weight neurotransmitters. Instead, neuropeptides diffuse away from sites of release and eventually are degraded by extracellular proteases. Since neuropeptides cannot be synthesized and repackaged in vesicles within the synaptic terminal, it is not surprising that the membrane of large, dense-core vesicles is also not recycled.

GASES SERVE IN RETROGRADE SIGNALING

Gas neurotransmitters differ in many ways from the other two neurotransmitter classes. For one, they are often synthesized in a dendrite or dendritic spine. Moreover, gases are exceptions to the rule that neurotransmitters are packaged within vesicles. Gases are released directly from the cytosol where and *when* they are synthesized. Remember that gases in solution diffuse freely through intra- and extracellular compartments and across membranes. Therefore, once synthesized, gases diffuse away in the gaseous equivalent of neurotransmitter release. Thus, synthesis plus release are a one step-process for gaseous neurotransmitters. Here, we briefly examine the synthesis (and release) and effects of one gas, *nitric oxide (NO)*.

Nitric oxide is formed from arginine and oxygen by *nitric oxide synthase (NOS)*. A common way of activating NOS is by the actions of calcium ions and calmodulin. *Calmodulin* is a calcium ion–binding protein that is ubiquitous in all cells. As we know, calcium ion concentrations can be increased by opening voltage-gated channels. As discussed in the next chapter, calcium ion concentrations can also be increased by opening ligand-gated channels. For example, calcium ion influx through a particular type of glutamate receptor activates NOS in a calcium-/calmodulin-dependent fashion, resulting in the synthesis and release of NO. Flexibility in NO signaling is achieved through a number of modulatory points, including a handful of different potential co-factors, each of which can be modulated by other second-messengers and through direct modulation of NOS activity.

The termination of NO signaling and its effects are still somewhat unclear. Clearly, NO can diffuse throughout the tissue. Yet, as a free radical, NO has a short lifetime—just a few seconds—before it participates in a chemical reaction. As you recall, a free radical is a molecule with an unpaired electron in an orbit by itself. Unpaired electrons readily participate in chemical reactions, so that free radicals are unstable, short-lived, and highly reactive molecules.

Nitric oxide is typically formed in the postsynaptic cell and then diffuses in all directions, including retrogradely to the presynaptic terminal. Retrograde signaling is important because it provides an avenue for presynaptic terminals to receive information about the state of the postsynaptic target. In this way, presynaptic terminals can "find out" about changes, including damage, that occur in the postsynaptic target cells.

A VARIETY OF MOLECULES CAN HAVE NEUROTRANSMITTER-LIKE EFFECTS ON NEURONS

Some molecules that are not packaged and released as neurotransmitters nonetheless cause postsynaptic effects that are similar to and in some cases even indistinguishable from the effects of neurotransmitters. For example, when mechanical trauma ruptures cell membranes, cytosolic contents and membrane components are released into the extracellular space. In this way, large increases in the local concentration of glutamate, protons, potassium ions, ATP, arachidonic acid, and many other molecules and ions occur. All of the released substances can either activate postsynaptic receptors or modulate receptor activation by traditional neurotransmitters. In the periphery, substances released from non-neural cells can also have neurotransmitter-like actions on peripheral neurons. Cytokines and histamine are released from various types of immune cells. Another source of neuroactive signaling molecules is blood. Substances such as bradykinin and serotonin, which are normally present in blood, may reach primary afferents after either rupture of a blood vessel or increased blood vessel permeability.

ADDITIONAL READING

Albrecht J, Sonnewald U, Waagepetersen HS, Schousboe A. Glutamine in the central nervous system: Function and dysfunction *Front Biosci.* 12: 332–343, 2007.

Alia-Klein N, Goldstein RZ, Kriplani A, Logan J, Tomasi D, Williams B, et al. Brain monoamine oxidase A activity predicts trait aggression. *J Neurosci.* 28: 5099–5104, 2008.

Boehning D, Snyder SH. Novel neural modulators. *Ann Rev Neurosci.* 26: 105–31, 2003.

Brunner HG, Nelen M, Breakefield XO, Ropers HH, van Oost BA. Abnormal behavior associated with a point mutation in the structural gene for monoamine oxidase A. *Science.* 262: 578–580, 1993.

Caspi A, Hariri AR, Holmes A, Uher R, Moffitt TE. Genetic sensitivity to the environment: the case of the serotonin transporter gene and its implications for studying complex diseases and traits. *Am J Psychiatry.* In press; epub ahead of print, 2010.

Committee on Genetics. Policy statement: Maternal phenylketonuria. *Pediatrics* 122: 445–449, 2008.

Couroussé T, Gautron S. Role of organic cation transporters (OCTs) in the brain. *Pharmacol Ther.* 146: 94–103, 2015.

Daws LC. Unfaithful neurotransmitter transporters: Focus on serotonin uptake and implications for antidepressant efficacy. *Pharmacol Ther.* 121: 89–99, 2009.

Ernst M, Plate RC, Carlisi CO, Gorodetsky E, Goldman D, Pine DS. Loss aversion and 5HTT gene variants in adolescent anxiety. *Dev Cogn Neurosci.* 8: 77–85, 2014.

den Ouden HE, Daw ND, Fernandez G, Elshout JA, Rijpkema M, Hoogman M, Franke B, Cools R. Dissociable effects of dopamine and serotonin on reversal learning. *Neuron.* 80: 1090–1100, 2013.

Fuller, RW. Pharmacology of brain epinephrine neurons. *Ann Rev Pharmacol Toxicol.* 22: 31–55, 1982.

Hariri AR, Holmes A. Genetics of emotional regulation: The role of the serotonin transporter in neural function. *Trends Cogn Sci.* 10: 182–191, 2006.

He Q, Xue G, Chen C, et al. COMT Val158Met polymorphism interacts with stressful life events and parental warmth to influence decision making. *Sci Rep.* 2: 677, 2012.

Mitchell JJ, Trakadis YJ, Scriver CR. Phenylalanine hydroxylase deficiency. *Genet Med* 13: 697–707, 2011.

Rudnick G. Vesicular ATP transport is a hard (V)NUT to crack. *Proc Natl Acad Sci.* 105: 5949–5950, 2008.

Sarter M, Parikh V. Choline transporters, cholinergic transmission and cognition. *Nature Rev Neurosci.* 6: 48–56, 2005.

Stein MB, Fallin MD, Schork NJ, Gelernter J. COMT polymorphisms and anxiety-related personality traits. *Neuropsychopharm.* 30: 2092–2102, 2005.

Uhe AM, Collier GR, O'dea K. A comparison of the effects of beef, chicken and fish protein on satiety and amino acid profiles in lean male subjects. *J Nutr.* 122: 467–472, 1992.

van Spronsen FJ. Phenylketonuria: A 21st century perspective. *Nat Rev Endocrinol.* 6: 509–514, 2010.

13.

RECEIVING THE SYNAPTIC MESSAGE

To come full circle in understanding neural communication, we now consider how a neuron receives messages. The message conveyed by a neurotransmitter depends on the complement of receptors present in the membrane of the cell receiving the message. This dependence is absolute: in the absence of matching receptors, neurotransmitter release is meaningless. Moreover, different types of receptors confer drastically different responses. For example, acetylcholine excites cells with nicotinic acetylcholine receptors and inhibits those expressing muscarinic acetylcholine receptors. Since the neurotransmitter acetylcholine is absolutely the same in both situations, it is the difference in the receptor expressed on the postsynaptic cell that dictates the response of the cell. The effect of a neurotransmitter on a target cell also depends on the signaling molecules present within the postsynaptic cell. To extend the example of cholinergic signaling, a single muscarinic receptor may couple to different signaling cascades, resulting in either an increase or a decrease in a second-messenger such as cyclic adenosine monophosphate (cAMP) and, ultimately, leading to opposing final consequences.

Given the dependence of a neurotransmitter's effects on postsynaptic biochemistry, you may be wondering why, in the previous chapter, glutamate was called an *excitatory* amino acid neurotransmitter and γ-aminobutyric acid (GABA) and glycine were said to be *inhibitory* amino acid neurotransmitters. The answer is that these monikers are shortcuts that happen to be largely accurate: glutamate virtually always causes excitation, and GABA and glycine almost always cause inhibition. Yet there are exceptions, and the shortcut is as regrettable as it is ingrained in the vernacular. The reality is that the effect of a neurotransmitter is not predictable from any property of that neurotransmitter. Rather, the receptor- bound and signaling pathways engaged by a neurotransmitter determine its effect.

As you recall, receptors that bind neurotransmitters come in two varieties: ionotropic and metabotropic. Two fundamental differences between ionotropic and metabotropic receptor functions stem from the receptor types' distinct physical structures (Fig. 13-1). The first difference has to do with speed of action and the second with the variety of neurotransmitter-elicited effects. Each of these is explored in brief.

When neurotransmitters bind to ionotropic receptors, the result is the rapid opening of an ion pore. *Because ionotropic receptors are also channels, channel openings are very rapid,* typically starting within a fraction of a millisecond and continuing for a few milliseconds at most. In contrast to ionotropic receptors, *metabotropic receptors bind a ligand but cannot form an ion-permeant pore. Instead metabotropic receptors can only affect ion channels indirectly* (Fig. 13-1B). The indirect route from metabotropic receptor activation to change in ion channel function requires time. Thus, metabotropic receptor-mediated affects are always slower to start and end than those caused by neurotransmitter binding to ionotropic receptors.

The "adrenaline rush" familiar to everyone depends principally on the actions of adrenaline, typically termed epinephrine in the United States (although the vernacular of an adrenaline rush remains), on a large number of peripheral targets, such as the heart and blood vessels, to increase heart rate and blood pressure. The onset of an adrenaline rush feels rapid but the time course of an adrenaline rush is in fact, measured in seconds to tens of seconds, orders of magnitude slower than the millisecond time scale of ionotropic receptor–mediated signaling. Furthermore, the feeling of an adrenaline rush *turns off* very slowly. The long-lasting time course of an adrenaline rush mirrors the kinetics of the metabotropic receptors that bind epinephrine

A. Ionotropic receptor

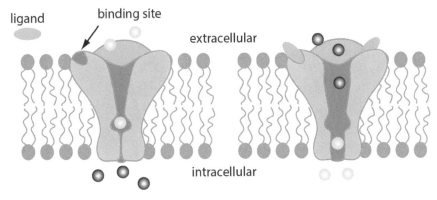

B. Metabotropic receptor

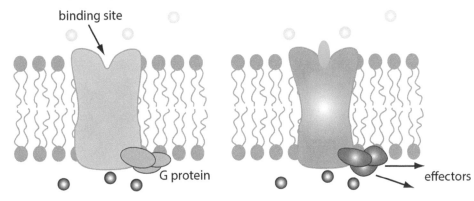

Figure 13-1 Different physical configurations underlie the functional properties of ionotropic (A) and metabotropic receptors (B). A: Ionotropic receptors form an open channel when bound to a neurotransmitter. Most ionotropic receptors require the binding of two neurotransmitter molecules (*blue ovals marked ligand*) for activation. The electrical consequences of ligand-binding to an ionotropic receptor are rapid and always involve channel opening that permits the passage of ions (*green and black balls*) through the channel pore. B: Metabotropic receptors are not able to form an open channel. When neurotransmitter binds to a metabotropic receptor, signaling occurs indirectly through second-messenger intermediaries and biochemical effectors (*right panel*). Here, a type of metabotropic receptor, a G protein-coupled receptor, commonly used by neurons, is illustrated. Metabotropic receptor activation can result in any number of effects through a variety of effector mechanisms. The critical point here is that metabotropic receptors only affect the electrical properties of a cell *indirectly* and thus slowly. No ions pass through a metabotropic receptor.

in the periphery. In contrast, sensing the sting of a needle or jerking one's leg in response to a knee tap depends on fast ionotropic receptor–mediated transmission. In keeping with the time course of ionotropic receptor–mediated transmission, the pricking sensation and the knee jerk reflex begin and end very quickly.

When neurotransmitters bind to ionotropic receptors, an ion pore may open but it will never close or change its kinetic properties. In other words, there is only one possible change that can occur when a neurotransmitter binds to an ionotropic receptor and that is ion channel opening. Neurotransmitters do not directly close ionotropic receptors nor do they alter receptor properties such as desensitization rate. In contrast, when neurotransmitters bind to and activate metabotropic receptors, all manner

of consequences are possible including channel-opening, channel-closing, changes in channel kinetics, and electrically silent effects that may involve gene regulation, cytoskeletal remodeling, and so on.

Although neurotransmitters do not alter the kinetic properties of ionotropic receptors, the kinetic properties of these receptors, as well as of metabotropic receptors, may change as a result of *allosteric modulators*. Allosteric modulators are substances that bind to a site distinct from the neurotransmitter-binding site and cause a conformational change that alters channel properties. An allosteric modulator may, for example, increase or decrease the probability of channel opening or change the time course of receptor desensitization. *Benzodiazepines* are clinically important positive allosteric modulators of the ionotropic $GABA_A$

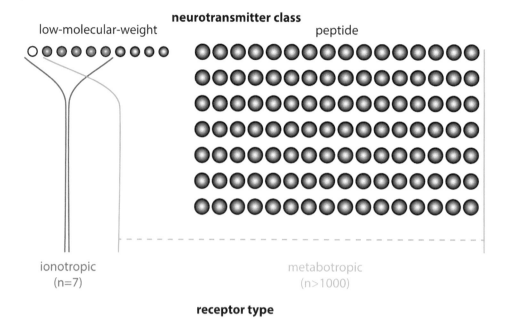

neurotransmitter class

low-molecular-weight   peptide

ionotropic   metabotropic
(n=7)   (n>1000)

receptor type

Figure 13-2 The alignment between different types of neurotransmitters and receptors. There are more than ten times more peptide neurotransmitters (*large spheres*) than low-molecular-weight neurotransmitters (*small spheres*) and more than 100 times more metabotropic receptor types than ionotropic receptor types. Peptide neurotransmitters only signal through metabotropic receptors, whereas low-molecular-weight neurotransmitters signal through metabotropic receptors only (*black spheres*), metabotropic and ionotropic receptors (*red spheres*), or in one case only through an ionotropic receptor (*empty sphere*).

receptor that boost the effects of GABA on the receptor. Allosteric modulators, which offer a nuanced way to influence channel function and are of increasing clinical interest, may affect either ionotropic or metabotropic receptors.

Of the hundred-plus neurotransmitters, about 90% are peptides, and only ten or so are low-molecular-weight neurotransmitters (Fig. 13-2). Of the thousand-plus receptors, fewer than ten are ionotropic. As we have seen, neural communication depends on a transmitter signaling through a matching or *cognate* receptor. The alignment of neurotransmitter to receptor is not random. Instead, members of the two primary (low-molecular-weight, peptide) neurotransmitter classes match up with members of the two types of receptors in a specific manner:

- Low-molecular-weight neurotransmitters bind to ionotropic and/or metabotropic receptors.

- Peptide neurotransmitters only bind to metabotropic receptors.

Table 13-1 lists individual (low-molecular-weight) and class (peptide) neurotransmitter to receptor alignments. From the receptor perspective, the few ionotropic receptors only bind to low-molecular-weight neurotransmitters (Fig. 13-2). Even within the low-molecular-weight class, only six of the ten neurotransmitters have a cognate ionotropic receptor. In contrast, there is a known metabotropic receptor

Table 13-1 ALIGNMENT BETWEEN NEUROTRANSMITTER CLASS AND RECEPTOR TYPE

NEUROTRANSMITTER	IONOTROPIC RECEPTORS	METABOTROPIC RECEPTORS
Low-molecular-weight neurotransmitters		
Acetylcholine	nACHR (nicotinic)	M_1–M_5 (muscarinic)
Glutamate	AMPA, NMDA	$mGluR_{1–8}$
GABA	$GABA_A$	$GABA_B$
Glycine	Glycine	None
Dopamine	None	D_1–D_5
Norepinephrine, epinephrine	None	$\alpha_{1–2}$, $\beta_{1–3}$
Serotonin	$5HT_3$	$5HT_{1–2, 4–7}$
Histamine	None	$H_{1–4}$
Purines (e.g., ATP)	P2X	P1, P2Y
Peptide neurotransmitters		
>100 peptides e.g., Tachykinins	None	>1,000 receptors
Substance P	None	NK_1
Neurokinin A	None	NK_2
Neurokinin B	None	NK_3

for every neurotransmitter known save one: glycine. The number of receptor types should not be confused with the number of receptors. For example, there are far more metabotropic receptor types than ionotropic receptor types but there are far more α-amino-3-hydroxyl-5-methyl-4-isoxazolepropionic acid (AMPA) receptors in the brain than there are receptors of any single metabotropic variety.

A LIMITED NUMBER OF IONOTROPIC RECEPTORS MEDIATE FAST SYNAPTIC TRANSMISSION

Although only about seven varieties exist, ionotropic receptors are workhorses, mediating fast synaptic transmission at virtually all central synapses in the brain and spinal cord. In the periphery, acetylcholine released from motoneurons acts on the prototypical ionotropic receptor—the *nicotinic acetylcholine receptor (nAChR)*—present in skeletal muscle, to excite skeletal muscle. Similarly, preganglionic motor neurons release acetylcholine, which acts on a different isoform of the nAChR to excite ganglionic (i.e., the *autonomic* ganglia) motor neurons. Although ionotropic receptors predominate in the central nervous system (CNS) and neuromuscular junction, acetylcholine and norepinephrine act exclusively on metabotropic receptors at the synapses between autonomic ganglionic motor neurons and target cells—cardiac muscle, smooth muscle, and glands.

When activated, excitatory ionotropic receptors (nAChR, AMPA, N-methyl-D-aspartate [NMDA], 5-hydroxytryptamine-3 [5-HT$_3$], P2X) conduct, or allow passage of, cations. Excitatory ionotropic receptors are nonselective with respect to the cation species, conducting sodium, potassium, and, in some cases, calcium ions. As we saw in Chapter 9, nonselective cation permeability depolarizes a cell toward a reversal potential of about zero millivolts. Two ionotropic receptors, the GABA$_A$ and glycine receptors, pass chloride ions primarily. The effect on membrane potential of increasing the permeability to chloride ions depends on the distribution of chloride ions inside and outside the cell. Since rest potential is usually a few millivolts more depolarized than the Nernst potential for chloride ions (E$_{Cl}$), opening GABA$_A$ and glycine receptors at most adult synapses results in a hyperpolarization and is inhibitory.

The seven major ionotropic receptors just listed can come in subtypes with distinct pharmacology, meaning that different drugs preferentially bind to and act at different subtypes. In addition to the major ionotropic receptors, there is at least one minor type of ionotropic receptor—a type of glutamate receptor preferentially activated by the ligand kainate. The kainate receptor will not be discussed here.

A class of ion channels termed transient receptor potential (TRP) receptors, warrants mention here. Several families of TRP receptors exist; these receptors are important to a number of somato- and chemosensory modalities including thermosensation, chemosensation, and mechanosensation. Under natural circumstances, TRP receptors are activated by heat, cold, stretch, or chemicals released by cell rupture or damage (see much more on TRP receptors in Chapter 17). For example, TRPV$_1$ is activated by heat above 43°C or by protons and is modulated by many of the products indicative of tissue damage. Furthermore, some, but not all, TRP receptors are either activated by or modulated by exogenous substances. In the case of TRPV$_1$, capsaicin, the active ingredient that produces the pungency of hot peppers, is an agonist: when capsaicin binds to TRPV$_1$, a cation pore opens. Other TRP receptors are activated or modulated by a number of compounds such as menthol, acrolein (a component of wood fire smoke and tobacco smoke), allyl isothiocyanate (the pungent ingredient in wasabi), and chlorine. In sum, TRP receptors are clearly ionotropic receptors, but their ligands are not neurotransmitters. We do not discuss TRP receptors further in this chapter.

In the following sections, we consider AMPA and NMDA, the two glutamate receptors, the nAChR, and the GABA$_A$ receptor in some depth. Although space does not permit discussion of the other ionotropic receptors, they, too, have important functions. The glycine receptor mediates inhibitory transmission, primarily in the spinal cord, but also in the brainstem. Patients with certain mutations impacting glycinergic transmission, including several that are known to alter the glycine receptor itself, have an exuberant, nonhabituating startle reflex. The 5HT$_3$ receptor, present in nociceptors innervating the gut and in many regions of the CNS, is an important mediator of nausea and vomiting. Thus, patients receiving chemotherapeutics are treated prophylactically with 5-HT$_3$ receptor antagonists to prevent the otherwise inevitable feeling of nausea and consequent vomiting. The ionotropic purinergic receptor family, P2X, mediates fast pain as well as visceral signals such as bladder-filling.

GLUTAMATE BINDS TO AND OPENS TWO FUNDAMENTALLY DIFFERENT IONOTROPIC RECEPTORS

When activated by glutamate, AMPA receptors mediate fast, excitatory transmission by forming a pore that conducts both sodium and potassium ions (Fig. 13-3). The rapid depolarization due to flux through AMPA receptors constitutes the majority of the excitatory transmission in the CNS.

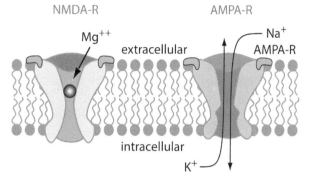

A. Glutamate released onto neuron at rest
(Mg^{++} block)

NMDA-R   AMPA-R

Mg^{++} Na$^+$
extracellular   AMPA-R

intracellular

K$^+$

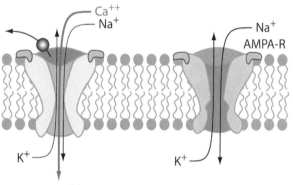

B. Glutamate released onto depolarized neuron
(relief of Mg^{++} block)

Ca^{++}
Na$^+$ Na$^+$
AMPA-R

K$^+$ K$^+$

release of Ca^{++} from internal stores,
activation of Ca^{++}-dependent kinases

Figure 13-3 Glutamate (*blue symbol*) elicits different effects depending on the state of the postsynaptic neuron. A: When released onto a neuron at rest, glutamate binds to both AMPA and NMDA receptors. However, only AMPA receptors pass current because the NMDA receptor pore is blocked by external Mg^{++} at rest potentials. The consequence of glutamate transmission in the presence of a Mg^{++} block is a small excitatory postsynaptic potential (EPSP), carried by an influx of sodium ions and tempered by an efflux of potassium ions. B: Neuronal depolarization pushes the Mg^{++} ion out of the pore and *relieves the Mg^{++} block*. Under these conditions, current flows through NMDA as well as AMPA receptors. Notably, the inward current carried by the NMDA receptor involves influx of both sodium and calcium ions. The calcium ion influx in turn triggers release of more calcium ions from internal stores, which in turn further depolarizes the cells and thereby perpetuates the relief of the magnesium block. Calcium ions also act as second-messengers, by for example activating kinases, and may thereby elicit numerous physiological changes.

The AMPA receptors not only open rapidly but also rapidly desensitize, meaning the receptor pore closes and is insensitive to ligand-gated opening for a period of time. Along with diffusion, uptake, and degradation, *rapid receptor desensitization is another mechanism that terminates neurotransmitter action at ionotropic receptors*. Because of their kinetic features, *AMPA receptor–mediated synaptic potentials are punctuated, starting and ending quickly, within milliseconds*.

Glutamate also binds to a second ionotropic receptor, the NMDA receptor. Activation of the NMDA receptor involves a unique hitch not seen with other receptors. Normally, a magnesium ion, Mg^{++}, blocks the NMDA receptor pore from the extracellular side. The magnesium ion is secured in place by electrostatic attraction to the inside of the negatively charged neuron (Fig. 13-3A). Membrane depolarization repels the positively charged magnesium ion, and the magnesium ion leaves the pore to re-enter the extracellular milieu (Fig. 13-3B). Once the magnesium block is relieved or removed, activation of the NMDA receptor by glutamate opens a nonselective cation pore and causes a depolarization.

As a result of the magnesium block, NMDA receptor activation alone does not result in a depolarization. This is because, in the absence of a coincident depolarization, the magnesium block occludes the NMDA receptor. Thus, even when the NMDA receptor binds glutamate and the NMDA pore opens, the pore is still blocked and no ion flux occurs (Fig. 13-3A). In contrast, when glutamate binds an NMDA receptor *at the same time* as a large depolarization occurs, typically through the activation of AMPA receptors, the magnesium block of the NMDA receptor is relieved and current flow through the open pore occurs (Fig. 13-3B).

Current through NMDA receptors is comprised of sodium, potassium, *and* calcium ions. The influx of calcium ions is highly consequential because it may trigger a cascading release of calcium ions from internal stores. Often, the result is a high concentration of free calcium ions, which serve as second-messengers and can exert a myriad of additional effects. Thus, the NMDA receptor is an exception to the rule that ionotropic receptors act only through direct channel opening. Opening the NMDA channel results directly in the recruitment of a second-messenger, in this case calcium ions. Calcium ions, in turn, interact with protein kinases, phosphatases, and other enzymes, leading to changes in membrane potential, excitability, gene expression, neuronal shape, and so on.

In sum, permeability of the NMDA channel to calcium ions and release of calcium ions from intracellular stores are important because they can result in a high concentration of free calcium ions that, in turn, can:

- Cause further depolarization, which consequently produces prolonged relief from magnesium block

- Act as second-messengers and, as such, alter enzymatic activity to modify ion channel activity, cytoskeletal proteins, and gene expression

The activation of NMDA receptors during the persistent relief from magnesium block produced by a depolarization allows additional NMDA receptor activation and more calcium ion entry, more release of calcium ions from internal stores, and so on. The changes in cell physiology consequent to the relief of the NMDA block play a critical role in the synaptic plasticity that is thought to underlie learning and memory.

LEARNING DEPENDS ON CHANGES IN SYNAPTIC STRENGTH

In the 1950s, we learned from Brenda Milner's work with patient HM that the formation and retrieval of declarative memories requires the hippocampus (see Chapter 7). The localization of memory formation to the hippocampus represents a neurobiological triumph and major milestone. Yet a macroscopic understanding of the pathways and circuits involved in learning—a goal not yet fully achieved—does not illuminate the cellular and molecular mechanisms of learning, the topic of this section.

As presciently proposed by Donald Hebb in the middle of the 20th century, the structural basis for learning occurs in the synapse. Hebb's idea was that if neuron A is repeatedly effective in exciting neuron B, over and over again, then something in the connection from A to B would change so that "A's efficiency" in activating B would increase. In other words, *learning involves a change in synaptic strength*, a change in the response of one neuron to a synaptic input from another neuron. The learning does not exist in either neuron A or neuron B but rather dwells in the *synaptic connection* between the two cells. Hebb's principle, often paraphrased as "neurons that fire together, wire together," has been the target of extensive experimental attention and ultimately has been fundamentally validated by modern neurobiology.

The breakthrough in subjecting Hebb's proposal to experimental analysis came from Terje Lømo and Timothy Bliss who demonstrated that high-frequency stimulation, or *tetanus*, of an input pathway to the hippocampus resulted in a sustained increase in the response of hippocampal neurons to that input (Fig. 13-4A). This phenomenon, now known as *long-term potentiation (LTP)*, lasts for a long time, for as long as synaptic strength has been experimentally monitored. LTP in the hippocampus requires depolarization of the postsynaptic neuron and the resulting calcium ion influx through the NMDA channel. An input that occurs while a postsynaptic cell is strongly depolarized will be augmented. The strong depolarization may arise from the response to

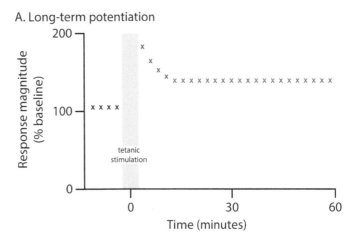

A. Long-term potentiation

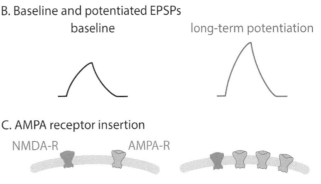

B. Baseline and potentiated EPSPs

C. AMPA receptor insertion

Figure 13-4 Long-term potentiation (LTP) is thought to constitute the cellular basis of learning. A: Tetanic stimulation results in a long-lasting increase in the response of a postsynaptic cell to a standard excitatory input. Tetanic stimulation produces an immediate but transient increase in the postsynaptic response (*blue x-s*) over the baseline magnitude (*black x-s*). Following this transient post-tetanic potentiation, the postsynaptic response remains stably elevated (*red x-s*), a plastic synaptic change known as LTP. B: After undergoing LTP, the response of a neuron increases in magnitude over the baseline response. C: A critical mechanism underlying LTP is the insertion of AMPA receptors into the postsynaptic membrane.

a tetanus at the same synapse (homosynaptic) or from the response to strong inputs at other synapses onto the same cell (heterosynaptic). In either case, NMDA receptor–mediated signaling onto a depolarized neuron strengthens that synaptic input, essentially binding a presynaptic input to a postsynaptic neuron more strongly (Fig. 13-4B).

Effective learning requires a process to undo learning, a process that we can think of as *forgetting*, when conditions change. Indeed, in *The Mind of a Mnemonist*, Alexander Luria wrote of S, a man with a uniquely lopsided capacity to make memories but no ability to forget. S's striking ability came with profound disadvantages. S locked all images and experiences into memory and therefore could not distinguish dreams from internal thoughts and images or external realities. We now think that LTP in the hippocampus is opposed by a putative cellular form of forgetting called *long-term depression (LTD)*.

The idea that LTP underlies learning and LTD serves forgetting holds for the hippocampus where declarative memories are formed (see Chapter 7). The same rules appear to also hold in the amygdala, where fear-based emotional memories are made. In other regions of the brain, slightly or even radically different cellular mechanisms support the formation of other types of memories. For example, in the cerebellar cortex, where motor memories are made, LTD supports learning and LTP supports unlearning. This role reversal arises because the cell that "learns" is inhibitory rather than excitatory. LTD decreases the excitation of inhibitory output neurons, with the ultimate effect that neurons targeted by cerebellar cortex neurons discharge at a *greater rate* after LTD in the cerebellar cortex.

As noted earlier, the NMDA channel is permeable to calcium ions. Elevated intracellular levels of calcium ions resulting from NMDA channel opening lead to important changes that are collectively considered as the top candidate for the cellular mechanism of hippocampal learning. The calcium ion influx leads to calcium ion release from internal stores. The resulting elevation in calcium ion concentration activates *Ca++/calmodulin-dependent protein kinase II (CaMKII)*. CaMKII is ubiquitous in the brain, representing 1–2% of all brain protein. CaMKII activation leads to trafficking, or movement, of cytoplasmic AMPA receptors into the membrane. AMPA receptor insertion is largely responsible for synaptic strengthening through LTP. Once there are more AMPA receptors in the postsynaptic membrane, a glutamatergic input will evoke a substantially larger response than it did prior to AMPA receptor insertion (Fig. 13-4C).

As with LTP, LTD also depends on calcium ions. However, whereas a high concentration of calcium ions is necessary for LTP, a low concentration can trigger LTD. In LTD, a low calcium ion concentration activates *Ca++-dependent phosphatases*, which in turn remove AMPA receptors from the plasma membrane of the postsynaptic cell. Internalization of AMPA receptors leads to a smaller postsynaptic response to a glutamatergic input.

It should be noted that the calcium ion-dependence of LTP and LTD in the cerebellum is switched so that LTD depends on a high concentration of calcium ions and LTP on a low concentration of calcium ions. Thus, the mechanisms of synaptic learning appear to parse according to ultimate effect—learning or unlearning—rather than by physiological go-between (LTP or LTD).

GLUTAMATE'S ACTIONS AT NMDA RECEPTORS ARE CRITICAL TO SYNAPTIC PLASTICITY

As we have seen, the NMDA receptor forms a molecular coincidence detector. A depolarization alone will not open the NMDA channel. Glutamate binding to the NMDA receptor will open the channel, but no ionic flux will occur in the absence of a depolarization to relieve the magnesium block. The NMDA channel only passes current if both depolarization and neurotransmitter binding occur together (Fig. 13-3). In other words, neither glutamate alone nor depolarization alone will open the NMDA receptor, but glutamate plus depolarization will. If a cell becomes sufficiently depolarized, the magnesium block will be relieved, making the NMDA channel open for ionic traffic.

INTERFERENCE WITH THE NMDA RECEPTOR CAN PRODUCE SEVERE PSYCHOLOGICAL DYSFUNCTION

NMDA receptors are widespread within the brain, present on the majority of neurons including those of the cerebral cortex. Furthermore, as coincidence detectors, NMDA receptors are required for synaptic plasticity. Given the NMDA receptor's ubiquity and critical role in learning, it is not surprising then that antagonizing normal NMDA receptor function has profound psychotropic effects. Here, we consider two drugs and one disease that reduce NMDA receptor–mediated communication.

Phencyclidine (PCP), colloquially referred to as "angel dust," binds to a site located within the pore of the NMDA receptor and prevents current from flowing through the

NMDA channel. *Ketamine*, or Special K, which is used for veterinary sedation and also abused by humans, acts as an NMDA receptor antagonist. Both phencyclidine and ketamine produce a dissociative effect (i.e., they disconnect subjective experience and external reality), creating a feeling of separation from one's own body. Phencyclidine and ketamine also produce hallucinations and disordered thought that are thought to resemble—and therefore are used to model—the cognitive experience of patients suffering from schizophrenia.

In *anti-NMDA receptor encephalitis*, a disease recognized only in the past decade, antibodies against the NMDA receptor gain access to the brain. The antibodies cause harm by stimulating receptor endocytosis, competing with glutamate for binding to the NMDA receptor, or both. Consequently, the number of NMDA receptors available for glutamate binding is reduced and glutamatergic transmission at the NMDA receptor depressed. As we saw earlier, blocking NMDA receptor–mediated transmission produces a psychotic break from reality, a state where paranoia, disordered thought, and hallucinations reign free. This is the clinical picture of anti-NMDA receptor encephalitis. Anti-NMDA receptor encephalitis is often paraneoplastic, with the responsible antibodies being secreted most commonly by an ovarian teratoma. Paraneoplastic cases are resolved by tumor removal. In the remaining cases, treatment is supportive coupled with therapies aimed at immune suppression or antibody removal through plasmapheresis.

In *My Month of Madness*, Susanah Cahalan, an American journalist, writes a gripping account of her experience with, and eventual recovery from anti-NMDA receptor encephalitis. Signs of her disease started mildly. An early symptom was an overblown, and in fact completely unwarranted, certainty that bugs infested her apartment. Normally a pack-rat, Ms. Cahalan found herself in an uncharacteristic cleaning frenzy, bagging or throwing out all of her belongings. Upon consulting an exterminator, she refused to accept the exterminator's assurances that no infestation existed, and she insisted on paying for a spray treatment. At the end of all of her anti-bug efforts, Ms Cahalan "still didn't feel any better." Ms. Cahalan's disease progressed to include further signs of paranoia along with amnesia, emotional lability, hemispatial neglect, hallucinations, and highly disordered thought best described as psychosis. She also suffered seizures, an objective symptom that worked to her advantage because it made it harder for physicians to brush her off as hysterical and commit her to psychiatric treatment. Nonetheless, some physicians did just that, albeit in the early days of the recognition of the disease. Ultimately, Ms. Cahalan ventured inordinately close, for a previously

healthy 24-year-old, to death before receiving a diagnosis and journeying back to health.

Anti-NMDA receptor encephalitis is now recognized as one of a growing family of *autoimmune encephalopathies* that result when antibodies against surface proteins cross the blood–brain barrier (BBB) to gain access to the CNS. Although more than half of the known antigens are receptors (NMDA, AMPA, mGluR, D_2, $GABA_A$, $GABA_B$, glycine), other antigens are surface proteins present at synapses and nodes of Ranvier. Of note, the disease symptoms develop rapidly and affect people of all ages, often afflicting young adults, adolescents, and even infants under 5 years of age. The broad range of symptoms observed in autoimmune encephalopathies includes disorders of mood and thought such as psychosis, abnormal sleep, motor abnormalities such as excess movements, seizures, and autonomic failures. The set of symptoms typical of each autoimmune encephalopathy is roughly aligned to the antigen involved. For example, in cases of anti-$GABA_A$ receptor encephalopathy, seizures are always prominent, whereas in anti-D_2 receptor encephalopathy, excess movements predominate. The latter is fitting given the concentration of D_2 receptors in the basal ganglia pathways (see Chapter 25). Regardless of the particular constellation of symptoms presented, autoimmune encephalopathy should always be considered when a previously healthy young person presents with acute psychiatric symptoms, seizures, or the like. Diagnosis is key to treatment since most patients find that their symptoms ameliorate with immunotherapy. Unfortunately up to 10% of patients with an autoimmune encephalopathy die. Hopefully, this figure will decrease as this disease class is more widely appreciated and physicians begin to recognize and treat patients earlier in the disease process.

NICOTINIC ACETYLCHOLINE RECEPTORS MEDIATE NEURONAL COMMUNICATION WITH SKELETAL MUSCLES

The most thoroughly studied and best-understood synapse is the *neuromuscular junction* (*NMJ*) or *endplate*, where a motoneuron axon contacts a skeletal muscle fiber expressing nAChRs (Fig. 13-5). An action potential in a motoneuron results in the release of thousands of acetylcholine molecules from each of hundreds of vesicles. Thus, it is estimated that one action potential in one motoneuron results in the release of *millions* of molecules of acetylcholine onto a single postsynaptic muscle fiber. Released acetylcholine

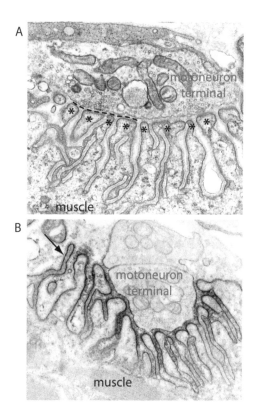

Figure 13-5 In a normal human neuromuscular junction or endplate, a motoneuron axon ends on a skeletal muscle fiber. A: The muscle contains junctional folds (*asterisks in A*) across from the many active zones within the axonal terminal. A basal lamina (*dashed line in A*) runs between the axonal plasma membrane and the muscle. B: At the top of each junctional fold, acetylcholine receptors are concentrated (*arrow in B*) and at the base of the folds, voltage-gated sodium channels are concentrated (not shown). Acetylcholinesterase is anchored to the basal lamina. Photomicrograph kindly provided by Andrew G. Engel, MD, Mayo Clinic.

diffuses across the synaptic cleft, itself densely packed with acetylcholinesterase, an enzyme that degrades acetylcholine (see Chapter 12), to reach the receptors. Although most of the acetylcholine molecules released are hydrolyzed by acetylcholinesterase, enough make it to the postsynaptic membrane to elicit a response in the muscle. This response is mediated by activation of nAchRs, which are crowded at very high density, more than 10,000 receptors per square micron. The receptors are concentrated on the muscle membrane at a location exactly opposite to axonal release sites. As is the case for AMPA receptors, activated nicotinic receptors form an open channel through which sodium and potassium ions pass. The extracellular acetylcholinesterase present in the synaptic cleft ensures that the effect of acetylcholine released by a single action potential is short-lived.

At an individual neuromuscular junction, a single action potential opens tens of thousands of channels and produces a depolarization in the target muscle fiber that typically reaches threshold for an action potential. Thus,

neuromuscular transmission enjoys a high safety factor, meaning that transmission from the motoneuron axon to muscle contraction succeeds more often than it fails in healthy individuals. The high safety factor ensures that essential functions such as breathing, moving about, and eating happen. It also follows that motor weakness at the neuromuscular junction is typically a sign that the synapse has been severely compromised.

In contrast to the neuromuscular junction, a typical hippocampal neuron (modern neurobiology's favorite model of a central neuron) integrates a large number of synaptic inputs from a variety of sources. At any single hippocampal glutamatergic synapse, a presynaptic action potential results in either no release or the release of only a single vesicle. Neurotransmitter contained in a single vesicle in turn opens fewer than a hundred AMPA channels. As a result, the postsynaptic neuron may respond with an excitatory postsynaptic potential (EPSP) but is unlikely to fire an action potential due to a single glutamatergic input. Central synapses, with a low safety factor, are ideal for situations that require the integration of a large number of synaptic inputs. In contrast, at the neuromuscular junction, there is only one input—from the motoneuron axon—and the safety factor is cumulatively high.

In patients with *myasthenia gravis*, the concentration of nicotinic acetylcholine receptors at the neuromuscular junction is compromised, resulting in muscle weakness. Myasthenia gravis is usually an autoimmune disease involving antibodies that attack the clustering or integrity of acetylcholine receptors present at the endplate. The pathological antibodies activate complement and thereby lead to the degradation of the postsynaptic membrane. Most myasthenic patients have antibodies directed against the nicotinic acetylcholine receptor, and a sizable minority has antibodies that recognize *muscle-specific kinase* (*MuSK*), which is critical to receptor clustering at the endplate. Congenital mutations in a variety of proteins involved in endplate formation and function are responsible for rare genetic forms of myasthenia. Regardless of the pathophysiology involved, patients present with muscle weakness, often of the eyelids. The affected muscles can be contracted but rapidly fatigue with repeated efforts by the myasthenic patient. This rapidly fatiguing weakness stands in marked contrast to the initial weakness that improves with continued use observed in patients with Lambert-Eaton syndrome (see Chapter 11). To increase the amount of acetylcholine available to bind to the diminished number of nicotinic receptors, patients with myasthenia gravis are treated with cholinesterase inhibitors (see Chapter 12).

Nicotinic acetylcholine receptors, like all other ionotropic receptors, are multimeric complexes, meaning that several subunits assemble into one functional receptor complex. For each subunit, there may be numerous genes as well as potential post-translational modifications. Therefore, there are a number of different subtypes of receptors depending on the particular subunit makeup. In the case of the nAChR, there are three primary subtypes:

- The *muscle nicotinic receptor*, present on all skeletal muscle, mediates the communication between a motoneuron axon and a skeletal muscle fiber.

- The *ganglionic nicotinic receptor* is present in all *autonomic* ganglia and mediates communication between an autonomic preganglionic neuron and a ganglionic neuron.

- The *neuronal nicotinic receptor* is present in the brain and mediates communication between two central neurons.

Nicotine activates all three subtypes. However, the muscle nicotinic receptor has only a low affinity for nicotine, and, therefore, nicotine produces primarily autonomic and psychotropic effects.

Nicotine's autonomic effects are sympathetic in nature, including elevations in cardiac output, blood pressure, and heart rate along with epinephrine release from the adrenal medulla. Nicotine's psychotropic effects include alertness, relaxation, reduced appetite, and enhanced focus of attention. The sympathetic and psychotropic effects interact so that, for example, the sympathoexcitatory effects of epinephrine enhance nicotine's psychotropic effects.

Nicotine is the major active ingredient in tobacco and is one of the most widely used drugs of the modern world. Many individuals who use tobacco develop a strong dependence or addiction to nicotine. Dependence on nicotine, a common and costly problem today, stems from nicotine's actions in the CNS. By replacing an addiction to cigarettes with a dependence on nicotine patches or gum, smoking cessation programs parse the addiction, separating a patient's dependence on the act of smoking and the full complement of tobacco ingredients from the dependence on nicotine per se. Patients who successfully quit smoking but continue to take in nicotine reduce their risk of lung disease but may still suffer from other negative consequences of the drug,

most notably adverse cardiovascular effects. Nicotine has little to no effect on skeletal muscle because it is a poor agonist at the muscle nicotinic receptor.

Distinct sets of receptor agonists and antagonists act selectively on the muscle, ganglionic, and neuronal subtypes of nicotinic acetylcholine receptors. *Curare* is a nicotinic receptor antagonist that blocks the muscle nicotinic receptor but not the ganglionic nicotinic receptor. It is a large, bulky plant alkaloid that does not gain access to the brain, precluding the possibility of its acting on neuronal nicotinic receptors. Curare came to the attention of the Western world when explorers saw South American natives using curare-tipped arrows on prey. Curare-injected prey lost control of their muscles, fell out of trees, and were then killed by the natives. Even if the natives had not killed them, the prey would have died eventually because curare would paralyze the diaphragm, the muscle needed for inspiration. The natives could safely eat the prey because curare is too large and charged to be absorbed across the gastrointestinal lining.

Although still invaluable as a research tool, curare itself is not used in medicine. Several related compounds with affinity for the muscle nicotinic receptor are used as *muscle relaxants* during surgery or brief, minimally invasive procedures. For example, *pancuronium*, pharmacologically similar to curare, is a nicotinic receptor antagonist that is used at low doses as a muscle relaxant for surgery. Pancuronium competes with endogenous acetylcholine released at the endplate and thereby decreases the postsynaptic response of the muscle. Nicotinic receptor *agonists* such as *succinylcholine* may also serve as muscle relaxants by depolarizing the muscle, leading to voltage-gated sodium channel (VGSC) inactivation. Nicotinic receptor agonists are often termed *depolarizing* neuromuscular blocking agents, whereas antagonists are called *nondepolarizing* for their opposing mode of action. As long as succinylcholine remains at the neuromuscular junction, muscle VGSCs do not recover from inactivation, thus preventing the muscle from firing action potentials. Within the emergency room, succinylcholine is used to relax upper airway muscles and allow a health professional to intubate a patient (place a tube into the trachea) without the patient gagging. The effect of succinylcholine is brief because the agent is hydrolyzed by plasma esterases within about 10 minutes. Nonetheless, use of any muscle relaxant acting on the neuromuscular junction should always be coupled with a means of artificially ventilating a patient, should the need arise.

Blocking the neuromuscular junction is desirable only when performed under controlled conditions. Clearly, blocking skeletal muscle contraction can be lethal if it blocks diaphragmatic contraction. Indeed, pancuronium is part of the lethal cocktail of drugs administered to prisoners executed in the United States since 1982. Until the early 21st century, the other drugs used included a barbiturate such as sodium pentobarbital and potassium chloride. Injecting potassium chloride causes cardiac asystole by the same mechanism that hyperkalemia does (see Chapter 10). The barbiturate produces a state of general anesthesia (see next section), rendering the condemned prisoner unconscious for his or her agonal moments. Since the early 2000s, the European Union, which forbids the death penalty in constituent nations, has successfully pressured pharmaceutical companies into not making barbiturates available for use in lethal injection. Barbiturates are currently difficult to obtain, and no general anesthetic has been used in recent prisoner executions in the United States. As a result, recently executed prisoners in the United States have had a prolonged dying experience with some apparent level of nervous system activity evident.

GABA BINDS TO AND OPENS THE IONOTROPIC GABA$_A$ RECEPTOR

When GABA binds to a GABA$_A$ receptor, the receptor changes conformation and forms a pore that is permeable to chloride ions. As detailed in Chapter 9, the reversal potential for chloride ions depends on the distribution of chloride ions, which in turn depends on the type of chloride transporters active in a cell. In most neurons in the adult nervous system, the KCC transporter, which you recall transports chloride ions out of the cell, dominates, so that the Nernst potential for chloride ions is about −70 mV. Since neurons typically have resting potentials of about −60 mV, activation of the GABA$_A$ receptor usually causes chloride influx and a hyperpolarization and thus inhibits most neurons.

As the predominant fast inhibitory receptor in the CNS, the GABA$_A$ receptor is central to the actions of many therapeutics including general anesthetics, anxiolytics, hypnotics, muscle relaxants, and anticonvulsants, as well as alcohol. Yet most clinical drugs that act on the GABA$_A$ receptor are neither receptor agonists nor antagonists. Instead, they are allosteric modulators that bind to a site distinct from where endogenous GABA binds and alter channel properties.

Benzodiazepines, a large class of drugs that includes anxiolytics, muscle relaxants, and hypnotics, bind to a site on the GABA$_A$ receptor distinct from the site where GABA binds (Fig. 13-6). A third site on the GABA$_A$ receptor binds barbiturates, including a number that are effective as anticonvulsants and general anesthetics. The

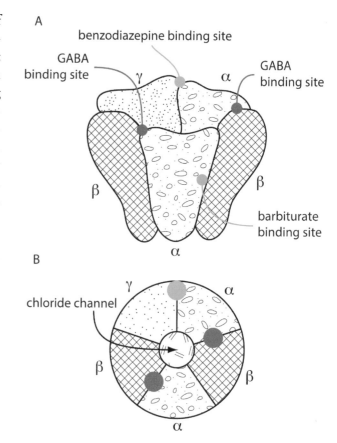

Figure 13-6 Five subunits—two α subunits, two β subunits, and one γ subunit—make up the GABA$_A$ receptor. Two γ-aminobutyric acid (GABA) binding sites are present at the α–β interfaces, and both have to be occupied for the pore, a chloride channel, to open. A site that binds benzodiazepines and a limited number of related compounds is located at the α–γ interface. General anesthetics act at a few sites within the lipid bilayer. For example, barbiturates that have both anticonvulsant and general anesthetic actions bind at the α–β subunit interface within the lipid bilayer. Other general anesthetics act elsewhere within intramembranous regions of the GABA$_A$ receptor. Panel A shows an oblique side view of the receptor and B shows a top-down view of the receptor.

affinity of a GABA$_A$ receptor for GABA increases when the receptor is also bound to a benzodiazepine and/or to a barbiturate. Alcohol and general anesthetics beyond barbiturates facilitate and may even act as an agonist at the GABA$_A$ receptor. Ultimately, benzodiazepines, barbiturates, alcohol, and general anesthetics result in more chloride ion influx. Because of the ubiquity of GABA$_A$ receptor distribution, positive allosteric modulators of the GABA$_A$ receptor cause widespread inhibition of brain function. Thus, for example, it is through inhibition of central neurons rather than neuromuscular junction blockade by which benzodiazepines act as muscle relaxants. By the same token, sedation resulting from elevated central inhibition is a common effect of every positive allosteric modulator of the GABA$_A$ receptor.

Like the nAChR to which it is closely related, the GABA$_A$ receptor is made up of multiple subunits. A highly diverse set of subunit isoforms results in a large number of possible subunit combinations. Different drugs bind preferentially to different subunit combinations that are expressed in different neurons so that, for example, one drug may have the predominant effect of inhibiting anxiety while a different drug primarily inhibits movement.

METABOTROPIC RECEPTOR-MEDIATED SIGNALING IS AMPLIFIED BY CYCLES OF G PROTEIN ACTIVATION

A large and increasing proportion of the modern medical pharmacopeia acts on metabotropic receptors. Current treatments for chronic pain, hypertension, glaucoma, and irritable bowel syndrome all target metabotropic receptors. Most metabotropic receptors involved in chemical neurotransmission are coupled to G proteins and therefore are called *G protein-coupled receptors* (*GPCRs*). Here, we focus on common mechanisms by which activation of G protein-coupled receptors results in ion channel modification before examining the roles of these receptors in autonomic function and therapeutic management.

Upon binding neurotransmitter, a GPCR undergoes a conformational change and activates associated *guanine nucleotide-binding proteins* (*G proteins*) present on the inner surface. Changes in the electrical properties of a cell result when the activated G proteins either directly affect ion channels or modify the activity of enzymes that synthesize second-messengers, which, in turn, affect ion channels, sometimes through the production of additional signaling molecules and effectors. As emphasized earlier, metabotropic receptor-mediated signaling requires time so that resulting changes in electrical properties occur relatively slowly.

G proteins associated with GPCRs are comprised of three subunits—α and the inseparable β-γ—located along the inner leaflet of the cell membrane. At rest, all three subunits are bound together with a guanine diphosphate (GDP) molecule bound to the α subunit (Fig. 13-7). Upon stimulation by an activated receptor, guanine triphosphate (GTP) is exchanged for GDP, and the α subunit dissociates from the β-γ subunits, which never dissociate under physiological conditions. The activated α subunit, bound to GTP, is free to diffuse throughout the cell and directly interact

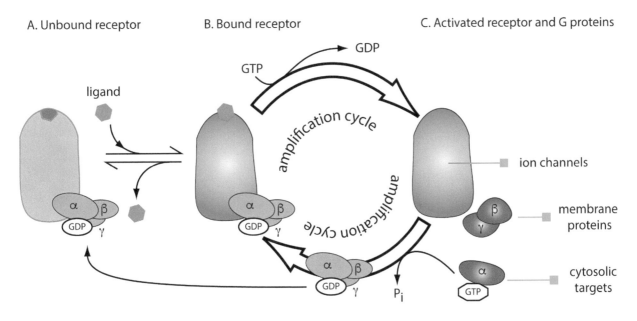

Figure 13-7 Metabotropic receptor activation lasts as long as a ligand is bound to the receptor. A: At rest, a metabotropic receptor is bound to a G protein, which is bound to guanine diphosphate (GDP). Three subunits—α, β, and γ—make up a G protein. The α subunit binds GDP in the resting state. When a ligand binds to a metabotropic receptor (B), the GDP that is bound to the α subunit is exchanged for a guanosine triphosphate (GTP; C), and the receptor and associated G protein are activated. The activated receptor can affect ion channels within the membrane. The β and γ subunits stay bound together and, when activated, can affect membrane-associated proteins. The activated α subunit, bound to a GTP molecule, diffuses throughout the cell and can affect a large variety of cytosolic targets, as well as distant membrane protein targets. When the α subunit hydrolyzes GTP into GDP, releasing a phosphate ion (P$_i$) in the process, it rapidly reassociates with the β–γ subunits. The G protein can then associate with either a receptor bound to a ligand or to an unbound receptor. If the G protein associates with a ligand bound receptor, another round of activation of the receptor, β–γ subunits, and α subunit occurs.

with channels or enzymes. Although activated receptors and β-γ subunits may produce effects on proteins within the cell membrane, the α subunit is responsible for the vast majority of metabotropic receptor-mediated changes in membrane excitability.

G protein activation is terminated when the α subunit itself hydrolyzes GTP to GDP, allowing the α subunit to reassociate with the β-γ subunits (Fig. 13-7). Yet, guanine exchange can reoccur, and the reassociated trimeric G protein can once again dissociate if the G protein binds to an activated (bound to agonist) GPCR. Thus, *for as long as a GPCR remains bound to an agonist, it can continue to activate G proteins over and over again.* This cycle greatly *amplifies* the effect of ligand binding, allowing many iterations of G protein activation per ligand binding event. In addition, each activated G protein can trigger the production of many molecules of a second-messenger, which can, in turn, lead to the production of additional second-messenger species or varieties. In this way, the binding of an agonist to a GPCR can set into motion a signaling cascade in which increasing numbers of second-messenger species and increasing numbers of molecules of each species are produced through successive waves of biochemical activity thereby greatly amplifying the effect of activation of a single receptor.

THE VARIETIES OF G PROTEINS, SECOND-MESSENGERS, AND EFFECTOR PATHWAYS PROVIDE GREAT FLEXIBILITY TO POTENTIAL EFFECTS OF GPCRS

Due to enormous variation in GPCRs, second-messengers, and potential effectors, a single neurotransmitter can have many different effects depending on the molecules present in the postsynaptic cell. It is not unusual for a neurotransmitter to exert opposing effects on two cells expressing the same GPCR coupled to different α subunits. For example, G proteins containing $G\alpha_s$ (stimulatory) stimulate cAMP production, whereas G proteins containing $G\alpha_i$ (inhibitory) inhibit cAMP production. In this way, a neurotransmitter that binds to a GPCR can either open or close an ion channel through opposing effects on the same second-messenger. Since metabotropic receptors that work through G proteins are found throughout the body, toxins and drugs that target G proteins have effects that are not limited to the nervous system (see Box 13-1).

G protein-coupled receptors produce highly diverse effects through myriad variations on several canonical

Two toxins—*pertussis* and *cholera*—wreak physiological havoc and, in the case of cholera toxin, cause death if left untreated. Pertussis toxin causes *whooping cough* primarily through effects on the respiratory epithelium. Cholera toxin causes cholera, still a major threat in developing countries (primarily in sub-Saharan Africa), by initially attacking the gastrointestinal epithelium. Pertussis toxin binds to and interferes with the function of certain isoforms of $G\alpha_i$, whereas cholera toxin blocks the function of certain $G\alpha_s$ isoforms. Both toxins cause exclusively or predominantly non-neurological symptoms in large part because their access to the nervous system is restricted, or at least delayed, by the blood–brain barrier. The whooping cough caused by pertussis toxin and severe diarrhea caused by cholera toxin reflect the access of toxin to vulnerable barrier tissues, as well as the ubiquity of G protein signaling in physiological function, neural and non-neural alike.

second-messenger systems. The best-described targets of the activated, GTP-bound, α subunit are:

- *Adenylyl cyclase*: Adenylyl cyclase activation leads to cAMP production, whereas adenylyl cyclase inhibition leads to a decrease in cAMP levels. The concentration of cAMP in turn modifies the activity of a number of cAMP-dependent protein kinases.

- *Phospholipase C*: Phospholipase C activation leads to production of diacylglycerol and inositol trisphosphate (IP_3), which in turn lead to activation of protein kinase C (PKC) and the release of calcium ions from internal stores, respectively.

- *Phospholipase A_2*: Phospholipase A_2 activation leads to production of arachidonic acid, which in turn leads to production of a variety of further signaling molecules, such as prostaglandins, prostacyclins, and leukotrienes.

Second-messengers that derive from the membrane—diacylglycerol and arachidonic acid—primarily stay associated with the plasma membrane, whereas soluble second-messengers such as calcium ions, cyclic nucleotides, and IP_3 exert effects throughout the cytosol as well as on membrane proteins.

A classic example of G protein-mediated effects involves the autonomic control of heart rate. Parasympathetic and sympathetic neurons influence heart rate through effects on cells in the sinoatrial node within the right atrium that pace cardiac contractions. Acetylcholine, released from parasympathetic nerves, binds to a muscarinic receptor, a metabotropic receptor named after muscarine, a plant compound that selectively activates these receptors. The activated muscarinic receptor activates a $G\alpha_i$-containing G protein, resulting in a reduction in cAMP production. The reduction in cAMP levels decreases the activity of cAMP-dependent protein kinase A (PKA) and, in turn, the phosphorylation state of calcium channels, which renders calcium channels less likely to open at rest potentials. Along with an increase in potassium channel activity produced by the activated β-γ subunits of the G protein, the decrease in calcium channel activity hyperpolarizes cardiac pacemaker cells, prolonging the interval between action potentials and therefore between heart beats. In contrast, norepinephrine, released from sympathetic nerves, acts at adrenergic receptors to activate a $G\alpha_s$-containing G protein that increases cAMP production and PKA activity, thereby increasing the phosphorylation state and consequently the activity of calcium channels. Thus, *two different neurotransmitters bind to different GPCRs and, through different G proteins, have opposing effects on a single effector molecule, cAMP, which leads to opposing effects on excitability.*

Another example of cyclic nucleotide signaling is exemplified by the process of *phototransduction*, changing light energy into electrical energy, in the retina. In the absence of light stimulation, *photoreceptors*, a special class of retinal cells that respond to light, have a relatively high concentration of cGMP, which directly binds to and opens cyclic nucleotide gated cation channels (see Box 13-2). In the dark, cGMP levels are high, and cyclic nucleotide gated channels are open. This means that, in the dark, photoreceptors have an inward cation current, carried by sodium and calcium ions, that depolarizes them to about –40 mV (Fig. 13-8A). Light stimulation activates *transducin*, a particular type of G protein contained within photoreceptors. The activated α subunit of transducin activates phosphodiesterase, which then degrades cGMP. The resulting decrease in cGMP concentration leads to less inward cation current and therefore membrane hyperpolarization (Fig. 13-8B). And, yes, this physiological trick is unusual in that sensory cells are typically depolarized by stimulation.

Like cGMP, cAMP also directly opens a number of cyclic nucleotide-gated channels, providing another avenue for cAMP signaling in addition to kinase activation. Furthermore, cAMP can act through a number of pathways beyond PKA and opening cyclic nucleotide gated channels. For example, cAMP can activate guanine nucleotide exchange factors, which in turn regulate the activity of small GTPases, soluble proteins such as *ras* that are small

Mutations in the cyclic nucleotide-gated cation channel present in retinal photoreceptors can impair vision. Some of these mutations lead to a form of *retinitis pigmentosa*, a disease in which the photoreceptors degenerate. Although it is straightforward to understand how mutations in the photoreceptor cyclic nucleotide-gated channel would impair phototransduction, it remains unclear why photoreceptors with mutated channels eventually die as a result of this deficit. Other mutations in the photoreceptor cyclic nucleotide-gated cation channel lead to a form of congenital *achromatopsia*. In this disease, the three types of photoreceptor responsible for seeing both color and high-acuity forms lack functional cyclic nucleotide-gated channels and therefore do not function at all. Patients with achromatopsia can see light and dark and general forms but cannot see colors or detailed forms (for more information, see Chapter 15).

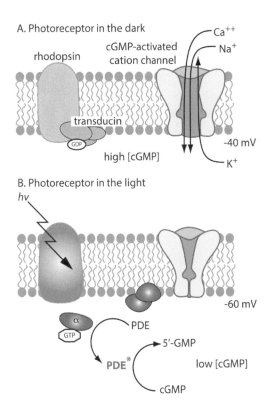

Figure 13-8 A: Photoreceptors have a "dark current," an inward current that persists in the absence of light. Cyclic nucleotide gated cation channels, activated by a high resting concentration of cyclic guanosine monophosphate (cGMP) carry the dark current. B: Light (*hv*) activates rhodopsin, which activates a G protein called transducin. The activated α subunit of transducin activates cGMP phosphodiesterase, which converts cGMP into 5'-GMP, thus lowering the concentration of cGMP in the photoreceptor. As a result of the decrease in cGMP concentration, cyclic nucleotide-gated cation channels close and the cell hyperpolarizes.

versions of the α subunit of membrane-bound G proteins and are present in the cytosol. The effects of such signaling are wide-ranging and include diverse electrically silent modifications of cellular physiology.

Just as cAMP acts through a number of signaling pathways, cGMP can act through pathways beyond those involving phosphodiesterase described earlier. For example nitric oxide (NO), the gas neurotransmitter introduced in Chapter 12, results in the activation of soluble guanylyl cyclase and consequently the production of cGMP from GTP. In the periphery, cGMP production activates protein kinase G, which phosphorylates proteins that change the contractile properties of smooth muscle and result ultimately in relaxation. Sildenafil, commonly known as Viagra, is an inhibitor of the cGMP-activated phosphodiesterase and is approved in the United States to treat erectile dysfunction. By inhibiting the cGMP-selective phosphodiesterase that is present in the penile corpus cavernosum, sildenafil prolongs relaxation of blood vessel walls and consequently the vasodilation underlying penile erection. Within the CNS, NO acts both by increasing cGMP levels and by initiating the *S*-nitrosylation (addition of an NO to the sulfur of a cysteine) of a number of cytosolic proteins including ion channels, transporters, cytoskeletal components, and enzymes. Thus, NO acts as a signaling molecule and engages the production of additional signaling molecules such as cGMP.

METABOTROPIC RECEPTORS ACTIVATED BY NOREPINEPHRINE AND ACETYLCHOLINE ARE KEY TO CLINICAL PHARMACOLOGY

Parasympathetic and sympathetic ganglion neurons release either acetylcholine or norepinephrine, both of which act on target cells exclusively through the activation of metabotropic receptors (Fig. 13-9). Acetylcholine acts at muscarinic receptors, whereas norepinephrine acts at adrenergic receptors (see Table 13-1). Since autonomic targets are always peripheral, there is no requirement that a drug cross the BB in order to affect autonomic function. It should be noted that the vesicles of both parasympathetic and sympathetic ganglion neurons contain and release two neurotransmitters beyond acetylcholine or norepinephrine: ATP and a peptide called *neuropeptide Y* (*NPY*). ATP, as you may recall, is present in virtually all synaptic vesicles. It binds to ionotropic P2X receptors and metabotropic P1 and P2Y receptors, which are widespread throughout the

body. As the name suggests, NPY is a neuropeptide whose cognate receptor is metabotropic. In sum, neurotransmission from autonomic ganglionic neurons is predominantly but not exclusively (remember the P2X receptors) mediated by metabotropic receptors.

Acetylcholine and norepinephrine, released from autonomic ganglion neurons, bind to a panoply of muscarinic and adrenergic receptors present on non-neuronal target tissues. By targeting cardiac muscle, glands, and smooth muscle tissues, autonomic neurons influence physiological function throughout the body. In many cases, this influence may operate simply by increasing or decreasing the blood flow to a tissue through an effect on the smooth muscle supplying blood vessel walls. Thus, *drugs that either mimic or antagonize the synapse from autonomic ganglionic neurons to target tissues can influence the function of virtually every tissue in the body.*

Drugs that either mimic or block neurotransmitter actions upon autonomic targets comprise an important part of the pharmaceutical arsenal used by cardiologists, ophthalmologists, diabetologists, pulmonologists, urologists, anesthesiologists, and virtually every other clinician, including general practitioners. Moreover, because of the widespread expression of muscarinic and adrenergic receptors, most drugs that modify autonomic transmission have multiple physiological effects. In some instances, this may be clinically desirable, as can be the case for so-called *β-blockers*, β adrenergic receptor antagonists that decrease both heart rate and cardiac contractility. In other instances, effects are undesirable and thus colloquially termed "side effects." As an example of the latter, a decongestant such as phenylephrine, an α adrenergic receptor agonist that constricts blood vessels in the nose and reduces nasal secretions may constrict blood vessels widely and thus cause hypertension. Side effects can sometimes be circumvented by lowering the dose, targeting the route of administration, and, in a few cases, by tailoring the drug to an isoform found in a restricted set of tissues.

THE BALANCE OF PARASYMPATHETIC AND SYMPATHETIC TONE VARIES ACROSS CONDITIONS AND THE LIFE CYCLE

In the common vernacular, the sympathetic nervous system is active during "fight or flight" and the parasympathetic nervous system is active during conditions of "rest and digest" (Fig. 13-9). Indeed, the effect of massive sympathetic stimulation is to enlist the body's energy

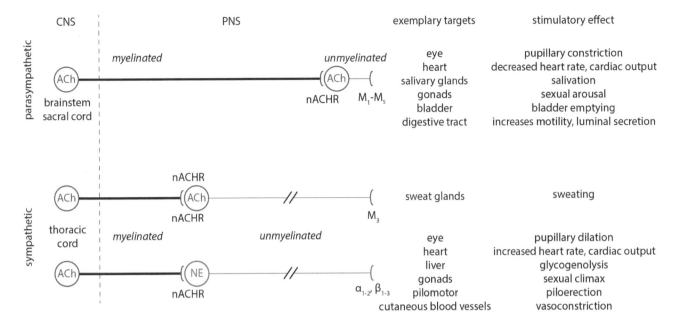

Figure 13-9 The anatomical and pharmacological organization of the parasympathetic and sympathetic pathways. All preganglionic neurons have a cell body in the central nervous system, synthesize and release acetylcholine, and send a long (parasympathetic) or short (sympathetic) myelinated axon to an autonomic ganglion. Neurons in autonomic ganglia express the ganglionic nicotinic receptor and send an unmyelinated postganglionic axon to a target that may be smooth muscle, cardiac muscle, or a gland. Parasympathetic ganglionic neurons utilize acetylcholine as a neurotransmitter. All sympathetic ganglionic neurons except those that innervate sweat glands utilize norepinephrine. The peripheral targets of autonomic ganglionic neurons express G protein-coupled muscarinic (parasympathetic) or adrenergic (sympathetic) receptors. Note that the fibers are not illustrated to scale; broken lines indicate a break in the illustrated fiber length.

resources to support activity and alertness. Extensive sympathetic activation greatly increases oxygen availability by increasing cardiac contractility, heart rate, and blood pressure and dilating the bronchi. Blood flow is diverted from the viscera involved in digestion to skeletal muscles to support protective movements, such as fleeing and fighting. At the same time, sweating prevents overheating. The sympathetically mediated constriction of cutaneous blood vessels and decrease in clotting time help prevent hemorrhage in the event of invasive wounds. The effects of parasympathetic activation largely oppose the effects of sympathetic activation. Energy is channeled into digestion and away from skeletal motor activity. Secretion of mucus, saliva, and tears is promoted. In sum, sympathetic activation promotes arousal and skeletomotor action, whereas parasympathetic activation promotes rest, inactivity, and digestion.

Most tissues—the heart, lungs, kidneys, pancreas, skin, hair follicles, bladder, dura, and so on—receive innervation from parasympathetic neurons, sympathetic neurons, or often from both. Despite the popular notion that sympathetic and parasympathetic functions diametrically oppose each other, there is a range of relationships between the effects of parasympathetic and sympathetic activation, from direct opposition to unopposed. As already discussed,

parasympathetic and sympathetic influences act in direct opposition to produce either a reduction or an increase in heart rate.

In contrast to the simplicity of opposing autonomic influences on heart rate, parasympathetic and sympathetic influences on ocular pressure are complex. The importance of ocular pressure is revealed by *glaucoma*, a disease that typically involves an increase in intraocular pressure (Fig. 13-10). Even in normal pressure glaucoma, involving no increase in pressure, decreasing intraocular pressure is beneficial. Therefore, therapy is aimed at decreasing the production of aqueous humor, increasing the drainage of aqueous humor, or both. To accomplish these ends, glaucoma can be treated by a muscarinic agonist, an α adrenergic agonist, or a β adrenergic antagonist. To understand how three different drugs can produce the same clinical outcome, we consider each drug in turn.

- *Muscarinic agonist*: When administered in eye drops, pilocarpine, an agonist at the M_3 receptor, mimics acetylcholine's actions on the ciliary muscle, leading to the muscle's contraction and an increase in the iridocorneal angle (Fig. 13-10). This in turn opens up the trabecular meshwork and increases drainage

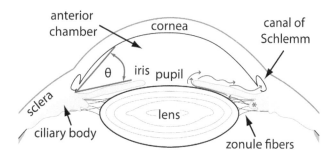

Figure 13-10 The ciliary body consists of ciliary muscles, which control pupillary size and lens shape, and the ciliary processes, which make aqueous humor. Aqueous humor is necessary to maintain the health of the lens and the anterior part of the eye, including the cornea and iris. Aqueous humor flows out from the ciliary processes through the zonule fibers. Aqueous humor flow follows a path between the iris and the lens, and then through the pupil to enter the anterior chamber. Aqueous humor bathes anterior tissues and flows through the trabecular meshwork, a spongy tissue that sits atop the iris, to exit the eye through the canal of Schlemm. The angle between the iris and the cornea, the iridocorneal angle, is larger in open-angle than in closed-angle glaucoma. Strategies at combating glaucoma are aimed at decreasing aqueous humor production or at increasing the iridocorneal angle to allow for greater aqueous humor drainage through the canal of Schlemm.

of aqueous humor from the eye, thereby decreasing pressure.

- *α Adrenergic agonist*: α-2 Adrenergic agonists such as apraclonidine, activate receptors on the ciliary body that activate $G\alpha_i$ and decrease cAMP production. As a result, the ciliary body produces less aqueous humor.

- *β Adrenergic antagonist*: β Adrenergic antagonists, colloquially know as β-blockers, prevent endogenous norepinephrine from binding to β adrenergic receptors on the ciliary body. Endogenous activation of β adrenergic receptors by norepinephrine activates a $G\alpha_s$ protein that increases cAMP production. Blocking the β receptor with a drug such as timolol results in less cAMP production and consequently less production of aqueous humor by the ciliary body.

Healthy individuals exist in the continuum between sympathetic and parasympathetic extremes, maintaining a balance of sympathetic and parasympathetic tone. The balance between sympathetic and parasympathetic activity varies not only with the moment-to-moment arousal state but also across longer time scales, such as health status, athletic conditioning, and age change. In young elite athletes, parasympathetic activity dominates to the extent that resting heart rates are often less than 50 beats per minute. With age, disease, and sedentary lifestyle, the balance in autonomic activity shifts toward sympathetic domination.

Most drugs that act on muscarinic receptors do not cross the BBB. Even those that do, such as atropine, act entirely or primarily peripherally to produce therapeutic effects. As a consequence, drugs that act on muscarinic receptors do not, as a rule, produce psychotropic effects. Muscarinic antagonists used to counteract motion sickness, such as scopolamine, are exceptions in that their site of action appears to be central, on chemoreceptive neurons of the medulla. However, as with other muscarinic drugs, scopolamine and related therapeutics do not produce psychotropic effects.

In contrast to the majority of muscarinic drugs, most commonly used adrenergic drugs act both peripherally and centrally, and many produce at least some psychotropic effects. To understand how the central and peripheral consequences of adrenergic drugs interact, consider the conundrum addressed by William James: *are we afraid because we are running from the bear, or do we run from the bear because we are afraid?* In other words, to what extent does the sense of the body generate emotion, and to what extent does emotion drive the physical accompaniments to emotion? The current consensus is that centrally generated affect and bodily expressions interact in both directions to produce the full emotional experience. For example, a person with a "pounding heart," reflective of elevations in heart rate and blood pressure, will have a difficult time maintaining an internal calm. Similarly, a person with a low heart rate and low blood pressure is unlikely to feel uncontrollable rage.

Panic attacks can be viewed as nature's version of "we are afraid because we are running from the bear." Massive sympathetic activation, marked by sweating, heart palpitations, rapid heart rate, dizziness, and even chest pain, occurs during a panic attack. As a result, the patient is unable to escape from affective feelings of fear, loss of control, and panic.

Under normal circumstances, an anxious body and an anxious mind occur together, as do a calm mind and body and so on. As an example of the interaction between body and brain, memory formation is enhanced when the body mounts a sympathetic reaction to an event. In other words, we remember deeply moving events that are accompanied by sympathetic excitation far more readily than we do mundane and banal occurrences. Reinforced learning of events that elicit emotional reactions serves to give cognitive and mnemonic weight to impactful events. Now consider the consequences of using a β-blocker such as propranolol to lessen the body's expression of emotion. β-Blockers prevent increases in heart rate and blood pressure and thereby render emotional events more neutral and therefore less memorable.

The effect of β-blockers on memory consolidation may be used to ameliorate the reaction to traumatic memories. Patients with *post-traumatic stress disorder* (*PTSD*), often react to stimuli reminiscent of a previous trauma with an emotional reaction and a generalized increase in sympathetic tone. To reduce the impact of such triggering events in PTSD, some therapists have paired recall of the traumatic event or exposure to triggers with administration of β-blockers. This allows reconsolidation of the traumatic memory without the ability to mount a generalized sympathetic reaction. The hope is that by repeatedly re-remembering a traumatic event while in a less sympathetically aroused state, individuals will become less anxious and upset when they recall that same event at a later time.

GAP JUNCTIONS PROVIDE A DIRECT ROUTE OF INTERCELLULAR COMMUNICATION

Gap junctions enable communication utilizing both electrical and second-messenger systems. These junctions are present throughout the body, including in nervous tissue, both peripheral and central. Within the nervous system, gap junctions are the physical substrate for electrical synapses, which differ from chemical synapses in several important ways:

- Both depolarizing and hyperpolarizing potentials are conveyed across an electrical synapse.

- There is no appreciable delay.

- Current carried by ions travels bidirectionally across many electrical synapses.

- The gap junction is a physical connection that allows molecules up to about 1 kilodalton to flow through. Thus, not only calcium and potassium ions but also small metabolites such as ATP and second-messengers such as IP_3 or cAMP may flow through gap junctions.

A gap junction is made up of two aligned hemichannels or half-channels, also termed *connexons*. Each hemichannel, made up of protein subunits called connexins, sits within the membrane of one cell. The gap between two cell membranes narrows to only 3 nm at the site of gap junctions, about 10-fold closer than apposing membranes at a classical chemical synapse. The hemichannels from adjacent cells align to form a pore that is up to 2 nm in diameter. Through this pore, ions travel down their electrochemical gradients.

By providing an open, albeit small, conduit between cells, gap junctions harken back to the idea of the brain as a many-celled syncytium. The structural continuity of two neurons connected by a gap junction compromises the physical discreteness of cells and is a formal violation of the neuron doctrine established by Ramon y Cajal (see Chapter 2). Yet the spirit of the neuron doctrine is not challenged by gap junctions because the neuron is clearly the fundamental unit of the nervous system.

Gap junctions often occur in association with chemical synapses, giving rise to mixed electrical–chemical synapses. Although gap junctions exist in neurons of the retina, inferior olive, hypothalamus, cerebellum, thalamus, and cerebral cortex, as well as in astrocytic glia, their contribution to normal CNS function remains poorly understood. This stems in large part from the absence of neurological diseases that are the primary result of connexin mutations in the CNS. From this fact, one may conclude—probably incorrectly—that gap junctions contribute relatively little to brain function.

Connexin mutations affecting peripheral tissues both non-neural and neural are associated with dramatic clinical presentations including several congenital neurological diseases. When connexins (gap junction proteins) present on myelin are affected, demyelination results. In fact, the most common gap junction–related disease involves peripheral demyelination caused by an inherited mutation; inherited demyelination diseases comprise the largest group of the heterogeneous set of Charcot-Marie-Tooth syndromes. Deafness is another common result of certain connexin mutations. Connexin mutations prevent supporting cells in the stria vascularis of the cochlea (see Chapter 16) from sharing nutrients and distributing potassium ions, resulting in cochlear sensory cells dying and consequent deafness.

COMMUNICATION OCCURS AMONG NEURONS USING DIVERSE MECHANISMS

The picture presented in this section on neural communication is of a presynaptic element releasing neurotransmitter to send a message to a postsynaptic element, which receives the message using a receptor for the released neurotransmitter. Even considering the very large number of neurotransmitters and the even larger number of receptors, this version of synaptic transmission oversimplifies neural communication in the following respects:

- As mentioned in Chapter 12, many neurons release multiple neurotransmitters.

- Cells that are postsynaptic in the classical sense (i.e., they express receptors but do not contain synaptic vesicles) may release neurotransmitters such as NO, leading to the term *retrograde signaling* for communication emanating from the "postsynaptic" element.

- Neural elements on both sides of a chemical synapse express receptors. Neurotransmitter binding to presynaptic receptors often regulates subsequent neurotransmitter release or even the packaging of neurotransmitters within vesicles within the presynaptic terminal.

- As mentioned earlier, many synapses are mixed, having both electrical and chemical components.

- Many—possibly most—postsynaptic elements express multiple types of receptors.

- The structural arrangement of synapses, with some located more proximally (closer to the cell body) than others, weights the inputs arriving at different synapses.

From the diverse mechanisms at each step of the synaptic process arises an enormous repertoire of potential messages that can be sent and received. The diversity in neural communication exists across different synapses and also across time, so that a single synapse may operate differently at different times. This plasticity of synaptic function resulting from experience is the fundamental component of learning.

THE OUTCOME OF SYNAPTIC ACTIVITY DEPENDS ON THE CONNECTIVITY OF THE CELLS INVOLVED

At each stage of our simplified synaptic communication, there is a critical output that serves as the input to the next stage in synaptic communication:

- A membrane potential reaches the threshold for an action potential.

- An action potential elicits calcium influx in a synaptic terminal that then triggers fusion of a synaptic vesicle and release of neurotransmitter.

- Neurotransmitter activates a receptor and thereby causes a change in the electrical properties and/or in the second-messenger status of the cell.

Even if we knew *everything* about each of these steps, we still could not predict the effect of the communication. To understand the result of synaptic communication, we need to understand the *identity* and *connectivity* of the neurons involved. The same pattern of action potentials sent from a neuron that innervates the cochlea or from a neuron that innervates a skeletal muscle conveys two vastly different messages. Therefore, we now embark on a tour of the basic connections of the human nervous system.

ADDITIONAL READING

Biel M. Cyclic nucleotide–gated cation channels. *J Biol Chem.* 284: 9017–9021, 2009.

Cahalan S. *Brain on Fire: My Month of Madness.* Simon and Schuster, 2013.

Hughes BW, de Casillas MLM, Kaminski HJ. Pathophysiology of myasthenia gravis. *Sem Neurol.* 24: 21–30, 2004.

Kaupp UB, Seifert R. Cyclic nucleotide-gated ion channels. *Physiol Rev.* 82: 769–824, 2002.

Kemp SF, Lockey RF, Simons FE. Epinephrine: The drug of choice for anaphylaxis. A statement of the World Allergy Organization. *Allergy.* 63: 1061–1070, 2008.

Laird DW. Life cycle of connexins in health and disease. *Biochem J.* 394: 527–543, 2006.

Leypoldt F, Armangue T, Dalmau J. Autoimmune encephalopathies. *Ann N Y Acad Sci.* 1338: 94–114, 2015.

Nathanson NM. A multiplicity of muscarinic mechanisms: Enough signaling pathways to take your breath away. *Proc Natl Acad Sci.* 97: 6245–6247, 2000.

Nickel R, Forge A. Gap junctions and connexins in the inner ear: Their roles in homeostasis and deafness. *Curr Opin Otolaryngol Head Neck Surg.* 16: 452–457, 2008.

Rocher J-P. Recent advances in drug discovery of GPCR allosteric modulators. *Medchem News.* 3: 7–13, 2011.

Söhl G, Maxeiner S, Willecke K. Expression and functions of neuronal gap junctions. *Nature Rev Neurosci.* 6: 191–200, 2005.

Trudeau MC, Zagotta WN. An intersubunit interaction regulates trafficking of rod cyclic nucleotide-gated channels and is disrupted in an inherited form of blindness. *Neuron.* 34: 197–207, 2002.

SECTION 4

PERCEPTION

Sensing the outside world is critical to both survival and reproduction. Sensory pathways work at an unconscious level to guide our movements, provide necessary information to homeostatic systems, and influence our mood. Thanks to sensory systems, we avoid walking into trees, we sweat when our body temperature increases, we spit out rotten-tasting food, and we smile when we hear the bobwhite calling her own name. In such circumstances, sensory systems operate automatically, outside of voluntary control or awareness. Yet sensory systems also allow us to gain *awareness* of our surroundings and our insides. The conscious awareness of either our environment or our own bodies that arises from activity in sensory pathways is termed *perception.*

In this section, we focus on the perceptual aspects of sensation. Visual, auditory, and somatosensory perception are of obvious importance to humans, and a chapter is devoted to each of these systems. We also devote a chapter to the vestibular system because the unpleasant symptoms that occur when the vestibular system stops working—vertigo, dizziness, nausea—hammer home the importance of the vestibular sense to our conscious life. We give short shrift to gustation and olfaction due to the relatively minor role they play in clinical medicine. Proprioception is largely ignored in this section because, rather than funneling into perception, it exists in service to the motor system. Proprioception is therefore discussed extensively in Section 5 on Motor Control. The vestibular system forms our bridge to the motor system because, when working normally, it is the driving force for maintaining balance and gaze.

14.

PERCEIVING THE WORLD

As introduced in the first chapter, we do not sense the world in the way that cameras, tape recorders, and gas chromatographs do. No faithful, pixel-by-pixel representation of the world exists in the brain. Instead, we use top-down expectations—remember the cortico-thalamic projections discussed in Chapter 7—to interpret features extracted from bottom-up sensory processing. The sensory information presented to the neocortex by sensory pathways includes select features mined from the stimulus and excludes or downplays other features. For example, the visual cortex does not get information regarding the amount of medium wavelength light, commonly perceived as green, in a given location. Instead, the retina passes on a comparison between the amounts of long- and medium-wavelength light, normally perceived as red and green, respectively. Only this comparison is available to build a perception of color; no information regarding absolute wavelength is ever presented to the visual cortex. Medium-wavelength light surrounded by medium-wavelength light is perceived as less green than medium-wavelength light surrounded by long-wavelength light (Fig. 14-1A). In sum, we perceive the gestalt of a sensory scene, and we do this *rapidly*.

The monumental feat of quickly achieving a "good-enough" representation of the outside world comes with a cost: loss of access to stimulus properties not deemed important by the nervous system. This can be illustrated by the ridiculously simple trick of reversing the directions of arrowheads on either end of a line. Lines with inward pointing arrowheads are perceived as longer than lines with outward pointing arrowheads (Fig. 14-1B). Essentially, four oriented lines alter the perception of a fifth line's length. This illusion is so powerful that it persists even after a person is fully aware that the lines are the same length (and even if you make the illusion yourself!). In other words, it is impossible *not* to see the illusion. Illusions such as these demonstrate in dramatic fashion that we simply do not have access to basic stimulus features. Instead, our neocortex is fed a constant diet of contextual information about the entire stimulus world.

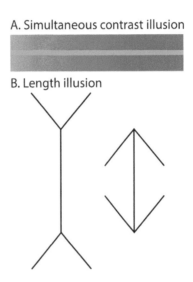

Figure 14-1 Sensory illusions demonstrate that perception is a context-dependent interpretation rather than an accurate representation of the stimulus. A: In the simultaneous color contrast illusion, the middle stripe of medium-wavelength is perceived as a brighter green when surrounded by progressively longer wavelength light. B: In a common adaptation of the Müller-Lyer illusion, a line bordered by inward facing arrows is perceived as longer than a line of identical length that is bordered by outward facing arrows.

Clearly, the brain's interpretations of the sensory scene are not only "good-enough" to survive through evolutionary time but are also of greater value than are decomposed and highly accurate representations of the world. Impressionist painters were on to something.

TRANSDUCTION, TRANSMISSION, AND MODULATION ARE COMPONENTS OF ALL PERCEPTUAL PATHWAYS

The starting point for all sensation is a *stimulus* (i.e., any change in the external environment or internal milieu). To transform a stimulus into perception, the brain uses pathways that share a common blueprint. Every

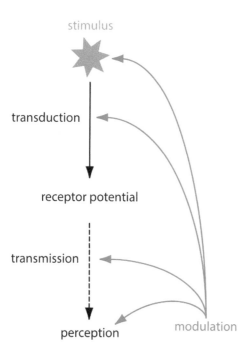

stimulus

transduction

receptor potential

transmission

perception

modulation

Figure 14-2 Sensory pathways leading to perception of a stimulus include three components: transduction, transmission, and modulation. The transduction of a stimulus into a receptor potential by a sensory receptor cell is a necessary first step in translating a stimulus into perception. Transmission carries the information regarding the stimulus through the nervous system to the cerebral cortex, the seat of perception and other cognitive functions. Stimulus information, carried by central neurons in the form of a series of action potentials, is refined as transmission ascends the neuraxis. Modulation can operate at multiple levels of the sensory pathway, from the periphery to the cerebral cortex to modify the neural interpretation of a stimulus, allowing different perceptions to result from the same physical stimulus under different circumstances. Modulation can even modify an incident stimulus.

perceptual pathway includes three predominant processing stages (Fig. 14-2):

1. *Transduction* refers to the conversion of stimulus energy, such as light or mechanical displacement, into a neural signal. This step is performed by a sensory cell that in many cases is a neuron and in many other cases is not.

2. *Transmission* carries the signal from the site of transduction to the cortex through an oligosynaptic pathway (i.e., a pathway involving several synapses). Ascending sensory transmission involves a minimum of three neurons: a neuron that projects to the thalamus, a thalamic neuron, and a neocortical neuron.

3. *Modulation* acts on transmission pathways at multiple levels, allowing context to modify sensation.

To sense the world either inside or outside of our bodies, we use sensory receptors to transform various types of energy into an electrical potential interpretable by the

nervous system. For example, as discussed in Chapter 13, photoreceptors transduce or convert light energy into a change in membrane potential. Mechanically sensitive sensory receptors are involved in sensing touch, sound, head acceleration and position, and organ distension. Examples of the latter include baroreceptors that sense blood pressure and afferents sensitive to mechanical deformations that sense bladder fullness. Chemoreceptors cells with specific receptors that respond to certain chemicals are critical to smell, taste, pain, and to visceral sensations, such as the partial pressure of oxygen in the blood.

After transduction, sensory information is transmitted from the site of the sensory receptor, up the neuraxis to the neocortex. All sensory information except olfactory input makes a stop in thalamus before reaching cerebral cortex (see Chapter 7). Only after processing by neocortex does transmitted sensory information give rise to perception. Although we do not entirely understand the mechanisms that give rise to perception, the experience of neurosurgical patients who receive intraoperative brain stimulation while awake provides compelling evidence that the cerebral cortex is in fact responsible for perception.

Stimulus information is represented in the pattern of action potentials that neurons fire. We term this *coding*. Coding is a critical concept because it is the way that meaning is represented in the nervous system. If a dim light and a bright light both elicit the same response from a cell, that cell cannot inform us as to the intensity of the light stimulus. In contrast, if a bright light causes a much larger response than does a dim light, then the cell's response *codes* for light intensity. Although sensory pathways code for information in the world around us, coding is not limited to sensory pathways. For example, neurons in motor pathways code for intended movements.

During neurosurgical procedures to remove an epileptic focus or a tumor, patients are often treated with local anesthetics and remain awake. The local anesthetics prevent the patient from feeling pain from the scalp, skull, and dura. Since there are no somatosensory receptors in the parenchyma, brain stimulation itself does not cause pain. Therefore, neurosurgeons partner with awake and verbal patents in many types of neurosurgical procedures. This approach is critical to preventing damage to language areas.

So, what happens when the brain is electrically stimulated? An extremely interesting general account of the effects of cortical stimulation is given in *The Cerebral Cortex of Man* by Penfield and Rasmussen (1950). In general, there are a limited number of outcomes to brain stimulation:

• Report of a sensation: "I feel a sensation in my hand" or "I see flashing lights in front of me."

- Simple movements like those made by a baby, a feeling of not being able to move, or a feeling of wanting to move: The neurosurgeon may see flexion or extension of a joint or the patient may report, "You paralyzed my hand" or "my hand wants to shake," or "my hand and arm contracted."

- Interpretation of a scene: "I hear an orchestra playing."

- Report of a memory or scene: "I heard an old friend call my name."

- Aphasia: To test for aphasia, a neurosurgeon may ask a patient to count during the procedure. A Broca-type aphasia is observed when the patient stops speaking. Afterward, the patient reports "you paralyzed my jaw" or something to that effect. To reveal other types of aphasia, a neurosurgeon may show a common item and ask the patient to name it. Stimulation may prevent the patient from speaking or from naming the object. For example, Penfield and Rasmussen reported that a patient, when shown a top, said, "one of those things that goes" during stimulation. When stimulation ended, the patient immediately said "top."

For our purposes here, the important outcome is the first listed. Sensory perceptions reliably occur when a region of sensory cortex is stimulated. Often, the sensations are abnormal. For example, patients report sensations of tingling or pins and needles rather than a squeeze of the arm or a gentle breeze. The abnormal sensations are likely the result of the artificial excitation of neurons by electrical stimulation. As one may imagine, the neurons excited by an electrode are a hodge-podge of those that are closest to the electrode and not necessarily the coherent group that would be excited by a natural stimulus under normal, physiological conditions.

Sensory pathways from stimulus to cerebral cortex are modulated in a myriad of ways by both local and descending influences. An example of local modulation is the mutual inhibition between two inputs that enhances the detection of stimulus edges. Another example is the *Land effect*, in which light of a single wavelength is interpreted as different colors depending on the wavelengths emitted from surrounding objects. Modulatory processes are also responsible for rendering the feel of an ice-cold drink as pleasurable on a hot day and unpleasant on a frigid winter day.

SENSE ORGANS STEER STIMULI TO SENSORY RECEPTORS

For transduction to occur, stimulus energy must reach a sensory receptor. We possess four specialized organs—eyes, ears, nose, and mouth—that guide stimulus energy toward appropriate sensory receptors (i.e., receptors that are able to transform the type of stimulus energy gathered into a receptor potential). Light is focused by the eye onto the retina, where photoreceptors transduce light into a change in membrane potential. The outer ear collects ambient sounds and steers them into the ear canal. Sniffing sucks volatile odorants into the nose, where they can bind to sensory receptors. Ingestion and chewing distribute tastants (i.e., substances that we taste) so that they can reach taste cells within oral tastebuds. Of note, somatosensory stimuli act on sensory receptors that are distributed all over the body surface and internal organs.

Once a stimulus reaches a sensory receptor, transduction occurs through mechanisms specific to each type of afferent. Transduction mechanisms for vision, hearing, somatosensation, and vestibular senses will be discussed in the following chapters. Importantly, *a stimulus only registers to the extent that we possess the machinery to transduce that stimulus into a neural potential.*

The type of energy transduced by a sensory receptor reflects sensory function in some but not all cases. Clearly, the conversion of light into a hyperpolarization by photoreceptors allows us to sense the visual world. Thus, light transduction and photoreceptor function align well. In contrast, mechanically sensitive sensory neurons called *hair cells* in the ear transduce mechanical displacements of less than a micron rather than the larger movements caused by sound and head motion. In other words, hair cells are sensitive to physical displacements that are thousands of times smaller than the physical movements caused directly by sound, head position, or head acceleration. It is the apparatus surrounding the hair cells that is responsible for transforming sound or head motion into mechanical displacements of less than a micron.

Animals react to only a subset of the entire spectrum of possible environmental stimuli. Humans cannot see the infrared emissions coming from a warm body, hear the ultrasonic vocalizations of bats, or navigate through the environment by sensing electrical fields. Yet these are biologically possible senses: some snakes perceive infrared emissions, bats and other animals detect ultrasound, and sharks navigate and find prey by sensing electrical fields. For any given animal, the capabilities of sensory organs and receptors simply have to match the stimuli that have been important through evolutionary time. Humans respond to vibratory frequencies, light wavelengths, and thermal stimuli that are of benefit to their terrestrial lives. It is of obvious utility that humans can hear frequencies contained in speech and of no particular import that fish are incapable of hearing frequencies in the speech range. Similarly, bats detect the high frequencies required for echolocation (or else they die), whereas humans suffer no adverse biological consequences as a result of not perceiving echolocation signals.

THE BRAIN PROCESSES SENSORY STIMULI USING A FOURIER-TYPE ANALYSIS

Fourier analysis is a powerful tool in sensory physiology because it allows us to break up complex stimuli into simple components. The basic idea behind Fourier analysis is that any signal consists of a number—often a large number—of component sinusoidal waves. Static noise, a pure musical tone, and clicks can all be reproduced by summing a finite number of sinusoidal waves with specific frequencies, amplitudes, and phases (Fig. 14-3A). Similarly, a picture has high, medium, and low spatial frequency components (Fig. 14-3B–D), and a moving scene has both spatial and temporal frequency components. In visual terms, low spatial frequencies convey the proverbial forest, the general scene, whereas high spatial frequencies are critical to our perception of the trees, the

A. Fourier analysis
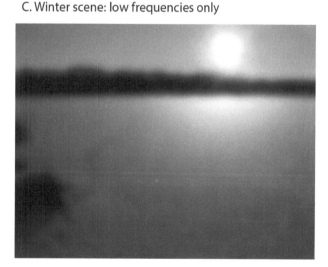

B. Original photograph of winter scene: all frequencies
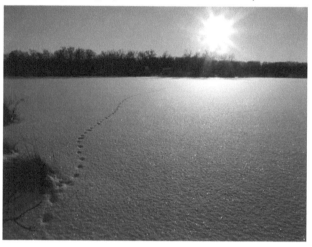

C. Winter scene: low frequencies only

D. Winter scene: high frequencies only
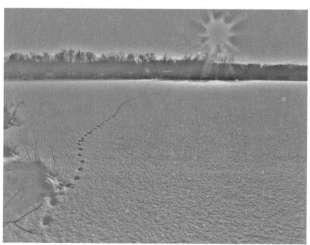

Figure 14-3 Using Fourier analysis, stimuli can be represented by the addition of a finite number of sinusoidal waves. A: Fourier analysis can reveal the component sin waves within a periodic signal, such as a square wave (*left*), as well as in nonperiodic noise (*right*). The bolded signals in the top traces can be formed by the addition of the sine waves below the equal signs. B–D: Most natural scenes contain a mixture of low and high spatial frequencies. Low-frequency components within the original image in B are shown in panel C, and high-frequency components are illustrated in D. Note the differences between the low- and high-frequency components in different features. Details, such as the fox tracks, the branch in the bottom left foreground, and the outline of tree tops, are primarily high spatial frequency features. Most of the color in this image is at low spatial frequency. Some features have both low- and high-frequency components that are prominent. For example, the sun has a high spatial frequency edge and a low spatial frequency change in color and luminance.   Photograph in B kindly provided by Gisèle Alma Perreault.

detail. Fourier analysis can be applied to auditory, mechanical, thermal, vestibular, and visual stimuli but not to chemical stimuli.

The fundamental idea that stimuli can be represented as the sum of a number of sinusoids is important because the nervous system appears to use a form of Fourier analysis to process sensory signals. One example of this principle in the periphery is the distribution of different component frequencies in a complex sound to different locations in the cochlea (see Chapter 16). The result is an auditory prism whereby auditory frequencies are mapped along the length of the cochlea. Fourier-type analysis also occurs in sensory pathways of the central nervous system (CNS). For example, high spatial frequency information is used for high-acuity vision, important in reading and perceiving the form of objects (see Chapter 7). In contrast, low spatial frequencies, important for detecting moving objects, are highly represented in the dorsal visual stream. Damage or disease within central visual pathways can preferentially impair high or low spatial frequency vision.

SENSORY RECEPTORS RESPOND PROBABILISTICALLY TO STIMULI

The activation of a receptor is *probabilistic* (i.e., stimuli with certain characteristics are most likely to excite the receptor). Stimuli with similar but not identical properties also excite the receptor but at a lower probability (Fig. 14-4). A *tuning curve*, such as that in Figure 14-4A, shows the combination of stimulus intensity and feature—wavelength, frequency, temperature, and the like—needed to excite a receptor. Such a tuning curve can be constructed for all sensory receptor types. Consider, for example, the *Pacinian corpuscle*, which is a type of somatosensory afferent that reacts to vibration. Pacinian corpuscles respond optimally to vibration at 300 Hz, meaning that vibration at 300 Hz will excite Pacinian corpuscle even when the skin is indented only by a minute amount. Pacinian corpuscles are also excited by vibration at frequencies other than 300 Hz but require that the skin is indented more than in the case of the 300 Hz vibration. Thus, the stimulus intensity (i.e., amount of indentation) needed to excite Pacinian corpuscles is minimal at the optimal response frequency and greater at other vibration frequencies.

Every sensory receptor responds to stimulation in some locations but not others. The range of locations where appropriate stimulation will excite a sensory receptor is termed the *receptive field*. For example, some cutaneous somatosensory afferents respond to indentation of the skin at the tip of

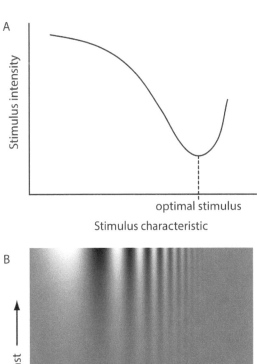

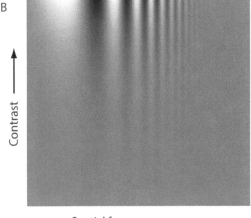

Figure 14-4 A: A stereotypical tuning curve for a sensory receptor. The stimulus intensity needed to excite the sensory receptor at each value of the appropriate stimulus property is plotted. For example, the amount of light, in candles or some other measure of light intensity, needed to excite a photoreceptor is least at a given wavelength, the optimal wavelength. Light at other wavelengths may excite the photoreceptor when presented at higher intensity than is needed for light at the optimal wavelength. Note that sensory receptors are often named for the stimulus that excites them at minimal intensity, their optimal stimulus; as an example, cone photoreceptors that respond to short wavelength light are called short-wavelength cones. Note that the tuning curve is not a step function but has some width. Consequently, sensory receptors respond to a range of stimuli. For sensory receptors with broad tuning curves, the probability of activation does not decrease rapidly as a stimulus characteristic deviates away from the optimal value. B: A black-and-white grating with continuously varied contrast (vertical direction) and spatial frequency (horizontal direction) illustrates the relationship between an optimal stimulus feature and intensity. The stimulus feature is spatial frequency, and the intensity varies with contrast. At optimal spatial frequencies, gratings are visible even at low contrast. However very-high-frequency gratings (all the way to the right) are not visible at any contrast level. Very-low-frequency gratings (all the way to the left) are only visible at high contrast values. If you draw a line at the boundary between the part of the gratings visible to you and the part that is at too low a contrast to perceive, the shape of that line will be similar to that of the tuning curve in A.   Panel B kindly provided by S. Murray Sherman.

the index finger (Fig. 14-5A) but not the tip of the thumb, whereas other afferents have reciprocal properties. Some cells in the auditory pathway respond to sound arising from

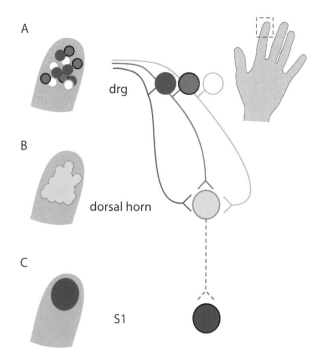

Figure 14-5 Individual dorsal root ganglion cells that respond to touch typically have punctate receptive fields (A). For example, the blue cell responds to stimulation of the index finger at any of the blue dot locations illustrated at the left, the red cell responds to stimulation of the red sites, and so on. Multiple touch-sensitive primary afferents converge onto one dorsal horn cell (B), which then has a larger, filled-in receptive field (*light gray region*). Within the dorsal column nuclei and thalamus, receptive fields are further modified by both excitatory convergence and lateral inhibition, so that the receptive fields of neurons in the somatosensory cortex (C) are smooth and well delineated (*dark gray area*) and may even be surrounded by a region that elicits an inhibitory response (not illustrated).

a particular location in space. Light from a specific region of the visual field hits photoreceptors, and region of space from which the incident light arose is the photoreceptor's receptive field. The small receptive fields of somatosensory afferents and photoreceptors summate to form larger, smoother, and better delineated receptive fields as sensory transmission ascends the neuraxis (Fig. 14-5B, C).

Since sensory receptors operate by probability, one might expect that perceptions will be misleading in some small proportion of cases. If a photoreceptor that responds optimally to short wavelength light may, on rare occasion, respond to light of medium wavelength, then why don't we perceive the blue sky as green every long once in a while? To understand why we never see the sky as green, consider that the receptive fields of many photoreceptors include portions of the sky. If the chance of just one short wavelength photoreceptor responding to medium wavelength is negligible, then the chance of two responding in this way is "negligible squared." The chance of all, most, or even a

handful of neighboring short wavelength photoreceptors being excited by medium wavelength light is zero. Because virtually all the input to the brain suggests that the sky region consists of short wavelength light, the brain ignores any lone dissenting input suggesting that the sky consists of medium wavelength light. Top-down expectations also help to squelch rogue sensory information. In sum, we reliably perceive a cloud-free sky on a sunny day as a solid blue.

THE BRAIN USES A COMBINATORIAL STRATEGY TO INTERPRET INPUT FROM SENSORY AFFERENTS

The *finite* number of receptor types yields a finite number of stimulus types represented by sensory afferents to the nervous system. In contrast, the world contains a continuum of stimuli with an infinite number of possible stimulus properties. This raises the paradox of how a restricted number of receptor types can represent a continuum of stimulus characteristics. In essence, the strategy used by the brain is to combine input from multiple receptor types. For example, we perceive a continuous spectrum of color despite having only three photoreceptor types that support color vision (see Chapter 15). Scenes that reliably stimulate only short wavelength photoreceptors are interpreted as violet, whereas objects that stimulate both short and medium wavelength photoreceptors are often viewed as aqua (depending on context). By using a fine combinatorial code, we can distinguish a range of colors, sounds, and textures using a limited number of sensory afferent types.

SENSORY RECEPTORS TRANSDUCE STIMULUS ENERGY INTO A CHANGE IN MEMBRANE POTENTIAL

Transduction produces a local change in membrane potential called a *generator receptor potential*. By changing a sensory cell's membrane potential, a generator potential alters the amount of neurotransmitter released from the cell. For example, the membrane potential of a photoreceptor in the dark is about −40 mV. At such a depolarized level, the photoreceptor releases neurotransmitter at a steady rate. When a light flashes, photoreceptors hyperpolarize and consequently release less neurotransmitter. To consider a more typical example, a hair cell in the cochlea has a membrane potential of about −50 mV in the absence of sound. Associated with this resting membrane potential is a moderate rate of neurotransmitter release. When stimulated, the hair cell depolarizes, which results in more transmitter release. Yet the hair cell never fires an action potential. In essence, this means that the hair cell, like other neuroepithelial sensory cells, communicates to a primary afferent neuron by releasing more or less neurotransmitter. The next cell in line from a neuroepithelial sensory cell, a primary afferent neuron, responds to the amount of transmitter released from the transducing cell by changing the rate of action potential discharge.

Some somatosensory neurons, such as Pacinian corpuscle afferents, possess the transduction machinery at their own peripheral terminals. In these cases, stimulation evokes a generator potential *within* the afferent terminal. If the generator potential is large enough, it triggers an action potential in the afferent. The action potential initiation site is typically just proximal to the terminal. For example, when vibration excites a Pacinian corpuscle, a depolarization occurs in the corpuscle-covered terminal, the site of mechanical transduction. Just proximal (toward the CNS and away from the periphery) to the corpuscle, a sufficiently large generator potential can trigger an action potential, which then travels through the Pacinian corpuscle afferent to enter the axon traveling up the dorsal columns of the spinal cord.

THE NUMBER OF SENSORY MODALITIES GREATLY EXCEEDS FIVE

The anachronistic notion of five senses—sight, hearing, touch, smell, and taste—is wrong by several times, not by one or two. The vestibular apparatus allows us to sense our head movement and position in space. Proprioceptive afferents sense joint angle and muscle length. Afferents carrying information about tissue damage, innocuous warming and cooling, and so on are distinct from other somatosensory afferents that code for touch, hair-bending, vibration, and so no. Interoceptors, sensory receptors that innervate viscera, such as the bladder, colon, stomach, and lung, are excited by a variety of internal stimuli such as organ distension or by the products of cell lysis. Under most conditions, interoceptors function to maintain homeostasis but can, in unfortunate conditions, also alert an individual to potential harm by signaling pain. Each modality has numerous distinct qualities that are coded for by distinct types of afferents. For example, four different types of photoreceptors each respond to slightly different preferred wavelengths and five different types of taste buds preferentially respond to salty, sweet, umami (a savory taste elicited by glutamate such as that contained within meat), sour, or bitter substances.

The question of what constitutes a modality is a judgment call. The number of modalities, could be as low as 20 or as high as hundreds depending on one's penchant for categorical splitting or lumping. There are 300–400 different *types* of olfactory receptors in humans. A splitter may consider each olfactory receptor type as a separate modality, whereas a lumper could categorize all olfactory receptor types into a single modality. Similarly, some might consider all of taste as a modality or all of somatosensation as one modality. However, most consider each taste—salty, sweet, umami, and so on—or each cutaneous percept—light touch, pain, pressure, vibration, and so on—as a modality. The latter approach has the advantage that it reflects the critical importance of distinct afferent types to distinct percepts. Yet one must be careful of the misleading conclusion that one afferent type equals one perception. In reality, activation of multiple afferent types contributes to normal perception, so that the loss of any one afferent type leads to abnormal or weird perceptions. One example of this is color blindness. Another example is the paresthesia accompanying a peripheral neuropathy that damages one or a few types of somatosensory afferents.

ADAPTATION ENABLES PRIMARY AFFERENTS TO CODE FOR A LARGE RANGE OF STIMULUS INTENSITIES

We are able to sense an enormous range of stimuli within each modality. We can hear a whisper, crashing cymbals, and a jackhammer. We can see the glow of an animal's eyes in the dark, a candlelit meal, and a sun-scorched desert landscape. We can feel the difference between glossy and matte paper, lose sleep over a pea in our bed, and feel the weight of a growing child. We can attend to a single bead of sweat and to the crash of water from a wave. A fundamental trait of sensory perception is responsible for our ability to respond to such a wide range of stimulus intensities. Rather than code for absolute stimulus intensity, we code for stimulus intensity relative to the background level of stimulation. For example, in a dimly lit lecture hall, we easily follow the light from a laser pointer but are unable to see that same light shone on the sidewalk on a sunny day. Likewise, we can feel the weight of a quarter if that is all we are holding but could only detect a role of quarters if we are also holding a textbook (Fig. 14-6). In other words, our ability to detect stimuli is proportional to the background level of stimulation.

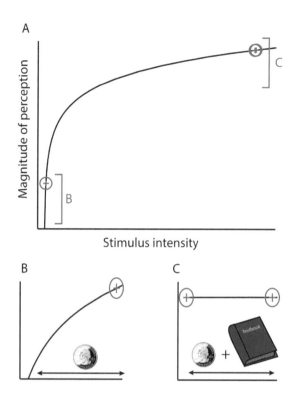

Figure 14-6 A generalized version of Weber's law. Perceptual magnitude is logarithmically related to stimulus intensity. The blue circle at the left, labeled *B*, shows the predicted perceptual outcome of holding a quarter alone. The two blue circles at the right, labeled *C*, show the predicted perceptual magnitude of holding a book alone or holding a book with a quarter on top. As illustrated in B and C, the change in perceptual magnitude elicited by a quarter alone is far, far more than the negligible change in perceptual magnitude elicited when a quarter is placed on top of a textbook. In fact, a quarter placed on a book is unlikely to be perceived at all.

Weber's law relates stimulus intensity to perception. For most stimulus modalities, Weber's law holds in the following form:

$$\Delta P = k * \ln\left(\Delta S / S_o\right)$$

where ΔP is the change in perceptual magnitude, k is a constant, ΔS is the change in stimulus intensity, and S_o is the background stimulus intensity. Weber's law tells us that a change in stimulus intensity is only perceived (i.e., $\Delta P \neq 0$) when that change is a large proportion of the background stimulation level. As a simple example of this principle, we see the glow of a candle far more easily in the dark than in sunshine. We feel the first drop of rain on a dry summer day but do not feel individual raindrops as we despondently run through a drenching rainstorm on the way to catch a bus. Thus, a low-intensity stimulus is perceived on a background of little to no stimulation but not on a background of strong stimulation (Fig. 14-6).

SENSORY TRANSMISSION TRAVELS A STEREOTYPICAL ROUTE

Specialized cells use specific molecules to accomplish transduction. In many cases, neuroepithelial cells carry out transduction, but, in other cases, neurons do. Beyond this one wrinkle, the path from transduction to perception is somewhat stereotyped (Fig. 14-7). After a stimulus is transduced, information about the stimulus is conveyed toward cortex. After the synapse between the sensory receptor and the primary afferent, the transmission of sensory information includes a minimum of three synapses. The minimum of three synapses includes:

- Primary afferent (located in periphery) to secondary sensory neuron (located centrally)
- Secondary sensory neuron to thalamic neuron
- Thalamic neuron to cortical neuron

The primary afferent, which either receives information from a transducing cell or performs transduction itself, synapses onto a secondary sensory neuron. For all sensory modalities except vision, the connection between the primary afferent and secondary sensory neuron involves a transition from the periphery to the CNS. The secondary sensory neuron itself projects to the thalamus. Thalamocortical projection neurons then project to sensory cortex. This basic pathway from primary afferent to secondary sensory neuron to thalamus to sensory cortex holds for cone-mediated vision and somatosensation.

SENSORY PATHWAYS TRANSMIT INFORMATION ABOUT LOCATION, TIMING, INTENSITY, AND TYPE OF STIMULUS

Sensory transmission conveys enough information about a stimulus that we can describe that stimulus in time and space. The following are components of sensory discrimination:

- Stimulus modality
- Stimulus location
- Time of stimulus: onset and offset
- Intensity of stimulus

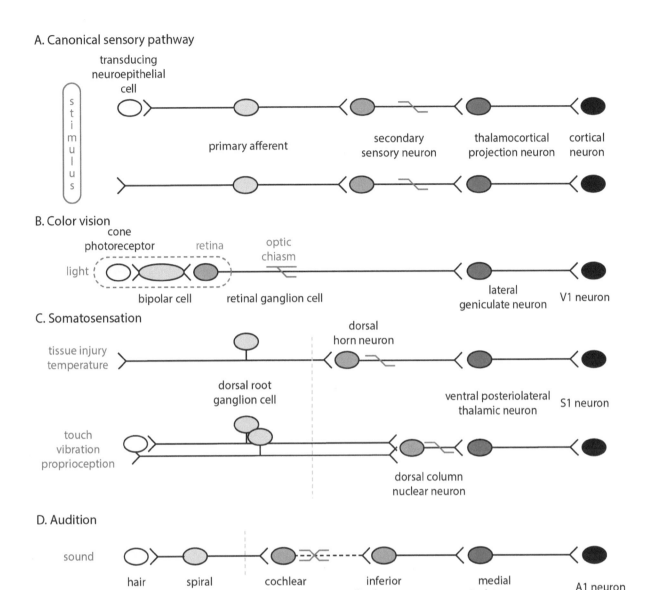

A. Canonical sensory pathway

transducing
neuroepithelial
cell

s t i m u l u s

primary afferent

secondary
sensory neuron

thalamocortical
projection neuron

cortical
neuron

B. Color vision

cone
photoreceptor

retina

optic
chiasm

light

bipolar cell

retinal ganglion cell

lateral
geniculate neuron

V1 neuron

C. Somatosensation

tissue injury
temperature

dorsal
horn neuron

dorsal root
ganglion cell

ventral posteriolateral
thalamic neuron

S1 neuron

touch
vibration
proprioception

dorsal column
nuclear neuron

D. Audition

sound

hair
cell

spiral
ganglion cell

cochlear
nucleus neuron

inferior
colliculus neuron

medial
geniculate neuron

A1 neuron

Figure 14-7 A: Sensory pathways include a primary afferent, a secondary sensory neuron, and a thalamocortical projection neuron that terminates in sensory cortex. Transduction is accomplished either by a neuroepithelial cell (*top*) or by a primary afferent (*lower*). Typically, the secondary sensory neuron crosses the midline (*red step symbol*), so that inputs from one side reach the contralateral thalamus and cortex. B: Light is transduced by retinal photoreceptors, which in turn synapse on retinal bipolar cells. Bipolar cells receiving input from cone photoreceptors, critical to form and color vision, synapse directly on a retinal ganglion cell. Information from rod photoreceptors, important for night vision, travels through several more synapses to reach the retinal ganglion cell (not illustrated). Retinal ganglion cells project out of the retina (*dashed oval*) to the lateral geniculate nucleus in the thalamus. Nasal retinal ganglion cell axons cross at the optic chiasm (*red step*), whereas temporal ganglion cell axons project ipsilaterally (*red line*). From the thalamus, a thalamocortical neuron projects to visual cortex (*V1 neuron*). C: In the case of somatosensation from the body, the primary afferent neuron is a dorsal root ganglion cell, the thalamic neuron is in the ventral posterolateral nucleus, and the cortical neuron is in somatosensory cortex (*S1 neuron*). Somatosensory transduction is either accomplished by the primary afferent itself or by a neuroepithelial cell. For noxious and thermal stimuli, the secondary sensory neuron is a spinothalamic tract neuron in the dorsal horn, which crosses the midline (*red step*) in the spinal cord. For light touch, vibration, and proprioception, the secondary sensory neuron is a dorsal column nuclear neuron that crosses the midline in the medulla (*red step*) and projects to the thalamus through the medial lemniscus. D: Sound is transduced by cochlear hair cells, which contact primary afferent neurons in the spiral ganglion. Spiral ganglion cells synapse in the cochlear nucleus, which in turn project bilaterally (*red steps*) either directly or indirectly (*dashed line*) via the superior olivary complex to the inferior colliculus. Inferior colliculus neurons project to the medial geniculate nucleus in the thalamus. From the thalamus, a thalamocortical neuron projects to auditory cortex (*A1 neuron*). In all panels, the blue dashed line shows the division between the peripheral (*left*) and central (*right*) nervous systems. Note that the visual system is entirely central since the retina is derived from the diencephalic vesicle (see Chapter 3).

A heuristic way to understand sensory systems is the idea of a so-called *labeled line* or *lemniscal pathway*. Labeled line pathways rely on neurons that receive input from one type of afferent passing that information on exclusively to one set of neurons (Fig. 14-8). In this way, neurons in the CNS are activated whenever one type of afferent is active but not when other afferent types are activated. In an idealized labeled line pathway, dorsal root ganglion cells that respond to touch would terminate on a set of dorsal horn cells that only receives input from afferents that signal touch. These dorsal horn cells would in turn excite a group of thalamic neurons that receive only touch-related input and so on, up to somatosensory cortex. In this way, activity in a somatosensory cortex neuron receiving touch-related input from thalamus would always signal touch. It is important to remember that the idea of a labeled line is only a construct. There are no pure labeled lines within the CNS. Yet, all sensory pathways employ *restricted connections*: taste input leads to a taste perception and not to a visual perception.

Just as modality is conveyed by the identity and connectivity of a neuron, stimulus location is also conveyed by neuronal identity and connectivity. As introduced in Chapter 7, the brain maps the external world. Neighboring parts of the brain process input from neighboring parts of the sensory world. For example, *retinotopy* refers to an arrangement in which adjacent bits of the neural tissue represent adjacent bits of the retina, which in turn means adjacent bits of the visual field. *Tonotopy* refers to the representation of adjacent sound frequencies or tones in adjacent regions of the cochlea or brain (see Chapter 16). In a similar vein, recall that *somatotopy* refers to the representation of adjacent areas of skin in adjacent regions of the spinal cord or brain. Thus, the theme of mapping, or adjacent representation of continuously distributed sensory "space," recurs in somatosensation, audition, and vision.

The timing and intensity of a stimulus are coded in the language of action potentials. Because the action potential is finite in duration and cannot occur continuously, the language of the neuron resembles a series of bullets fired from a machine gun rather than the continuous flow of water from a hose. As stimulus intensity increases, the number of action potentials elicited and the frequency of discharge both increase. In addition, the number of *cells* recruited by a stimulus reflects the intensity of that stimulus. At every level of a sensory pathway, far fewer neurons respond to weak stimuli than to strong stimuli.

THE BRAIN INTEGRATES INFORMATION ABOUT STIMULI FROM MULTIPLE SENSORY SYSTEMS

We refer to the visual, auditory, somatosensory, gustatory, and other sensory systems as though each is a discrete pathway. Yet the reality is that stimuli in the world stimulate multiple sensory systems. In one experiment, people were asked to concentrate on counting the number of taps applied to their fingertips and to ignore anything else going on in the testing room. Nonetheless, when, for example, five flashes of light accompanied four taps to the fingertip, people reported *feeling five taps*. As described in Chapter 16, visual clues are critical to understanding speech, even for those with normal hearing. Dubbing highlights both our ability to ignore mismatches between sensory systems and the problems that can result from such mismatches. When watching a well-dubbed movie in which speech starts and stops as mouth movements start and stop, the clear sound track overrides the visual input that signals words other than those that we hear. In contrast, when a sound track is poorly synchronized to the visual film, we find it very disconcerting when an actor's lips are moving and no words are heard, or when an actor's lips are still while words are heard.

Ultimately, sensory pathways are important because they allow us to interpret our world. The sensory pathways described up to this point are capable of producing a decent description of the world around and within us. However, we do not see visual objects as accurately as a good camera or

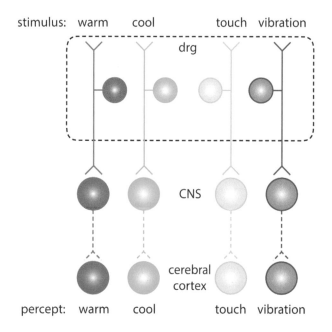

Figure 14-8 Labeled line or lemniscal pathways are principally responsible for signaling sensory modalities particularly in the somatosensory and auditory systems. Input from distinct sets of afferents largely stays separate as it travels up the neuraxis. The ultimate result of lemniscal transmission is that perceived modalities reflect afferent modalities to a great degree. drg: dorsal root ganglion.

record sounds as well as a good voice recorder. Discriminating the world pixel by pixel or note by note is not our strength. Instead, we excel at *interpreting* what arrives at the doorsteps of our sensory systems. As any experienced birdwatcher knows, most birds are identified from a general impression and shape rather than from a laundry list of anatomical features. Similarly, we use the ensemble of clues from multiple senses to identify the person walking down the street, understand a lecture, or ensure that a baby's bottle is warm enough. The case of Dr. P. described in Chapter 1 dramatically shows us that, without the ability to either understand or act upon the meaning of what we sense, the ability to describe stimuli is not particularly valuable or useful.

ADDITIONAL READING

Adrian ED. *The Basis of Sensation*. London: Lowe and Brydone Printers, 1928.

Bresciani JP, Dammeier F, Ernst MO. Vision and touch are automatically integrated for the perception of sequences of events. *J Vis.* 6: 554–564, 2006.

Cabanac M. Physiological role of pleasure. *Science.* 173: 1103–1106, 1971.

Cohen YE, Knudsen EI. Maps versus clusters: Different representations of auditory space in the midbrain and forebrain. *Trends Neurosci.* 22: 128–135, 1999.

Jousmäki V, Hari R. Parchment-skin illusion: Sound-biased touch. *Curr Biol.* 8: R190, 1998.

Penfield W, Rasmussen T. *The Cerebral Cortex of Man. A Clinical Study of Localization of Function*. New York: The Macmillan Company, 1950.

15.

SEEING THE WORLD

THE BRAIN RAPIDLY PROCESSES INPUT TO ARRIVE AT AN INTERPRETATION OF THE WHOLE VISUAL SCENE

We and other primates are extremely visual animals. We use sight for tasks critical to survival such as identification of food, obstacles, family members, and rivals. Sometimes small differences in the visual appearance of objects—think of the difference between a scrumptious mushroom and its evil and poisonous twin—carry great import. At other times, visual details, such as the lines in a sidewalk, are simply optical details that we detect but ignore. Using information gained through vision drives behavior, enables survival, and richly colors the conscious life of sighted individuals. Whereas half or more of human neocortex participates in vision, far more restricted regions are involved in somatosensation and hearing.

Visual pathways enable a rapid *interpretation* of the optical world. Rather than encoding the intensity and wavelength of light at every pixel in the visual field, the brain processes information to detect and abstract pertinent features for object identification and localization. Ultimately, assessment of visual objects motivates behavior, hopefully leading to approach or avoidance as best serves an individual's goals.

The visual system does not act like a camera. Whereas a camera encodes detected light and stores a pixel-by-pixel copy of the visual scene on film, the visual system utilizes parallel circuitry to achieve rapid *comprehension* of a visual scene rather than a detailed recapitulation of the scene. Figure 15-1 illustrates the inexact correspondence between the optics of a scene and the resulting visual perception. Although fewer than half of the letters in the text are depicted normally, most people are able to "read" the text almost normally by rapidly and unconsciously substituting correct letters for errant ones. Remarkably, letter substitution typically occurs without awareness of the substitution rule used. In essence, we don't see lines and edges or even letters. Instead, as those who solve acrostic puzzles know,

15И'7 17 4M4Z1ИG 7H47 Y0U C4И
R34D 7H15 3V3И 7H0UGH 0ИLY 4
M1И0R17Y 0F 7H3 "L3773R5" 4R3
C0RR3C7? 7H3 И30C0R73X 15
4M4Z1ИG! 4ИD D0 Y0U И071C3
7H47 R34D1ИG 7H15 B3C0M35
M0R3 4U70M471C 45 Y0U G0
4L0ИG? 7H15 15 7RU3 3V3И
7H0UGH R1GH7 И0W Y0U 4R3
UИL1K3LY 70 B3 C0И5C10US 0F
WH1CH 5YMB0L5 4R3 R3PL4C1ИG
WH1CH L3773RS

Figure 15-1 People are able to read substituted text even when numbers or reversed symbols are substituted for more than half of the original letters. In this case, only 42% of the original letters remain.

we perceive words, phrases, and even sentences from the minutest clues.

The raw material for all visual processing consists of photons, more photons, and still more photons. Yet the output of the visual system is not numbers of photons, edges, or even forms. From the totality of photons that impinge on the retina, we perceive *meaning*. The flood of photons is boiled down to identifying objects and assessing their salience in order to guide behavior. Thus, the visual system interprets the whole of the visual message, the *gestalt* of the optical image, as it relates to an individual's goals and circumstances.

THE VISUAL PATHWAY TRAVERSES THE BRAIN

Before starting in on the details of visual processing, it is helpful to consider an overview of the pathways involved in visual perception (Fig. 15-2). Light enters the visual system through the eye and is refracted or bent by the cornea and lens. In order for light to be perfectly focused in the retina, the refractive power of the cornea and lens must

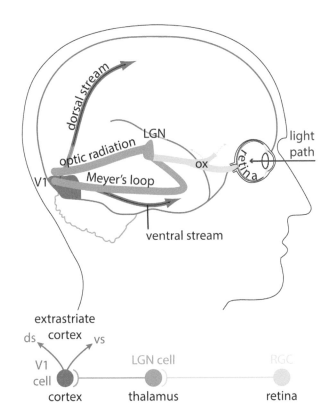

Figure 15-2 The visual pathway on the right side of the brain is illustrated. Light is focused by the eye to hit the retina at the back of the globe. In the retina, photoreceptor cells transduce light into electrical energy. Retinal ganglion cells (*RGC*) from the left nasal hemiretina travel through the optic chiasm (*ox*) to join retinal ganglion cells from the right temporal hemiretina that bypass the chiasm. These retinal ganglion cells, carrying information about the contralateral visual field, project to the lateral geniculate nucleus (*LGN*) of the thalamus. Lateral geniculate neurons (*LGN cell*) then project to the primary visual cortex (*V1*). From primary visual cortex, there are two polysynaptic pathways: a dorsal stream (*ds*), concerning visual motion and depth, and a ventral stream (*vs*), concerning object recognition. Both visual streams involve areas of extrastriate cortex. Dashed lines from the chiasm indicate contralateral projections that are not fully drawn here. The connections displayed at the bottom of the panel represent the minimal circuit supporting vision. Omitted from this diagram are visual pathways involved in circadian rhythm entrainment, orientation movements, eye movements, and pupillary control.

match the length of the eye. The eye's refractive power, built for distance viewing at rest, is adjusted during near viewing so that light from near objects is focused onto the retina. Because the most common visual impairment is refractive error, we will spend some time examining how light travels through a normal eye and through the eyes of individuals with refractive error.

After traveling through the eye, light hits the *photoreceptors* of the outer retina. Retinal photoreceptors transduce or transform light into a neural response, a process termed

phototransduction (see Chapter 13). After a single photon is absorbed, the photopigment must be biochemically regenerated through a *visual cycle* before that molecule can respond to another photon. A large number of molecules all need to be in working order for phototransduction and the visual cycle to occur normally. Furthermore, the outer retina where phototransduction occurs is an environment of high-energy light, high oxygen concentration, and free radicals. Not surprisingly then, the outer retina is vulnerable to a number of genetic mutations as well as age-related damage.

Moving on from photoreceptors, optical information is processed by retinal circuitry (not covered here) and then traverses the visual pathways described in Chapter 7. Most of our visual field is *binocular*, and only a small temporal crescent is *monocular* (Fig. 15-3). Since light from most of the visual field strikes both eyes, a small hole in the visual field, termed a *scotoma*, will not be obvious as long as it is in the binocular part of the visual field and as long as both eyes are open. In fact, all of us possess a scotoma in each eye. The fact that we are not aware of this physiological scotoma, the so-called *blind spot*, is a tribute to low peripheral acuity and to the brain's power to "guess" at what an image should look like and fill it in accordingly.

Retrochiasmal damage in the visual pathways can produce a scotoma. Even when viewing the world with only one eye, small scotomas often escape notice as the brain "fills in" the blank area. For this reason, computerized visual field testing, always performed on one eye at a time, requires the detection of points of light throughout the visual field. Such testing is typically necessary to uncover scotomas outside of central vision. Scotomas may signal pathology such as a stroke, retinal damage, a tumor, or the onset of a migraine; in the latter case, the scotoma is transient.

Development of the visual system is as critical to seeing as are the structure and connections of the eye, retina, primary visual cortex, and so on. Babies don't innately understand how the firing in their brains links to lighted objects; they use their multimodal experience to make connections between optical stimuli and cortical firing patterns. Babies *learn* to see. In fact, they *must* learn to see and they must do so during a restricted period of time. In humans, learning to see must happen during the first few years of life, the *critical period* for vision. If the visual experience of a baby or infant is disrupted during the critical period, vision does not develop normally (see further discussion in section). In such cases, adult vision is irreversibly compromised and cannot be rescued.

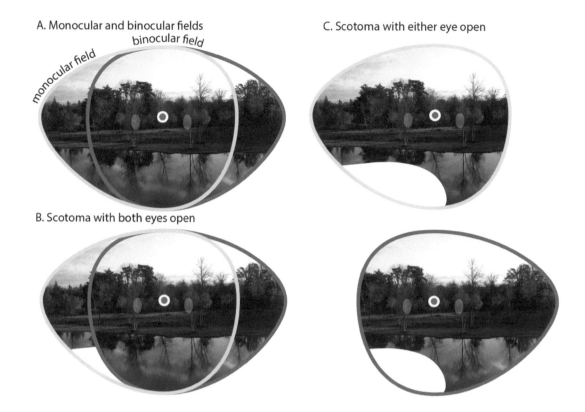

A. Monocular and binocular fields

monocular field

binocular field

C. Scotoma with either eye open

B. Scotoma with both eyes open

Figure 15-3 A: The visual field with both eyes open combines a large central binocular field and monocular crescents on either side. The point of fixation is indicated by the white-encircled red dot. The two blind spots, where retinal ganglion cell axons collect into the optic nerve, are shown as two lightened spots on either side of the fixation point. B: A scotoma will not affect binocular vision and is rarely noticed in a monocular field. C: A large peripheral scotoma *may* be noticed with either eye open alone but can reliably be discovered using visual field testing.

Ultimately, neural processing of optical information transforms incident light into ideas about the world and also provides a continuously updated guide for our physical interactions with the world. Identifying and interpreting objects in the world depends on *high-acuity vision*. Today, high-acuity vision is required for reading, playing video games on hand-held devices, driving, and so on. The ability to detect, follow, and ultimately act upon moving objects requires motion detection, a neural talent that is shared with vertebrates who depend on catching moving prey and avoiding predators for survival. Modern humans are highly dependent on high-acuity vision and it is impairment of this aspect of visual perception that most often motivates an individual to seek help. Therefore, this chapter emphasizes the mechanisms and pathways that support high-acuity or *form vision*.

Remember that visual perception is only one end point for information coming into the eyes. Additional functions that use input from the eye either always operate without conscious visual perception or *can* operate without conscious awareness. Such functions include circadian entrainment (see Chapter 27), pupillary reflexes (see Chapter 5), and eye movements; all topics discussed in other chapters.

CENTRAL LOCATIONS WITHIN THE VISUAL FIELD ARE OF DISPROPORTIONATELY HIGH IMPORTANCE

Visual acuity is greatest in the center of the visual field and falls off rapidly more peripherally. By supporting food, predator, and mate identification through evolutionary time, central vision has been a key to biological success. The evolutionary importance of high-acuity vision is reflected in several brain features evident in the human. First, as mentioned in Chapter 7, a disproportionate amount of neocortical territory is devoted to processing optical input from the center of the visual field. For example, the central 10 degrees of the retina (~1–2%) occupies more than 50% of primary visual cortex.

A second feature that facilitates high visual acuity is the high density of *cone photoreceptors* (*cones* for short) in the very center of the retina, which receives light from the very center of the visual field, the area of space that we "are looking at" (see Fig. 7-14). As described in detail later, cone photoreceptors support our ability to detect the form or shape of objects. Without cones, visual acuity is extremely poor and reading typically sized print impossible. Cones

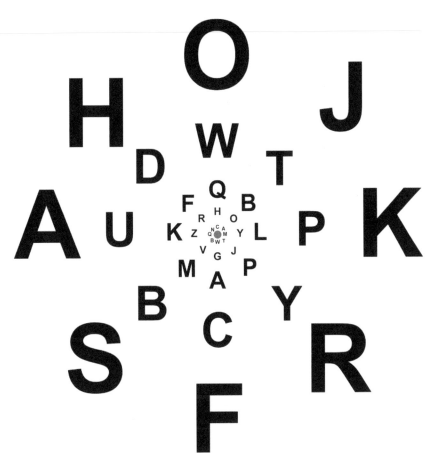

Figure 15-4 Visual acuity decreases dramatically in the peripheral visual field relative to the center of the visual field. Even as you fixate on the central red dot, you probably can read the surrounding letters. The size of the peripheral letters is increased to make up for the diminution in acuity at eccentric retinal positions.   Modified from Antis SM. A chart demonstrating variations in acuity with retinal position. *Vision Research* 14: 589–92, 1974, with permission of the publisher, Elsevier.

are extremely densely packed within the very center of the retina, an indented or pitted region called the *fovea* (Latin for "small pit"). In the fovea, not only are cones densely packed, but the cone also is the only retinal cell type present. All other retinal neurons are off to the side. Essentially, the distribution of cones increases visual resolution selectively at the center, analogous to the center of a photograph having thousands of times more pixels per unit area than the periphery of the same photograph. The density of cones falls off with increasing *eccentricity* (distance from the center) but is still high for roughly the central 5–10 degrees of the retina, an area called the *macula* or the *area centralis*. The area centralis contains a concentration of yellow-tinted carotenoid pigments that must be acquired from the diet and that filter out ultraviolet light, much as sunglasses do.

A third feature that supports high-acuity vision is provided by motor pathways. Because of the rapid decline in acuity away from the retinal fovea, we have a dedicated system to keep our fovea fixated on the part of the visual field of interest at any moment in time (see Chapter 19). An elaborate *gaze control* system, also known as the *oculomotor system*,

controls head and eye movements and minimizes slippage of the retinal image (i.e., the optical landscape that is projected onto the retina). In other words, gaze control allows light from objects to hit the same place on the retina even as the objects and viewer move in the world. By maintaining fixation, healthy individuals are able to perceive a steady visual image when so desired. Fixation, *smooth pursuit*, and the *vestibulo-ocular reflex* are types of eye movements that keep light from an object of interest focused on the macula. Other eye movements, exemplified by ballistic shifts in eye position termed *saccades*, serve to *shift* the point of fixation. Eye movements are critical to vision. Without proper yoking of the two eyes' positions, the same visual scene will not hit the foveae of both eyes. In such a case, the two eyes will pass along different scenes to the rest of the visual system, resulting in *diplopia* or double vision (see Chapter 5).

To appreciate the differences in acuity across the visual field, spread your fingers out over a page of this textbook placed at arm's length. Fixate on a spot just above your middle finger. Which text can you read? I think that you will find that you can only read the text that immediately surrounds your middle finger. Even text around your index and ring fingers will be difficult to read, and that surrounding your pinky and thumb is surely not legible. One of the most challenging parts of this task is to not cheat by shifting your gaze, highlighting the effort needed to suppress eye movements toward objects of interest. Figure 15-4 illustrates the polar skew in visual acuity in a different way. Even as you fixate on the central red dot, you will find that you are able to read the peripherally placed letters because letters at progressively more eccentric retinal positions are larger in size in this illustration. The size of the letters is increased just enough to counteract the diminution in acuity at eccentric retinal positions.

EYE LENGTH, CORNEA, AND LENS COMBINE TO FOCUS LIGHT ON TO PHOTORECEPTORS

The eye is the required portal for sight. Light that enters the eye through the pupil is focused to a point in the outer retina (Fig. 15-5B). Three anatomical features are critical to focusing light to just the right point in the retina:

- The length of the eye
- The cornea
- The lens

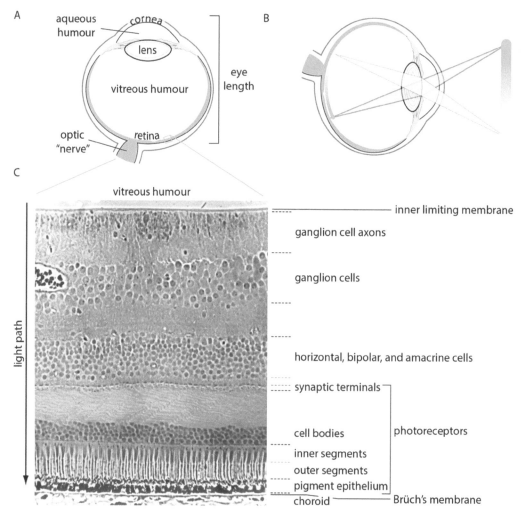

Figure 15-5 **A:** This cartoon shows a horizontal cross-section through the right eye as viewed from above. To reach the neural retina, light must pass through the transparent parts of the eye. Incident light bends upon encountering each interface: air to cornea, cornea to aqueous humor, aqueous humor to lens, lens to vitreous humor and, finally, vitreous humor to retina. Yet, the largest changes in refractive index occur at the cornea and at the lens, and, consequently, light bends principally at these two interfaces. The output of the retina travels through the optic nerve. **B:** The cornea and lens effectively focus the cone of light arriving from any one spot in the visual field onto one spot on the retina. All images on the retina are reversed in both the horizontal (shown, this eye is simply rotated 90 degrees clockwise from its orientation in A) and vertical (not shown) planes with respect to the source within the visual field. **C:** A cross-section through the human retina shows a laminated structure. Incident light arriving from the vitreous humor passes through a layer of ganglion cells and a second layer of retinal cells (a mixture of horizontal, bipolar, and amacrine cells) before reaching the photoreceptors. Photoreceptors are oriented with synaptic terminals closer to the vitreous humor and outer segments, where phototransduction takes place next to the pigment epithelium.   Photograph in C reprinted from Boycott BB, Dowling JE. Organization of the primate retina: Light microscopy. *Phil Trans R Soc B* 255:109–84, 1969, with permission of the publisher, The Royal Society.

The length of the eye, from cornea to retina, must exactly match the total refractive power of the eye in order for light from distant objects to be perfectly focused on the retina. Although the cornea and the lens both refract incoming light, *the cornea does the bulk of the focusing achieved by the eye*, producing about two-thirds of the total refractive power. Using the cornea alone, we would see forms in the world, but those forms would not be in fine focus. The additional refraction produced by the lens provides a fine focus, rendering forms sharp and crisp rather than blurry—at least ideally. Eye length is matched to the total refractive power of the eye for *far* vision, such as occurs when looking at the horizon. High-acuity vision of near objects is afforded by the near triad, which includes *accommodation*, adjusting the eye's refractive power through modifying the shape of the lens (see Chapter 5).

The resting refractive power of the eye allows light from objects located anywhere between the horizon and a distance of 20–23 feet (7 meters) away to be perfectly focused on the outer retina. However, light from objects at depths inside of optical infinity will be focused to a point behind the retina, and the perceived image will be blurry. Accommodation fixes this problem by increasing the refractive power of the eye through a change in the shape of the lens.

Lens opacities called *cataracts* are the leading cause of blindness in many countries. They greatly impair acuity and can ultimately cause total blindness. Cataracts can arise as a congenital condition, or they may develop with age. Steroids such as prednisone and cortisone can actually cause cataracts. In Western countries, surgeries to remove the lens from the lens capsule and place a clear implant within the capsule are both available and successful in the vast majority of cases. Unfortunately, surgery is far less available in developing countries. Consequently, in developing countries, cataracts are often the leading cause of blindness both in older individuals who develop cataracts as they age and in children

born with congenital cataracts. Adding to the urgency of this situation for those born with congenital cataracts, surgery during adulthood is useless because developmental and irreversible harm to visual acuity has already occurred.

The corneal surface should curve spherically in all directions. However, sometimes, the cornea is more cylindrical in that the radius of curvature is not uniform across all orientations. This causes a condition known as *astigmatism*. As a result, lines in one orientation may be distorted or blurred. Most astigmatisms can be corrected with appropriate lenses.

ACCOMMODATION ALLOWS FOR FOCUS ON NEAR OBJECTS

The near triad, consisting of convergence of the two eyes, pupillary constriction, and lens accommodation, allows for near vision (see Chapter 5). The near triad is engaged automatically whenever fixation is shifted from a far target to a near one. Upon switching from near back to far vision, the near triad is simply turned off. In other words, *far vision is not actively produced*. The eyes relax back toward the neutral position rather than being actively abducted out of the converged state; the ciliary muscle relaxes, allowing the lens to flatten; and activation of the pupillary constrictor muscle ceases, allowing the pupil to widen. As you recall, all components of the near triad are supported by axons that travel in the third cranial nerve (see Chapter 5). The near triad includes both rapid changes afforded by skeletal muscle (convergence) and slow changes dependent on slow muscle (accommodation and pupillary constriction).

Accompanying convergence, the incident angle at which light hits the cornea increases, which in turn increases the total refractive power of the eye (see Box 15-1). The total

---

Box 15-1 **LIGHT BENDS WHEN IT HITS AN INTERFACE BETWEEN DIFFERENT MEDIUMS**

As you know from common experience (see Fig. 15-6), light bends when it crosses an interface that involves a change in *refractive index*. Looking from air into water is just such an interface. As light travels into and through the eye, there are three interfaces where the refractive index changes:

- Air to cornea: *Large increase* in refractive index at *concave* surface

- Aqueous humour to front surface of lens: *Small increase* in refractive index at *concave* surface

- Back surface of lens to vitreous humour: *Very small decrease* in refractive index at *convex* surface

The outcome of light traversing the eye's interfaces is that light bends toward the eye's axis, miniaturizing the optical image on the retina.

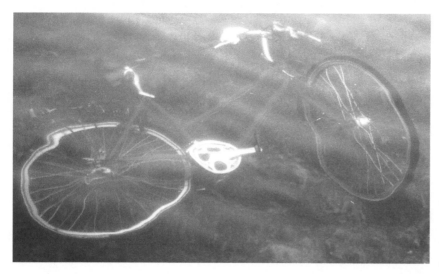

Figure 15-6 Light traveling from water to air is bent. When the water surface is uneven, as is the case here, light is bent unevenly. Because of this uneven refraction, a perfectly round bicycle wheel and its straight spokes are haphazardly bent and curved.

The angle at which light bends at a refractive interface depends on (1) the change in the refractive index at the interface and (2) the angle at which incoming light hits the interface. To illustrate how the size of the difference in refractive index impacts the angle of refraction, compare light coming in at a 45-degree angle (with respect to the eye's axis) to either the cornea or the lens.

- Air to cornea, outgoing angle: $32°$, $\Delta = 13°$

- Aqueous humour to lens, outgoing angle: $41°$, $\Delta = 4°$

Thus, the larger the change in refractive index, the greater the bend in the light path. Because both of these interfaces involve light transitioning from a lower to a higher refractive index, light is bent toward the vertical axis.

Incident angle also has a strong impact on refraction angle. Consider light arriving at the cornea at a 30-degree angle. This light will leave the cornea at roughly 27 degrees, a bend of only a few degrees. In contrast, we saw that light with a 45-degree incident angle is bent by more than 10 degrees by the cornea.

Light of different wavelengths refracts at slightly different angles, producing *chromatic aberration*. This is illustrated in Figure 15-8. Incident sunlight carries a range of wavelengths, including wavelengths normally perceived as violet, yellow, and red. As mixed wavelength light passes through the cornea and subsequently the lens, long wavelength light (red) is bent less than short wavelength light (violet, blue), resulting in photons of mixed wavelengths being focused to a mixture of depths (see Fig. 15-8A, B). In the case of the human eye, light of a wavelength commonly perceived as yellow is focused to the site of phototransduction, whereas longer wavelength light is focused to a more distant plane and shorter wavelength light to a nearer plane. To put short wavelength light into focus, we relax accommodation, looking farther away, and we accommodate in order to put long wavelength light into focus. Because we practice this all the time, we learn that "red" objects require accommodation and "blue" objects require a relaxation of accommodation. Artists employ this trick by using "warm" (long wavelength) colors to indicate close objects and "cool" (long wavelength) colors to indicate distant objects (see Fig. 15-8C, D).

refractive power of the eye is further increased by lens accommodation, which leads to a rounding up of the front edge of the lens (Fig. 15-7A). Just as for eyeglass lenses, a lens with a more spherical profile creates greater refraction due to the increased curvature. Together, convergence and accommodation increase the refractive power sufficiently so that near objects are in fine focus.

Narrowing the pupillary diameter is advantageous to near vision because it restricts the cone of blur that is possible (Fig. 15-9). Essentially, light from a more restricted range of locations can access the retina through a constricted pupil than through a dilated pupil. Additionally, objects at a range of depths will all be in focus through a constricted pupil just as they are in a photograph taken

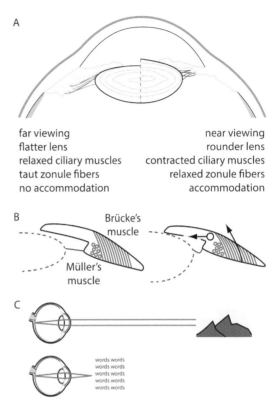

far viewing | near viewing
flatter lens | rounder lens
relaxed ciliary muscles | contracted ciliary muscles
taut zonule fibers | relaxed zonule fibers
no accommodation | accommodation

Figure 15-7 A rounding up of the lens—accommodation—changes the refraction for light hitting the lens, biasing the eye's fine focus to near objects. A: During far viewing (*left*), there is no accommodation and the ciliary muscles are relaxed. Zonule fibers are taut when the ciliary muscles are relaxed. The taut zonule fibers pull on the lens, rendering it flattish. For near viewing (*right*), accommodation is accomplished by contraction of the ciliary muscles, which moves the ciliary body anteriorly and medially. As a result, the zonule fibers relax and this allows the lens to adopt a more rounded, relaxed shape. B: There are two sets of ciliary muscles critical to changing lens shape. Müller's muscles are circumferential fibers that are located medially; when they contract, the ciliary body moves medially and forward. Brücke's muscles are radially oriented, like the spokes on a wheel, and pull the ciliary body forward and medially when they contract. Contraction of both types of ciliary muscles moves the ciliary body closer to the lens and thus allows the zonule fibers to relax, which in turn allows the lens to ball up. C: When looking at mountains, or anywhere at optical infinity, incident light arrives along parallel paths. In contrast, during near viewing, incident light arrives along convergent angles. The changes in lens shape, zonule fiber length, and so on that are illustrated here are hugely exaggerated because the difference is barely perceptible even when exaggerated many fold.

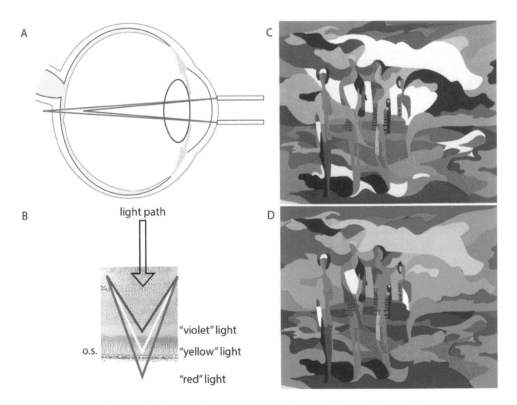

Figure 15-8 A–B: Incident white light (*black outlined rectangles*) carries a range of wavelengths, including wavelengths normally perceived as violet, yellow, and red light. As white light passes through the cornea and subsequently the lens, long wavelength light (*red*) is bent less than short wavelength light (*violet, blue*), resulting in an image of mixed wavelengths being focused to a variety of distances. In the case of the human eye, light of medium wavelength, commonly perceived as yellow, is focused to the level of the photoreceptor outer segments, whereas longer wavelength light focuses to a more distant plane and shorter wavelength light to a nearer plane. Thus, to put long wavelength light into focus we accommodate, as though we were focusing on something near. Because we practice this all the time, we learn that long wavelength objects require accommodation and short wavelength objects require a relaxation of accommodation. The result is that we *perceive* short wavelengths to be farther away than long wavelengths located at the same distance. C–D: Artists use the perceptual trick resulting from chromatic aberration to either lend a perception of depth (D) or to flatten an image (C). Warm colors—red and orange—are perceived as in the foreground, whereas cool colors—blue and violet—create a perception of depth. Paintings in C and D kindly provided by Jane S. Mason.

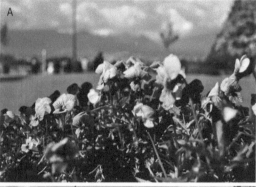

A1. wide aperture/pupil

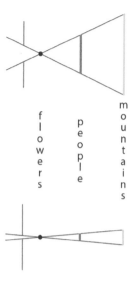

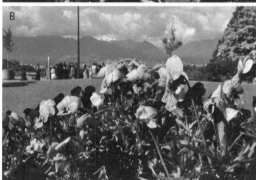

B1. narrow aperture/pupil

Figure 15-9 Two photographic images, one obtained through a pinhole aperture (B), show the effect of a narrow camera aperture, or pupil, on depth of field. A: When the aperture of a camera is open, focus is restricted to a narrow depth of field. Only some of the foreground flowers are in focus. The people in the street and the clouds and mountains in the far distance are all blurry. A1: A wide aperture allows a circle of blur from multiple depths to enter. B: Narrowing the aperture of a camera, like constricting the pupil, has a profound effect on depth of field. In this photograph, taken through a pinhole aperture, the flowers, people, mountains, and clouds are in focus. B1: Virtually all of the light entering through a narrow aperture arises from a narrow cone of space, resulting in minimal blur at any depth. The result is a large depth of field. Photographs kindly provided by Claude V. Perreault.

with a pin-hole camera (Fig. 15-9). The visual system evolved to serve near vision involving a range of near focal planes—think of picking berries from a bush—and not within the context of the single flat page or screen that is so ubiquitous in modern life. Pupillary constriction is thus a critical part of the near triad.

THE LENS INEVITABLY BECOMES FIXED IN SHAPE BY MIDDLE AGE

As we age, it takes longer and longer to change our lens shape by less and less. The loss of lens elasticity with age is as sure of happening as are death and taxes so that all of us lose the ability to accommodate if we live for at least five decades. The inability to bring near objects into focus is termed *presbyopia* (ancient Greek for "old man eye"). To understand the effect of presbyopia, consider the change in the *near point of accommodation*, which is *the closest depth at which objects appear in focus*, across the life span. For children without refractive errors, the near point of accommodation averages less than 3 inches (~7 cm). By the age of 36 years, the near point is almost double that of a child. In the fifth decade, the near point averages almost 10 inches (25 cm), and, at 50, the near point is at arm's length. By 60 years of age, the nearest point

that can be viewed is typically the better part of a yard (or meter) away.

The loss of lens elasticity ultimately leads most people to hold reading material farther and farther away in order to read the letters. When holding pages at arms' length no longer suffices, "reading glasses" become absolutely necessary for near vision. Some myopic individuals escape the need for reading glasses, at least for some time, because of their long eyes.

A DEVELOPMENTAL PROGRAM DICTATES EYE GROWTH TO A LENGTH THAT SUPPORTS FOCUS OF DISTANT IMAGES

Emmetropia is the ideal condition that occurs when the eye, with relaxed ciliary muscles, focuses light from far objects onto the outer retina, to the photoreceptor outer segments where phototransduction occurs (Fig. 15-5C). In an emmetropic individual, the retina is located at just the right distance from the cornea so that light from far objects arrives at the photoreceptor layer when the lens is not accommodated (Fig. 15-10A). The process by which the eye grows to the length that exactly matches the refractive power of the eye is called *emmetropization*.

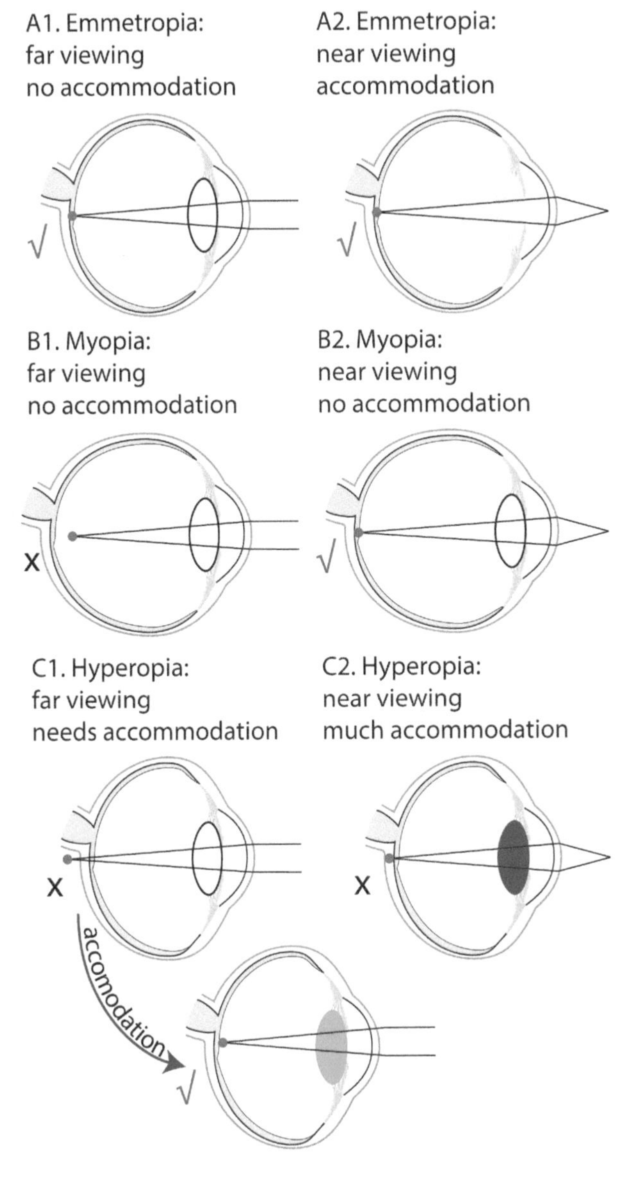

A1. Emmetropia:
far viewing
no accommodation

A2. Emmetropia:
near viewing
accommodation

B1. Myopia:
far viewing
no accommodation

B2. Myopia:
near viewing
no accommodation

C1. Hyperopia:
far viewing
needs accommodation

C2. Hyperopia:
near viewing
much accommodation

Figure 15-10 Aberrant eye length is the leading cause of refractive vision problems. Ideally, the eye grows to a length that matches the refractive power of the lens and cornea, so that light is focused on the retina without any accommodation (A1). This condition is emmetropia. The increased refraction afforded by accommodation brings near objects into focus in emmetropic people (A1). B: When the eye is too long, far objects come into focus somewhere in the vitreous humor (B1), but near objects come into focus on the retina, even with no or very little accommodation (B2). C: When the eye is too short, far objects come into focus behind the eye (C1). Hyperopic individuals may engage the near triad while looking at far objects and thereby increase the refractive power of their eyes. This can result in far objects coming into focus. However, even with maximal accommodation, near objects cannot be properly focused upon without corrective lenses (C2).

Emmetropization is vision-dependent in that it depends on the quality of the images focused on the retina. Yet it occurs independently of the brain. Thus, emmetropization appears to involve *local* interactions between the retina,

which somehow detects the blur from out of focus images, and the sclera.

Any minute error in the length of the eye will change the refractive power needed and thereby produce a measurable defect in vision. Luckily, most refractive errors can be corrected with lenses. The most typical consequence of defective emmetropization is *myopia* in which the length of the eye, from cornea to retina, is too long so that far images are focused short of the photoreceptor outer segments (Fig. 15-10B). However, when viewing near objects, incident light arrives at a greater angle. As a result, light from near objects is perfectly focused in myopic people, even with little or no accommodation. Therefore, individuals with long eyes see near, but not far, objects in focus and are colloquially termed "near-sighted."

Myopia is a condition that affects a large proportion of the human population in industrialized nations. The risk of developing myopia appears to depend on both an inherited vulnerability and an environmental factor. The importance of the environment is clearly seen from the explosion in myopia over the past several decades. For example, 30% of Taiwanese 12-year-olds were myopic in 1986, and that proportion doubled by 2000. An explosive increase in the incidence and severity of myopia has occurred in many South and East Asian countries. In affected countries, such as Singapore, the majority of people are myopic, and myopia is considered epidemic. *The key environmental factor appears to be time spent outdoors.* Children who spend more time outdoors have a lower chance of developing myopia than do children who spend more time indoors. The mechanism by which time outdoors protects against myopia is not clear but is under active investigation. It is possible that a certain amount of time spent viewing distant scenes is necessary for normal emmetropization. Alternatively, the intensity and quality of light that children are exposed to outside may be a key factor in preventing myopia. Regardless of the mechanism, time spent outdoors is protective. Send kids outside to play!

In people with short eyes, distant images arrive at the retina out of focus because the theoretical focal point is located somewhere past the ideal spot in the outer retina (Fig. 15-10C). This condition, far rarer than myopia, is known as *hyperopia*. When viewing images at a distance, hyperopic individuals can correct for refractive errors by employing accommodation. However, at short distances, accommodation is insufficient to bring near objects into focus. Therefore, hyperopia is sometimes called "far-sightedness." The majority of cases of both myopia and hyperopia can be effectively treated with appropriate corrective lenses.

PHOTORECEPTORS SIT AT THE END OF THE LIGHT PATH TO INTERACT DIRECTLY WITH THE PIGMENT EPITHELIUM

After passing through the length of the eye, light finally hits the neural retina, a thin, layered, and nearly perfectly transparent structure at the back of the eye. The retina's transparency allows light to travel, without significant distortion or diminution, to the outer retina where photoreceptors are located. Even upon reaching photoreceptors, light passes through the synaptic terminals and somata before arriving at the photoreceptors' outer segments, where light-sensitive molecules are densely packed. Although it may seem puzzling that the light-sensitive part of photoreceptors lies in the deepest part of the retina and farthest away from the light source, this arrangement is necessary because photoreceptors *require direct interactions with the pigment epithelium*, the non-neural outer layer of the retina, for biochemical regeneration of photopigment that permits continued function.

The pigment epithelium is a single layer of retinal cells containing pigments called *ocular melanins*. The choroid, a vascularized epithelial tissue deep to the pigment epithelium is also pigmented, appearing black or nearly so (Fig. 15-11A). The dark backing of the eye functions like the darkened interior of a camera: light is absorbed and therefore does not bounce around. This means that light does not reflect off the back of the eye and return to "hit" photoreceptors for a second time. Unfortunately, individuals with *ocular albinism*, an inherited condition, are unable to synthesize the pigment found in the choroid and pigment epithelium. As a consequence, light bounces around within an albino's eye and can hit photoreceptor outer segments multiple times. This leads to diffuse and unfocused light and consequently extremely poor acuity; albino individuals are legally blind.

Beyond the optical advantages that they confer, *pigments at the back of the eye absorb a great deal of energy by absorbing light*. This prevents some of the cellular damage that would otherwise be caused by the dangerous combination of light and oxidation. The most damaging light in this regard is higher frequency or shorter wavelength

lights, mostly blue, violet, and ultraviolet light. The lens filters out most of the ultraviolet light and the retinal pigment epithelium absorbs a good portion of the remaining damaging light energy. The pigment epithelium also ferries nutrition and waste between the choroidal blood vessels and the neural retina.

Due to the critical interactions between the pigment epithelium and the neural retina, any separation between the two, a condition termed *retinal detachment*, has dire consequences. Severe myopia, associated with a long eye and therefore a thinly stretched retina, is a risk factor for retinal detachment. Retinal detachment can occur for a number of reasons including physical trauma or as a complication of *diabetes mellitus* or cataract surgery. There also appears to be a hereditary component, with a high risk of retinal detachment running in some families.

Once started, detachments have the tendency to spread, with the retina peeling off like paint from a wall. Therefore, it is critical that patients seek medical care immediately if they experience large floaters or flashes of light. If caught soon enough, treatments now exist that can repair retinal detachment. In one approach, a the sclera is buckled in order to push the retinal epithelium toward the retina. Coupled with freezing any frankly detached part of the retina, scleral buckle surgery has a high degree of success.

PHOTORECEPTORS COME IN TWO VARIETIES

As you may already be aware, photoreceptors come in two varieties: rods and cones. Both rods and cones have an outer segment, the segment closest to the pigment epithelium at the back of the eye where phototransduction occurs; an inner segment where energetic housekeeping occurs; a cell body containing the nucleus; and a synaptic terminal (Fig. 15-11A). The outer segment of both cell types contains rows and rows of *discs*, membranes that house the visual pigments responsible for phototransduction.

Among the important differences between rods and cones is the far greater sensitivity of rods than cones to light. As a result, only rods mediate vision under the dimmest light conditions, such as those on a moonless night in the country, termed *scotopic* conditions. In light bright enough to see vibrant colors, rod responses are saturated and cannot signal any further differences in luminance. Therefore,

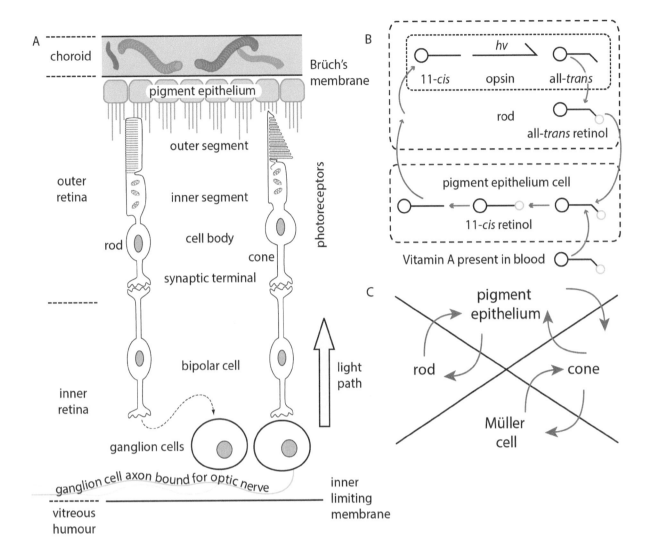

Figure 15-11 A: The retina is a layered half-globe structure at the back of the eye. The part of the retina closest to the back of the eye is the outer retina, and the layers closest to the inside of the globe, occupied by vitreous humor, comprise the inner retina. After light passes through the vitreous humor, it first passes through a layer of ganglion cell axons and cell bodies. The ganglion cells, which are the output of the retina, send an axon toward the optic disk. The unmyelinated ganglion cell axons collect at the optic disk and become myelinated as they form the optic nerve. As a result, myelin does not interfere with the path traversed by incoming light. After passing through layers of ganglion cells and bipolar cells, and through the cell bodies and inner segments of photoreceptors, light finally reaches the outer segments of the photoreceptors. Within the outer segments, stacks of membranous discs either continuous with the plasma membrane (cones) or located completely intracellularly (rods) house an enormous number of rhodopsin molecules (*red dots*), each ready to catch a photon. Photoreceptor outer segments are embedded in the microvilli—thin processes of retinal pigment epithelial cells. Pigment epithelial cells contain melanin pigments that absorb light, minimizing the number of photons that can reflect off the back of the eye and stimulate photoreceptors on the rebound, thereby diffusing the image. Deep to the pigment epithelium is the choroid. The inner layer of the choroid is Brüch's membrane. The choroid is heavily pigmented and therefore can absorb the small amount of light that makes it through the sclera, vitreous humor, and retina. With age, Drusen, hard accumulations of extracellular material, accumulate between Brüch's membrane and the pigment epithelium. Too much Drusen interferes with nutrient and waste exchange between the choroid and the retina and is a major contributor to age-related macular degeneration. B: When a molecule of rod rhodopsin catches a photon (*hv*), 11-*cis* retinal is converted into all-*trans* retinal and the rhodopsin molecule is activated. Rhodopsin kinase is an enzyme that inactivates rhodopsin containing all-*trans* retinal. All-*trans* retinal is then transported out of the opsin and converted into all-*trans* retinol by retinal dehydrogenase. Note that all-*trans* retinol is synonymous with vitamin A and is available both from the photoreceptor and from blood. All-*trans* retinol is transported out of the rod and into the pigment epithelium. Within the pigment epithelium, all-*trans* retinol is isomerized into 11-*cis* retinol and then into 11-*cis* retinal. It is 11-*cis* retinal that is then transported out of the pigment epithelium and back into the rod, where it is inserted into an opsin and available for photoisomerization. C: Although pigment epithelium is the exclusive source of reisomerization (*red lines*) for rods, both pigment epithelium and Müller cells contribute to reisomerization of retinal for cone cells.

during bright, colorful conditions, termed *photopic* conditions, vision depends exclusively on cones. During intermediate light or *mesopic* conditions, present in a dimly lit restaurant or at dawn and twilight, when colors are visible but appear muted, both rods and cones respond to light and contribute to vision.

MODULATORY MECHANISMS ALLOW US TO SEE IN DIFFERING LIGHT CONDITIONS

One of the most remarkable features of vertebrate vision is the wide range, *about 10 log units*, of intensities over which it operates. Think of the difference between navigating among the furniture in a dark room, reading outside on a bright summer day, or walking in a winter wonderland of snow. As predicted by Weber's law (see Chapter 14), we are sensitive to small changes in dim light while being insensitive to those same small changes in bright light. In bright light, a much brighter light is needed to elicit the same response as a dim light in the dark. In essence, rather than responding to light at some absolute level of intensity or even to a change in light intensity of a set magnitude, *the visual system reacts to stimuli that are different enough from the background to stand out*. Put in other words, the visual system supports responses to any stimulus with a sufficient stimulus-to-background intensity ratio.

Part of the flexibility in reacting to light intensity over such a large range derives from having two different systems: one based on rods, which operate alone during scotopic conditions, and one based on cones, which operate alone during photopic conditions. Additionally, adaptation, a general feature of all sensory systems, enables the retina to show high sensitivity to light at low-stimulus intensities and a far lower, nonsaturating sensitivity at high-stimulus intensities. In the dark, sensitivity is increased, and, in the light, sensitivity is diminished. As an example of the former, a dark-adapted retina, one that has been in total darkness for at least 40 minutes, is *exquisitely* sensitive to light, supporting detection of just a few photons. Jeremy Nathans calculated that a person adapted to the dark can detect a flash of light containing "the potential energy [equivalent to that] lost by dropping a single *Escherichia coli* [bacterium] 2 mm" (Nathans 1994).

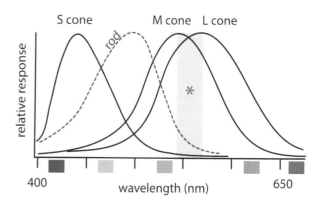

Figure 15-12 Humans have four different types of photoreceptors (three types of cones and the rods) that respond optimally to different wavelengths of light. The three cones respond best to different peak wavelengths but have broad tuning curves. As a consequence, they respond, with higher or lower probability, to a range of wavelengths. Thus, the response of any single cone type does not unambiguously signal wavelength. The color swatches are approximate representations of the colors typically perceived at selected wavelengths. The gray area (*asterisk*) within the overlap between L and M absorption curves represents the approximate range of wavelengths that is filtered out by EnChroma sunglasses.

RODS AND CONES USE A DERIVATIVE OF VITAMIN A TO TRANSDUCE LIGHT

All of our photoreceptors contain the same light-absorbing molecule or *chromophore: retinal*. Retinal is derived from the alcohol retinol or *vitamin A*, which must be ingested through the diet. Retinal fits within a protein called an *opsin*, and the retinal-containing opsin forms a metabotropic receptor (see Chapter 13) called rhodopsin. You should be aware that the word rhodopsin is used in a somewhat

confusing manner. It is the only term for the specific photopigment contained in rods. Rhodopsin is also the generic (and most commonly used) term for any retinal-containing opsin, including that in cones.

The particular opsin in each rhodopsin determines the optimal wavelength of light that the rhodopsin absorbs (Fig. 15-12). One opsin is contained in the single type of rods, whereas three different iodopsins are contained in each of three different types of cones:

- Rod opsin or rhodopsin (peak absorption of light with wavelength of ~496 nm)

- Cone opsin in L (for long wavelength) cones (~560 nm)

- Cone opsin in M (medium wavelength) cones (~530 nm)

- Cone opsin in S (short wavelength) cones (~420 nm)

For all rhodopsins, the ligand is not a neurotransmitter but rather light.

Retinal exists in two conformations: 11-*cis* and all-*trans*. In the dark, retinal is in the 11-*cis* conformation (Fig. 15-11B). When rhodopsin *catches* or absorbs a photon, retinal changes its conformation to all-*trans*, and rhodopsin becomes activated. This change in conformation triggered by light is termed *photoisomerization*. Activated rhodopsin, like other activated metabotropic receptors, activates a G protein, which in this case is called *transducin* (see Chapter 13). In fact, each activated rhodopsin activates hundreds of transducin molecules. The activated α subunit of transducin then activates phosphodiesterase E, which hydrolyzes cyclic guanosine monophosphate (cGMP), leading to a decrease in the cytoplasmic concentration of cGMP. As long as phosphodiesterase E is bound to the activated α subunit of transducin, it continues to hydrolyze cGMP into guanosine monophosphate (GMP). Recall that photoreceptors have a resting, *in the dark*, inward current that uses a nucleotide-gated ion channel, the cGMP-gated ion channel. By decreasing the concentration of cGMP, light decreases the number of open cGMP-gated ion channels. Since cGMP-gated ion channels carry inward current, closing them leads to a *hyperpolarization*. Mutations in the genes for proteins involved in phototransduction are among a large heterogeneous group of genetic causes of *retinitis pigmentosa* (see the next section).

For rhodopsin to respond to light, retinal must be in the 11-*cis* form. Therefore, after photoisomerization, a mechanism to switch retinal from all-*trans* back to 11-*cis* is needed (Fig. 15-11B, C). This means separating the retinal from the opsin, isomerizing the retinal to 11-*cis*, and returning it to an opsin, all of which takes energy. In fact, not only the energy necessary for isomerization but also energy for transport is required because photoreceptors cannot isomerize all-*trans* retinal into the 11-*cis* form. Other retinal cells perform this isomerization.

There is a remarkably large response to just one photon. This results from two steps of amplification in the light-evoked signaling cascade:

1. Activation of transducin

2. Conversion of cGMP to GMP

Thus, *one* photon that activates *one* rhodopsin molecule leads to the activation of *hundreds* of G proteins (transducin molecules), a measurable reduction in the local concentration of cGMP and, ultimately, the closure of *hundreds* of cGMP-gated cation channels.

Vitamin A, the substrate for retinal synthesis, is an absolute requirement for normal vision. Individuals deficient in vitamin A develop a number of eye and skin problems. Often, the earliest symptom associated with vitamin A deficiency is *night blindness*, an impairment of vision in scotopic conditions due to a lack of retinal in *rods*. Persistent vitamin A deficiency will eventually cause total blindness when cones also stop functioning due to the lack of available retinal. Persistent vitamin A deficiency also impairs tear production, resulting in severe *xerophthalmia* or dry eyes, and causes a number of changes in the cornea that eventually lead to the irreversible destruction of the cornea. Vitamin A deficiency is a major problem and cause of blindness in poorer nations. Moreover, although not an issue among the well-nourished, populations whose nutritional intake does not regularly include fresh vegetables and fruits are at risk of vitamin A deficiency. Notably, vitamin A deficiency is on the rise within the United States due to poor nutrition.

RETINITIS PIGMENTOSA IS A DEGENERATIVE DISEASE OF PHOTORECEPTORS

Retinitis pigmentosa is a diverse family of genetic diseases that cause a progressive loss of photoreceptor function, resulting ultimately in the death of photoreceptors and blindness. The disease is named for the pathological appearance of pigmented blotches in the retina. The majority of retinitis pigmentosa disease initially impacts rod vision, with night blindness and loss of peripheral sight comprising typical early symptoms. Eventually, sometimes at a much later time point, cones die and central high-acuity vision is lost.

A large number of varied mutations are associated with retinitis pigmentosa, which is relatively common, affecting 1 in 4,000 people worldwide. Some of these mutations, for example those in the genes for rod opsin, rod cGMP-phosphodiesterase subunits, proteins involved in retinal recycling, or proteins important in vitamin A metabolism make some sense in that they have functions critical to photoreceptor physiology. Consider a defect in the cGMP-phosphodiesterase subunit. An inability to activate cGMP-phosphodiesterase would lead to persistently high levels of cGMP and, in turn, constitutively open cGMP-gated ion channels, which would in turn cause excessive cation influx. Cation influx, likely including influx of calcium ions, may injure and eventually kill rods. As another example, mutations in the rod opsin gene, accounting for 25% of retinitis pigmentosa cases, appear to interfere with metabolism or the structure of the outer segments or may cause harmful intracellular protein aggregates. Interestingly, just as high levels of intracellular calcium ions can kill photoreceptors, it appears that excessively low levels of calcium ions can also kill photoreceptors. This susceptibility may explain why continuous light exposure causes blindness in animals. Recall that light reduces the influx of cations, including calcium ions, into photoreceptors so that continuous light would be expected to be accompanied by a very low concentration of resting calcium ions.

In contrast to the "sensible"—or within the realm of sensible—mutations just mentioned, some mutations associated with retinitis pigmentosa affect universal processes with no particular or exclusive connection to photoreceptor function. For example, mutations in genes that code for enzymes that splice out introns or for a particular pH-regulating enzyme (carbonic anhydrase IV) are associated with retinitis pigmentosa. An understanding of such associations remains to be elucidated.

Patients with retinitis pigmentosa benefit from aggressive treatments to optimize vision—visual aid devices, cataract removal, and so on. Although no well-established and effective treatment exists for all or even a large proportion of patients, a number of genetic therapies aimed at restoring absent proteins coded for by genes with recessive mutations or aimed at inactivating defective proteins coded for by genes with dominant mutations are being pursued with some success.

PHOTORECEPTORS DEPEND ON THE VISUAL CYCLE

People with healthy vision are extremely sensitive to light, able to detect just a handful of photons. Not only is visual sensitivity high, but, in addition, the rate of *false positives* (i.e., the detection of light when none is present) is very low. Coupling high accuracy with high sensitivity means that (1) a dark environment is perceived as dark and (2) minimal light within a dark environment is correctly detected as light. High sensitivity and high accuracy are successfully accomplished when:

- One photon leads to a response (high sensitivity).

- After absorption of one photon, a sensory cell is no longer responsive to light (high accuracy).

As a result of this arrangement, photopigment must be regenerated—made responsive to light once again—thorough biochemical means. This is termed the *visual cycle*. The visual cycle is a key concept because it is the reason that phototransduction in rods and cones is completely dependent on an intact and healthy retina. Healthy rods and cones in isolation cannot support vision. Two cell types participate in the visual cycle: retinal pigment epithelial cells and the *Müller cells*, a type of glial cell found only in the retina. Without functioning pigment epithelial and

Müller cells, vision is lost because phototransduction does not occur because photopigment is not regenerated.

It is interesting to contrast this arrangement with the arrangement in invertebrates, where one photon leads to a visual response and a second photon returns the photopigment to a responsive state. Vertebrates depend on a complex biochemical cycle to recycle "spent" photopigment and regenerate fresh photosensitive molecules. There are two different cycles (Fig. 15-11C). Retinal pigment epithelial cells participate in the "rod cycle" that is the only option for rods (Fig. 15-11B). Cones may use the same cycle but also use a "cone cycle" that involves the Müller cell. The cone cycle is fast, regenerating photopigment in 2–3 minutes for use by cone photoreceptors. In contrast, to fully regenerate the photopigment of rods requires roughly 40 minutes in the dark. A person who has been in the dark for 40 minutes has a full complement of photopigment available to catch photons. Such a person is said to be "dark-adapted" and, in this state, is able to detect a single photon.

DISCS ARE PHAGOCYTOSED BY THE PIGMENT EPITHELIUM EVERY 10 DAYS

The retina is particularly oxygen rich because it extracts about *half of the oxygen* arriving in the choroidal arteries. Coupled with the high concentration of oxygen, photon bombardment renders the retina highly susceptible to oxidative damage. To minimize oxidative damage of photoreceptors, discs and their component molecules are renewed every 10 days. This renewal ensures against molecules "going bad" and errantly failing to function or functioning inappropriately in the absence of light. The disc renewal cycle operates on discs of both rod and cone outer segments.

The opsins contained in photoreceptor discs are synthesized in the inner segment and then incorporated into the plasma membrane at the base of the outer segment. Discs form from this plasma membrane, either budding off in the case of rods or simply forming repeated invaginations in the case of cones (Fig. 15-11A). As newer discs form, the older ones move outward, toward the tip of the outer segment. The oldest discs contain the highest concentration of free radicals and proteins damaged by light and oxygen. Each day, the pigment epithelium phagocytoses the tips of the outer segments containing the last several rows of discs. The pigment epithelium's central role in the disc renewal cycle is another reason why retinal function is completely dependent on being in contact with a healthy pigment epithelium.

AGE-RELATED MACULAR DEGENERATION RESULTS IN SEVERE DEGRADATION OF CENTRAL VISION

Age-related macular degeneration is a heterogeneous disease that results in the deterioration of the central portion of the retina—the macula—and, consequently, a loss of central vision. In roughly 10% of affected individuals, an excess of *angiogenesis*, or blood vessel formation, in the choroid produces *wet* macular degeneration (Fig. 15-13). Yet, in most cases, *dry* macular degeneration results from a disruption of the delicate but required partnership between the pigment epithelium and photoreceptor outer segments. Discs within the photoreceptor outer segments are vulnerable to damage from both free radicals and from light. The pigment epithelium defends against these vulnerabilities by phagocytosing the oldest discs on a daily basis, absorbing damaging blue light, and neutralizing oxidative damage through the production of antioxidants.

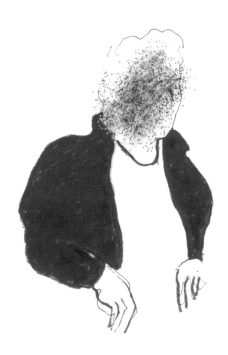

Figure 15-13 An artist's rendition of vision with wet macular degeneration shows central vision obscured by blood while peripheral vision is preserved. As blood vessels overgrow, they become fragile and can break or leak, bleeding into the vitreous humor. This picture was drawn soon after an initial episode of bleeding. Fortunately, treatment does exist for those with wet macular degeneration. Because the disease is due to the actions of vascular endothelial growth factor or VEGF, antibodies against VEGF introduced into the vitreous can be highly effective in preventing disease progression. Drawing kindly provided by Jane S. Mason.

Unfortunately, with age, lipofuscin accumulates to toxic levels in the pigment epithelium. The resultant culling of pigment epithelial cells means that each remaining pigment epithelial cell now needs to phagocytose more outer segments, clear more damaged proteins, and neutralize more free radicals. Pigment epithelial cells die from this cellular stress, leaving behind yellow deposits called *Drusen* that are pathognomonic for macular degeneration. The macula is most severely affected, perhaps because it is lipofuscin-rich and more energetically active than the peripheral retina. Age-related macular degeneration is the most common cause of blindness in industrialized countries, and most existing therapies are aimed simply at preventing progression.

MULTIPLE CONE TYPES ALLOW FOR COLOR VISION

Color vision depends on the presence of at least two different photoreceptor types that respond maximally to light of different wavelengths. Humans with normal color vision have in fact three different cone types containing three different photopigments. As introduced above, S, M, and L cones maximally absorb short, medium, or long wavelengths, respectively.

The absorption spectra of L and M cones are very similar (Fig. 15-12) because the protein sequences of the two iodopsins are very similar. The genes for these similar iodopsins sit next to each other on the X chromosome, and one probably arose from the other through gene duplication in an early primate. Having two cones with similar but distinct absorption spectra in the medium- to long-wavelength range may have facilitated picking out ripe yellow and red fruit from the surrounding green vegetation.

The absorption peaks for cone iodopsins do not do justice to the *response profiles* of cones to different wavelength light. The absorption spectra are broad, meaning that wavelengths far from the peak still elicit a response (Fig. 15-12). For example, an S cone with an absorption peak of about 420 nm may respond to wavelengths as long as 540–550 nm. Furthermore, a cone's response bears no information about the wavelength of the captured light. Consequently, regardless of the incident wavelength that excites a cone, the cone's response is the same. Thus, a cone response is a cone response is a cone response and is not an indicator of wavelength.

Multiple cones are needed to perceive colors from light of different wavelengths. If we only had information from M cones, a banana could be perceived as the same color as a piece of turquoise. Yet we easily tell the difference between yellow and turquoise. In part, this is because light with a wavelength of 590 nm, perceived as yellow, stimulates L cones near maximally whereas light with a wavelength of 510 nm, perceived as aqua, stimulates L cones poorly. Thus, the ratio of L cone to M cone responses, abbreviated as the L/M ratio, is critical to distinguishing between different wavelengths longer than 550 nm, about the longest wavelength light to which S cones respond appreciably.

Two other bits of information in addition to the L/M ratio are used by the brain to estimate the wavelength of incident light. First, the combined responses of L and M cones, abbreviated as L + M, provide an estimate of overall luminance. Second, retinal circuitry calculates the difference between the response of S cones and the overall luminance, abbreviated as S − (L + M). Short-wavelength light, commonly perceived as blue, will result in a positive value of S − (L + M), whereas light with a wavelength greater than about 500 nm will result in a negative value of S − (L+M). Thus, the value of S − (L + M) is an indication of how close a wavelength is to the peak wavelength of either the S cone or the L and M cones.

In sum, retinal circuitry transforms information from the three types of cones into three channels of information that the brain then uses to assign the percept of color to different wavelengths in the visual scene (Fig. 15-14):

- L/M ratio

- L + M or luminance channel

- S − (L + M) cone channel

Light of any wavelength produces a unique combinatorial signature from comparing activation in the three channels rather than in the three cones. Thalamic and, ultimately, cortical circuits build on the same three channels of wavelength information initially set up by retinal circuitry in order to decipher color information from the visual world. Additional modulatory information about form, motion, expectation, and a myriad of other factors can alter the color perceived even when the wavelength of an object remains steady (Fig. 14-1A).

COLOR PERCEPTION IS TRULY AN INDIVIDUAL EXPERIENCE

Color blindness refers to a group of disorders in which one or more of the cone pigments are defective. To understand these disorders, recall that the genes for medium- and

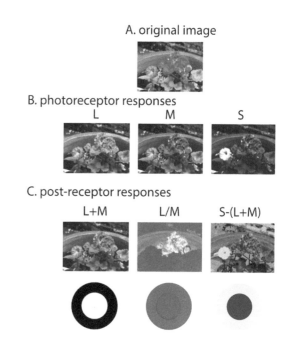

A. original image

B. photoreceptor responses
L   M   S

C. post-receptor responses
L+M   L/M   S-(L+M)

Figure 15-14 An analysis of how photoreceptors and ganglion cells of the three color channels would respond to an image of violet and red flowers with green foliage (A). B: The maximal responses of the three cone types are in white. S cones respond almost exclusively to the violet bloom. L and M cones respond similarly to both the green foliage and the red flowers. C: Information from the three cones is fed into three channels of color information. The L + M channel carries luminance information gained from the sum of L and M cone inputs. The L/M channel carries the ratio of L to M responses. This channel, unlike the responses of either L or M cones, clearly highlights the areas perceived as red over those that we perceive as green. The final channel, S-(L + M), carries the blue/violet signal. In the bottom row, the center-surround receptive field organization of retinal ganglion cells is shown. One class of ganglion cells, M ganglion cells, have opposing responses to light and dark and carry the luminance (L + M) channel. Another class, P ganglion cells, have opposing responses to medium-and long-wavelength light (L/M channel). Finally, K ganglion cells carry the S-(L + M) channel with opposing responses to yellow and violet/blue. This figure is modified from Shevell SK, Kingdom F. Color in complex scenes. *Ann Rev Psychol* 59:143–66, 2008, with permission of the publisher, Annual Reviews.

long-wavelength iodopsins are arranged in tandem on the X chromosome. Since males have only one X chromosome and females two, far more males—about 2% of the Caucasian population—than females lack either medium- or long-wavelength iodopsin. Without a medium- or long-wavelength iodopsin, different wavelengths over about 550 nm cannot be discriminated. Such *dichromatic* individuals can discriminate short-wavelength light from light of longer wavelengths but cannot distinguish between what most perceive as red, orange, yellow, and green.

The M and L iodopsin genes are 98% identical at the nucleotide level. Therefore, homologous recombination often occurs between them. As a consequence, many individuals make a hybrid M-L iodopsin that moves the peak absorbance of either opsin toward that of the other.

In these individuals, the L-M channel has a narrower range, and, as a result, long-wavelength lights are poorly distinguished.

The most common types of color blindness are:

- *Deuteranopia* refers to a loss of M cone function. Deuteranopes can distinguish short-wavelength light from longer-wavelength light, which activates the intact L cones, but wavelengths above 550 nm all activate the same L cone population and thus are perceived as one color.

- Individuals with *protanopia* have no L cone function. Like deuteranopes, protanopes can distinguish short-wavelength light from longer-wavelength light. However, wavelengths greater than 550 nm only activate M cones and therefore are indistinguishable.

- *Deuteranomaly* is the most common type of color blindness, affecting about 5% of males. In affected individuals, L cone function is normal whereas M cones contain a hybrid opsin with its peak absorption shifted toward longer wavelengths. Therefore, deuteranomaly results in *anomalous trichromacy*, with the distinction between wavelengths over 550 nm often, but not always, compromised.

- *Protanomaly* involves a hybrid L iodopsin with an absorption shifted toward shorter wavelengths and normal M cone function. Affected individuals, like those with deuteranomaly, are trichromats who often have a compromised ability to distinguish between wavelengths over 550 nm.

Recently, EnChroma has made sunglasses that filter out wavelengths in the overlap between the peak absorption wavelengths of the M and L cones (Fig. 15-12). Using these sunglasses, people with deuteranomaly and protanomaly can distinguish between medium and long wavelengths and thereby distinguish wavelengths that were not previously distinct to them. Fields of red poppies are transformed from a foliage and blossom sameness to a scene where blossoms pop out from the background foliage. Note that the glasses are *sun*glasses. Recall that luminance, overall brightness, is measured by the total excitation of M and L cones. By filtering out wavelengths in the heart of the M and L cone region, the overall luminance of a scene is greatly diminished. Therefore, the EnChroma approach only works in photopic conditions. Some individuals have had highly emotional reactions to the visual images enabled by EnChroma sunglasses, highlighting the link between perception and affect.

Additional variations in color vision exist but are far rarer than those just listed. For example, some individuals lack both M and L cone function and are consequently monochromats, dependent solely on S cone function for photopic vision. Another rare variation is the loss of S cone function, termed *tritanopia*. Since the short-wavelength iodopsin is coded by a gene on an autosomal chromosome, men and women are equally unlikely to suffer from tritanopia.

An inability to distinguish between long wavelengths puts a person at risk for mistaking a red traffic light for a green one. Such a potentially lethal error is a particular concern at night, when there is no surrounding context to differentiate red from green light. Additionally, different colors may appear to go together well only in the eyes of individuals with different iodopsin complements. Therefore, the next time you are tempted to "correct" a boy's drawing of red grass or a man's garish (to you) outfit, remember that you and he may be living in differently colored worlds. Finally, deficits in color vision diminish the vibrancy and excitement of certain scenes, such as the turning of the leaves in autumn.

Even beyond actual deficits in color vision, the large number of M and L iodopsin variations means that few of us share precisely the same perception of color. Indeed, the philosophical take-home message is that, as we all search for proverbial greener grass, we many not find it at the same wavelength.

ROD- AND CONE-DEPENDENT VISION DIFFER MARKEDLY

Key differences between rods and cones drive profound differences between the types of vision supported by the two types of photoreceptors. The key differences between rods and cones and between rod- and cone-supported vision include:

- *Rods are more sensitive to light than are cones.* Rods can respond to a single photon hit, whereas cones have a higher threshold.

- *Rods have slower responses to light than do cones*, making them poor at resolving temporal changes such as flicker. For instance, rods can only detect flicker at 12 Hz or less, whereas cones detect flicker at rates up to about 55 Hz.

- Rods do not support high-acuity vision and cannot support reading. Rod vision during scotopic conditions is sufficient only to make out rough shapes. In contrast, cone-mediated vision allows detection of fine visual details and is used for reading.

- Cones support color vision. Rods support vision along a grayscale.

- Rods and cones are distributed differently throughout the retina, so that cones are concentrated in the center of the visual field and rods in the periphery (Fig. 15-15). Thus, *highest acuity vision is at the point of fixation, also known as* foveation. On the flip side, the best approach to detecting dim lights, such as a faint star, is to look slightly (about 15 degrees) to the side of the object of interest. In this way, light from the dim object hits the peripheral retina at the location of the highest density of rods.

In sum, rod-supported vision is excellent for detecting low levels of light but not for tasks that require high acuity, such as reading. Cone-supported vision cannot operate in scotopic conditions but supports high-acuity vision as well as, of course, color vision.

Congenital achromatopsia is a rare inherited disease in which cones do not respond to light. Mutations in genes for the cone cGMP-gated cation channel and the cone isoform of transducin are two of several causes. Individuals with congenital achromatopsia view the world through rods alone. Consequently, these individuals have very poor visual discrimination in time (flicker) and space (form). As a consequence of vision's dependence on normal development and the low-resolution information provided by a coneless retina, cortical circuits never mature normally. Therefore, individuals with congenital achromatopsia see the world in low resolution. Since the development of normal eye movements depends on focused images, people with congenital achromatopsia also have abnormal eye movements. In sum, individuals without cones suffer far more from a lack of high visual acuity than from a lack of color perception.

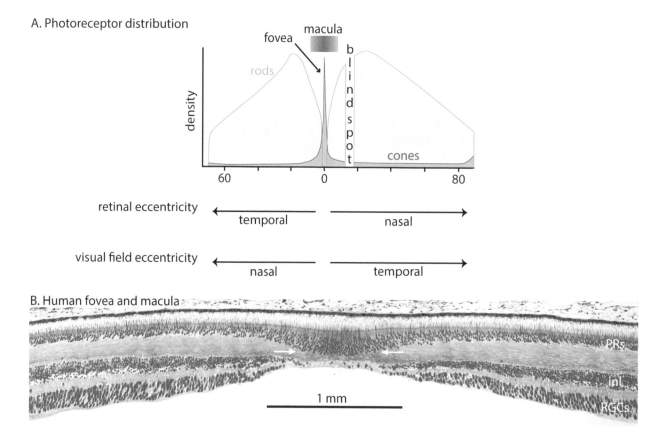

A. Photoreceptor distribution

B. Human fovea and macula

Figure 15-15 The spatial distribution of rods and cones across the retina. A: The only region where cones outnumber rods is within the fovea, which is located at the sharp peak of cones. In fact, in the very center of the fovea, no rods are present, and cones reach their maximal density. The fovea forms the center of the macula. Outside of the fovea, even within the macula, rods outnumber cones. The optic disc, where retinal ganglion cell axons collect to exit through the optic nerve, is in the nasal part of the retina and receives light from the temporal visual field. The optic disc contains no photoreceptors at all, and thus no light is transduced in this area, termed the *blind spot*. B: A stained section through the human macula shows the concentration of photoreceptors (*PRs*), all cones, and absence of ganglion cells (*RGCs*) in the fovea (between *white arrows*). The inner nuclear layer (*inl*), housing bipolar, horizontal, and amacrine cells, is also excluded from the fovea. Note that the region of retina presented here covers roughly the central 4.5 degrees of the visual field, comprising nearly the entirety of the macula. Photograph in B kindly provided by Anita Hendrickson, PhD, University of Washington.

Outside of the macula, our ability to make out visual detail is poor because there are relatively few cones (Fig. 15-15). Rods are concentrated in the peripheral retina, the retina outside of the macula and in the retina as a whole, rods far outnumber cones by about 30 to 1. Excluded from the fovea, rods reach their highest density at an eccentricity of about 15 degrees. Consequently, the best strategy to find a dim star on a dark night is to look just slightly away from its expected location.

MOST TYPES OF GANGLION CELLS CONTRIBUTE TO NONPERCEPTUAL FUNCTIONS OF VISION

Most retinal ganglion cell types do not participate in perception. Many contribute to eye movement control through projections to the midbrain, including the superior colliculus. As we know, the superior colliculus uses visual, auditory, and somatosensory input to guide orienting movements. For example, as we orient to a chipmunk scurrying across our path, we turn our body and shoulders and move our eyes. The superior colliculus is critical to all three turning movements:

1. Superior colliculus neurons *orient the body* through the *tectospinal tract* (*tectum* is another term for superior colliculus; tectospinal refers to neurons that project from the superior colliculus to the spinal cord).

2. Superior colliculus neurons contact neurons in the vestibular nuclei, which project to the cervical cord through the medial vestibulospinal tract to *orient the shoulders*.

3. Superior colliculus neurons can initiate *eye movements* through projections to the pontine horizontal gaze center and the midbrain vertical gaze center (see Chapter 6).

Orienting movements mediated by retinal projections to the superior colliculus occur outside of conscious control and therefore without conscious planning. In other vertebrates, the superior colliculus sits at the top of the visual hierarchy, but, in mammals, the expanded cortex dedicated to visual processing greatly surpasses the superior colliculus in functionality and flexibility.

A class of ganglion cells which itself is photosensitive was discovered at the turn of the millennium. The photosensitivity of *intrinsically photosensitive retinal ganglion cells* (*ipRGCs*) stems from a pigment called *melanopsin*, which is related to the photopigment used by insects. Ambient light excites melanopsin-containing ganglion cells in a sustained manner, for hours on end. Intrinsically photosensitive ganglion cells contribute to—indeed, are critical for—at least two functions:

- Light entrainment of the circadian rhythm
- Control of the pupillary light reflex

Photosensitive ganglion cells project to the *suprachiasmatic nucleus* in the hypothalamus, a nucleus that, as its name suggests, sits just dorsal to the optic chiasm. Suprachiasmatic neurons coordinate circadian rhythms, so that we are active during the day, sleep at night, release growth hormone during the night, and so on. By sensing light from the sun during the day, photosensitive ganglion cells entrain or align our endogenous rhythm to the Earth's circadian revolution and ensure that our internal circadian clock has a period that aligns with the Earth's rotation. Although temperature can entrain many animals, humans are nearly entirely dependent on vision and therefore on intrinsically photosensitive retinal ganglion cells for circadian entrainment (see Chapter 27).

Photosensitive ganglion cells also mediate the pupillary light reflex through projections to the pretectum, a region in the rostral midbrain just ventral to the superior colliculus (see Chapter 5). Overall changes in luminance are sensed by intrinsically photosensitive ganglion cells. When luminance visible to one eye increases, photosensitive ganglion cells in that eye trigger pupillary constriction in the same eye (the direct pupillary reflex) and in the contralateral eye (the consensual pupillary reflex). The pretectum is a necessary way-station for pupillary reflexes, while you will remember that the Edinger-Westphal nucleus contains the preganglionic parasympathetic neurons that control pupillary constriction.

VISUAL CORTEX PROCESSES CHANNELS OF VISUAL INFORMATION IN PARALLEL

To achieve visual perception, the brain uses a tactic of processing component features of a visual image in parallel before integrating those components back together to form a meaningful message. The primary visual cortex sends specific types of low-level visual information to particular cortical regions that focus on pieces of the puzzle such as form, texture, color, or motion. Cortical regions specialized for specific visual attributes can be considered intermediary within the visual hierarchy. Intermediate visual areas receive very elementary feature information, mostly concerning edges and their orientation, from primary visual cortex. They send out slightly higher level feature information such as texture to parietal and temporal cortical regions involved in putting the entire visual image back together again.

Patients with selective deficits in the intermediate levels of visual processing are rare. This may be because they truly are not out there, and it may be that such patients do not seek medical help. To support the latter possibility, imagine that a small area critical to processing local texture is lesioned by a stroke. The loss of texture information may in fact not prevent recognition of objects for which the patient retains size, shape, and color information. Alternatively, strokes in the area where the occipital and parietal lobes meet, particularly bilateral ones, are certainly less frequent than, for example, middle cerebral artery strokes.

Although few patients with small lesions in mid-level visual hierarchy are known, the experiences of those who exist are instructive. The largest group of such patients have an acquired inability to see colors, a deficit termed *achromatopsia*. This acquired form is distinct from congenital achromatopsia, the photoreceptor-based disease discussed earlier. Patients with achromatopsia cannot recognize colors—everything looks gray to them—even though there is no damage to color processing in the retina, lateral geniculate nucleus, or primary visual cortex. Thus, achromatopsia represents a deficit in the recognition or interpretation of a viewed object rather than a problem with the view itself.

Patients with deficits in perceiving motion are very rare—so rare that no medical name exists for this disorder. The most famous such patient, LM, was severely impaired by her inability to see smooth movement trajectories. In place of natural movement, LM saw objects jump unexpectedly and unpredictably from one place to another. The lips of a talking person looked like they were hopping about and liquid flowing into a container looked frozen in air. Moving cars appeared as sequential snapshots that appeared in new places unexpectedly, making it extremely tricky to distinguish the direction of traffic. As a consequence, LM experienced understanding speech, filling a measuring cup, and crossing the street as anywhere from confusing to frightening.

The rare impairments in the understanding of selective visual attributes described here provide a dramatic peek into ordinary brain processes that thankfully work so well in most of us.

DORSAL AND VENTRAL STREAMS PROCESS VISUAL INPUT IN PARALLEL

After the primary visual cortex, form, texture, and color information is sent ventrally toward the inferotemporal cortex, while motion and depth information primarily funnels into the dorsal stream bound for parietal cortex. The dorsal stream is very important in guiding movements, both those that we generate ourselves and those of others. For example, when we see a particularly delectable piece of fruit, the dorsal part of the dorsal stream helps us understand where that fruit exists in the world and where it will be by the time we reach out to grab it. As we walk along a rocky path, the dorsal stream is critical to understanding where objects are in the world and how we can avoid stumbling on obstacles. The ventral portion of the dorsal stream is also concerned with movements but primarily in understanding others' movements. Using more ventral regions of the dorsal stream, we may grasp the trajectory of another person's swinging fist or realize that the person approaching with outstretched hand intends to shake our hand.

The dorsal parietal cortex appears critical to spatial navigation and visually guided movements, including the use of *tools*. Lesions in this area can cause *ideomotor apraxia* in which individuals cannot execute certain movements such as dressing, setting the table, or cutting an apple (see Chapter 23). Patients with ideomotor apraxia have no motor deficits per se and no sensory visual deficits. Yet they cannot guide their movements using vision. This ventral part of the dorsal stream, centered around the temporoparietal junction, is thought to contribute to understanding others' actions.

The ventral stream is critical to understanding that a smooth red sphere with a thin brown cylinder coming out of the indented top is an apple. In other words, we recognize what optical images represent using the ventral stream. Of particular interest is the *fusiform face area*, a discrete region within the inferotemporal cortex that specializes in recognizing faces, both generically and individually. Thus, the fusiform face area is responsible for recognizing any face as a face and also for identifying individual faces.

As introduced in Chapter 7, *visual agnosia*, arising from damage to the inferotemporal cortex, is a condition marked by a failure to recognize and interpret visual images for their meaning. Agnosia refers to a class of disorders in which objects cannot be recognized or interpreted using a particular sense—in this case vision—although no deficit exists in the sensory pathways. Thus, there is nothing wrong with a patient's eye, retina, lateral geniculate nucleus, or primary visual cortex, and the input to the ventral stream is normal. Nonetheless, patients with visual agnosia experience difficulty in identifying objects using sight even while retaining the ability to identify the same objects using other senses. As described in Chapter 1, Oliver Sacks's patient Dr. P. could not identify a rose by looking at it but immediately recognized the rose by smell.

Visual agnosia is a heterogeneous group of disorders. Some patients show deficits in recognizing all objects, others in recognizing a subset of objects, such as tools. In the latter category, *prosopagnosia* is a particularly intriguing disorder involving the failure to recognize faces. Some *prosopagnostic* patients recognize no faces, including their own, and in fact do not know that they are looking at a face, with faces appearing as just another round object. Other patients may know that they are looking at a face but cannot identify the individual, even when that individual is a family member. Still other prosopagnostic patients may recognize faces but cannot interpret expressive social cues.

The late Oliver Sacks wrote of his own experiences with prosopagnosia in several of his books, including his final one, *On the Move: A Life*. With prosopagnosia, everyday events such as a planned meeting with a friend who "should" be recognizable become challenges that require planning and forethought. Unexpectedly running into a friend or acquaintance often develops into an awkward moment, with the prosopagnostic individual feeling embarrassed and the ignored friend feeling offended. As it turns out, the ability to recognize faces appears to exist on a continuum, with a few who are as exceptional at the task as prosopagnostics are poor. Online tests have been available for some time that test the ability to recognize famous people as well as to distinguish between isolated faces stripped of identifiable features such as hairstyle, skin color, and voice. Most people appear to have middling abilities of face recognition that, when coupled with nonfacial cues, are good enough to enable smooth social interactions.

In sum, prosopagnosia and the other visual agnosias provide a compelling glimpse into the biological categorization of visual objects, a categorization often obscured by classification systems imposed by dominant cultural norms.

WE NEED TO PAY ATTENTION IN ORDER TO SEE

Optical input washes over us unless we attend to what we are looking at. Every day we blink thousands of times and yet we do not perceive the back of our eyelids . . . until now that I have called attention to the blank scene accompanying each blink. It is commonplace that we fail to notice a friend's new hairdo or glasses. Our poor *attention* to visual scenes is central to our abysmal reliability as eyewitnesses. However, when we pay attention to what we are seeing and practice attentive viewing, we can quickly become experts at seeing particular details or types of objects. Such *visual learning* is the central theme in the child's game of "Where's Waldo?" As we find Waldo in one, two, and then three scenes, we become expert at finding the red-and-white striped shirt, blue pants, and floppy hat associated with Waldo. We then start to find Waldo more quickly. In a similar way, we can become expert in visually recognizing, even after only a brief glance, classmates, fossils, birds, airplanes, trees, cars, and so on.

The parietal cortex controls the application of attention to the outside world. Attention is multimodal, meaning that it uses visual, auditory, and somatosensory information, and in fact all sensory input. Curiously, the parietal cortex controls attention asymmetrically. Lesions in the right parietal cortex, typically ventral parietal and temporoparietal regions, can result in the loss of or complete failure to recognize the left side of the world. This condition is called *hemispatial neglect* and is perhaps the single brain disorder that is the most difficult for a healthy individual to imagine or conceptualize. *Anton syndrome*, which, as is true of hemispatial neglect involves anosognosia, may be a runner-up.

Hemispatial neglect results from right hemispheric damage, typically in the ventral parietal lobe caudal to the somatosensory strip and extending caudally toward the temporoparietal junction. The prevailing view is that the right parietal cortex is responsible for applying attention to both left and right parts of the world, whereas the left parietal cortex preferentially applies attention to the right part of the world. Thus, because of the right hemisphere's participation in both left- and right-sided attention, a left hemisphere lesion is not symptomatic whereas a right-sided lesion is.

In patients with hemispatial neglect, the left half of the world simply does not exist. *Neglect dyslexia* can occur in a global or local form. In the global form, patients only read the right half of a page or screen, whereas in the local form, patients read only the right portion of words. The latter involves confusions between words such as light, night, right, tight, bright, and straight. Patients with hemispatial neglect may get into car accidents with the left side of their cars without recognizing it. For example, the late journalist Robert Novak ran into a pedestrian, presumably approaching from the left side, and did not stop. Only blocks later, when confronted by a bicyclist approaching from the right did Mr. Novak stop. Days after this incident, it was announced that Mr. Novak had a brain tumor in the right parietal lobe. Mr. Novak died a little over a year later. There is no treatment for neglect per se. Rather, patients with neglect are treated for the underlying cause—usually a tumor, as in Mr. Novak's case, or a stroke.

The nonexistence of the left half of the world extends beyond perception to action. Patients with hemispatial neglect cannot look to the left or turn to the left. Perhaps the idea of looking to the left is as incomprehensible to the patient with hemispatial neglect as is turning the eyes to look inside one's head is to a healthy individual. As a stroke patient with hemispatial neglect recovers, nonexistence may yield to indifference and eventually to a return to a functional relationship with the left half of the world.

Neglect reminds us in dramatic fashion that vision, indeed perception, is not passive but requires active motor engagement and attention for full appreciation, recognition, and understanding of the outside world.

WE LEARN TO SEE BY VIEWING THE WORLD IN FOCUS

Our ability to interpret points of light—photon hits distributed over the retina—as objects and color and motion and the impetus to move is learned. To learn the trick of converting optical source code into interpretable information we need practice, lots of practice. As babies, we open our eyes upon awakening and start practicing. We move our hand in front of our face and learn how the hand image corresponds to the hand trajectory. Throughout infancy, the experiment of vision continues day in and day out, with the trial-and-error interpretation of millions of scenes and events. Now imagine that, during the practice years, our optical image is obscured, blurred, stretched, or somehow not in correspondence with the physical world. In this case, the daily visual experiments of infancy "won't work." If there is no rhyme or reason to the relationship between the optical image and the tangible world, the brain cannot set up the correct neural circuits to allow for interpretation of new incoming optical images. A person who grows up in a figurative "visual fun house," where images are randomly and unpredictably stretched this way or that, cannot learn the rules that transform photic input into accurate mental images. Therefore, even if this person is placed as an adult into a normal environment and has perfect refractive correction, so that images form crisply on the retina, the brain lacks the capacity—circuits fine-tuned through visual experience—to interpret optical images. Thus, this person will be severely visually impaired and possibly blind.

Not only does vision depend on normal development but also on development that occurs during a *critical period* of an individual's life. The critical period is a developmental phase that favors facile learning of a given natural process. In humans, the critical period for vision is thought to be the first 4 years or so of life. Significant learning also occurs outside of the critical period but occurs optimally and most effortlessly during the critical period. Another example of a critical period is learning a language, which is easiest before the age of 3. Language learning becomes progressively more difficult, albeit not impossible, to learn as a person ages. Although individual differences are commonplace in adult language-learning abilities, all of us learned a language as babies without study or effort, and none of us as adults could learn a new language without both study and effort. A young child can even pick up a second language through apparently effortless absorption from the environment. Similarly, we automatically learn the *language of visual perception* as babies.

Because of the importance of early learning to visual perception, developmental disruption of vision causes permanent, severe, and largely untreatable visual impairment. It produces permanent impairments in visual acuity and eye movements. People with congenital cataracts that are not corrected early in life fail to develop normal vision even if those cataracts are later removed. *Strabismus* (i.e., any misalignment of the eyes) also prevents normal development of visual function. The impairment of adult vision solely as a result of abnormal development is a condition termed *amblyopia. In amblyopia, impaired vision is a consequence of abnormal development and persists even if the original optical problem is resolved.* The most common form of amblyopia results from *anisometropia,* a condition in which the eyes have different refractive errors due to different eye lengths. Anisometropia causes babies to see different images in the two eyes. Thus, the cortex "sees" unmatched, unaligned images, and cortical circuits do not develop correctly. Whenever visual development is impaired, visual acuity is greatly reduced, particularly at high spatial frequencies. Furthermore, one may imagine that it would be difficult to learn where to look if the world appears too blurry. Indeed, eye movements are abnormal in people whose vision is impaired during the critical period, a time when eye movement circuits are also developing.

The story of Mike May dramatically highlights the importance of learning to see at a young age. May was blinded by corneal scarification caused by a chemical accident at the age of 3. More than four decades later, May received a corneal transplant, making his eye patent to light again and opening the possibility of vision. At the time of May's accident at age 3, circuits supporting color and motion vision were more developed than were those for form vision. Therefore, May immediately recognized colors and correctly remembered the color names, names that he had learned before his accident. May discovered that he could kick and catch a moving ball—visually guided movements—without effort. Yet, even years after corrective surgery, May's form vision remains sketchy. May can read 1-inch-high letters that are about 6 inches (15 cm) away. He can see forms such as the moon, buildings, shadows, signs, and people. However, he has difficulty interpreting the forms. Cracks in the sidewalk, steps, and curbs form images that appear indistinguishable to May. He has to use cognitive tricks to tell women from men and to recognize individuals, including family members. May's story provides a fascinating window into vision and into all the visual knowledge that we employ to *accomplish seeing.*

ADDITIONAL READING

Anstis SM. A chart demonstrating variations in acuity with retinal position. *Vision Res.* 14: 589–592, 1974.

Barton JJS. Disorders of face perception and recognition. *Neurol Clin.* 21: 501–520, 2003.

Berson DM. Strange vision: Ganglion cells as photoreceptors. *Trends Neurosci.* 26: 314–320, 2003.

Dowling JE. *The Retina: An Approachable Part of the Brain.* Boston: Belknap Press, 1987.

Fain GL. Why photoreceptors die (and why they don't). *BioEssays.* 28: 344–354, 2006.

Hartong DT, Berson EL, Dryja TP. Retinitis pigmentosa. *Lancet.* 368: 1795–1809, 2006.

Husain M, Nachev P. Space and the parietal cortex. *Trends Cogn Sci.* 11: 30–36, 2007.

Kurson R. *Crashing Through.* New York: Random House, 2007.

Maida JM, Mathers K, Alley CL. Pediatric ophthalmology in the developing world. *Curr Opin Opthalmol.* 19: 403–408, 2008.

Morgan IG. The biological basis for myopic refractive error. *Clin Exp Optometry.* 86: 276–288, 2003.

Nathans J. In the eye of the beholder: Visual pigments and inherited variation in human vision. *Cell.* 78: 357–360, 1994.

Riddoch MJ, Humphreys GW. Visual agnosia. *Neurol Clin.* 21: 521–548, 2003.

Rodieck RW. *The First Steps in Seeing.* Sunderland, MA: Sinauer Associates, 1998.

Rodriguez AR, Barton JJ. The 20/20 patient who can't read. *Can J Ophthalmol.* 50: 257–264, 2015.

Sacks O. *On the Move: A Life.* New York: Vintage Books, 2015.

Sacks O. *The Mind's Eye.* New York: Vintage Books, 2010.

Strauss O. The retinal pigment epithelium in vision. *Physiol Rev.* 85: 845–881, 2005.

Shevell SK, Kingdom FAA. Color in complex scenes. *Annu Rev Psychol.* 59: 143–166, 2008.

Trevino SG, Villazana-Espinoza ET, Muniz A, Tsin ATC. Retinoid cycles in the cone-dominated chicken retina. *J Exp Biology.* 208: 4151–4157, 2005.

Walls GL. *The Vertebrate Eye and Its Adaptive Radiation.* New York: Hafner Publishing Company, 1967.

16.

AUDITION

COMMUNICATION PORTAL

HEARING IS THE MAJOR HUMAN
PORTAL FOR INTERPERSONAL
COMMUNICATION

We care a great deal about hearing because most of us communicate through spoken language. Congenital deafness or hearing loss acquired during adulthood profoundly changes the course of one's life by severely reducing the ability to connect with others. The most devastating part of hearing loss or deafness is the social isolation, to one degree or another, that results. As Ludwig Van Beethoven wrote in 1802, when the great composer was already hard of hearing, "I [am] compelled to keep myself apart and conduct my life in solitude. . . . Not for me the invigorating company of my fellow man, the refinements of conversation, the mutual outpourings of human sentiment. I am utterly alone . . . , condemned to the life of an exile." Helen Keller, deafened and blinded by illness before the age of 2, wrote that "deafness is a much worse misfortune" than blindness.

There is no uniform or even predominant reaction to hearing loss or deafness, a heterogeneity attributable to the wide variety of personal histories and circumstances associated with the loss. Probably the most important factor is whether an individual loses hearing before or after developing language, termed pre- or postlingually, respectively. A system of communication must be provided to prelingual deaf babies both in order to combat social isolation and for normal brain development. Along with the age at which hearing loss occurs, the quality of an individual's past experience with spoken language, temperament, community support, and available resources all influence the response to hearing deficits. Individuals with poor hearing prior to deafness have a very different experience from those who become deaf after enjoying normal hearing. As with the differences in experiences, affected individuals cope differently with the inherent challenges of living with hearing loss or deafness. A number of superbly written memoirs, listed at the end of this chapter, are worthwhile reading for anyone interested in understanding the varied effects of hearing impairments on human lives.

As you recall, dysfunction of sensory systems leads to positive signs such as a perception of pins and needles in the case of somatosensation. In the case of hearing, *tinnitus* or ringing in the ear almost always accompanies hearing loss and may even be the first sign of impending deafness, as was the case with the great composer Ludwig van Beethoven. Now that cochlear implants can restore hearing to deafened individuals, we have learned that along with the return of hearing comes a resolution of tinnitus. Moreover, the congenitally deaf, who have never had hearing, do not experience tinnitus. Thus, tinnitus is linked mechanistically to the *loss of hearing*; fix the hearing, and the tinnitus will resolve as well.

HEARING REQUIRES SOUND
CONDUCTION FOLLOWED
BY SENSORINEURAL PROCESSING

The ear consists of three parts: outer, middle, and inner (Fig. 16-1). The outer and middle ears conduct airborne sounds to the inner ear, which serves our vestibular sense of head position and motion as well as hearing. We will consider vestibular function in Chapter 18 and restrict ourselves to hearing here.

Hearing involves two steps that are vulnerable to damage or disease: conduction and sensorineural processing. These steps are accomplished peripherally by the outer and middle ears and the inner ear, respectively. This categorization is used clinically to describe hearing loss and thus is important to understand:

- *Conduction* refers to the ushering of airborne sounds through the external and middle ear and to the

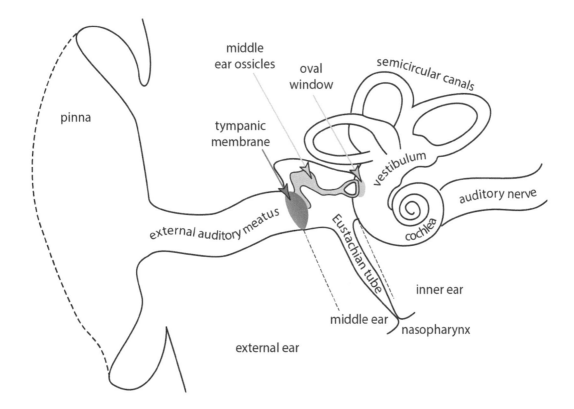

Figure 16-1 The ear is divided into external, middle, and inner compartments. The external ear includes the pinna and the external auditory meatus or ear canal. The tympanic membrane forms the border between the external and middle ears. The middle ear is a closed chamber with only one way out, the Eustachian tube. At rest, the Eustachian tube is closed at the pharyngeal end. The middle ear ossicles (*shown all together in ochre*) physically convey vibrations of the tympanic membrane to the inner ear via the oval window. The oval window opens onto the fluid-filled cochlea, which contains the hair cells that support hearing. The auditory nerve contains the axons of spiral ganglion cells that carry cochlear input into the central nervous system. The spiral ganglion cells are located within the cochlea itself (not shown).

threshold of the inner ear. Importantly, conduction involves amplification of the stimulus magnitude. Therefore, although the intensity of incoming sound inevitably decreases before arriving at the inner ear, it does not decrease by as much as would occur without the *amplification* accomplished within the external and middle ear. This amplification is passive or mechanical, dependent solely on the physical properties of the external and middle ears. The ultimate result of conduction is that airborne pressure waves are transformed into fluid pressure waves within the fluid-filled spaces of the cochlea.

• *Sensorineural* transduction and processing include transduction by cochlear hair cells and an *active* amplification step called *cochlear amplification* that is also accomplished by hair cells. Hair cells (non-neural sensory cells) transmit information across a synapse to *spiral ganglion neurons*. The ultimate output from the spiral ganglion cells consists of trains of action potentials. The axons of spiral ganglion cells travel

through the vestibulocochlear nerve to serve as the afferents to the central nervous system (CNS).

The conductive step in audition serves to capture airborne sounds and transform those sounds into fluid pressure waves. The external and middle ear are responsible for the capture, conduction, and air-to-fluid transformation of sound. As sound travels through the external ear, its intensity increases (Fig. 16-2). This amplification step is beneficial because almost half of the sound intensity that arrives at the *tympanic membrane*, the border between the external and middle ear that is commonly referred to as the eardrum, does not make it through to the cochlea. Airborne pressure waves move the tympanic membrane, which in turn moves a series of *ossicles*, tiny bones in the middle ear. Movement of the chain of ossicles results in the *stapes*, the final ossicle in the chain, beating upon the *oval window* of the fluid-filled cochlea within the inner ear (Fig. 16-1). Because of this arrangement, about 60% of the sound energy that reaches the tympanic membrane makes it through to the cochlea. In sum, stimulus magnitude is increased by travel through

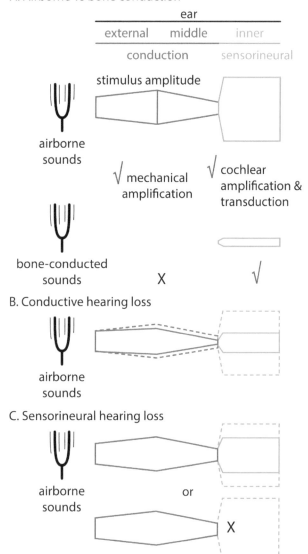

A. Airborne vs bone conduction

ear

external   middle   inner

conduction   sensorineural

stimulus amplitude

airborne
sounds

√ mechanical
amplification

√ cochlear
amplification &
transduction

bone-conducted
sounds

X   √

B. Conductive hearing loss

airborne
sounds

C. Sensorineural hearing loss

airborne
sounds

or

X

Figure 16-2 A: Airborne and bone-conducted sounds are processed differently by the ear. In this diagram, the amplitude of the stimulus is denoted by the height of the polygons. Airborne sounds are amplified by passing through the external and middle ear. These sounds arrive at the inner ear as pressure waves within the cochlea. Within the inner ear, an active process, cochlear amplification, further amplifies the pressure wave, which is then transduced into a graded potential in the hair cell. The final step of sensorineural processing within the inner ear is the synaptic transmission from the hair cell to spiral ganglion cells. Bone-conducted sounds reach the inner ear directly, without passing through the external and middle ears. Although cochlear amplification, transduction, and synaptic transmission all still occur, the starting stimulus is small because it has not been amplified by normal conduction. B: Conduction hearing loss occurs for a variety of reasons, including impacted earwax or a punctured eardrum. As a result, the stimulus delivered to the inner ear is smaller in magnitude (*solid lines*) than what would be delivered if conduction were normal (*dotted lines*). The consequence is that the ultimate effect of cochlear amplification is correspondingly reduced. There are practical or surgical solutions for most types of conduction hearing loss. C: Age-related hearing loss is due to a loss of cochlear amplification (*top panel*) or to a diminution of synaptic transmission from the hair cells to the spiral ganglion cells (*bottom panel*), with the external and middle ear working normally. When cochlear amplification is diminished or even abolished, the result is a profound hearing loss. Sensorineural hearing loss is typically treated with a *hearing aid*, which boosts the conduction amplification prior to the inner ear. The delivery of a larger stimulus to the inner ear mitigates the loss of cochlear amplification but does not replace it. Most congenital forms of deafness occur because of a deficit in either transduction or synaptic transmission (x in bottom panel). The only treatment for this type of sensorineural deafness is a cochlear implant.

the external ear and decreased by conduction through the middle ear.

The cochlea, the portion of the inner ear important for hearing, is fluid-filled with *perilymph*, similar to extracellular fluid elsewhere, and *endolymph*, a potassium ion (K^+)-rich fluid that fills the space around the sensory end organ. Sound at different frequencies is distributed in the form of waves of fluid pressure to different parts of the cochlea. This distribution is the basis for the gross *tonotopy* of the cochlea. Sensory cells in the cochlea itself then amplify pressure waves of different frequencies to fine-tune the tonotopic map. The pressure waves move the stereocilia of the hair cells, the stimulus for sensory transduction. Graded potentials in hair cells lead to a change in the amount of neurotransmitter released from the hair cell onto spiral ganglion afferents. Finally, spiral ganglion cells carry sound

information from the cochlea, through the vestibulocochlear nerve, to the cochlear nuclei of the rostral medulla.

Central processing of cochlear input transforms sound information into hearing but also alerts us to unexpected sounds and to the location of sound sources. Most important to the human experience, the CNS allows us to interpret meaning from acoustic sounds, including speech. In this chapter, we focus on the latter process. Within the nervous system, auditory information from the two ears is combined almost immediately (see Fig. 6-12). As a result, central auditory pathways above the cochlear nuclei carry redundant auditory information. Consequently, lesions within the brainstem and thalamus do not produce symptomatic difficulties for humans. Therefore, we describe ear function in some detail and then skip from the auditory nerve to cortex to consider how we make sense of the sounds that we hear and to consider in particular how we both produce and understand speech.

Corresponding to the exclusively peripheral vulnerability of hearing, hearing problems, including both deafness and hard of hearing conditions, are classified into two major categories: *conductive* or *sensorineural*. This classification of hearing loss reflects the division of labor between the external and middle ear on one hand and the inner ear on the other. External and middle ear deficits lead to conductive hearing loss, whereas cochlear problems with the *stria vascularis*, hair cells, spiral ganglion afferents, or their synaptic connections produce sensorineural hearing loss. After stepping through the mechanisms of hearing, we will examine the clinical tests that can distinguish between the two types of hearing loss.

PRESSURE WAVES ARE THE STIMULUS FOR HEARING

The stimulus for sound is a pressure wave. The pressure must act on something to produce a sound; no sound arises from a vacuum. In the case of airborne sounds (the stimulus for hearing), sound acts on the molecules of the atmosphere. Sound produces alternately *compression*, an increase in pressure, and *rarefaction*, a reduction in pressure. As with visual and mechanical stimuli, auditory stimuli can be broken down into component sine waves, sometimes a few and, more typically, a great number. The amplitude and frequency of the component sine waves greatly influence perceived *loudness* and *pitch*.

Sound waves dominated by a periodic component are perceived as *tonal* whereas those without a dominant frequency sound are perceived as *noisy*. The lowest frequency with power is called the *fundamental frequency* (f_0) and is typically perceived as the pitch of the sound. For example, single tones are perceived as whistles whose pitch varies directly with the frequency of the tone. Tones can also be accompanied by harmonics that consist of sounds at integer multiples of the fundamental frequency. For example, middle C in Western music has a frequency of about 261.6 Hz. Therefore, when a person plays middle C on a piano, the pressure waves that come out have power at frequencies of $2*f_0$ (= 1st harmonic = 523), $3*f_0$ (= 2nd harmonic = 785), $4*f_0$ (= 3rd harmonic = 1,047), and so on, as well as at the fundamental frequency. The perceived pitch of tones with harmonics depends not only on the fundamental frequency but also on the relative power of the various harmonics.

The difference between the fundamental frequencies of speech and the frequencies used to transmit speech by telephone highlights the importance of harmonic frequencies to perception (Fig. 16-3). The fundamental frequency of speech averages about 130 Hz for men and 200 Hz for women. Yet these frequencies are below the frequencies transmitted by telephone (300–3,400 Hz). Thus, speech comprehension relies heavily on the harmonics of the fundamental frequencies involved and can even be supported by the harmonics alone. The range of frequencies used to understand direct conversations (100–5,000 Hz) is broader than the *voice range* used in telephony. In a similar way, appreciation of speech depends on a range of frequencies

Figure 16-3 The frequency ranges (*brown lines at top*) used to understand speech, including several phonemes; transmit speech by telephone; and appreciate orchestral music are illustrated along with the fundamental frequencies of speech and orchestral instruments (*dashed lines delimited by asterisks*). In the graph below are idealized audiograms for normal hearing and presbycusis (age-related hearing loss). To generate an audiogram, sounds of varied frequencies and amplitudes are played into an ear and the patient presses a button every time that she detects a sound. In this way, audiograms for each ear show the minimum threshold for perceiving tones of different frequencies. Note that audiograms are customarily shown with an inverted intensity scale. Normally, the detection threshold is close to 0 dB, defined as the typical detection threshold. In presbycusis, age-related hearing loss, perceptual thresholds for higher frequencies are elevated so that a shout as loud as a jet engine is needed for a person to detect sound frequencies that should be easily detected when spoken at the intensity of a whisper. The approximate intensity in decibels of a whisper, conversation, and rock concert are shown by the italicized words.

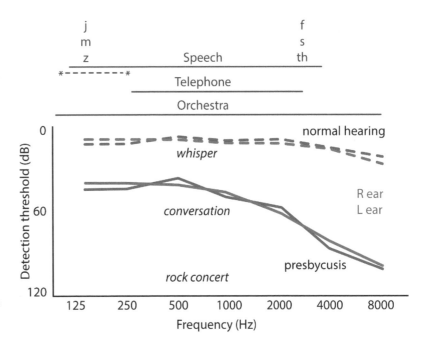

that is far wider and greater than the range of speech fundamental frequencies.

Although perceived pitch increases as fundamental frequency increases and decreases as fundamental frequency decreases, pitch is influenced by features of incident sound beyond simply the fundamental frequency. Auditory illusions take advantage of these additional influences on pitch perception. For instance, a sound that has power at 523, 785, 1,047, and so on will be perceived as a middle C even if the fundamental frequency of middle C (261 Hz) is not present at all in the acoustic stimulus. Nonacoustic factors can also influence our perception of pitch.

The *loudness* of a sound is related to the amplitude of the pressure wave. Our auditory system is extremely sensitive. In fact, we would hear blood whooshing through capillaries if they were nearby. As it turns out, the capillaries supplying the inner ear are located far enough away from the hair cells that we do not hear blood pulsing within. Our ability to "hear the ocean in a seashell" is in fact due to the extreme sensitivity of our auditory system. You can imitate this by simply cupping your hand or a large glass over your ears. The whoosh that you hear is your perception of the resonating motion of air molecules amplified by passage through the external ear.

Pitch and loudness are not enough to describe the rich variety of sounds that we perceive. An additional aspect of sound is *timbre*. Because of a difference in the sound envelope, the middle C produced by a guitar, an oboe, and a human voice are distinguishable. The distinction of sounds with different timbres but the same fundamental frequency depends on three factors:

- *The frequencies present*: The number of harmonics present and the power in each of these harmonics varies across sounds with different timbres. In addition to variation in the harmonics, there may be *inharmonics*, frequencies that are noninteger multiples of the fundamental frequency.

- *The envelope waveform*: The form of the sound envelope, including the rise and decay times of a sound, differs across sounds with different timbres.

- *Vibrato*: Natural sounds such as the human voice have a modulated or changing fundamental frequency.

The human auditory system is optimized for speech. Yet we respond to sounds in a variety of frequency ranges and at variable intensities. Even within speech sounds, there is variation in the frequency of different phonemes. For example, sounds such as the /f/ and /s/ of "fear" and "sum" are far higher in frequency than are sounds such as the /z/ and /m/ of "zoo" and "mind" (Fig. 16-3).

THE EXTERNAL EAR FUNNELS AND AMPLIFIES SOUNDS

The outer ear or pinna collects sound and funnels it into the external auditory meatus (Fig. 16-1). In an analogous way to an organ pipe or a flute, the external auditory meatus acts as a *resonance tube*, meaning that sound waves bounce back and forth in the canal and summate through constructive interference. The result is that *the amplitude of pressure waves increases by 5–10 dB as the waves travel through the external ear* (see Box 16-1). To appreciate the acoustic amplification

---

Box 16-1 **DECIBELS ARE A RELATIVE MEASURE OF SOUND PRESSURE**

The *bel* is a term, named after Alexander Graham Bell, that describes the relative amplitude, or loudness, of one sound in comparison to a standard sound. The bel is an enormous unit and is virtually never used. Instead we talk of *decibels*, which are tenths of bels and are abbreviated as *dB*. Decibels are typically computed for sound pressure as:

$$dB = 20 \log \frac{P_1}{P_0}$$

where P_1 is the sound whose loudness is being measured and P_0 is the standard sound pressure.

The standard sound pressure (P_0) used to define bels is that of a just-detectable sound. Thus, a sound that exerts 10 times the sound pressure ($P_1 = 10*P_0$) at the human threshold for sound will be a 20 dB sound ($P_1/P_0 = 10$; log [10] = 1). The range of sound intensities in modern life extends from less than 10 dB—the soft breathing of a sleeping infant—to 130 dB or more—a nearby siren. The loudness of a sound decreases as one moves away from the sound source and as obstacles are interposed between the sound source and the ear. A jet engine located a football field away produces a roughly 150 dB sound but when aloft at 30,000 feet, or about 9,000 meters, the same engine sounds far less loud. Similarly, very close to a jackhammer, sound levels are greater than 100 dB but are greatly reduced by simply covering the ears. Hearing damage can occur with long-term exposure to sounds as soft as 80 dB and more rapidly upon exposure to sounds of 120 dB or higher, levels reached at some live music performances, as well as at some construction sites.

provided by a tube, compare what you hear when you blow into air (nothing) versus when you blow into a beer bottle (a tone). The increase in sound wave ampltitude is a result of constructive interference at the resonating frequency. The resonating frequency depends primarily on the length of the tube. You can easily remember this by thinking of the register of various wind instruments: the sound of the very short piccolo is far higher than the bass tones of the long and winding contrabassoon. The geometry of the human auditory canal is such that frequencies of 2,000–5,500 Hz, the core frequency range of human speech, resonate within the canal (Fig. 16-3). This means that the amplitude of sound waves with frequencies of 2,000–5,500 Hz is selectively increased, whereas sound waves outside of this frequency range are either unaltered or decreased in amplitude (through destructive interference).

Sebaceous glands lining the ear canal produce *cerumen*, or earwax, which has the positive effect of lubricating the external auditory meatus. However, cerumen can build up, obstructing the ear canal and impairing hearing by blocking airborne pressure waves from accessing the tympanic membrane. With enough accumulation, cerumen may become impacted and difficult to remove. Impacted cerumen occurs fairly commonly, particularly among nursing home residents and intellectually disabled individuals who may not adequately care for themselves. Impaired hearing due to impacted cerumen decreases social communication and can therefore cause great distress to individuals, particularly those in vulnerable populations.

Removal of impacted cerumen is accomplished mechanically using some kind of manual scoop or by irrigation with saline or a *ceruminolytic*, a compound that breaks down cerumen. Although aggressive treatment of impacted cerumen is warranted, care should be taken because treatment options can produce several potential complications, such as perforation of the tympanic membrane.

The external auditory meatus ends in the conically shaped *tympanic membrane* or eardrum. Pressure waves that enter the ear canal cause movement of the tympanic membrane. As a result, the membrane oscillates back and forth at the frequency of the incident wave. The tympanic membrane is the bridge between the external ear and the middle ear.

THE MIDDLE EAR TRANSFERS ENERGY FROM AIR TO THE FLUID-FILLED INNER EAR

The middle ear is a closed bony chamber with one outlet, the *Eustachian tube* (Fig. 16-1) that leads to the throat (see Box 16-2). The middle ear forms the bridge between the external ear

---

Box 16-2 THE EUSTACHIAN TUBE IS THE ONLY POTENTIAL OUTLET FROM THE MIDDLE EAR

The Eustachian tube runs from the middle ear to the pharynx, or upper throat. On the pharyngeal side, the Eustachian tube normally sits in a closed position (Fig. 16-1). During swallowing, pharyngeal muscles pull on and then elevate the soft palate and in so doing, pump the contents of the tube. Opening and closing the mouth using large jaw movements can approximate the effect of swallowing. In either case, the Eustachian tube is not opened in the sense that it affords free passage from the middle ear to the throat all at once. Rather, swallowing propels the tubular contents, both gaseous and fluid, through the tube, in both directions. After enough iterations, this action allows equilibration between the pressure and contents within the middle ear and within the pharynx. Pharyngeal pressure is equivalent to atmospheric pressure. Thus, when descending rapidly from a higher to a lower altitude, as during an airplane landing or an elevator descent, the pressure in the middle ear is lower than the atmospheric pressure of the lower altitude. To equilibrate these pressures, we chew gum or repeatedly open and close our mouth.

In an upright adult, the middle ear is located just above the pharyngeal exit point of the Eustachian tube, whereas in a supine person, the reverse is true. This means that, normally, as we move around, fluid accumulated in the middle ear drains through the Eustachian tube and exits into the throat during swallowing. Certain conditions hamper the drainage of middle ear fluid. Some people simply have a congenitally narrow Eustachian tube. In individuals born with a *cleft palate*, the insertions of the muscles surrounding the Eustachian tube are changed in such a way that greatly hinders or prevents *milking*, meaning pumping, of the Eustachian tube contents. When mucus cannot be drained, infections in the middle ear, termed *otitis media*, worsen; in the most severe instances, these can cause rupture of the tympanic membrane. The middle ear and the tympanic membrane receive a dense innervation from nociceptors, and, consequently, middle ear infections are painful, sometimes severely so. Although the tympanic membrane often regrows spontaneously, it sometimes fails to do so; in such cases, surgical replacement, *tympanoplasty*, can be used to restore function.

In infants and children, the muscles that surround the Eustachian tube compress the tube but in adults, these same muscles are stretched away from the tube. This difference in muscle anatomy combined with a shallower tube trajectory in children renders drainage from the middle ear more difficult in children than in adults. Therefore, early in the course of a respiratory infection, mucus may move from the pharynx *to* the middle ear chamber, particularly when an individual is supine, as during sleep. Eventually, inflammation associated with infections can keep the Eustachian tube in a closed position at the pharyngeal end.

The anatomical features of the Eustachian tube peculiar to infants, combined with an inability to be instructed on how to swallow, cause prelingual infants to have a very difficult time equilibrating pressure in the pharynx and middle ear. The discomfort resulting from unequal pressures is likely a major reason why babies and infants cry during airplane rides, particularly during takeoffs and landings.

and the cochlea within the inner ear. On the external ear side is the tympanic membrane, and on the inner ear side is the *oval window*, the input portal to the cochlea. By virtue of transmission through the middle ear, the energy transfer from airborne pressure waves to fluid pressure waves (in the cochlea of the inner ear) is maximized.

Sound waves arrive through *air*, but the cochlea, where sensory transduction occurs, is a *fluid*-filled structure. When sound waves traveling through air hit water, they are reflected back into the air and, for the most part, do not enter water. Indeed, when we put our heads under water, we are deaf to even the loudest airborne shouts. The middle ear solves this problem. Airborne sound waves move the tympanic membrane, which moves middle ear ossicles, and the latter movement sets up fluid movements in the inner ear. Consequently, we lose less than half of the energy contained within incident sound when that sound transfers through the middle ear: about 40% of the sound energy present at the tympanic membrane is lost at the level of the cochlea. A 40% loss is a vast improvement over the roughly 99% loss of sound energy that would occur if airborne sound encountered water directly.

The three ossicles in the middle ear are, from outside to inside, the *malleus, incus,* and *stapes* (Fig. 16-4A). The malleus attaches to the internal surface of the tympanic membrane on the distal (relative to the brain) side and to the incus on the proximal side. The incus attaches to the stapes, the inner-most middle ear bone. The stapes moves the oval window of the cochlea back and forth. The ossicles in the middle ear are so light that minute vibrations of the tympanic membrane are enough to move them.

The physical arrangement of the three ossicles amplifies sound pressure primarily because the area of the tympanic membrane is roughly 15 times greater than the contact area between the stapes and the oval window (Fig. 16-4B). Since

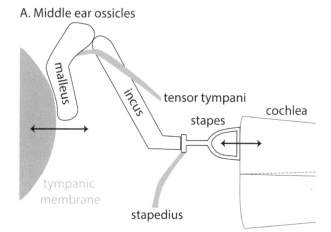

A. Middle ear ossicles

B. Amplification due to reduction in surface area

C. Tensor tympani action

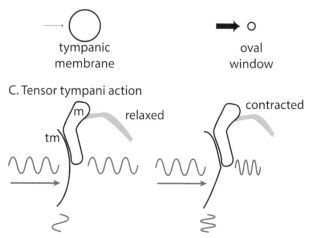

Figure 16-4 A: The three ossicles of the middle ear form a physical link between the tympanic membrane and the cochlea. The malleus attaches to the back of the tympanic membrane and to the incus. The incus then attaches to the stapes, which pushes on the oval window of the cochlea. The two middle ear muscles (*blue*), the tensor tympani, and the stapedius, attach to the neck of the malleus and the head of the stapes, respectively. B: Most of the amplification achieved by the middle ear results from the transfer of the force exerted on the large tympanic membrane onto the far smaller oval window. The increase in sound pressure, proportional to the width of the arrows, is about 15 times greater on the oval window than on the tympanic membrane. C: When the tensor tympani contracts, it pulls the malleus (*m*) and stretches the tympanic membrane (*tm*). Stretching the tympanic membrane results in higher frequency and slightly lower amplitude vibrations (*red sine waves*) of the eardrum in response to any given displacement, thus changing the characteristics of the stimulus that arrives at the cochlea.

the entire force of the sound on the eardrum is focused onto the small stapes, the pressure—force per unit area—is amplified by about 15 times. The mechanical advantage of the decrease in surface area from the tympanic membrane to the stapes is primarily responsible for the efficiency of sound transfer from the tympanic membrane to the cochlea.

In *otosclerosis*, the stapes forms a bony attachment to the temporal bone that circles the oval window. If stapes movement is restricted or blocked altogether, conductive hearing loss results, usually in both ears, and is accompanied by tinnitus. About half of the cases of otosclerosis are sporadic, occurring for reasons that we cannot identify. The other half of otosclerosis cases are inherited, with most produced by an autosomally inherited dominant mutation. Although most familial cases of otosclerosis show a dominant pattern of inheritance, the penetrance of the disease is only about 40%, meaning that 60% of the individuals who inherit the mutation do not develop the disease. It appears likely that mutations in several different genes, including some inherited through a recessive pattern, can give rise to otosclerosis.

Patients with otosclerosis typically present with hearing loss in their twenties. Luckily, a straightforward surgical treatment exists for this condition: replacement of the frozen stapes with a prosthetic device that acts like a piston on the inner ear. Often, postsurgical swelling transiently impairs conduction through the eighth cranial nerve, with the result that patients often experience transient hearing loss and/or vertigo, the latter reflective of vestibular damage. With time, these deficits usually resolve. An additional potential complication is facial palsy. The facial nerve courses through a canal in the wall of the middle ear, adjacent to the oval window and normally separated from the middle ear chamber by a thin sheath of bone. However, in some people, the facial nerve canal is *dehiscent*, meaning that the nerve is not covered by a thin layer of bone but actually enters the middle ear chamber, sometimes coursing near the oval window. In individuals with this condition, which is typically present bilaterally, facial palsy is a particular risk with any middle ear surgery. This consideration is important when surgical intervention on both ears is required or when a surgical redo is needed.

TWO MUSCLES MODULATE SOUND TRANSFER THROUGH THE MIDDLE EAR

As its name suggests, the *tensor tympani* muscle modulates the tension of the eardrum. The tensor tympani stretches from the malleus to the side of the Eustachian tube. When the muscle contracts, the malleus is pulled medially, and this in turn pulls on and therefore tightens the tympanic membrane (Fig. 16-4C). Just as is the case when a drumhead is tightened, tightening the tympanic membrane increases the frequency and decreases the amplitude of vibrations. Recall from Chapter 5 that the trigeminal nerve innervates the tensor tympani along with the muscles of mastication. The tensor tympani contracts during both chewing and speech. Chewing and speech set up pressure waves that arise from either the meeting of teeth in bites or from the larynx; these waves travel through bone to the inner ear. When the tensor tympani contracts, the frequency of incoming airborne sounds increases, allowing for better differentiation between external (airborne) and internal (traveling through bone) sounds. In other words, incoming speech is transformed to a higher frequency and is thus easier to distinguish from the lower frequencies of one's own chewing or speaking sounds. Tensor tympani contraction is neither a reflex nor a voluntary action; it is a centrally commanded (skeletal) muscle contraction that automatically accompanies the specific noise-producing actions of speech and mastication.

In response to loud sounds, the second middle ear muscle, the *stapedius*, contracts reflexively and thereby pulls the stapes back away from the oval window. When the stapedius is contracted, the stapes cannot hit the oval window as forcefully, and this reduces the amount of pressure that is communicated to the cochlea. In response to loud noises—higher than about 70–80 dB—the stapedius contracts within about 100 ms, resulting in an attenuation of ensuing sounds by up to 40 dB. The end result is that loud environments produce less stimulation of the cochlea through the reflexive activation of the stapedius muscle.

THE SENSORY REGION OF THE COCHLEA SITS WITHIN THE CENTER OF A U-SHAPED FLUID-FILLED TUBE

The three-dimensional anatomy of the inner ear is complicated because the bony cochlea forms a spiral, wide at its base and narrow at the apex. Yet, if we unroll the spiral and look at the flattened cochlea, the essential organization is fairly simple (Fig. 16-5). At the base of the fluid-filled cochlea is the oval window upon which the stapes presses. The stapes moves the oval window toward and away from a U-shaped, perilymph-filled cochlear compartment composed of two different regions joined by a narrow canal. The region adjoining the oval window is the *scala vestibuli* or the vestibular canal. The scala vestibuli runs from the oval window at the base of the cochlea to the tip of the cochlear spiral, where it connects through the *helicotrema* to the *scala tympani* or the tympanic canal. At the basal end of the scala tympani is the *round window*, a membranous structure similar to the oval window. Because of the connection at the helicotrema, there is no actual divider between the perilymph-filled scala vestibuli and scala tympani.

Between the scala vestibuli and scala tympani runs the *cochlear duct*, the sensory region of the cochlea. The cochlear duct spirals up the center of the bony cochlea but

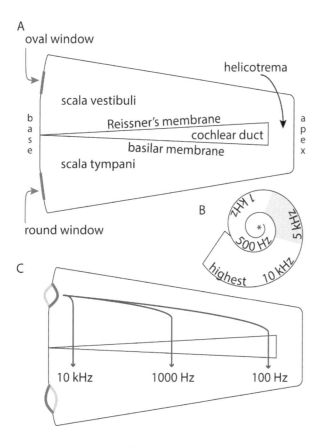

the *basilar membrane*, and the separation between the scala vestibuli and the cochlear duct is *Reissner's membrane*. Like the scala vestibuli and scala tympani, the cochlear duct is filled with fluid but the fluid in the cochlear duct is endolymph rather than perilymph (see more later). Importantly, *the cochlear duct is flexible, so that pressure waves move the cochlear duct up and down* (i.e., toward the scala vestibuli or toward the scala tympani) at the frequency of incoming sound.

INPUT AT THE OVAL WINDOW IS TRANSFORMED INTO A WAVE OF MOVEMENT ACROSS THE COCHLEAR DUCT

When the stapes hits the oval window, a pressure wave travels up the scala vestibuli and then across the cochlear duct to the scala tympani before traveling down the scala tympani to the round window (Fig. 16-5C). Because the cochlea is surrounded by unyielding bone, two pressure valves are needed to support any movement of the fluid within. Just as liquid does not come out of a single pinhole in a soda can, *movement of the oval window only produces a pressure wave because a second compressible portal, the round window, exists*. Compression at the oval window results in rarefaction at the round window, and rarefaction at the oval window produces compression of the round window.

Airborne sounds that arrive at different frequencies set up movements of the oval window at corresponding frequencies. The movement of the oval window in turn sets up a pressure wave at a given frequency that travels through the cochlea. Pressure waves of decreasing frequencies cross the cochlear duct at increasingly more apical points along the cochlear spiral (Fig. 16-5B, C). Thus, pressure waves at the highest frequency represented in the human cochlea (20,000 Hz) move the cochlear duct at the base of the spiral; pressure waves with low frequencies (less than 200 Hz) move the cochlear duct closest to the helicotrema.

An important mechanism of tonotopy is the flexibility of the stiffest part of the cochlear duct, the basilar membrane. Recall that the basilar membrane forms the border between the cochlear duct and the scala tympani. At the base of the cochlear spiral, the basilar membrane is narrow, and, at the cochlear apex, the basilar membrane is wide (Fig. 16-5A). Note that the dimensions of the bony cochlea and those of the cochlear duct are inversely arranged:

Figure 16-5 A: The inner ear is illustrated in a simplified diagram of the unrolled cochlea. The scala vestibuli, cochlear duct, and scala tympani are all fluid-filled compartments within the cochlea. Reissner's membrane separates the cochlear duct from the scala vestibuli, and the basilar membrane separates the cochlear duct from the scala tympani. The helicotrema is a narrow channel that connects the scala vestibuli and scala tympani at the apex of the cochlea. Movement of the oval window sends a pressure wave through the scala vestibuli. The pressure wave crosses through the cochlear duct and then moves down the scala tympani to impact the round window. B: A rough outline of the tonotopy in the cochlea is illustrated on a cartoon of the bony cochlea viewed from the apex (*asterisk*). The shaded region shows the area where most speech processing occurs. C: Compression at the oval window results in rarefaction at the round window (*red arcs*). Conversely, rarefaction at the oval window results in compression at the round window (*dim brown arcs*). Pressure waves of different frequencies pass through the cochlear duct at different locations along the base-to-apex axis. The highest frequency sounds, about 20 kHz, displace the cochlear duct at the base, and the lowest frequency ones, about 5–10 Hz, at the apex. Note that the bony cochlea is wide at its base and narrow at the apex but that the orientation of the cochlear duct is reversed, narrow at the base and wide at the apex.

has the opposite orientation, with a narrow base and a wide apex (Fig. 16-5A). The cochlear duct separates the scala vestibuli and scala tympani for most of their lengths, ending just short of the cochlear apex, where the helicotrema joins the two canals. The cochlear duct shares one wall with the scala vestibuli and one wall with the scala tympani. The wall between the cochlear duct and the scala tympani is

- The narrowest part of the cochlear duct is located at the widest part of the bony cochlea.

- The wide base of the cochlear duct is located at the narrow apex of the bony cochlea.

The narrow basilar membrane at the base of the cochlea is stiffest and therefore moves maximally in response to high-frequency pressure waves. In contrast, at the apex of the cochlea, the wide basilar membrane is relatively loose and bends maximally in response to low-frequency pressure waves. Consequently, the basilar membrane moves maximally in response to sounds of progressively lower frequencies as one moves from the base of the cochlea to its apex. This topographic arrangement of maximal pressure wave excursion along the length of the cochlea follows a tonotopic organization. The tonotopy of the basilar membrane dictates a tonotopic neural response to sound so that the apical cochlea responds best to low-frequency sounds and the basal cochlea responds best to sounds of high frequency. The frequency that produces the greatest movement of the basilar membrane, and consequently the greatest hair cell response at any one point within the cochlea, is termed the *characteristic frequency*.

HAIR CELLS IN THE ORGAN OF CORTI TRANSDUCE SIGNAL USED FOR HEARING

A small region, pie-shaped in cross-section and located on the basilar membrane side of the cochlear duct comprises the *organ of Corti*, the site of sensory transduction within the cochlear duct (Fig. 16-6). Dividing the organ of Corti from the rest of the cochlear duct is the *tectorial membrane*, which emanates outward from the *modiolus*, the central pillar of the cochlear spiral. Sensory hair cells sit atop the basilar membrane and extend cellular extensions termed *stereocilia* into the *scala media*, the fluid chamber of the organ of Corti.

Hair cells are mechanosensitive sensory cells present in both the cochlea and vestibulum. Cochlear hair cells have three rows of stereocilia on their apical surface (Fig. 16-7). These stereocilia are in fact neither cilia nor "hairs" but

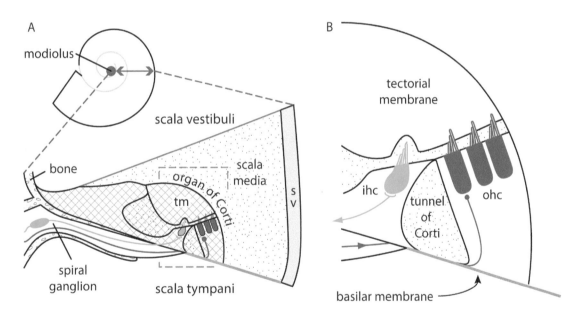

Figure 16-6 A: The organ of Corti occupies the inner portion of the cochlear duct extending outward from the modiolus, the central pole around which the cochlea turns. At the outer edge of the cochlear duct is a specialized tissue, the stria vascularis, which pumps potassium ions into the scala media to form endolymph. Endolymph is a potassium ion-rich fluid that fills the scala media, the fluid-filled portion of the cochlear duct. The organ of Corti contains two types of hair cells, inner and outer, and the tectorial membrane (*tm*). Spiral ganglion cells (*blue*) innervate a single row of inner hair cells (*blue*) and carry afferent input from the inner ear to the cochlear nuclei in the hindbrain. Efferents arising from cells in the pons (*maroon*) innervate three rows of outer hair cells (*maroon*). Outer hair cells serve as the cochlear amplifier. B: The stereocilia of outer hair cells (*ohc*) are embedded in the tectorial membrane. When a sound elicits a pressure wave in the cochlea, the basilar membrane moves up and down at the frequency of the incident sound. If the frequency of basilar membrane movement matches the characteristic frequency of the hair cells at the cochlear location, the outer hair cells themselves will move up and down. The movement of outer hair cells serves as an independent resonator, which amplifies the movement of the basilar membrane. The stereocilia of inner hair cells (*ihc*) float within the endolymph and respond to pressure waves produced by basilar membrane movement and the movement of endolymph. The responses of inner hair cells are conveyed to spiral ganglion cells through a synapse.

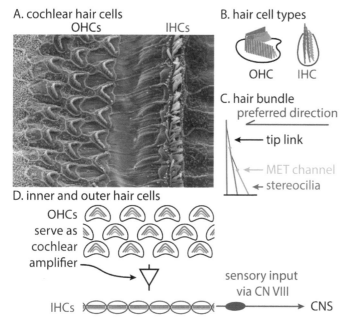

A. cochlear hair cells
OHCs   IHCs

B. hair cell types
OHC   IHC

C. hair bundle
preferred direction
tip link
MET channel
stereocilia

D. inner and outer hair cells
OHCs
serve as
cochlear
amplifier

sensory input
via CN VIII

IHCs   CNS

Figure 16-7 Cochlear hair cells come in two varieties: the more numerous outer hair cells (OHCs) and the inner hair cells (IHCs) that send sensory input to the central nervous system (CNS) via spiral ganglion cells. A: A colorized scanning electron micrograph showing a top view of outer (*left three rows*) and inner (*right row*) hair cells. The stereocilia have been colored red. B: All cochlear hair cells have three rows of stereocilia, but they are arranged as an arrowhead in the outer hair cells and in a straight line in the inner hair cells. C: A schematic side view of three stereocilia showing the tip-links that attach from the taller stereocilia to a MET channel on the neighboring shorter stereocilia. The preferred direction, defined as the direction of hair bundle movement that leads to hair cell depolarization, is deflection toward the tallest stereocilia (*brown arrow*). D: Outer hair cells alter the basilar membrane displacement in response to incoming pressure waves. In this way, they serve as the cochlear amplifier to both amplify and narrow the tuning of the stimulus delivered to the inner hair cells. The inner hair cells synapse onto spiral ganglion cells that in turn provide sensory input to hindbrain cochlear nuclear neurons. Scanning electron micrograph in A reprinted with permission from Levitan IB, and Kaczmarek LK. *The Neuron: Cell and Molecular Biology* (4 ed.). New York: Oxford University Press, 2015.

instead are long extensions from the cell body that contain an inner actin skeleton. Nonetheless, the stereocilia are called the *hair bundle*. Stereocilia are arranged from short to tall, with thin proteinaceous *tip-links* linking shorter stereocilia to their taller neighbors. When the hair bundle is bent toward the tallest stereocilium, the tip-links pull on the *mechanoelectrical transduction* or *MET channel* to increase the probability of its opening. The MET channel is a nonspecific cation channel through which sodium, potassium, and calcium ions pass, thus depolarizing the hair cell. The direction of hair bundle deflection that causes cell depolarization—toward the tallest stereocilia—is the *preferred direction*. When the stereocilia are bent away from the tallest stereocilia (the *nonpreferred direction*), the probability that the mechanoelectrical transduction channel will close increases, thus hyperpolarizing the cell. Cochlear hair cells are aligned so that all the hair cells in a patch of cochlea share a response to hair bundle stimulation.

Cochlear hair cells come in two varieties: *inner* and *outer hair cells* (Fig. 16-7). The human cochlea contains about 3,500 inner hair cells arranged in a single row close to the modiolus and about 12,000 outer hair cells arranged in three rows farther from the modiolus (Fig. 16-6). Although both inner and outer hair cells are sensitive to basilar membrane displacement, the functional significance of inner and outer hair cell activation differs in fundamental ways. *The inner hair cells are the source of auditory information bound for perceptual pathways* and comprise the input to the auditory afferents in the eighth cranial nerve. Outer hair cells do not contribute input to central auditory pathways but are critical to normal hearing because they fine-tune

and amplify inner hair cell responses. In short, the *outer hair cells serve as the cochlear amplifier*, a topic that we now examine in more detail.

OUTER HAIR CELLS FINE-TUNE THE FREQUENCY RESOLUTION OF THE COCHLEA

Although outer hair cells do not send a message to the CNS, they are critical to auditory perception through their role as the cochlear amplifier. *Electromotility*, the basis for outer hair cell cochlear amplification discovered by William Brownell in the mid 1980s, is one of the most intriguing stories of basic neurobiology to emerge over the past half century. An overview of cochlear amplification is as follows:

- Outer hair cells respond to incoming pressure waves with changes in membrane potential (depolarization when the hair bundles are deflected in the preferred direction and hyperpolarization when stimulated in the nonpreferred direction).

- *Prestin*, a molecular motor contained exclusively in outer hair cells, alters its conformation so that the length of the outer hair cells changes with every cycle of hyperpolarization and depolarization (Fig. 16-8). You are encouraged to seek out one of the many "dancing hair cell" videos (set to a variety of musical tastes) available on the Internet; these videos are of greater worth than many, many words.

- The lengthening and shortening of outer hair cells pivots the basilar membrane, amplifying its excursion and the fluid movement within the organ of Corti. The end result is a facilitation of the stimulus magnitude presented to inner hair cells.

- Outer hair cells selectively amplify a section of the basilar membrane corresponding to a narrow range of frequencies. In this way, outer hair cell motility improves cochlear tuning, facilitating discrimination between stimuli of similar frequencies.

Prestin is a protein, evolved from a family of anion transporters, that is only present in the outer hair cells of mammals. In response to changes in membrane potential, prestin changes conformation within the plasma membrane between long and short forms. Because prestin serves, by itself, as a motor, electromotility is fast—orders of magnitude faster than skeletal muscle contraction. This means that the outer hair cell shortens and lengthens in response to sinusoidal deflection of the hair bundle at physiological frequencies. The shortening and lengthening of the outer hair cell pulls the basilar membrane up and down, thereby amplifying the excursion of the basilar membrane within the organ of Corti (Fig. 16-8). Thus, *outer hair cells boost the stimulus that reaches the inner hair cells.*

Without outer hair cells, inner hair cells would only respond to high-intensity stimulation at the characteristic frequency. For example, a hair cell that normally responds to its characteristic frequency presented at less than 10 dB would, in the absence of outer hair cells, require a stimulus

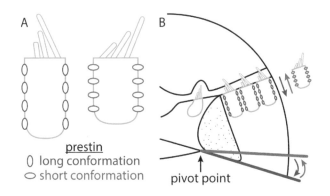

prestin
0 long conformation
○ short conformation

pivot point

Figure 16-8 Outer hair cells show electromotility because of a transmembrane protein called *prestin* that serves as a molecular motor. A: When an outer hair cell depolarizes, it shortens compared to its hyperpolarized length because of a change in prestin's conformation. B: Changes in outer hair cell length (*straight arrows*) move the basilar membrane up and down (*arcing arrows*) at a pivot point and thereby amplify fluid pressure waves in the cochlear duct. Ultimately, movement of the hair cell greatly increases the displacement of the basilar membrane over what it would be from passive mechanisms alone.

of more than 80 dB. People with deleterious mutations in the prestin gene are deaf (not hard of hearing), dramatic evidence that the boost in stimulus magnitude provided by the electromotile outer hair cells is absolutely essential for cochlear function. Salicylates, metabolized from aspirin, impair outer hair cell function, possibly by interfering with electromotility. Associated with the consequent loss of hearing is tinnitus. When caused by high doses of aspirin, both hearing loss and tinnitus often reverse upon discontinuing aspirin intake. Since salicylates and prestin mutations both act through adverse effects on outer hair cell motility, they do not affect vestibular function.

Outer hair cells also improve frequency discrimination. To understand how this occurs, we start with Georg von Békésy who won the Nobel Prize for Physiology or Medicine in 1961 for showing that the cochlea acts as a *sound prism*, fanning out fluid waves of different frequencies to different locations along the cochlear spiral. Von Békésy worked on cochlea from cadavers, and the passive dispersal of pressure waves in these dead cochlea produces only a crude level of frequency discrimination that fails to match human psychophysical performance. For example, a pressure wave with a frequency of 500 Hz moves the basilar membrane of a dead cochlea across a wide stretch corresponding to characteristic frequencies of roughly 450–550 Hz. On the other hand, we can distinguish between tones at very close frequencies, for example between tones with frequencies of 500 Hz and 501 Hz. The outer hair cells increase the resonance of the basilar membrane and thereby provide the added resolution to cochlear tonotopy.

Outer hair cells use resonance matching to effectively amplify basilar membrane oscillations. The mechanism of natural resonance amplification is a potentially powerful force that has caused bridges to collapse, glass to shatter, and car doors to vibrate. To understand this, we first need to understand that everything has a natural resonant frequency or frequencies. Drinking glasses resonate at higher frequencies than do car doors. Regardless of the particular frequency, adding energy in the form of pressure waves or sound at an object's resonant frequency has the effect of greatly increasing the object's oscillatory movements at that frequency. Thus, a very loud bass sound from a radio can shake an automobile door. In the same way, belting out a tone at the resonant frequency of a wine glass will first lead to the glass's vibrating and ultimately to its shattering. Unfortunately, this same principle has led to the demise of at least two bridges, one from wind and one or more from the rhythmic marching of soldiers at the bridges' natural resonant frequencies. A number of structural fixes—wider, heavier spans and mechanical dampeners—are commonly used today to avoid bridge collapse due to winds at the bridge's resonance frequency. To prevent bridges from collapsing under marching soldiers, soldiers have broken cadence when crossing bridges for at least the past century and a half.

Amplification of basilar membrane displacement is greatest for pressure waves at the characteristic frequency of the inner hair cells at that cochlear location. As a result of intrinsic differences in membrane stiffness, the resonant frequency of the basilar membrane varies progressively from the basal turns of the cochlea to the apex. Basally, the basilar membrane has the highest resonant frequency, and apically the resonant frequency of the basilar membrane is lowest. The movement produced by stimulated outer hair cells produces the greatest amplification of basilar movement at the location with the matching resonant frequency. Thus, even if outer hair cells across a wide area are stimulated by a pressure wave, the effect of the movement produced by the outer hair cells is greatest at one particular location. In this way, the gross tonotopy of the initial pressure wave combines with the independent resonance created by the outer hair cells to generate a very fine tonotopy in the cochlea.

One of the most peculiar features of outer hair cells is that they do not transmit information to the CNS. Even stranger, outer hair cells actually *receive input from the CNS*! Moreover, the pontine neurons that contact outer hair cells use acetylcholine, the transmitter common to all motor output neurons (see Chapter 12). These features fit with the *motor* function of outer hair cells, which we can think of as very small, incredibly fast "muscles." Acetylcholine released from cochlear efferent terminals opens nicotinic receptors on outer hair cells, initiating calcium ion entry; downstream effects including hyperpolarization of the outer hair cell and suppression of electromotility. This chain of events is protective, reducing noise-induced cochlear trauma, presumably by decreasing cochlear amplification but possibly by additional mechanisms as well. Remarkably, the connection from pontine neurons to outer hair cells allows the CNS to influence the most peripheral aspect of hearing, the stimulus itself.

OTOACOUSTIC EMISSIONS RESULT FROM OUTER HAIR CELL ACTIVATION

Consider how sound reaches outer hair cells. Now imagine that that pathway is reversed, so that activation of an outer hair cell initiates a sequence of events that ends with a sound coming out of the ear. Let us go through this step by step. Let's say that outer hair cells in a patch of cochlea are activated. This activation sets up a local resonance at the characteristic frequency. The resonance produces movement of the basilar membrane and the resulting fluid wave travels to the oval window and moves the middle ear muscles in reverse. First, the stapes moves, and this moves the incus, which in turn moves the malleus. The malleus is attached to the crown of the tympanic membrane, and so movement of the malleus moves the tympanic membrane. Movement of the tympanic membrane produces sound in a manner analogous to the production of sound from a woofer; this sound comes *out of the ear* as an *otoacoustic emission*. Otoacoustic emissions may be low in amplitude, but they can be picked up by a microphone placed into the ear canal.

Otoacoustic emissions can occur spontaneously but can also be elicited by playing a tone into the ear. Tone-evoked otoacoustic emissions start with the activation of outer hair cells by the incoming tone. Then, the rest of the reverse pathway just described ensues, and the result is an emission of the same frequency as the tone that was originally played into the ear. Since otoacoustic emissions depend on healthy outer hair cells, *the presence of evoked otoacoustic emissions can be used as an early test for cochlear health*. This test is particularly useful for testing the hearing of babies, young children, and nonverbal individuals.

THE ENDOCOCHLEAR POTENTIAL IS CRITICAL TO HEARING

Human cochlear hair cells respond to sounds that can range from 20 Hz to 20 kHz (20,000 Hz; 1 kHz is 1,000 Hz)! In fact, the highest frequency sound that mammals such as bats can hear is more than 100 kHz. Adult humans hear sounds that range in frequency up to 12–16 kHz, a maximum that progressively decreases with age (see Box 16-3). In contrast, fish hear frequencies below 1 kHz, and birds are primarily sensitive to frequencies of no more than 5–10 kHz. To place the challenge of high-frequency responses in context, first consider the relatively easy job of responding to sinusoidal stimulus at 10 Hz. A 10 Hz stimulus moves the hair cell stereocilia bundle in one direction for 50 ms, an ionotropic ion channel "eternity." Now consider a 20 kHz stimulus, which changes direction every 25 microseconds (μs). In that 25 μs time period, the hair cell stereocilia must physically move and an ion channel in the hair cell membrane must open for a hair cell to respond.

A critical feature that permits the mammalian cochlea to respond to high-frequency stimuli is the *endocochlear potential* (*EP*), which is produced by the *stria vascularis*. Disruption of the EP or mutations that prevent proper stria vascularis formation result in deafness. The EP decreases from its most positive value (+90–100 mV) at the cochlear base (serving high frequencies) to a minimum value of about +70–75 mV in the apex of the cochlea (serving low frequencies), highlighting the EP's importance to high-frequency stimulus transduction.

The stria vascularis, a layered structure lining the outside wall of the cochlea (Fig. 16-6A), operates as a battery that generates the EP in the cochlear endolymph. The stria vascularis also pumps out potassium ions into the endolymph. Yet, it is the EP rather than the K$^+$-rich makeup of endolymph that is critical to hearing. Combined with the slightly elevated resting potential of the hair cell (~ 50 mV), the EP produces a driving force of more than 100 mV for ions entering MET channels present on the stereocilia.

When MET channels open, potassium (and sodium) ions from the endolymph flow into the stereocilia because of the strong electrical driving force (more than 100 mV) existing between cochlear endolymph and the internal potential of the hair cell, at about −50 mV. The influx of cations into the stereocilia depolarizes the entire hair cell and opens calcium channels in the cell body. The hair cell depolarizes. Particularly fast potassium channels, present in the membrane of the hair cell soma, are activated

by depolarization and are responsible for repolarizing hair cells *quickly*. Rapid repolarization of hair cells allows the hair cell membrane potential to follow sounds with frequencies of up to 3,000 Hz or so (Fig. 16-9A). For example, vibration of the basilar membrane at 1 kHz alternately moves the basilar membrane sinusoidally up and down every millisecond. Because of the fast repolarization mechanisms in hair cells, hair cells show a sinusoidal response of alternating depolarization and hyperpolarization with a period as short as 1 ms. However, hair cells cannot follow the sinusoidal movements at frequencies greater than

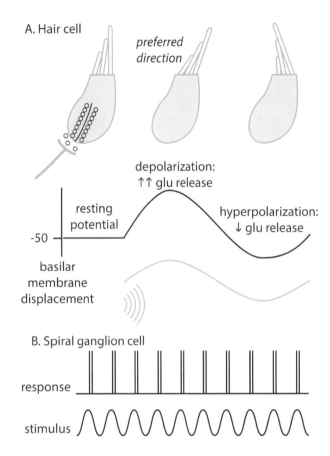

Figure 16-9 Hair cells, like other non-neuronal sensory cells, use graded potentials and synapse onto spiral ganglion cells that fire action potentials. A: The resting (in silence) potential of hair cells is about −50 mV due to open MET channels at rest. When a sound occurs and a pressure wave moves the basilar membrane up and down (*gray*), the stereocilia of the hair cell are bent. When the stereocilia bend toward the tallest stereocilium (middle), the preferred direction, the hair cell depolarizes; when the stereocilia bend away from the tallest stereocilium, the hair cell hyperpolarizes. When the membrane potential is depolarized above the resting potential, release of neurotransmitter is increased. The release of more glutamate (*glu*) vesicles increases the probability of an action potential in the postsynaptic spiral ganglion cell. Note that neither tip-links nor MET channels are illustrated here. B: In response to a pressure wave of 3 kHz or less (stimulus), a spiral ganglion cell fires one or more action potentials in response to each cycle. The number of action potentials fired per cycle is greater as the amplitude of the stimulus increases.

3 kHz or so. Sounds above frequencies of 3 kHz produce a sustained depolarization of hair cells at the corresponding tonotopic location.

Compromise of the EP is a common cause of deafness. Genetic causes of deafness stem from mutations in genes for connexins, the gap junction building blocks; channels and transporters found in the stria vascularis; and several transmembrane proteins with as of yet undiscovered functions. In fact, mutations in genes coding for connexins are the most common genetic cause of deafness. The diuretics furosemide (sold as Lasix in the United States) and ethacrynic acid can impair stria vascularis function, thereby compromising the EP and impairing hearing, either reversibly or permanently. It is important to recognize that hearing loss associated with damage to the EP is not associated with deficits in vestibular function. These forms of hearing loss or deafness are termed nonsyndromic (syndrome derives from Greek for "to run together") in that they do not *run* with symptoms in vestibular or other functions.

SEVERAL OTOTOXIC DRUGS HARM COCHLEAR HAIR CELLS

Both outer and inner hair cells respond to incoming pressure waves with a change in cellular membrane potential. For outer hair cells, the important consequence of this change in potential is electromotility (Fig. 16-8), whereas the critical consequence of a change in potential for the inner hair cell is a change in the amount of neurotransmitter released onto spiral ganglion neurons (Fig. 16-9A). Thus, the outer hair cells' role in sensory transduction may be considered indirect because they modify the stimulus presented to the inner hair cells but do not send messages to the brain. The inner hair cells are the conduit for sensory information from the cochlea bound for the brain. Regardless of their indirect or direct roles, both outer and inner hair cells are needed for normal hearing. Moreover, both types of hair cells use tip-links connected to MET channels to respond to pressure waves, a reliance that renders them sensitive to certain antibiotics and chemotherapeutics.

Aminoglycoside antibiotics and the chemotherapeutic agents cisplatin and carboplatin can kill hair cells. These ototoxic drugs appear to enter hair cells through open MET channels. Ototoxic drugs may have a predilection to kill either cochlear or vestibular hair cells or may be toxic to hair cells in both parts of the inner ear. The antineoplastic agents neomycin, kanamycin, and amikacin act primarily in the cochlea and primarily on outer hair cells. The mechanisms of toxicity are diverse. In the case of ototoxic antibiotics,

affected cells die through caspase-dependent apoptosis. The cochlear hair cells most at risk for ototoxicity are outer hair cells in the basal turns of the cochlea. Loss of basal outer hair cells leads to a loss of hearing in the high-frequency range and an accompanying tinnitus.

Although the proportion of patients suffering ototoxic hearing loss is relatively small, the consequences for affected patients can be devastating. Often, the patient taking an antibiotic or chemotherapeutic is an older individual who, upon losing hearing, lacks the resources to compensate by learning sign language or lip-reading or using a cochlear implant. Fortunately, the prescription of some ototoxic compounds can be avoided when alternative therapeutic approaches exist. When prescription of a potentially ototoxic compound is warranted, close monitoring of serum levels should be used to prevent audiologic or vestibular damage. Since genetic factors may predispose some to ototoxic damage, patients with a family history should be particularly carefully managed.

STIMULUS FREQUENCY IS CODED BY BOTH LABELED-LINE MECHANISMS AND DISCHARGE PATTERN

Each inner hair cell is innervated by, on average, eight afferents from the spiral ganglion. The spiral ganglion cells have somata that sit just inside the organ of Corti within the bony cochlea (Fig. 16-6A). When a pressure wave arrives, hair cells respond by releasing their neurotransmitter, which is glutamate, in a pattern that reflects the incident sound (Fig. 16-9A). Consider a 500 Hz tone. Close to the apex of the cochlea, the basilar membrane will resonate at 500 Hz, and the inner hair cells there will respond with alternating depolarizations and hyperpolarizations every 2 ms (equal to the period of a 500 Hz stimulus). Glutamate release mirrors the hair cell's membrane potential. As a result, the postsynaptic auditory afferents in the eighth cranial nerve tend to fire every 2 ms (Fig. 16-9B). The location of the hair cell and the identity of the auditory afferent brand the stimulus as having a characteristic frequency of 500 Hz. In addition, the afferent fires action potentials that occur with a frequency of 500 Hz.

Hair cell location, afferent identity and firing pattern all combine to effectively code sound frequencies up to 3 kHz. However, above 3 kHz, auditory afferents cannot follow the stimulus by firing an action potential once per period of stimulation. Therefore, auditory afferents coding for sounds at frequencies above 3 kHz employ a labeled-line mechanism rather than discharge pattern for coding.

Hair cells, in both the cochlea and vestibulum, have a resting potential of about −50 mV that is due to MET channels open at rest, even in complete silence. Because of their elevated resting potential, hair cells can signal pressure waves in either the preferred or nonpreferred direction. This fits with the fact that it is the frequency of pressure waves rather than the direction of hair bundle deflection that carries meaning in the auditory system. The elevated resting potential in hair cells leads to ongoing release of glutamate and therefore a resting discharge in the spiral ganglion cells, even in conditions without sound. Thus, the hair cell-to-spiral ganglion cell is a much-trafficked synapse with, as it turns out, its own version of synaptotagmin called *otoferlin*. Otoferlin serves as the calcium ion sensor that triggers neurotransmitter release from hair cells. In people with otoferlin mutations, pressure waves are transduced normally but no sound-related activity occurs in the auditory nerve fibers, causing nonsyndromic deafness.

As discussed in Chapter 6, auditory inputs are represented bilaterally in the CNS above the cochlear nuclei. Because of this architecture, auditory pathway neurons that are third-order or more carry information about sound arriving at both ears. Neurons in the inferior colliculus and in the medial geniculate nucleus carry bilateral auditory information, as do auditory cortex cells. Thus, despite the fact that central neurons involved in hearing pathways greatly outnumber hair cells (see Fig. 16-14), no singular central lesion can produce deafness, which is always caused by a peripheral lesion.

COCHLEAR FUNCTION DEPENDS ON A LARGE NUMBER OF GENE PRODUCTS

The genetic analysis of congenital deafness in humans has provided important clues to understanding the molecular mechanisms of hearing. In the reverse direction, molecular investigations into the basic mechanisms of hearing have led to the discovery of novel genetic causes of deafness. The rich interplay between human deafness and molecular mechanisms of hearing is rooted in the large number of molecules involved in cochlear function. About 1% of the coded genes in the human genome contribute to peripheral hearing function, and many of the molecules serve no other known function. As a result, most congenital deafness disorders are nonsyndromic, with hearing as the only affected system. Genetic mutations cause nonsyndromic congenital deafness through effects on multiple targets:

• *Ionic homeostasis within the cochlear duct*: Defects in connexins, the gap junction building blocks; a potassium channel found in the stria vascularis; transporters; and several transmembrane proteins with as of yet undiscovered function are all associated with deafness. Connexins are critical to both the formation of endolymph and the clearance of potassium ions from the interstitial fluid surrounding hair cell somata. Mutations in genes coding for connexins that are specifically found in the inner ear are the most common genetic cause of deafness.

• *The tectorial membrane*: Proteins including collagens and tectorins are integral components of the tectorial membrane. A set of anchoring proteins are involved in securing the tectorial membrane within the organ of Corti.

• *Hair-cell stereocilia*: The actin core of the stereocilia is stabilized and extended by interactions with several proteins, including a number of myosin isoforms and a protein "glue" called harmonin.

• *Prestin*: The molecular motor of the outer hair cells forms the basis of the cochlear amplifier.

• *Synaptic transmission from the inner hair cell to spiral ganglion afferents*: As introduced earlier, otoferlin serves as the calcium ion sensor that triggers neurotransmitter release from hair cells. In people with otoferlin mutations, sound is transduced normally, but no sound-related activity occurs in the auditory nerve fibers.

In addition to the nonsyndromic deafness disorders, deafness can be part of a syndrome, meaning that a group of symptoms run together. The most common syndrome of deafness along with vestibular impairment and blindness is *Usher syndrome*. Patients with Usher syndrome have a defect in any of about 10 genes. The syndrome has varying severity, afflicting some patients with deafness and others only with a hearing loss. In the most severe cases, patients are born deaf, quickly develop balance problems, and start losing vision by the age of 10 years.

A continued dialog between scientists and physicians is critical to the effective application of appropriate therapies to particular forms of congenital deafness. For example, if and when hair cell regeneration becomes a realistic therapeutic option, it will have to be used on individuals with hospitable cochlea. In other words, hair cell regeneration would be an inadvisable therapy for people whose deafness stems from a defective stria vascularis and consequently an ionic environment that cannot support hair cell function.

TWO TESTS ARE USED TO DIAGNOSE HEARING LOSS

Recall that hearing loss can be divided into conductive and sensorineural depending on whether conduction through the external and middle ears or processing in the inner ear are responsible for the deficit (Fig. 16-2). The *Rinne test* and *Weber test* can be easily performed with a tuning fork and can be sufficient to determine the type of hearing loss suffered by a patient (Table 16-1).

The Rinne test is used to diagnose or rule out a conductive hearing loss. A vibrating tuning fork is placed in the air, just beside the ear or on the mastoid process just behind the ear. The patient is asked which location produces a louder sound. A tuning fork held in the air produces an airborne pressure wave that reaches the cochlea through the normal channel of traveling through the external ear. In contrast, when a tuning fork is placed on the skull, the pressure wave bypasses the external and middle ears to reach the cochlea directly through bone conduction. Because of the conductive amplification provided by the external ear, the tuning fork's vibration that arrives via air is perceived as louder than the same vibration arriving by bone conduction. Therefore, a person with normal hearing will perceive the air-conducted sound to be louder than the bone-conducted sound. To confirm this result, one can keep the vibrating tuning fork on the mastoid until it can no longer be heard through bone conduction. At that point, move the tuning fork to a point just outside the pinna. A person with normal conduction will hear an airborne sound.

Sensorineural hearing loss decreases the perceived loudness of sound on the affected side or sides, regardless of whether that sound arrives via bone or air. Thus, sensorineural hearing loss cannot be detected by the Rinne test because an affected individual will resemble a person with normal hearing in perceiving airborne sound as louder than bone-conducted sound. To detect sensorineural hearing loss, the Weber test is used on a person with a normal Rinne test.

The Weber test is performed by placing a vibrating tuning fork on the vertex of the head (Fig. 16-10A). Normally, we hear the sound of the tuning fork as equally loud on either side (Fig. 16-10B). In an individual with sensorineural hearing loss, the perceived sound is, of course, greater on the unaffected side (Fig. 16-10C). In an individual with conduction hearing loss, the perceived sound is greater on the affected side (Fig. 16-10E). We can return to Weber's law (see Chapter 14) to understand this result. An individual with conductive hearing loss hears only the bone-conducted sound produced by the tuning fork and does not hear background sounds—traffic, people talking, birds singing—that are conducted through the external and middle ear on the affected side. The perceived sound of the vibrating tuning fork on the vertex of the head will thus be greater on the side without background stimulation, the side with conductive hearing loss.

The Rinne and Weber tests can only detect sensorineural hearing loss that is unilateral or strongly asymmetrical. To identify bilateral hearing loss, as occurs often in age-related hearing loss and several other conditions, an audiological examination is needed. In an audiological examination, the intensity threshold for detection of tones at different frequencies played into each ear through headphones is measured in a quiet environment.

The treatment options for conductive and sensorineural hearing loss are quite different. In general, practical solutions or surgical remedies exist for many forms of conductive hearing loss. In contrast, the strategy used for sensorineural hearing loss is to employ a hearing aid to boost the intensity of the stimulus coming into the cochlea, essentially an end-around strategy that does not address the actual cause of the hearing problem. Indirect though it may be, increasing the stimulus intensity of incoming sounds effectively improves the hearing of millions with hearing loss.

Table 16-1 **THE RINNE AND WEBER TESTS PROVIDE A QUICK METHOD FOR DETECTING UNILATERAL CONDUCTIVE OR SENSORINEURAL HEARING LOSS**

CONDITION	RESULT OF RINNE TEST	RESULT OF WEBER TEST
Normal	Airborne louder than bone for each ear	Loudness is equal on left and right
Unilateral conduction hearing loss	Bone louder than airborne on affected side	Louder on affected side
Bilateral conduction hearing loss	Bone louder than airborne for each ear	Loudness is equal on left and right
Unilateral sensorineural hearing loss	Airborne louder than bone for each ear	Louder on unaffected side
Bilateral sensorineural hearing loss	Airborne louder than bone for each ear	Loudness is equal on left and right

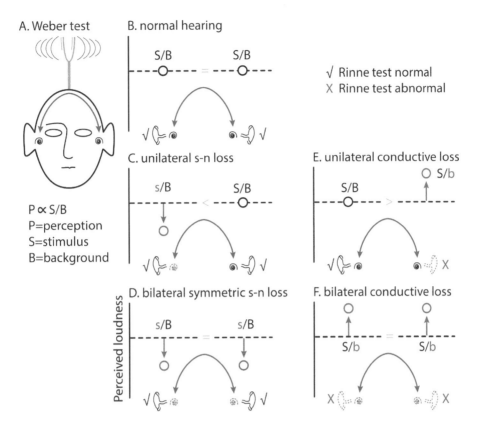

Figure 16-10 A: The Weber test involves placing a vibrating tuning fork at the vertex of the head. The pressure waves travel through bone to the cochlea on either side. B: This should produce a sound that is perceived as equally loud on the two sides. However, an individual with unilateral sensorineural hearing loss will perceive the sound as louder on the unaffected side (C), whereas an individual with unilateral conductive hearing loss will perceive the sound as louder on the affected side (E). Bilateral and symmetric hearing loss of either type (D, F) as well as normal hearing (B) will result in a perception that the sounds are of equal intensity on the two sides (=). The Weber test alone also fails to distinguish one-sided conductive hearing loss (E, louder on the affected side) from one-sided sensorineural hearing loss (C, louder on the unaffected side). The Rinne test can disambiguate results from the Weber test.

NOISE-INDUCED SENSORINEURAL HEARING LOSS IS COMMON TODAY

A revealing study more than a half-century ago showed that Mabaan tribespeople in the Sudan, a premodern and reproductively isolated population that had not been exposed to modern noises, suffered from minimal hearing loss as they aged. Seventy-year-old Mabaans had the hearing of 20-something Americans. At the time of the study, Mabaans and Americans likely differed in genetics, diet, and also noise exposure. Although it is clear that noise exposure is one factor that drives hearing loss in (loud) modernized societies, not all individuals exposed to loud noises lose their hearing to the same extent. In fact, age-related hearing loss or *presbycusis* (ancient Greek for "old man hearing") does not occur with the inevitability of presbyopia, with some individuals retaining normal hearing into their tenth decade and others suffering from severe sensorineural hearing loss in their forties or younger. This difference suggests that presbycusis does not arise from a programmed aging process that occurs at a consistent rate in all people (as is the case in presbyopia) but arises from accumulated damage combined with particular (and unfortunately largely unknown) genetic, nutritional, and environmental factors.

Noise is the cochlea-damaging stimulus that we know the most about. Extremely loud noises can lead to stereocilia being sheared off from the outer hair cells, which have their stereocilia embedded in the tectorial membrane. This is an irreversible loss because new hair cells are not made in the mammalian cochlea. However, noise exposure that acutely kills outer hair cells is rare. Far more common are the loud, but not immediately deafening, noises of modern life. These sounds, in the 70–120 dB range, can cause irreversible damage to the organ of Corti. Such noises are now commonplace everywhere: in rural (farming and mining machinery) and urban (nightclubs, subways, construction sites) environments, in the home (ear buds, television) and outside the home (restaurants, stadiums, movies, symphonies).

Susceptibility to noise-induced damage differs between individuals. For example, people with mutations in a potassium channel that is found in the stria vascularis are highly vulnerable to a severe form of noise-induced hearing loss. However, in most cases, it is unclear whether a person's level of susceptibility stems from genetic, environmental, and/or nutritional factors. Regardless of the cause, individual variation in noise susceptibility means that there is no one noise threshold above which all individuals suffer damage; noise levels that may harm one person's hearing may not harm another's (Fig. 16-11). The cumulative number of insults to auditory pathways increases with age, and this, combined with the inability of cochlear cells to repair themselves, appears to account for the greater incidence of hearing loss in older individuals.

Loud noises, such as the sound of exploding firecrackers or the roar of a stadium crowd, may transiently impair people's hearing, a hearing loss often accompanied (unsurprisingly) by tinnitus. The hearing issues can be quantified as a temporary elevation in hearing thresholds (as measured by an audiogram), which is also accompanied by a reduction in otoacoustic emissions, reflecting impaired outer hair cell function. Since hearing thresholds and otoacoustic emissions recover days or weeks after a rock concert or fireworks display, it was originally thought that this temporary noise-induced hearing loss was without permanent consequences. However, more recent studies in nonhuman mammals tell us that loud noises cause irreversible damage to auditory afferents. The damage happens immediately and is mediated by excitotoxicity. In response to moderate to loud noises, strongly depolarized inner hair cells release excessive glutamate onto afferent terminals. The afferent

terminals swell in response to all that glutamate and then rupture. It is this damage to spiral ganglion afferent terminals that leads eventually to permanent noise-induced hearing loss. No regeneration of hair cells, spiral ganglion cell afferents, or the synaptic connection between them occurs. With absolutely no natural repair processes present within the mammalian cochlea, damage to the cochlea accumulates over time without mitigation, becoming increasingly problematic with age.

Noise-induced hearing loss is often *hidden* in the sense that it is not detected by an audiogram. Yet, people with hidden hearing loss perform poorly on a speech-in-noise test, which assesses how well a person hears spoken words. The difference in test sensitivity is understandable since audiograms are tests of tone detection, a task that is far easier than understanding speech, which requires far more information than simply whether a sound is present or not. Thus, people's ability to verbally communicate in the world is better reflected by the results of a speech-in-noise-test than those of an audiogram. Hidden hearing loss is widespread today and is not limited to the aged population, now being observed in younger people. The clinician should remember that a person who reports difficulty in verbal communication (or is reported to have hearing loss by a loved one) but has a normal audiogram may have hidden hearing loss due to cochlear damage.

Outer hair cell and cochlear afferent damage is concentrated in the basal turns of the cochlea and therefore presbycusis typically involves a preferential loss of high-frequency hearing. Losing high-frequency auditory information severely impairs the ability to understand speech (see Fig. 16-3). Individuals with presbycusis detect that speech is occurring but cannot make out the words. The ability to comprehend verbal speech is exacerbated by a noisy background, strongly accented speech, and a high-pitched voice. Hearing aids amplify sounds across all frequencies, or in some cases across the frequencies of human speech, but they cannot restore *sensitivity* to high frequencies. As mentioned earlier, hearing aids work on the conductive side of hearing, whereas presbycusis and most other forms of hearing loss are sensorineural. Thus, hearing aids are an imperfect treatment that help but do not restore normal hearing.

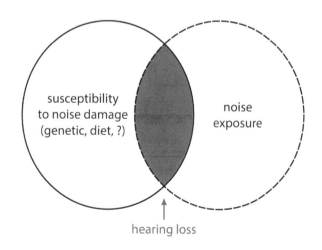

Figure 16-11 Hearing loss occurs when people who are susceptible to noise damage are exposed to loud noises. The relative sizes of the circles and the area of overlap are only illustrative and are not meant to represent measured values. The relative proportions of people with susceptibility to noise damage, noise exposure, and both are not known at present.

COCHLEAR IMPLANTS CAN PROVIDE AUDITORY PERCEPTION TO SOME DEAF INDIVIDUALS

When sensorineural hearing loss is profound and hearing aids cannot provide any improvement, a person is deaf.

In such cases, the only available therapeutic option is a cochlear implant. Cochlear implants allow children with congenital or acquired deafness and adults with acquired hearing loss to participate in and communicate with the hearing world. The dramatic therapeutic success of cochlear implants is demonstrated by the ability of recipients to talk on a telephone. Telephone communication is viewed as the gold standard of hearing loss treatment efficacy because it means that hearing is restored to a level at which acoustic information alone supports language comprehension.

Cochlear implants receive and process sound, emphasizing frequencies present in human speech (Fig. 16-12). Different frequencies of incoming sound are separated through Fourier analysis, and corresponding regions of the cochlea are accordingly stimulated so that, for example, when high-frequency sounds occur, the cochlea is stimulated close to the base. Most cochlear implants operate by producing a constant rate of electrical pulses that are amplitude-modulated to reflect the frequencies contained in incident sound. Remarkably, in the early days of cochlear implants, some individuals achieved fairly reliable speech recognition with only one channel of stimulation! In truth, the reasons for the remarkable efficacy arising from implants with a single channel remain unclear. Although some cochlear implants employ more than 20 channels of stimulation, each consisting of an electrode located at a specific site in the cochlea, it appears that five to eight channels is sufficient to allow for speech perception in most patients.

A cochlear implant will not restore hearing to all who are deaf. Although the device's electrode array takes the place of both the hair cell and the hair cell-to-spiral ganglion cell synapse, it uses the patient's auditory nerve and central auditory pathways, both of which must be functional for therapeutic effect. A second prerequisite for a cochlear implant is either experience with language or an age of less than 3 years, preferably about 1 year old. For a baby who is deaf at birth or who loses hearing prior to language acquisition, cochlear implants must be provided early, and the earlier the better. Providing a prelingually deafened adult with cochlear implants will not restore hearing for the same reason that individuals without early sight can never achieve high-acuity vision (see Chapter 15). Humans are not born knowing how to interpret sensory inputs. During a critical period, babies learn how to interpret sensory input and thereby see, hear, and use language. In the case of speech comprehension, the critical period ends at about 3 years of age, after which time cochlear implants are no longer effective for prelingually deaf individuals.

A cochlear device does not magically lead to language development. Infants learn language from the words and

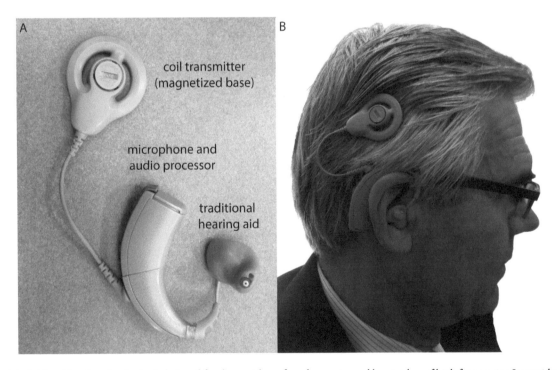

Figure 16-12 A hybrid cochlear hearing device is designed for those with profound sensorineural hearing loss of high frequencies. It provides electrical stimulation of the basal cochlea for high-frequency sounds in combination with a traditional hearing aid for amplification of low-frequency sounds. A: The hybrid device resembles a traditional cochlear implant in having a magnetized coil transmitter connected to an audio processor and microphone but differs by leaving the apical cochlea undisturbed. B: The entire device can be attached during the day and removed at night.

language that they hear. The vocabulary of a school-aged child is directly related to the richness of the child's linguistic environment. The linguistic environment in families of lower socioeconomic status and less education is on average more impoverished than that of wealthier, well-educated families. The result is that children raised in different environments emerge with substantially different vocabulary sizes. The issue is not limited to education or socioeconomic class; depressed individuals speak less and thereby provide babies with a poorer language environment. Regardless of the environment, all children receiving cochlear implant surgery have missed out on critical months, or even years, of language exposure prior to surgery. However, there is good news. Educating parents about the impact of linguistic environment on language development and helping them expand their linguistic interactions with their children effectively mitigates and can even obliterates school-aged vocabulary and academic achievement disparities related to educational and class background.

Even for postlingually deafened individuals, a cochlear device may not miraculously and instantaneously restore speech comprehension. The electrical pulses emitted by the cochlear implant are not the same as native auditory perception, and so postlingually deafened individuals have to relearn how to hear by deciphering the meaning of the new electrical activity. The facility of this relearning process depends on the quality of hearing prior to a patient becoming deaf. A person with years and years of normal hearing is more likely to comprehend speech quickly. For example, Tom Rice had normal hearing until he was roughly 20–30 years old and employed hearing aids starting at age 30. A few decades later, Rice's hearing had degraded to the point where he had to either retire from his meeting-intensive job (which he did not want to do) or get a cochlear implant. He received a cochlear implant, and the effect was "instantaneous"—his hearing returning the moment the device was activated. Despite this remarkable success, Rice is aware that his hearing is not the same as it used to be. For example, the /t/ sound at the end of "boat" did not sound like a /t/ at first. Rice recognized this despite not having heard the sound for a long time, and he seamlessly learned to reassign the new sound to /t/. Rice no longer notices the difference in this new sound, exemplifying the flexibility of the human brain to interpret and comprehend auditory input if language was initially learned in the early years of life.

In individuals who have always had difficulty hearing, learning to interpret auditory input with a cochlear implant is neither a simple nor a quick task. Michael Chorost was born hard of hearing and only learned to talk when he received hearing aids at the age of 3, at the closing of the critical window. As evocatively described in his book *Rebuilt: My Journey Back to the Hearing World*, Chorost lost all residual hearing one summer day in his mid-thirties. Months later, he received a cochlear implant. Chorost worked hard for months learning to interpret the input from his new device, concluding that successful use of the implant required him to become an expert "athlete of perception." He had to actively practice hearing, devise tricks, and learn rules. As with vision, hearing—particularly speech comprehension—is learned, and learning the new language of a cochlear implant as an adult can be a challenging process.

SIGN LANGUAGES PROVIDE DEAF CHILDREN WITH A NECESSARY MODE OF COMMUNICATION

It is critical that congenitally deaf children have the opportunity to acquire language. Without a mode of communication, prelingually deaf children suffer enormously from social isolation. These children must be given the opportunity to learn to communicate, either through immersion in a sign language community or through cochlear implants. Given that roughly 90% of congenitally deaf individuals are born to hearing parents, sign language must often be learned outside of the home at a school for the deaf. Among the congenitally deaf, experiences vary depending on whether one grows up signing within a deaf community or receives cochlear implants and grows up hearing. The experience of significant but not total hearing loss late in life is vastly different again.

Sign languages, of which there are many, are stand-alone languages. They are not signed versions of the local spoken language. For example, American Sign Language (ASL) is not a signed version of English. It is called American because it is the sign language used in the United States; moreover, it is different from British sign language although English is the spoken language in both Britain and America. ASL and other sign languages have their own grammar, syntax, and semantics, possessing lexical richness and sophistication on a par with any spoken language. Yet one key difference exists: namely, that no widely accepted or commonly used written system for sign language exists. For native signers who have never spoken or heard language, learning to read and write a spoken language, such as English, is a daunting challenge. They must learn a foreign language at the same time as they learn a phonetic representation of sounds that they have never experienced. Consequently, prelingually deaf signers are not fluent in written language. Virtually all of our written accounts of the signing community come from hearing children of deaf parents, postlingual deaf individuals who learned to sign as a second language, sign interpreters, and the like.

Even deaf individuals who learn sign language face challenges. One residual problem is the inability to overhear conversations. As Michael Chorost writes, "Social norms are not taught, they are overheard [and] the one thing even the most skilled deaf people cannot do is overhear." A second problem for the signing deaf is the impossibility of hearing nonlinguistic sounds that signal impending dangers, such as approaching vehicles or falling objects. Within the medical context, most physicians do not understand sign language, and sign interpreters are not widely available. Furthermore, health professionals may fail to appreciate that speakers of sign language are rendered mute by trauma or treatment that restricts arm movements.

Speaking combined with lip-reading, termed *oralism*, can allow deaf people to communicate with the hearing population and lessen the social isolation often associated with hearing loss. However, oralism is only possible in postlingually deafened individuals. The memoirs of David Wright, an English poet deafened at age 7, and Henry Kisor, an American journalist deafened at age 3, provide invaluable insight into the experience of deafness within the oralism tradition. Note that learning either lip-reading or sign language becomes progressively more difficult with age. Thus, people who lose their hearing in their advanced years typically do not learn to read lips or sign and consequently fail to overcome their new disability, suffering immensely from social isolation.

SPEECH PRODUCTION REQUIRES VIBRATION OF THE GLOTTIS WITH CONTROL OVER THE SHAPE OF THE VOCAL TRACT

The most important function of audition is to facilitate communication through spoken language. Before jumping from the auditory nerve to the cortex to discuss the mechanisms of speech *comprehension*, we take a brief detour to understand speech *production*.

The first step in speech production is *phonation*, which means pushing an air stream through the glottis, between the vocal folds of the larynx (Fig. 16-13). The glottis is pushed open when the lungs push air at a sufficient pressure. After being pushed open, the vocal folds collapse to a closed position, and then the glottis is pushed open again by the air pressure exerted by the lungs, and so on. In this

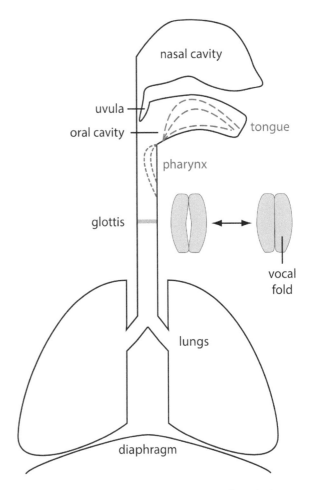

Figure 16-13 A schematic of the human vocal tract. Air from the lungs is placed under pressure from contraction of the diaphragm. When a sufficient pressure is reached, the vocal folds are pushed apart and the glottis opens (*left inset*). The pressure quickly dissipates and the glottis closes (*right inset*). The glottis opens and closes at a frequency that is the fundamental frequency of speech, 100–250 Hz or so. Phonation at the fundamental frequency is then filtered by the vocal tract to produce articulated speech. The shape of the vocal tract can be modified by muscles (*dashed lines*) of the pharynx, or upper airway, that are innervated by cranial nerves IX and X. Movements of the tongue (cranial nerve XII) and lips (not shown, cranial nerve VII) modify the shape of the last portion of the vocal tract, the oral cavity. The position of the uvula, another influence on the shape of the vocal tract, is controlled by muscles of the soft palate, which are innervated by cranial nerve IX.

way, the glottis opens and closes many times in a second to produce the fundamental frequency of speech. The tension in the vocal folds and the distance between them determine the fundamental frequency, which averages about 120 Hz for men and about 210 Hz for women.

The fundamental frequency of speech is the raw material for what we actually hear. But the semantic content of speech depends on filtering by the vocal tract (Fig. 16-13). The vocal tract is fundamentally a curved tube consisting of the space between the larynx and the lips and the nostrils. The length and shape of the vocal tract influence the frequency of the vocalizations. Just as the very long contrabassoon has a low frequency range and the very short piccolo has a very high frequency range, our vocalization frequency depends *in part* on the length of our vocal tract. The short vocal tract length of babies and children, along with laryngeal factors, contributes to the high-pitched sounds that young people produce.

The shape of the vocal tract is even more important than simply the length of the vocal tract in the articulation of sounds. When filtered by different configurations of the vocal tract, the same phonation produces different sounds. For example, we lift our tongue caudally and purse our lips to articulate the "oo" sound in "who," while we narrow our pharynx, depress our tongue, and open our lips to say the "ah" sound in "hot." As these two examples illustrate, the movements involved in language articulation are complex and precise, arguably the most intricate volitional movements that humans make. It is no surprise then that even small lesions in motor areas related to cranial nerves innervating muscles that change the shape of the vocal tract (VII, IX, X, XII) or muscle weakness can produce dysarthria (see Chapter 5).

VERBAL COMMUNICATION INVOLVES PROSODY AS WELL AS SEMANTIC CONTENT

The nonsemantic characteristics of speech along with accompanying body and facial movements, termed *prosody*, convey the emotional content of verbal communication. Nonsemantic, acoustic features of speech, posture, gestures, and facial expressions are all components of prosody. Prosody exists in all verbal languages, albeit in different forms. The acoustic features used to signal prosody in nontonal languages such as English and other Indo-European languages include:

- *Frequency*: The same words spoken at a high frequency convey a different meaning than when spoken at a low frequency.

- *Loudness*: A whisper and a shout impart very different meanings.

- *Timing*: Speaking in a rapid slur and in a slow deliberate fashion lends different meanings to the same sentence.

For example, "Good morning" said in a low and steady voice is recognized as a greeting by rote, a virtual automatism that has little personalized meaning and does not give the listener pause. In contrast, a slowly articulated "Good morning" in an up-and-down melodic voice is nearly as eloquent as saying, "Wasn't last night fun? I am so happy to see you this morning." In tonal languages, such as Mandarin Chinese, many sub-Saharan languages, and Navajo, one syllable can have several different semantic meanings depending on intonation. Individuals who speak tonal languages use pitch to convey semantic meaning while employing timing and loudness to impart prosody.

The fundamental frequency of speech and its modulation are a big part of prosody. Heard in isolation, the fundamental frequency sounds like a hum and does not involve articulated words. It changes from the beginning to the end of a sentence in a manner that differs depending on whether the utterance is a statement, question, or exclamation. The fundamental frequency of synthetic voices is typically unchanging rather than modulated and therefore can be identified instantly as "artificial." While containing no semantic content, the fundamental frequency carries communicative value and social meaning, as do other nonsemantic characteristics of speech such as speed, intensity, and tonal alignment (e.g., which syllable in a word is emphasized).

Prosody changes according to a speaker's emotional state. Words accompanied by an eye roll communicate a different emotional message than the same words said with a frown or a grin. When we respond to a friend's simple "hello" with "what's wrong?" we are intuitively and instantly understanding mood through prosody rather than semantic content. Dogs may perceive the word "walk" and cats may recognize their name when so inclined but communication with pets is often dominated by prosodic rather than semantic content.

Prosody exerts a great influence on the meaning that is communicated by spoken words. In fact, people and pets alike trust prosody over semantics. Given the emotional power of prosody, it is no surprise that prosody is a significant social signal. In the course of a dialogue, the fundamental frequencies of interacting speakers may change and either converge or diverge. Phonetic convergence may serve as a social lubricant. In one application of this principal, the fundamental frequencies of American celebrities in conversation with a talk show host, Larry King, were studied. King adapted his fundamental frequency to that of some guests—Bill Clinton, Barbra Streisand, Elizabeth Taylor, Tip O'Neill—but not to that of others—Dan Quayle, Jimmy Carter, or Spike Lee. This result was interpreted as an example where convergence signaled respect. Remarkably, in US presidential candidate debates from 1960 to 2000, the nominee who changed his fundamental frequency less was always the nominee who won the popular vote, although not the winner of the office in 2000.

Even with perfect articulation, the sounds of speech are not unambiguous. No reliable silence occurs between words or syllables. A single phoneme, such as /t/ or /d/, is pronounced differently depending on the phonemes that come before and after. Anyone who has tried to learn a new language as an adult has encountered the common confusion between acoustically similar consonant pairs such as /d/ and /t/ or /p/ and /b/. In face-to-face conversation, knowledge of a language's lexicon, a speaker's lip movements, and expectations usually are enough to resolve acoustic ambiguities. In the case of letter codes with no inherent meaning, easily understood words such as "alpha, bravo, charlie, delta" are substituted for the ambiguous phonemes.

Although the sounds of speech do not unambiguously reflect words, we customarily understand speech with high accuracy, particularly when the speaker's mouth is visible. Facial movements, particularly of the lips, are one of the most important clues used to decipher the ambiguous sounds. A well-known auditory illusion, the *McGurk effect*, takes advantage of the comparable weights placed on auditory and visual cues to interpret speech. In this illusion, an auditory /ba/ combined with a visual /ga/ produces the illusion of having heard /da/. The utility of lip movements to speech comprehension reaches its zenith in *lip reading*. Particularly in individuals with postlingual hearing loss, with or without cochlear implants, lip reading is central to accurate speech interpretation. David Wright, the South African poet who lost his hearing after contracting scarlet fever at 7 years old, wrote, "One would think that deafness must have been self-evident from the first. On the contrary it took me some time [months] to find out what happened. . . . One day I was talking with my cousin and he, in a moment of inspiration, covered his mouth with his hand as he spoke. Silence! Once and for all I understood that *when I could not see I could not hear* [emphasis added]." In sum, speech comprehension makes use of all available sensory cues—auditory, lip movements, and facial expression.

Spoken language evolved as an interaction between two people: speaker and listener. The listener carries into the interaction expectations concerning what the speaker may want to communicate. We easily understand the sentence, "Did you eat breakfast yet?" spoken by a significant other, early in the morning, and at home. In contrast, we are unlikely to correctly "hear" the exact same sentence spoken by a boss, in the afternoon, and at the office—in other words, when it is out of context. Context places enormous constraints on the possible interpretations of what we hear. For example, we hear "call me" when a person holds their hand next to their face in the universal sign for a telephone while elevating their eyebrows and saying, "Molly," "text me," or any number of other misleading words.

Even when we rely entirely on acoustic information, context is critical to our understanding of what we hear. The interpretation of one acoustic component is often noticeably delayed until more acoustic components are available to provide additional clues. Comprehension may even depend on playback that occurs many seconds after hearing an initial remark. Translating spoken words from one language to another perfectly illustrates the difficulties of understanding verbal speech. Translators do not translate words, one by one, in the order spoken. Instead, they have to hear a complete thought—a phrase or entire sentence—before being able to interpret the meaning of each sequential word.

Auditory cortex and related neocortical regions are the substrate for language comprehension. As with any type of sensory interpretation, the task of interpretation is more difficult than a simple point-to-point mapping of the acoustic input. Information from the cochlea, arriving through ascending auditory pathways, must be processed into meaningful and interpretable information as phonemes, syllables, and then words. Because comprehension of spoken language depends so heavily on nonacoustic input, visual and contextual information is combined with auditory information. Eventually, there must be a hookup between a spoken word and a semantic representation. Whereas expertise in music or bird calls is optional, processing word sounds (speech) into lexical ideas is universal among humans, suggesting that neural circuits exist that are specialized to make the connection between auditory input and language or meaning. Such processing requires an enormous number of neurons, far more than are required at earlier stages of auditory processing (Fig. 16-14).

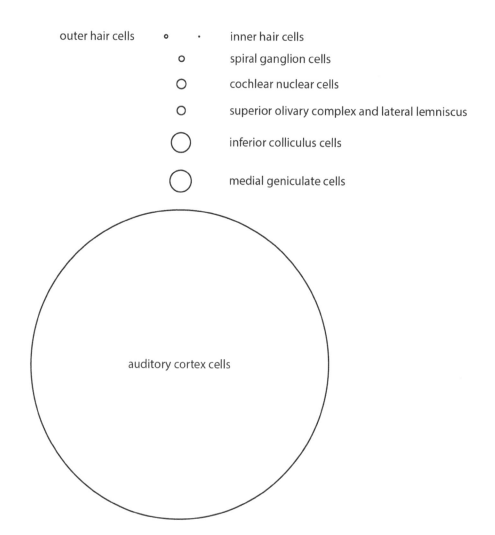

outer hair cells ∘ · inner hair cells

∘ spiral ganglion cells

○ cochlear nuclear cells

○ superior olivary complex and lateral lemniscus

◯ inferior colliculus cells

◯ medial geniculate cells

auditory cortex cells

Figure 16-14 The area of each circle is proportional to the number of cells contained in the labeled region. The number of inner hair cells is less than a third of the number of outer hair cells. The number of cells in central auditory pathways in turn dwarfs the total number of hair cells. The greatest number of cells is found in the auditory cortex.

SPECIFIC BRAIN REGIONS ARE CRITICAL TO LANGUAGE PRODUCTION AND COMPREHENSION

As you know, an impairment of language is termed *aphasia*. An inherently human problem, aphasia reflects a breakdown within a complex set of neocortical circuits that support language per se, leaving intact component sensory and motor functions required for spoken words, written text, or signing. Two main types of aphasia are recognized:

- *Broca's aphasia* or *nonfluent aphasia*

- *Wernicke's aphasia* or *fluent aphasia*

Since the late 19th century, the dominant model for language production and comprehension—and their failures—has been that the left hemisphere contains a temporal-parietal region specialized for comprehension (Wernicke's area) and a frontal area for language production (Broca's area). According to this model, Wernicke's area is responsible for speech comprehension and directly communicates to Broca's area, which is responsible for speech production. The model explains that damage to Wernicke's or Broca's area produces fluent or nonfluent aphasia, respectively.

While the 150-year-old model of language circuits forms a useful and still largely accurate scaffold for understanding language processing in the brain, incorporation of new knowledge into this model leads to an important new perspective on circuits supporting language in the brain. Recall that visual pathways divide into a ventral stream for visual recognition and a dorsal stream that feeds visually guided motor acts. In a similar vein, outputs from auditory processing areas diverge to form a ventral pathway dedicated to speech recognition and a dorsal pathway that connects to motor areas used to produce speech (Fig. 16-15).

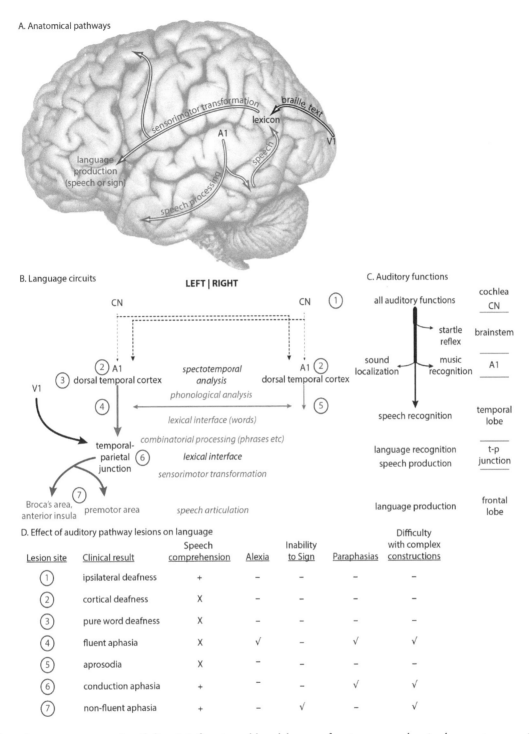

A. Anatomical pathways

sensorimotor transformation

braille text

lexicon

A1

V1

language production (speech or sign)

speech

speech processing

B. Language circuits

LEFT | RIGHT

CN   CN   ①   all auditory functions

②A1   spectotemporal analysis   A1②

③ dorsal temporal cortex   dorsal temporal cortex

V1

phonological analysis

④   ⑤

lexical interface (words)

combinatorial processing (phrases etc)

temporal-parietal junction ⑥   lexical interface

sensorimotor transformation

⑦

Broca's area, anterior insula   premotor area   speech articulation

C. Auditory functions

cochlea / CN

startle reflex — brainstem

sound localization   music recognition — A1

speech recognition — temporal lobe

language recognition / speech production — t-p junction

language production — frontal lobe

D. Effect of auditory pathway lesions on language

Lesion site	Clinical result	Speech comprehension	Alexia	Inability to Sign	Paraphasias	Difficulty with complex constructions
①	ipsilateral deafness	+	–	–	–	–
②	cortical deafness	X	–	–	–	–
③	pure word deafness	X	–	–	–	–
④	fluent aphasia	X	√	–	√	√
⑤	aprosodia	X	–	–	–	–
⑥	conduction aphasia	+	–	–	√	√
⑦	non-fluent aphasia	+	–	√	–	√

Figure 16-15 The auditory system serves primarily linguistic functions, although language functions can employ visual or somatosensory inputs. A: Speech sounds arrive in the auditory cortex (A1) and are processed phonologically in the ventral auditory pathway (*red*). The temporal-parietal junction serves as the mental lexicon where sensory inputs are connected to linguistic meaning. Inputs from visual cortex (V1) carrying information about visible text and Braille to the temporal-parietal junction are critical for reading. The dorsal auditory pathway (*blue*) transforms auditory signals into motor commands. Within the frontal cortex, production of language, typically verbal but also signing, depends on Broca's area ventrally and the premotor area dorsally. B: Circuits that serve linguistic functions (*italicized text*) are diagrammed. Primary auditory cortex receives polysynaptic (*dashed lines*) input from both ears, but contralateral input dominates. While commissural connections (*horizontal red arrow*) are present early in the ventral auditory pathway, the remainder of the pathways function in the dominant hemisphere, typically the left. C: The anatomical regions that support several auditory functions are illustrated. Music recognition and sound localization depend on cortical pathways distinct from those critical to speech comprehension, whereas the brainstem is responsible for the startle reflex. D: For auditory and language deficits produced by several lesions at brainstem and cortical locations (*circled numbers in panel B*), the resulting clinical condition is listed. Speech comprehension is intact (+) after a unilateral cochlear nucleus lesion or a lesion of the dorsal pathway but is impaired (X) after lesions of the ventral pathway. The presence (check mark) or absence (–) of language impairments such as alexia is noted. Abbreviations: A1, primary auditory cortex; CN, cochlear nuclei; t-p junction, temporal-parietal junction; V1, primary visual cortex.

In the ventral pathway, sounds are processed in parallel into very fast acoustic features (e.g., the s-t of "mast" versus the t-s of "mats"), phonemes, syllables, and syllabic sequences. The ventral auditory pathway interprets speech sounds by processing them into auditory chunks of varying sizes. Acoustic and phonological processing occur bilaterally within the dorsal temporal gyrus and dorsal portion of the middle temporal gyrus. As further explored later, these phonological characteristics are mapped onto semantic representations of words, and, ultimately, the ordered words of a phrase or sentence are mapped into meaning. Lexical processing of speech employs regions of the posterior and anterior temporal cortex that are progressively more left-lateralized so that the right (nondominant) hemisphere may support limited word comprehension but not sentence comprehension.

Connecting sensory input with a semantic meaning is a veritable magic trick performed by the brain. Lexical processing occurs in stages at the word, multiword, phrase, and sentence levels. People can have difficulty in comprehending speech from words on up or may understand words but be unable to parse the meaning of words strung together into a sentence. A common language difficulty is the comprehension of simple but not complex constructions. For example, a patient may be able to identify who did the licking in "Fluffy licked Sparky" but unable to do so when told "Sparky was licked by Fluffy" or "Sparky, licked by Fluffy, became very clean."

Lexical brain circuits serve written text and braille as well as speech, transforming all types of input into language, meaning, and concepts. The central node for the lexical interface shared by auditory, visual, and somatosensory modalities appears to be located in the temporal-parietal junction of the left hemisphere. Auditory input arrives here from the ventral pathway. Interestingly, comprehension of braille as well as visible text depends on input that arises in *visual cortex* and reaches the same lexical interface that serves spoken words. In one illustrative case, a congenitally blind braille reader suffered a bilateral occipital stroke that wiped out her visual cortex. Thereafter, braille "felt flat" although normal somatosensory discrimination—was a bump present or not?—remained intact. Since the lexical interface transforms inputs of any type into linguistic output, lesions in this area compromise all types of language comprehension, leading to *alexia*, a failure in reading comprehension, as well as fluent aphasia.

Ventral auditory pathways in both hemispheres participate in understanding the spoken word but do so differently. One major difference is in the time domain, with the right hemisphere integrating speech inputs over longer time scales than the left. Clinically, this difference may be connected to the finding that *aprosodia*, a difficulty in understanding the prosody of speech, results most typically from right-sided (nondominant hemisphere) lesions. Since prosody alone distinguishes the rote "how are you?" from the targeted concern of a slowly articulated "how are *you?*" it is not surprising that aprosodic patients experience difficulty in social interactions.

The ventral auditory pathway starts out as a generic auditory processor concerned with spectrotemporal features that form the foundation for all downstream auditory functions. Bilateral (and thus rare) lesions of auditory cortex can produce *cortical deafness*, which is similar to cortical blindness; subcortical auditory functions such as the auditory startle reflex are preserved, whereas all cortical auditory functions are impaired. After this common start, the ventral auditory pathway diverges into separate streams, one of which is dedicated to speech. We know this in part because *pure word deafness*, which is essentially agnosia selective for auditory speech, can result from dorsal temporal lobe lesions. Patients with pure word deafness have cortical pathways that allow them to localize sounds and recognize music but they cannot gather meaning from speech, which they perceive as noise or speech in an unintelligible and alien language. This problem is specific to auditory language and does not extend to other auditory functions (music, sound localization) or other modalities of language (reading, sign language). In sum, word deafness is a failure of auditory interpretation *specific to speech*; it is to spoken language what visual agnosia is to viewed objects (see Chapter 15). *Amusia* (a loss of music recognition with preserved sound localization and speech recognition) can also result from temporal lobe lesions, suggesting that the ventral auditory pathway diverges into at least three separate streams (for speech, music, and sound localization).

For speech production, the dorsal auditory pathway, which starts in auditory regions of the temporal lobe, passes on to the temporal-parietal junction and then to frontal cortex. The frontal regions of greatest importance are the premotor area and a large region in the ventral frontal cortex encompassing Broca's area and the anterior insula (Fig. 16-15). The dorsal pathway is strongly lateralized, with the left hemisphere responsible for lexical speech production. For this reason, nonfluent aphasia results from a lesion in the dominant (usually left) hemisphere. As with the mental lexicon, the dorsal pathway is shared across modalities, in this case output modalities. Thus, Broca's area and related regions in frontal cortex participate in language expression, regardless of whether that expression takes the form of speech or signing. Lesions in the dorsal pathway render deaf signers unable to sign just as they make speakers mute.

Auditory input to the dorsal pathway is critical for learning to speak as a baby and also for continuously monitoring one's own articulation thereafter. Just as songbirds model their songs after songs that they hear from a "tutor" bird, babies learn spoken language from those around them. Adults cannot recall the intense motor learning associated with learning to speak as babies but can appreciate the challenge when trying to say a multisyllabic word in an unfamiliar language for the first time. Indeed, verbal learning persists throughout life as new vocabulary or foreign languages are acquired. Beyond learning to speak or acquiring new vocabulary, matching our actual speech to our intended speech requires auditory input to the dorsal pathway. This accounts for the common observation that speech quality degrades after hearing loss when one's own speech can no longer be monitored through auditory feedback.

Deficits in speaking with prosody can result from either left or right hemisphere lesions. In addition, several diseases also involve aprosodic speech. For example, individuals afflicted with depression or schizophrenia often speak with minimal modulation of fundamental frequency, facial movements, and hand gestures. More so than having rigid and separate respective roles in speech production, the two hemispheres cooperate to produce normal-sounding speech. For example, in order to emphasize a particular word, the articulation process, predominantly dependent on the dominant hemisphere, must be coordinated with prosodic production in the nondominant hemisphere. Because of the tight link between prosody and lexical content, a selective deficit in prosody can be difficult to tease out. One approach to testing for prosody per se is asking an individual to repeat a prosodic intonation using simple sounds rather than words. For example, a person who may not be able to intone "What a cute baby" in the typical sing-song may be able to copy the tone and prosody used while saying "ba ba ba ba ba." Thus, reducing the articulation demands may reveal either normal or impaired prosody.

APHASIA IS A DISORDER OF LANGUAGE

Patients with different forms of aphasia perform differently on tests of spontaneous speech, naming, comprehension, repetition, reading, and writing. Using the pathways described earlier, we can understand how differing symptoms result from lesions in different locations.

In Broca's aphasia, also known as nonfluent aphasia or *motor aphasia*, patients typically string together a few nouns without connecting prepositions or articles. Their speech lacks prosody and sounds strained and labored. Patients with Broca's aphasia are frustrated by their inability to communicate through either speaking or writing (or signing in the case of native sign language speakers). They comprehend spoken and written language relatively well, although there may be deficits in understanding all but the simplest constructions.

Broca's aphasia is typically caused by damage to frontal lobe regions centered around Broca's area, which sits anterior to the tongue and larynx motor areas of the dominant hemisphere. A stroke in the superior division of the left middle cerebral artery is the most common cause of Broca's aphasia. Because of this location, right-sided volitional paralysis of the arm and face may accompany Broca's aphasia. Leg hemiparesis is rarer, and visual field disturbances are not typically present.

Patients with Wernicke's aphasia, also known as fluent aphasia, produce speech (and writing) that sounds normal except that it does not make sense. *Paraphasias*, incorrect words or syllables, of the semantic (horse for dog) or phonemic (log or dop for dog) type, are common. Patients have difficulty following spoken commands or pointing to objects, evidence of impaired language comprehension. The deficits in Wernicke's aphasia are caused by a failure in lexical mapping of words, phrases, and sentences onto meaning. This lexical failure extends to reading comprehension, which is compromised along with verbal understanding. Examining a Wernicke's patient is typically frustrating for the examiner because normal, two-way communication with the affected patient is severely compromised.

Wernicke's aphasia typically results from damage in the temporal lobe or temporal-parietal junction on the dominant side. Because of this lesion location, patients typically do not experience contralateral hemiparesis, as is the case for patients with Broca's aphasia. They often do have a visual field deficit, most commonly a right-sided upper quadrantanopia due to interruption of Meyer's loop (see Chapter 7). Some patients may have some degree of anosognosia, which you recall is a failure to recognize one's own deficits even when those deficits are quite evident to others. This latter issue leads some patients to think that a conversation is going well and may account for the relative lack of frustration expressed by many patients with Wernicke's aphasia.

The primary deficit in patients with *conduction aphasia*, a rarer form of aphasia than the other two, is impaired verbatim repetition of speech. Although patients can accurately respond to or paraphrase what they hear, they produce numerous phonemic paraphasias and transpositions (way-hall instead of hallway) when asked to repeat a sentence word by word. Patients are aware of their errors and try repeatedly to correct themselves. Although conduction aphasia has been traditionally attributed to lesions of the arcuate fasciculus that connects Wernicke's and Broca's areas, this explanation now appears incorrect. Instead, damage to neocortical regions around the temporal-parietal junction important for phonological transformation into lexical content is now thought to produce conduction aphasia.

FROM HEARING LOSS TO APHASIA

Hearing loss due to inner ear or nerve problems is associated with substantially different personal experiences, treatment options, and chances for improvement than are aphasias caused by cortical lesions. Unfortunately, hearing loss due to peripheral pathology does not improve without intervention. It is fortunate, then, that effective interventions exist for most patients with inner ear dysfunction. Cochlear implants can provide language for many children with congenital or prelingually acquired deafness. For children who cannot benefit from a cochlear implant or whose parents opt against the surgery, sign language provides a rich form of communication, albeit within a smaller and more restricted community. Hearing aids ameliorate the challenges of acquired hearing loss, with cochlear implants an available option for many with profound hearing loss. Although hearing aids do not restore perfect hearing, and some hearing loss is recalcitrant to available treatments, most hearing loss secondary to inner ear damage is manageable.

We started this chapter by emphasizing that hearing's primary job is to serve our social natures by enabling communication through language. And it is precisely this primary mission that is compromised by cortical lesions that produce aphasia of any type. Unfortunately, treatment options directed at aphasia are limited to rehabilitation, which can be effective but requires intense effort from both patient and therapist. The good news is that damage from cortical insults such as stroke or brain tumors tends to ameliorate over time (see Chapter 8). Yet the most meaningful difference between hearing loss and aphasia relates to the effect of the condition on a person's self-image and social identity. Only intractable and untreatable hearing loss impacts the self in the profound way that any magnitude of aphasia does.

ADDITIONAL READING

Chorost M. *Rebuilt: My Journey Back to the Hearing World*. Boston: Houghton Mifflin, 2005.

Cohen LH. *Train Go Sorry: Inside a Deaf World*. Boston: Houghton Mifflin, 1994.

Dallos P. Cochlear amplification, outer hair cells and prestin. *Curr Opin Neurobiol*. 18: 370–376, 2008.

Ealy M, Smith RJH. The genetics of otosclerosis. *Hearing Res*. 266: 70–74, 2010.

Eisen MD, Ryugo DK. Hearing molecules: Contributions from genetic deafness. *Cell Molec Life Sci*. 64: 566–580, 2007.

Fettiplace R, Hackney CM. The sensory and motor roles of auditory hair cells. *Nat Rev Neurosci*. 7: 19–29, 2006.

Gregory SW, Gallagher TJ. Spectral analysis of candidates' nonverbal vocal communication: Predicting U.S. presidential election outcomes. *Soc Psychol Q*. 65: 298–308, 2001.

Gregory SW, Webster S. A nonverbal signal in voices of interview partners effectively predicts communication accommodation and social status perceptions. *J Personality Social Psychol*. 70: 1231–1240, 1996.

Hamilton R, Keenan JP, Catala M, Pascual-Leone A. Alexia for Braille following bilateral occipital stroke in an early blind woman. *Cog Neurosci*. 11: 237–240, 2000.

Hickok G, Poeppel D. The cortical organization of speech processing. *Nat Rev Neurosci*. 8: 393–402, 2007.

Huttenlocher J, Haight W, Bryk A, Seltzer M, Lyons T. Early vocabulary growth: Relation to language input and gender. *Dev Pschol*. 27: 1236–1248, 1991.

Kisor H. *What's that Pig Outdoors? A Memoir of Deafness*. New York: Penguin Books, 1990.

Liberman MC. Hidden hearing loss. *Sci Am*. 313: 48–53, 2015.

Liberman MC. Noise-induced hearing loss: Permanent versus temporary threshold shifts and the effects of hair cell versus neuronal degeneration. *Adv Exp Med Biol*. 875: 1–7, 2016.

McCarter DF, Courtney AU, Pollart SM. Cerumen impaction. *Am Fam Physician*. 75: 1523–1528, 2007.

Pardo JS. On phonetic convergence during conversational interaction. *J Acoust Soc Am*. 119: 2382–2393, 2006.

Poeppel D. Pure word deafness and the bilateral processing of the speech code. *Cog Sci*. 25: 679–693, 2001.

Rizzi MD, Hirose K. Aminoglycoside ototoxicity. *Curr Opin Otolaryngol Head Neck Surg*. 15: 352–357, 2007.

Rosen S, Olin P. Hearing loss and coronary heart disease. *Bull NY Acad Med*. 41: 1052–1068, 1965.

Ross ED, Monnot M. Neurology of affective prosody and its functional–anatomic organization in right hemisphere. *Brain Lang*. 104: 51–74, 2008.

Rybak LP, Ramkumar V. Ototoxicity. *Kidney Int*. 72: 931–935, 2007.

Sacks O. *Seeing Voices*. London: Picador, 2012.

Sakaguchi H, Tokita J, Müller U, Kechar B. Tip links in hair cells: Molecular composition and role in hearing loss. *Curr Opin Otolaryngol Head Neck Surg*. 17: 388–393, 2009.

Seif S, Dellon AL. Anatomic relationships between the human levator and tensor veli palatini and the Eustachian tube. *Cleft Palate J*. 15: 329–336, 1978.

Stenross B. *Missed Connections: Hard of Hearing in a Hearing World*. Philadelphia: Temple University Press, 1999.

Walker LA. *A Loss for Words: The Story of Deafness in a Family*. New York: Harper Perennial, 1986.

Warren RM. *Auditory Perception*. 3rd ed. Cambridge: Cambridge University Press, 2008.

Wright D. *Deafness: An Autobiography*. New York: Harper Perennial, 1993.

17.

FROM MOVEMENT TO PAIN

SOMATOSENSATION IS AN UMBRELLA TERM FOR VARIED SENSORY PATHWAYS

Somatosensation is a far more varied system than either audition or vision. One striking result of this greater heterogeneity is that no one suffers from a complete absence of somatosensation. We do not even have a word for such a condition. In contrast, both the absence and severe impairment of vision and hearing are relatively common, with almost 1 in 20 people suffering from deafness, severe hearing impairment, blindness, or low vision even with correction. There are two primary reasons for the difference between vision and hearing on one hand and somatosensation on the other. First, light and sound arrive through portals—our eyes and ears—whereas somatosensory afferents cover the body surface and canvass the viscera and other deep structures. Second, the transducing pathways for light and sound are limited so that dysfunction of any of a large number of molecules knocks out function. In contrast, as described later in the chapter, there are at least a dozen known transduction pathways (and surely more yet to be discovered) involved in somatosensation. The only condition that renders a person anesthetic is a traumatic injury rostral to the sensory trigeminal complex. Although Jean-Dominique Bauby, introduced in the first chapter, had just this injury due to a stroke that left him locked-in, the injury occurs rarely and is survived even less often. Even rarer still are individuals who lose somatosensation secondary to a viral infection; two such patients have been described.

Somatosensory modalities run the gamut from finely discriminated perceptual modalities, such as the sense of touch, to poorly discriminated perceptual modalities such as visceral pain, to modalities that do not reach conscious perception at all, such as blood pressure or oxygen tension. As an example of a finely discriminated form of somatosensation, tactile pathways from our fingertips allow us to discriminate, without looking, glossy from matte paper, burlap from flannel, and flannel from brushed cotton. In contrast, a variety of visceral stimuli such as an overly distended stomach from eating too much, a peptic or duodenal ulcer, gallstones, or appendicitis all elicit essentially the same result: a report of abdominal pain, moaning, and holding the abdomen.

Under normal circumstances, the somatosensory system contributes more to shaping movements than to forming our detailed perception of the world. Somatosensory input from muscles and joints drives fundamental motor reflexes, input from our fingertips determines the firmness of our hand grip, and input from the oral cavity determines whether we chew, suck, or swallow. Even acutely painful events, such as stubbing a toe, that are certainly *perceived* are quickly forgotten and thus only briefly contribute to our conscious experience of the world. From this perspective, somatosensation closely resembles the vestibular sense, which is most critical to postural and orienting movements (see Chapter 18). In this regard, somatosensation contrasts sharply with audition and vision, which are so important to our perceptual world.

Because chronic pain is a common reason for individuals to seek medical help, we concentrate on the mechanisms underlying the transition from acute injury to chronic pain. Once the transition to chronic pain has been made, dramatic changes in the perceptual quality of normally unremarkable stimuli occur. We may feel constant awareness of a body part or sense an abnormal, and usually bothersome, feeling such as numbness or pins and needles. Positive signs arising from somatosensory dysfunction can be very unpleasant, as is the case with spontaneous feelings of pain or *allodynia* (i.e., pain elicited by a normally innocuous stimulus such as a light touch). A mild and transient form of allodynia is common, resulting from injuries such as a sunburn, open blister, or bruise. Luckily, in these cases, the pain goes away with time.

Unfortunately, allodynia is a steady hallmark of many conditions of chronic pain. For example, a patient with a neuropathy may feel the touch of clothing as exquisitely painful. A person with a headache may experience the pulsation of a blood vessel as a jackhammer pounding on the skull. As one can imagine, allodynia causes great distress and significantly decreases quality of life. *Spontaneous pain* often occurs in chronic pain conditions. Spontaneous pain can have a variety of qualities from lancinating and electrifying to throbbing and aching. It is unclear whether spontaneous pain is indeed spontaneous or is triggered by stimuli, such as intestinal peristalsis or body temperature, that normally do not elicit any perception. A final symptom of chronic pain is *hyperalgesia*. Hyperalgesic patients have enhanced pain perceptions so that, for example, a stimulus that ordinarily produces pain rated as 3 on a scale of 1 to 10 now produces a pain rated as 9.

As has been emphasized from the first chapter, damage to somatosensory pathways produces positive signs, and it is these signs that typically impel individuals to seek medical help. Therefore, our exploration of the mechanisms and pathways involved in touch perception is slanted toward understanding the contribution of the dorsal column–medial lemniscus pathway to the generation of paresthesias. Second, we examine and contrast the properties of superficial and deep pain along with the differences between superficial, escapable pain and deep, inescapable pain. Third, we look in some detail at the peripheral and central changes triggered by acute injury or disease that lead to long-lasting, chronic pain. Finally, endogenous modulation of somatosensation is briefly considered.

CUTANEOUS MECHANORECEPTIVE AFFERENTS RESPOND TO A DIVERSE RANGE OF INNOCUOUS STIMULI

As touched upon in Chapter 4, several types of primary afferents respond to superficial stimuli with different characteristics. Afferents innervating the skin can be divided into two classes, each of which is itself diverse and can be divided into several subclasses. Mechanoreceptors that support the fine discrimination of mechanical stimuli form a class of Aβ fibers. Aβ sensory fibers respond to innocuous mechanical stimuli including light touch, hair movement, and vibration. The second major class of cutaneous afferents is comprised of Aδ and C fibers; this class includes nociceptors and thermoreceptors that respond to tissue damaging stimulation and innocuous thermal stimuli, respectively. In

addition, there are Aδ and C fiber mechanoreceptors that do not support tactile discrimination but instead contribute to pleasurable and crudely discriminated forms of touch or stroking.

Initially, we focus on Aβ mechanoreceptive afferents. Aβ mechanoreceptors are large neurons with large-diameter, well-myelinated axons. Consequently, action potentials are conducted rapidly along the processes of Aβ afferents (Fig. 17-1A). Mechanoreceptors involved in *perception* fall primarily into two groups:

- Low-threshold mechanoreceptors are excited by touch or skin deformation. Different types of mechanoreceptors are tuned to mechanical stimuli of different temporal frequencies.

- Pacinian corpuscle afferents respond to vibration. Note that Pacinian corpuscles are located deep in the hypodermis and yet are so sensitive that they sense superficial vibration over a wide area of the body surface.

Activation of members of one class of afferents is *roughly* aligned with a perceptual modality. For example, vibration excites Pacinian corpuscle afferents and also typically leads to the perception of vibration. Similarly, excitation of a

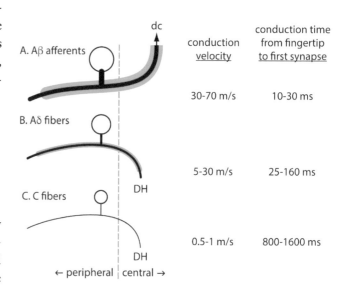

Figure 17-1 Aβ, Aδ, and C fibers differ in the caliber, or width, of their axons (*black*) and in the amount of myelination surrounding their axons (*blue*). As a result of the different caliber axons and myelination, action potentials conduct at different speeds (middle column) along the three fiber types. In the right hand column are given the approximate times required for an action potential to travel from the fingertip to the first central synapse in a woman of average height. In the case of Aβ fibers (A), the first synapse is in the dorsal column nuclei. In the case of Aδ and C fibers (B–C), the first synapse is in the dorsal horn. The dotted line shows the edge of the central nervous system.

low-threshold mechanoreceptor normally elicits a sensation of touch. Identifying the most typical percepts resulting from strong activation of different classes of somatosensory afferents provides a useful way to learn and think about the basic organization of somatosensory inputs.

A one-to-one connection between receptor class and percept is a simplification. In reality, *no single receptor class is dedicated to one percept, and no single percept relies on a single receptor class.* This is nicely illustrated by *wetness*, a compound sensation that requires activity in more than one afferent type. Low-threshold mechanoreceptors and cold-sensitive thermoreceptors both respond to wetness, and it is the combination of activity in the two afferent types that gives rise to a perception of wetness. As a result, water at skin temperature does not register as wet. For example, when swimmers enter a heated pool, they are often unable to discriminate the water line by feel alone. The ability to sense wetness is further compromised in competitive swimmers who shave their body hair and therefore receive neither mechanical nor thermal stimulation from entering a heated pool.

The dependence of wetness perception on both mechanical and thermal input means that tissues not innervated by both thermoreceptors and low-threshold mechanoreceptors cannot support the sensation of wet. Most of our deep tissues, including our viscera, are not innervated by low-threshold mechanoreceptors, such as those innervating skin. For example, our esophagus is innervated by cold thermoreceptors but not by low-threshold mechanoreceptors. Consequently, a cold drink traveling down our esophagus elicits a perception of cold but not of wet. An exception to the general rule that we cannot sense wetness in deep tissues is our ability to discriminate between gaseous, liquid, and solid contents in the anal canal. Essentially, we sense phase—solid, liquid, or gas—in part by using the compound sensation of wetness derived from inputs from mechanoreceptors and thermoreceptors. In fact, we are able to detect small changes in temperature of less than 1°C within the anal canal.

Detecting the phase of the contents of the anal canal allows us to distinguish between flatus (gas), diarrhea, and stool and to accordingly direct our actions. In fact, we automatically and regularly sample the contents of the rectum by relaxing the inner anal sphincter to allow rectal contents to enter into the anal canal. When afferents supplying the anal canal are damaged, the sensory arm of the sampling process is damaged, and a *sensory* form of fecal incontinence can result. Individuals with idiopathic fecal incontinence may be unable to detect the small changes in the temperature of sampled contents that normal people detect.

MOST LOW-THRESHOLD INFORMATION ASCENDS IN THE DORSAL COLUMN–MEDIAL LEMNISCUS PATHWAY

Aβ sensory afferents carry information about tactile inputs, vibration, and proprioception and conduct action potentials rapidly at speeds of 30–70 m/s. Aβ afferents enter the spinal cord through the medial portion of the dorsal root (Fig. 17-2), the portion of the root closest to the dorsal column. The axons immediately enter the dorsal column and turn to ascend rostrally. As Aβ fibers enter at progressively more rostral segments of the spinal cord, they extend the dorsal column laterally. Therefore, axons in the most medial part of the dorsal columns carry information that entered in the most caudal segments (see Chapter 4). Recall that sensory afferents innervating the perineal region, not the feet, arise from the most caudal dorsal root ganglia and thus enter the spinal cord most caudally and travel most medially. This topographic arrangement means that in the cervical cord, axons in the most medial parts of the dorsal columns carry information from the perineum. Axons located in progressively more lateral positions carry information from the feet; distal legs; proximal legs; lower trunk; upper trunk; hands, distal to proximal; shoulders; neck; and back of the head.

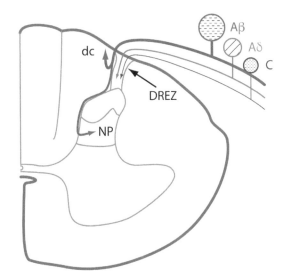

Figure 17-2 Aβ fibers enter the spinal cord more medially than do Aδ and C fibers. Aβ fibers send their main axon up the ipsilateral dorsal column (*dc*) toward the dorsal column nuclei (not shown). Aβ fibers also give off collaterals that contact nucleus proprius (*NP*) neurons. In this way, tactile input carried by Aβ fibers reaches the dorsal horn. Aδ and C fibers enter in the dorsal root entry zone (DREZ), just lateral to the entry point of Aβ fibers. DREZ lesions have been used to neurosurgically treat intractable pain. Unfortunately, although they provide temporary relief, the relief does not last and is typically replaced by neuropathic deafferentation pain.

Primary afferents travel through the dorsal columns to terminate in the dorsal column nuclei located in the caudal medulla. Thus, large-diameter afferents that innervate the foot extend from a peripheral terminal in the foot to a central terminal in the caudal medulla at the base of the skull. These primary afferents are easily the longest neurons and indeed are the longest cells in the body. Unfortunately, nerve length makes for nerve vulnerability because of two factors. First, a greater amount of surface area is exposed to potentially harmful substances in a long than a short nerve. Second, damage to an axon or to its myelin wrapping at any one spot disables function of the entire axon. Therefore, the greater length of nerves innervating the feet is associated with a greater risk of either failure or significant slowing of action potential conduction.

Because of the vulnerability of long nerves, neuropathies caused by toxins or metabolic disorders primarily affect distal function. Most nontraumatic *peripheral neuropathies* initially produce symptoms in the feet. One of the most common of these neuropathies, *diabetic neuropathy*, is prevalent in individuals with diabetes mellitus and usually causes symptoms that occur first in the feet. Since both sensory and motor axons are vulnerable, diabetic neuropathy usually affects all types of nerve fibers: sensory, somatomotor, and autonomic. Thus, a typical case of diabetic neuropathy is an individual with diabetes who complains of pain and abnormal sensations arising from the feet, pain when walking, weakness in the feet and ankles, and sores on the feet that do not heal. Nonsymptomatic abnormalities, changes that patients do not complain of, are often present in shorter nerves. For example, individuals may be insensitive to the sensation produced by placing a vibrating tuning fork on either the hands or feet. More information, at more cost, can also be gained from a nerve conduction study. Abnormalities may never develop into problems or may become problematic after further disease progression.

Upon reaching the dorsal column nuclei, primary afferents terminate. Dorsal column nuclear cells send an axon across the midline to reach the thalamus. The crossing of axons arising from dorsal column nuclear cells is often referred to as the *sensory decussation*. It is very important to remember that *below the sensory decussation, tactile, vibratory, and proprioceptive information travels on the same side as the stimulus, whereas above the sensory decussation, this information travels contralateral to the stimulus.* After crossing the midline, the axons of dorsal column nuclear cells travel in the medial lemniscus, a pathway that we followed in our tour through the brainstem (see Chapter 6). The

medial lemniscus terminates in the thalamus carrying tactile information from the contralateral body.

Recall that low-threshold touch, vibration, and proprioceptive information from the face and oral cavity terminates in the main sensory nucleus, the trigeminal analog to the dorsal column nuclei. Neurons in the main sensory nucleus project to the medial portion of the ventrobasal complex of the thalamus through a pathway very similar to the medial lemniscus, with the exception that the trigeminal dermatome is represented both ipsilaterally and contralaterally.

In sum, somatosensory information from the head reaches the ventral posteromedial nucleus, and somatosensory information from the body terminates in the ventral posterolateral nucleus. Thalamic neurons in both lateral and medial parts of the ventrobasal complex send axons through the posterior limb of the internal capsule that project to the somatotopically organized primary somatosensory cortex (see Chapter 7).

LOW-THRESHOLD MECHANORECEPTORS GUIDE GRIP AND OTHER ACTIONS

The somatosensory cortex supports the perception of touch. In addition, the dorsal column–medial lemniscus pathway is critical for *stereognosis*. Stereognosis is the process by which we use low-threshold tactile input to detect the size, shape, texture, hardness, and other qualities of an object. Using touch alone, we can distinguish a key from a bobby pin from a pencil from a chopstick and so on. In fact, we can distinguish these objects simply by running our fingertips over them. Accurate stereognosis requires information from proprioceptors as well as from cutaneous mechanoreceptors. To understand why this is so, consider holding a baseball in your hand. The baseball stimulates low-threshold afferents all over the glabrous (smooth and nonhairy) surface of your palm and fingers. Similar tactile information arises when you place your hand flat on a table top or flat on a wall. Yet we easily distinguish among a baseball, a table top, and a wall. We do so by using proprioceptive information regarding the *position of the hand*. The hand curves around a baseball, is horizontally flat when touching the table top, and is vertically flat when positioned against a wall.

We use stereognosis to guide our grip of objects. As objects vary, so do grips. Heavy objects require a firmer grip than do light objects. A bottle requires a wider grip than a pencil. In sum, somatosensory information, principally from the dorsal column–medial lemniscus pathway, is used to ensure that a grip is appropriate to both the object and the goal for that object. Without somatosensory feedback from proprioceptors and cutaneous mechanoreceptors, a person is unable to match grip force to a target object, either dropping the object because of inadequate force or crushing it. Thus, clumsiness can result from a somatosensory loss as well as a motor loss.

Neuropathy is a general term for a disorder involving peripheral nerves. Individuals with a neuropathy affecting the hands often complain of dropping things. Motor weakness due to affected motoneuron axons typically contributes to such clumsiness. However, damage to sensory afferents can also contribute to clumsiness by impairing the sensory guidance of grip. Faulty information about the size, weight, or slipperiness of an object will result in a correspondingly faulty grip and consequently the dropping of an object. Neuropathies may preferentially affect selected populations of peripheral axons such as large, well-myelinated axons or small unmyelinated axons. Afferents that convey information used to recognize body position include low-threshold mechanoreceptors from the skin, as well as joint and muscle afferents. All of these afferents have large, well-myelinated axons that are only slightly smaller in diameter than the axons of motoneurons. Thus, when present in nerves supplying the hands, large-fiber neuropathies, those that preferentially affect large-diameter axons, may cause clumsiness through impairment of sensory as well as motor function.

NOCICEPTION IS THE SENSATION THAT NORMALLY LEADS TO A PERCEPTION OF PAIN

We now turn our attention to pain. The brain supports two reactions to pain. First, like other sensory inputs, painful stimulation elicits sensory discrimination. Using sensory discrimination we know what type of pain—burning, lancinating, stabbing, aching and so on—occurred, where, and when. Second, painful stimulation elicits an emotional reaction with motivational implications. As Sherrington put it more than a century ago, pain is "curiously imperative," demanding an immediate and well-motivated reaction. The emotional suffering accompanying pain perception, typically termed the affective component of pain, feeds our motivation to react to and thereby remove ourselves from painful stimuli.

The bipartite nature of pain is accompanied by disparate cortical representations of pain. As one might expect, the primary somatosensory cortex is responsible for sensory discrimination of pain. In contrast, the affective component of pain depends on the anterior insula. Patients with anterior insular lesions can report sensory discriminative details about painful stimulation but have no or little affective reaction. In other words, these patients do not care about pain, a condition termed *asymbolia for pain*.

Regarding pain, we have a definitional problem. How do we know what is painful and what is not? The gold standard is a person's subjective verbal report of feeling pain. That gold standard cannot be used for babies and other nonverbal individuals. Nor can verbal reports be acquired during general anesthesia. Consequently, we use the term *nociception* to refer to the sensory pathway that normally results in a perception of pain. The advantage of the term nociception is that it is noncommittal regarding whether or not the final step, pain perception, occurs. Thus, a noxious stimulus activates nociceptive neurons in nociceptive pathways even in instances when pain perception is blocked. One such condition is opioid analgesia (i.e., the relief of pain by an opioid such as morphine).

The experience of pain involves both a discriminative aspect and an affective component. Both components of pain depend on the initial transduction of peripheral stimuli and on transmission from nociceptors to dorsal horn cells. The pathways supporting the discriminative and affective components of pain start to diverge at the point that nociceptive dorsal horn cells project to brainstem and diencephalic targets (Fig. 17-3). As we know, some nociceptive neurons in the superficial dorsal horn send an axon across the midline and into the ventrolateral funiculus to form the spinothalamic tract. The spinothalamic pathway ends in the ventrobasal complex of the thalamus; thalamic neurons in turn project to primary somatosensory cortex where sensory discrimination for pain and temperature occurs.

Several additional pathways arise from nociceptive dorsal horn cells. The spinohypothalamic tract conveys nociceptive information to the hypothalamus and may be important in coordinating autonomic and endocrine reactions to pain. Pathways from the dorsal horn that ultimately reach the anterior insula and anterior cingulate are critical to the affective component of pain. Individuals with damage to the anterior insula can sense pain (i.e., they can describe its sensory characteristics), but they do not care about it. The course of the pathways involved in pain affect is controversial but certainly involves both areas in brainstem and regions of thalamus outside of the ventrobasal complex.

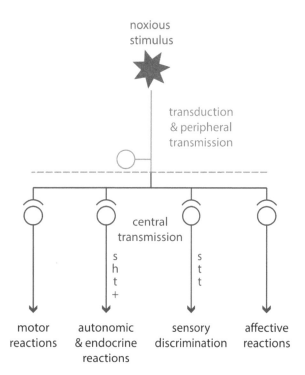

noxious
stimulus

transduction
& peripheral
transmission

central
transmission

s
h
t
+

s
t
t

motor
reactions

autonomic
& endocrine
reactions

sensory
discrimination

affective
reactions

Figure 17-3 Nociceptors are the common entry into pain pathways. However, pain pathways diverge upon entering the central nervous system (*dashed line*). Nociceptive information important for motor reactions, such as withdrawals and escape, reaches the ventral horn and brainstem. Nociceptive information used for autonomic and endocrine reactions travels through multiple tracts including the spinohypothalamic tract (*sht+*). The spinothalamic tract (*stt*) carries nociceptive information important for sensory discrimination to the somatosensory cortex. Nociceptive information critical to affective, motivational, and emotional responses reach the anterior insula and cingulate cortex through a number of pathways.

SMALL-DIAMETER FIBERS INCLUDE NOCICEPTORS AND THERMORECEPTORS

Nociceptors and thermoreceptors are small-diameter, lightly myelinated Aδ and unmyelinated C fibers that conduct action potentials either slowly or *very* slowly, respectively (Fig. 17-1). We focus on five classes of small-diameter fibers that contribute to the perceptions of pain and temperature:

- *High-threshold mechanoreceptors* are lightly myelinated Aδ fibers that respond to sharp, well-localized mechanical stimuli, such as a needle prick.

- *High-threshold thermoreceptors* are lightly myelinated Aδ fibers that respond rapidly to noxious heat.

- *Polymodal nociceptors* are a heterogeneous class of unmyelinated C fiber afferents that respond to tissue-damaging stimuli of multiple types: thermal (hot or

cold), mechanical, or chemical such as capsaicin, the active ingredient in hot chili peppers.

- *Thermoreceptors* are unmyelinated afferents excited by innocuous cool or innocuous warm temperatures.

- *Pruriceptors* include a group of unmyelinated C fiber afferents that respond to histamine, the prototypical itch stimulus. Histamine produces a sensation akin to that of a mosquito bite. Most pruriceptive afferents also respond to at least some forms of noxious stimulation.

Small-diameter Aδ and C fibers exist that code for modalities other than pain, temperature, or itch. For example, C-fiber mechanoreceptors respond to movements of the downy hair. These afferents may signal a form of crude touch, signaling the presence of a stimulus while not providing much discriminative information.

Itch, or *pruritus*, is defined as a sensation that elicits the desire to scratch. Pain, on the other hand elicits guarding, shaking, and biting. Yet pain and itch are both unpleasant somatic sensations, and they share overlapping ascending pathways. Moreover, most pruriceptive primary afferents and perhaps all pruriceptive dorsal horn cells also respond to noxious stimulation. Importantly, spinothalamic tract neurons that respond to pruritic, or itch-producing, stimuli also respond to noxious stimuli. Thus, at the neuronal level, there is virtually a complete overlap of pruriceptive pathways with nociceptive pathways. This conclusion is confirmed by individuals who received an anterolateral cordotomy, a neurosurgical lesion of the ventrolateral white matter of the spinal cord that has been performed to alleviate intractable pain. After an anterolateral cordotomy, individuals sense neither pain nor itch on the contralateral side below the level of the lesion. The strong overlap between itch and pain pathways has led some to consider itch as a form of pain. According to this view, itch is no more different from a sharp, lancinating, cutting pain than is a dull, throbbing, aching pain.

There are also several differences between itch and pain. First and foremost, people recognize these two sensations as definitively different and call them by different names. This counts for a great deal and is arguably the bottom line for some. Second, as mentioned earlier, stimuli that give rise to pain or itch elicit different motor responses. Third, the production of pain by intense scratching relieves itch. Another example of itch–pain antagonism is that opioid analgesics that alleviate pain can cause itch. In fact, itch induced by opioid drugs can be the factor that limits use of analgesics to treat pain. Finally, naloxone, an opioid receptor antagonist that antagonizes the pain-relieving effects of morphine, is antipruritic (i.e., it reduces itch sensation).

Itch is a nontrivial clinical issue. Not surprisingly, it is the primary complaint of patients seeking dermatological help. Many patients with itch due to bites, poison ivy, or allergic reactions find relief by taking antihistamines that antagonize the peripheral effects of histamine. However, a portion of the patients who seek medical help for itch have *central itch*, a form of itch that does not depend on a peripheral stimulus, such as a mosquito bite. Since central itch is not caused by a peripheral stimulus, such as the release of histamine, it is also unfortunately unaffected by antihistamines. The causes of central itch are varied. Individuals with hepatic failure often suffer from central itch. The itch produced by opioid administration is also a type of central itch. An astonishing case of severe itch was the topic of an article by Atul Gawande in *The New Yorker*. After a bout of herpes zoster (discussed later), a woman developed an unrelenting itch. The itch was so imperative that she scratched all the way through her skull and dura. Although this outcome is rare, perhaps even singular, the take-home message is that itch can be a significant clinical problem.

Most somatosensory afferents are very specific, only responding to one type of stimulus such as warming but not cooling, cooling but not warming, hair-bending but not touch, and so on. Polymodal nociceptors stand in stark contrast to this type of specificity. Polymodal nociceptors are highly nonspecific in their response profile because they respond similarly to noxious heat or to cutting the skin or pinching. Yet, nociceptors are specific enough to serve a protective purpose. In other words, regardless of the specifics, any stimulus that causes tissue damage or is likely to do so imminently activates nociceptors. Thus, *nociceptors are specific to physical injury or the threat thereof*. Befitting this specificity, nociceptor activation leads to protective reactions.

LARGE- AND SMALL-DIAMETER SENSORY FIBERS DIFFER IN SIGNIFICANT WAYS KEY TO THEIR INVOLVEMENT IN DIFFERENT DISEASES

The division between mechanoreceptors and nociceptors is a meaningful biological distinction. Most mechanoreceptors are large-diameter, well-myelinated afferents, whereas nociceptors and thermoreceptors are either very thin, unmyelinated or thin, lightly myelinated afferents. Moreover, the molecules involved in both the function and development of the different afferent classes are distinct. For example, certain growth factors or growth factor receptors are required for the development of unmyelinated and lightly myelinated afferents but not for the development of well-myelinated afferents. The differing molecular signatures of afferent classes also render different afferent types more or less susceptible to various environmental insults. Hypoxia, local anesthetics, hyperglycemia, the high glucose levels commonly experienced by diabetics, and chemotherapeutic agents often preferentially affect peripheral axons of a certain diameter.

Individuals lacking a subset of the molecules necessary for small-diameter primary afferent development are born with a congenital neuropathy called *hereditary sensory and autonomic neuropathy* (*HSAN*). There are several different forms of HSAN. All involve the loss of small-diameter fibers that share a common molecular vulnerability to developmental misprogramming. In one type of HSAN, also known as *congenital insensitivity to pain*, small-diameter nociceptors and thermoreceptors do not develop. As a result, patients cannot sense pain or temperature. In many patients, there is also a loss of small-caliber sympathetic fibers innervating sweat glands, resulting in patients' inability to sweat, a condition termed *anhidrosis*. Patients with such a congenital insensitivity to pain often present when they suffer injuries without crying or during teething at the latest, when parents discover that their child has chewed off a digit.

Sensory afferents are not the only peripheral axons susceptible to dysfunction. Motor axons serving skeletal muscle and autonomic axons can also fall victim to errant development or toxic environments. Recall that among all types of peripheral axons, the axons involved in touch are relatively small in diameter. The largest diameter axons belong to motoneurons that innervate skeletal muscles and proprioceptive afferents that innervate muscles and joints. Thus, the term "large-fiber neuropathy" refers to neuropathies that affect motoneurons and proprioceptive afferents and have primarily motor consequences. In contrast, small-fiber neuropathies may affect any combination of mechanoreceptors, nociceptors, and thermoreceptors. In addition, the motor fibers innervating autonomic targets are unmyelinated and therefore also affected in individuals with a large-fiber neuropathy.

The effect of chemotherapeutics on sensory neurons is illustrative. Single chemotherapeutics cause neuropathies at rates of up to 30–40%. Combination regimens may lead to neuropathy in up to 70% of patients treated! For most chemotherapeutic drugs, the development of neuropathy limits the dose and course of treatment. Chemotherapeutics produce toxicity through a variety of mechanisms. Platinum-containing drugs, such as cisplatin, cause peripheral neurons, especially those in the dorsal root ganglion, to re-enter the cell cycle and then undergo apoptosis or programmed cell death. Other drugs, such as taxanes, prevent microtubule disassembly and thereby disrupt both anterograde and retrograde axonal transport, leading to a dying back of the peripheral terminal. Most chemotherapy-induced neuropathies produce primarily sensory symptoms by damaging sensory neurons, predominantly the largest sensory neurons, mostly Aβ fibers. Damage to large, well-myelinated Aβ sensory fibers results in depressed motor reflexes, which depend on large-diameter muscle and joint afferents, as well as paresthesia, dysesthesia, or frank pain. The latter set of positive sensory signs reflects the most common result of damage to sensory pathways. Neurotoxic damage to motor and autonomic axons also occurs but leads to symptoms more rarely than does sensory neuron damage. Currently, decreasing the dose, frequency, or rate of chemotherapeutic infusions represents the only defense against inducing neuropathy. Although some remission of neuropathic symptoms can occur early on, symptom severity typically stabilizes thereafter. Efforts are now aimed at developing prophylactic adjuvants that, when administered with chemotherapeutic drugs, will protect against the development of a neuropathy. Although no clear success has yet been achieved, these efforts clearly hold great potential and hope.

DIFFERENT SPEEDS OF ACTION POTENTIAL CONDUCTION UNDERLIE FIRST AND SECOND PAIN

Because action potentials conduct at very different speeds in Aδ and C fibers, the perceptions initiated by activity in these two fiber types occur at different times (Fig. 17-1). Consider that a woman of average height steps on a thorn with a bare foot. The thorn will excite both high-threshold Aδ fiber mechanoreceptors and C fiber polymodal nociceptors. Since the high-threshold mechanoreceptors have lightly myelinated axons, with conduction velocities of 5–30 m/s, the message that the thorn has impaled the foot will reach the spinal cord in 30–200 ms. In contrast, the unmyelinated axons of polymodal nociceptors conduct action potentials at a far slower rate, 0.5–1 m/s. Consequently, input from polymodal nociceptors takes 1–2 *seconds* to reach the spinal cord from the foot. The delay between 200 ms and 1 or 2 seconds is perceptible and forms the basis for *first pain* and *second pain*. In general, first pain causes a fast, sharp, well-localized sensation, whereas second pain causes a less well-defined aching or burning pain. The

sensations of sharp and shooting versus aching and burning pain roughly reflect the perceptual consequences of Aδ or C fiber activation, respectively.

DEEP PAIN IS POORLY LOCATED IN SPACE AND TIME

Sir Thomas Lewis was an early 20th-century cardiologist who first described interactions between pain afferents and the peripheral circulation. Although recognized today mostly for his vast contributions to cardiology, Lewis's work on pain remains highly influential today. Lewis lamented that we use the same word, *pain*, to refer to all varieties of pain, which in fact differ extensively from each other. This semantic sloppiness is most evident when we contrast deep pain from superficial pain. Superficial injuries such as a burn, scratch, or a mosquito bite elicit an acute perception of pain (or itch in the latter case). We even sense the landing of a mosquito or fly on our arm or the moist track of a drip of sweat. In marked contrast to our ability to discriminate in place and time superficial stimuli, we are horrible at detecting and describing deep somatic stimuli.

Consider the striking differences between a paper cut and a penetrating injury. As everyone knows, paper cuts are peculiarly distracting, demanding our attention even when very small. Contrast the paper-cut experience with the experience of individuals who have been stabbed or shot, many of whom first become aware of their injury because of a feeling of warm blood on the skin not because of wounded deep tissue. Remarkably, there have been several instances in which a nail gun has backfired, driving a nail into the person rather than into the targeted object. In one case, a man immediately sought medical assistance because his cheek, where the nail penetrated, hurt. After having his cheek sewed up, the man went about his business until a week later when he visited a dentist for a toothache. The dentist took an x-ray that revealed that a nail had shot through the man's teeth and jaw and was now lodged in his frontal cortex. Note that the injured man did not all of a sudden become aware of the nail in his head or the hole in his tooth and jaw. Rather, the man complained of a toothache, a completely inaccurate depiction of the problem reflective of our greater sensitivity to persistent deep pain, borne of infection and the like, than to acute deep pain.

The contrast between our exquisite sensitivity to the lightest cutaneous stimulus and our incredible insensitivity to severely damaging deep stimuli corresponds to the contrasting behavioral strategies used in reaction to the two types of stimuli. Superficial pain perceptions, arising primarily from the skin, signal potential danger and serve as a call to action (Fig. 17-4). Superficial damage is *escapable* and calls for an immediate response. In marked contrast, there are a limited number of deep stimuli that we can do something about. We can void when our bladder or colon fills, and we can vomit when we feel nauseated. Outside of these instances, internal events are essentially *inescapable*. We are stuck with deep pain or at least we have evolved as animals that are stuck with deep pain. Modern medicine may provide us with treatment options in many cases, but our nervous system has not evolved to take advantage of this recent development. Like other animals, we react to deep tissue damage by inactivity and a retreat from social interactions until sufficient recuperation or death occurs. Using this framework, we can understand persistent pain as a form of inescapable pain. Indeed, animals, including humans, react to persistent pain as we do to deep pain—with social retreat and quiet immobility.

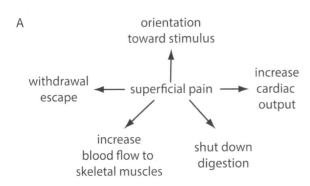

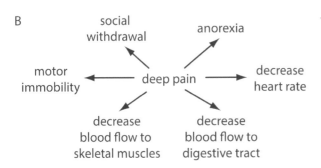

Figure 17-4 A: Superficial pain is a call to action. The motor responses to superficial pain include withdrawing from a noxious stimulus, orienting toward the noxious stimulus, and escaping from the situation. The motor activity elicited by superficial pain is supported by increased cardiac output and increased blood flow to skeletal muscles. B: Deep pain is inescapable. Animals, including humans, respond to deep pain by becoming immobile, withdrawing from social interactions, and not eating (anorexia). Cardiac output is decreased, and resources are shifted away from growth and toward the immune system.

Normally, we are not aware of our viscera. We do not perceive blood pulsing through vessels, urine traveling through the ureter, or the expansion of alveoli accompanying every sigh. We can sense distension of some of the hollow viscera, such as the colon, bladder, and even stomach. Yet, even this sensation is very crude. Although the uncomfortable sensation of a distended stomach is indicative of having eaten far too much, we cannot perceive small differences in visceral distension. We cannot, for example, perceive the difference in stomach distension after having eaten two or three slices of apple.

Although the hollow viscera support nonpainful sensations such as urgency, the nonhollow viscera and other deep structures only support a perception of pain. In other words, we do not feel tickle or pressure or warmth or coolness from our pancreas or our dura; we either feel nothing or we feel pain. Several visceral conditions can give rise to a perception of pain:

- *Excessive distension*: Failing to empty the bladder or colon can result in distension of these hollow viscera. This produces an acute perception of visceral pain.

- *Inflammation*: Inflammation of any viscera can produce a chronic feeling of pain. Examples include pericarditis, colitis, and appendicitis.

- *Frank tissue damage*: When the viscera is damaged by a disease process, as occurs with a peptic or duodenal ulcer, pain results.

- *Occlusion*: Occlusion of a blood vessel, such as occurs in sickle cell anemia, or a channel such as the ureter, as occurs in kidney stones, is painful.

Thus, the viscera normally give rise to either no sensation or to feelings of fullness in the case of some hollow organs. Yet, when any of the viscera are diseased or damaged, pain can result. The afferents responsible for these very different perceptual conditions are quite different from the complement of cutaneous afferents described earlier.

VISCERAL AFFERENTS DIFFER SUBSTANTIALLY FROM CUTANEOUS AFFERENTS

Most viscera are innervated by two different nerves. For example, thoracic dorsal root ganglion cells reach the bladder through the hypogastric nerve, whereas sacral dorsal root ganglion cells reach the bladder through the pelvic nerve. The bulk of the fibers in the hypogastric nerve are sympathetic fibers destined for pelvic viscera, whereas the bulk of fibers in the pelvic nerve are fibers destined for pelvic parasympathetic ganglia. For this reason, the afferents in the hypogastric nerve are sometimes referred to as *sympathetic afferents* and those in the pelvic nerve as *parasympathetic afferents*. These terms have utility. Yet it is important to remember that all of these afferents have their cell bodies in dorsal root ganglia.

Visceral afferents come in two varieties that roughly align to the sympathetic–parasympathetic division described earlier. Low-threshold afferents traveling in parasympathetic nerves respond to low-intensity stimulation and are critical to the normal function of the viscera (Fig. 17-5). Information about small changes in the state of the target viscera is carried through these low-threshold afferents to autonomic efferent pathways that maintain homeostasis. Neither the low-threshold visceral information nor the automatic adjustments to visceral function reaches consciousness or contributes to perception. In contrast, afferents traveling in sympathetic nerves have high thresholds for activation and thus function as nociceptors that are only activated by injurious stimuli. The excitation of sympathetic afferents leads to a brief perception of acute visceral pain. Finally, viscera are innervated by silent nociceptors. As their name suggests, silent nociceptors are normally silent, neither spontaneously active nor responsive to any natural stimuli. However, in response to an inflammatory stimulus, silent nociceptors become active. When visceral silent nociceptors are sensitized by inflammation, peripheral and central nociceptive pathways are altered (more on this later). As a result, low-intensity visceral input, which normally contributes to visceral reflexes but not to perception, now contributes to perception, leading to a persistent perception of visceral pain (Fig. 17-5C).

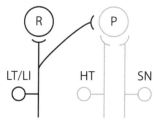

A. Normal conditions: no pain

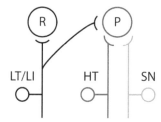

B. Brief noxious stimulation: acute pain

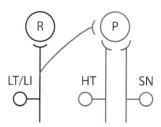

C. Inflammation and central sensitization: chronic pain

Figure 17-5 A: Under normal conditions, in the absence of visceral pain, low-threshold afferents (*LT/LI*) respond to low-intensity stimuli. The responses of low-threshold afferents drive neurons involved in visceral reflex control (*R*). Input from low-threshold afferents also reaches neurons that project to pathways that ultimately result in perception (*P*). However, the input from low-threshold afferents is normally insufficient to excite perception-related neurons. B: A brief noxious stimulus excites high-threshold visceral nociceptors (*HT*), which in turn leads to the excitation of perception-related neurons. The result of this activity is acute visceral pain. C: After inflammation and central sensitization, silent nociceptors (*SN*) start to fire spontaneously. The increase in activity in both high-threshold visceral nociceptors and silent nociceptors sensitizes the perception-related pathway. As a result, low-threshold input excites the perception-related pathway. The result is that normal visceral sensations important for homeostasis are now perceived as painful.   Modified from Cervero F, Jänig W. Visceral nociceptors: A new world order. *Trends Neurosci* 24:374–78, 1992, with permission of the publisher, Elsevier.

SPECIFIC TRANSDUCTION MOLECULES CONFER AFFERENTS WITH PARTICULAR RESPONSE PROFILES

The task of transducing the variety of somatosensory stimuli to which we are sensitive is accomplished by a variety of transduction molecules that are present in somatosensory afferents. Instead of there being one transduction molecule—rhodopsin and the mechanoelectrical transduction (MET) channel in the case of light and sound,

respectively—a number of receptors are capable of transducing somatosensory stimuli. Each receptor responds to some subset of somatosensory stimuli.

Many of the channels involved in somatosensory transduction that have been identified to date belong to a family of ionotropic channels called *transient receptor potential* or TRP channels. TRP channels may be sensitive to (1) temperature, (2) mechanical stimulation, or (3) chemical substances such as camphor, menthol, or capsaicin. Moreover, most of the TRP channels involved in somatosensation respond to at least two stimulus types, and some respond to all three stimulus types. Transient receptor potential channels can thus be considered the perfect molecular substrate for neurons that respond to multiple stimulus modalities. Fittingly, polymodal nociceptors also contain one or more types of TRP channel.

At least nine TRP channel subtypes respond to temperature within differing but overlapping ranges. The task of responding to the normal range of environmental and internal temperatures is divided up between types of TRP channels so that the entire complement of TRP receptors can support sensations of cold, cool, warm, and hot. For example, one TRP channel subtype, $TRPV_1$, is critical to sensing mild to moderate noxious heat, whereas another transduces intensely noxious heat, and still another member of the TRP family of channels opens at temperatures that are normally perceived as warm. $TRPM_8$ channels respond to temperatures normally perceived as cool, whereas $TRPA_1$ channels respond to temperatures normally perceived as cold.

Although most types of TRP channels respond to more than one type of stimulus, $TRPA_1$ channels are particularly promiscuous in their response profile. They respond to cold and also to irritants such as acrolein and other components of smoke, smog, and exhaust. In fact, $TRPA_1$ receptors are activated by chemicals that can covalently bind to cysteine, a varied group that includes nicotine, formaldehyde, and the active ingredients in mustard, wasabi, garlic, and cinnamon, as well as many air pollutants. $TRPA_1$ also opens in response to reactive oxygen species, such as hydrogen peroxide, which are produced by cells in oxidative stress.

The $TRPV_1$ channel, which is activated by heat, also opens in response to *capsaicin*, the ingredient responsible for the spicy hot sensation produced by chili peppers. Because of this response, $TRPV_1$ is often referred to as the capsaicin receptor. $TRPV_1$ is present in trigeminal afferents that innervate the oral cavity of humans and most other mammals. When we eat hot chili peppers, the burning sensation that we feel is due to capsaicin's actions on the $TRPV_1$ receptor. Mammals with the $TRPV_1$ receptor find capsaicin innately aversive, meaning that mammals avoid eating capsaicin. The preference for capsaicin and other hot substances expressed by some humans is an example of a learned taste preference. As it turns out, birds do not have a $TRPV_1$ receptor. This biology has led to the addition of capsaicin to bird-feed mixtures as a defense against backyard squirrels gobbling up food intended for songbirds. The birds do not sense the capsaicin and happily eat the food offered. On the other hand, squirrels will avoid bird food laced with capsaicin.

Of great clinical importance is the presence of $TRPA_1$ and $TRPV_1$ in sensory afferents that innervate the entire length of the airways from nose to lungs, including the nasal mucosa, pharynx, glottis, trachea, and bronchi. Activation of these TRP channels elicits an immediate protective reaction, coughing, and also suppresses breathing, which in turn decreases exposure to airborne irritants. We can view the airways as the lungs' "skin," their exposed and superficial barrier from the outside world. In this same vein, coughing in reaction to airborne irritants can be thought of as a protective withdrawal, essentially the lungs' version of yanking your hand away from the hot fire.

Acute exposure to agonists at $TRPA_1$ and $TRPV_1$ receptors is effectively countered by coughing and brief episodes of *apnea*, or not breathing. However, the protective effect of coughing goes awry in the face of chronic exposure to irritants. Chronic exposure to pollution, smoke, and products of oxidative stress, such as hydrogen peroxide and other reactive oxygen species, causes repeated activation of the TRP channels found in airway afferents. Chronic activation of sensory afferents, in turn, causes a hypersensitivity to airborne irritants through mechanisms analogous to those implicated in the pathogenesis of persistent pain syndromes. The end result is a decreased threshold for coughing, so that frequent coughing becomes pathological rather than protective. Additional signs of pulmonary disease are airway inflammation, bronchoconstriction, and excessive mucus production, all of which contribute to the primary symptoms of coughing and dyspnea, or shortness of breath.

The incidence of asthma, chronic obstructive pulmonary disease, and reactive airway dysfunction syndrome have all greatly increased, particularly in industrialized and polluted regions. The inflammation and sensory afferent hypersensitivity caused by chronic exposure to airborne irritants likely mediates this recent increase in pulmonary diseases. This perspective allows us to understand why certain compounds or environments exacerbate breathing problems. For example, cold, below about 15°C, activates $TRPA_1$ receptors and worsens asthmatic symptoms. Similarly, hypochlorite, the volatile agent arising from chlorinated pools and disinfectants such as bleach, also activates $TRPA_1$ receptors and greatly exacerbates asthma. Less well appreciated agonists at the $TRPA_1$ receptor include volatile compounds from cinnamon, wasabi, garlic, onions, and mustard. The critical importance of TRP channels in general and $TRPA_1$ in particular to pulmonary disease has led to efforts to develop TRP receptor antagonists into novel therapeutics for asthma and other pulmonary diseases.

TRP channels are also strongly modulated by a number of substances. For example, protons modify the responses of $TRPV_1$ channels to temperature, and menthol similarly modulates $TRPM_8$ channel responses. In the latter case, menthol raises the threshold for temperature activation of TRPM$_8$ channels so that a higher temperature is capable of opening the channel. The perceptual result of this is that warmer temperatures are perceived as cool.

The responses of TRP channels to multiple stimuli indicative of tissue damage reflect the diversity of injurious stimuli, as well as the singular meaning of such damage. In other words, *TRP channels respond to several types of damaging stimuli without distinguishing between the properties of the different stimuli.* TRP channels are the quintessential nociceptive receptor type—a jack-of-all-trades, or at least of-many-trades, an injury-in-any-form-sensing molecule. A further expansion of the injury-sensing repertoire of single nociceptors arises from the multiple TRP channels present within individual neurons.

Many additional transducing molecules outside of the TRP channel family contribute to nociception, some of which have been identified and a number of which assuredly have not. Most notably, acid-sensing ion channels (ASICs) are ionotropic channels activated by protons; ASICs accumulate extracellularly during injuries such as ischemia and also after tissue-damaging mechanical stimulation.

NOCICEPTORS ARE RESPONSIBLE FOR MUCH OF THE INFLAMMATION RESULTING FROM TISSUE DAMAGE

An important distinction cuts across the functional classes of nociceptors outlined earlier. Most Aδ and C fiber afferents contain neuropeptides that play important roles in normal everyday function and in the response to injury. Small-diameter afferents that contain neuropeptides are typically referred to as *peptidergic afferents*. A minority of Aδ and C fiber afferents and all Aβ fiber afferents do not contain neuropeptides and are nonpeptidergic. The importance of this distinction will become evident in the following discussion.

Dorsal root ganglion neurons are peculiar in that they send out a single process that bifurcates into two long processes, one of which extends to a peripheral target and one of which enters the central nervous system (CNS). The process that extends peripherally is dendrite-like in that it receives input but axon-like in that it conducts action potentials. In the case of many primary somatosensory afferents including high-threshold mechanoreceptors and polymodal nociceptors, the peripheral process ends in a spray of terminals connected by short branches to the main or parent process (Fig. 17-6A). The receptive field of somatosensory

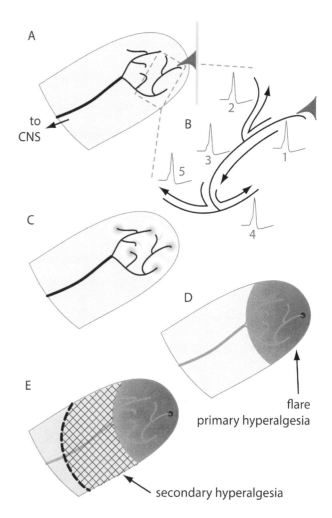

Figure 17-6 Peptidergic nociceptors end in a spray of terminals. When a thorn stimulates one ending of a nociceptor (A), an action potential is elicited. B: The initial action potential (*1*) is conducted back to the first branch point. At each branch point, the action potential invades the sister branch (*2, 4*) as well as the parent fiber (*3, 5*). C: When an action potential reaches the ending of a peptidergic nociceptor, peptides including substance P, calcitonin gene-related peptide (CGRP), and neurokinin A are released into the periphery (*blue spheres*). D: CGRP released from nociceptors causes a secondary vasodilation or flare. In addition, the inflammatory soup that is triggered by the release of neuropeptides sensitizes nociceptors, causing primary hyperalgesia in the flare zone. E: The barrage of nociceptor activity initiates central sensitization, which results in a zone of secondary hyperalgesia.

afferents with such a spray of terminals consists of a series of punctate spots.

The sensory function of primary afferents is served by action potentials that travel from the peripheral receptive field to a terminal in the dorsal horn where neurotransmitter is released. However, recall from Chapter 10 that action potentials travel in one direction only because of the refractory period. Therefore, when an action potential arrives at a branch point, it *invades*, or travels down, the parent axon but also can invade the sister branch (Fig. 17-6B). In this way, an action potential at one branch ending can reach all of the other branch endings of the parent neuron, a process that is termed the *axon reflex*.

The axon reflex has important consequences in the case of peptidergic nociceptors. An injury such as a sting or mechanical injury breaks opens blood vessels and cells and also activates nociceptors. The direct damage is localized and forms a small red spot, often referred to as a *bleb*. If this bleb, which occurs without any contribution from nociceptors, were all that occurred, we simply would not care about bee stings, scrapes, and cuts. The reason that we do care about initially mild injuries, the reason indeed that they are injuries rather than passing nothings, is because of the amplification of the injury set in motion by peptidergic nociceptors.

The end result of the amplification provided by peptidergic nociceptors is the *triple response* described by Sir Thomas Lewis, mentioned earlier. In order to understand the changes in microcirculation that occur at and around a region of cutaneous tissue damage, Lewis ran the end of a key firmly against the skin. He saw that a line of red appears within about 10 seconds. This red line is equivalent to primary vasodilation, a signature of direct tissue damage. The area on either side of the line then develops a flare, or *secondary vasodilation* in modern parlance. The leaked blood within the region of flare renders the skin both red and hot in under a minute. Within just a few minutes, a *wheal*, a raised region signifying an edematous reaction, develops due in part to plasma extravasation. These three reactions—flare (rubor), heat (calor), and wheal (tumor)—constitute the triple response of Lewis. Of great import to the clinician is that the triple response is accompanied by some degree of localized pain (dolor). We now examine our current understanding of the mechanisms of the triple response with an eye toward preventing the resulting pain.

The amplification of tissue damage by nociceptors is termed *neurogenic inflammation*, and it occurs because of (1) the axon reflex and (2) the peptides released by nociceptors. This process starts when an action potential occurs at the ending of a peptidergic nociceptor. Neurotransmitters including neuropeptides are released *from* the nociceptor and *into the periphery* (Fig. 17-6C). In other words, peptidergic afferents serve efferent (directed toward the periphery) as well as the expected afferent (signaling events from the periphery to the CNS) functions. This surprising reversal of the direction of information transfer is the key step involved in neurogenic inflammation and the generation of the triple response.

The afferent-released neuropeptides calcitonin gene-related peptide (CGRP), substance P, and neurokinin

A are particularly important. Each of these peptides has one or more important effects (Fig. 17-7). CGRP causes the vasodilation of blood vessels. This causes the flare or secondary vasodilation (the primary vasodilation is the central bleb) that extends around the bleb marking the site of an injury (Fig. 17-6D). The range of the flare represents the territory under the influence of all of the terminals belonging to stimulated nociceptors. Thus, through the axon reflex, action potentials invade all of the branches of all of the nociceptors activated by an injury. Neuropeptides are released from branch endings, and the released CGRP in turn dilates all nearby blood vessels, resulting in the flare.

Substance P and neurokinin A render blood vessels more permeable, so that plasma leaks out of the vessels and into the local tissue. The leaking of plasma from blood vessels, termed *plasma extravasation*, results in swelling or

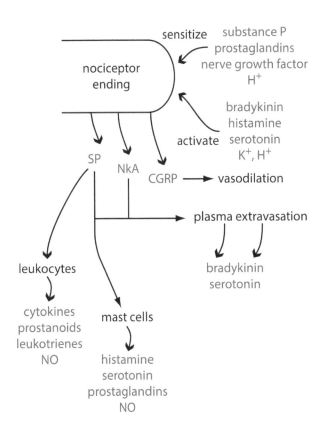

Figure 17-7 Pathways important in neurogenic inflammation and primary hyperalgesia. Nociceptors release substance P (*SP*), neurokinin A (*NkA*), and calcitonin gene-related peptide (CGRP). CGRP elicits vasodilation, whereas substance P and neurokinin A trigger plasma extravasation of a number of compounds, including bradykinin and serotonin. Substance P also promotes the recruitment of leukocytes into the damaged tissue and the degranulation of leukocytes and mast cells. Substances released from leukocytes and mast cells add to the inflammatory soup (*red*) within the damaged tissue. Substances present in inflamed tissue increase the activity and sensitivity of nociceptors. The perceptual consequence is primary hyperalgesia.

edema. Among the proteins that leak out of the now highly permeable venules is a potent pain-producing, or algesic, peptide called *bradykinin*. Substance P stimulates mast cells located deep in the dermis to *degranulate*, meaning that the chemical contents of secretory vesicles or granules in the mast cells are released. As a result, histamine, serotonin, prostaglandins, and nitric oxide join the mix of chemicals present in injured skin.

Substance P promotes the movement of white blood cells from blood vessels into damaged tissue and the resulting release of a dizzying array of signaling molecules including cytokines, prostaglandins, thromboxanes, leukotrienes, and nitric oxide.

After an initial injury and subsequent neurogenic inflammatory reaction, damaged tissue is bathed in an *inflammatory soup* (Fig. 17-7). This soup in turn dramatically increases the activity and sensitivity of nociceptors throughout the region of the inflammatory environment, outlined by the extent of the flare. Consequently, individuals experience spontaneous pain as well as exaggerated pain in response to even the slightest provocation. The increase in activity and sensitivity among regional nociceptors is a process termed *peripheral sensitization*. The connections between features of peripheral nociceptor activity after *sensitization* and perception are thought to consist of:

- Spontaneously active nociceptors producing spontaneous pain

- Responses to stimuli that ordinarily do not excite nociceptors contributing to allodynia

- Exaggerated responses to noxious stimulation leading to hyperalgesia

The collective results of peripheral sensitization are primary hyperalgesia. Although termed hyperalgesia, primary hyperalgesia also involves spontaneous pain and allodynia. As is familiar to everyone from experiences with cuts, scrapes, stings, burns, and the like, even the lightest touch of an inflamed area can elicit pain, an example of allodynia. Another common example of allodynia is the pain produced by warm water on sunburned skin; water of the same temperature would be experienced as neutral or even pleasant on uninjured skin.

Some of the most important components of inflammatory soup that contribute to the sensitization of polymodal nociceptors are *prostanoids*, a class of chemicals that included prostaglandins, prostacyclins, and thromboxanes. The synthesis of prostanoids is the target of *nonsteroidal anti-inflammatory drugs*, commonly abbreviated as NSAIDs, such as acetylsalicylic acid or aspirin. Critical to their analgesic, or pain-relieving, effect, NSAIDs block the synthesis of prostanoids by inhibiting cyclooxygenase enzymes. Since prostanoids have short half-lives, in the seconds to minutes range, inhibiting their synthesis quickly reduces the concentration of prostanoids even in inflamed tissue. The reduction in prostanoids reduces both inflammation and the pain that normally accompanies inflammation. Since there are plenty of inflammatory mediators within damaged tissue, it is understandable that inhibition of prostanoid synthesis alone often does not abolish inflammatory pain. It is, in fact, a testament to the power of prostanoid-mediated nociceptor sensitization that NSAIDs such as acetaminophen, ibuprofen, naproxen, and acetylsalicylic acid provide as much pain relief as they do.

In sum, the inflammatory soup released in response to injury serves an organism well in two respects. First, the soup promotes the immune fight against infection and thus is anti-infective. Second, the inflammatory soup produces peripheral sensitization and thereby hyperalgesia that reduces use of the body part. Less use of an injured body part means that there is less chance for reinjury.

NOCICEPTORS NORMALLY SERVE AN EFFERENT FUNCTION

As noted earlier, the axon reflex is a remarkable physiological trick that allows nociceptors to serve an *efferent* function that ultimately recruits immune and circulatory resources to the site of an injury and also to the surrounding region, which may be particularly vulnerable to damage. *Hyperemia*, or increased blood flow, may aid in clearing tissue of harmful substances. Certain components of the inflammatory soup actually *protect* targeted tissue. Yet nociceptor activation and sensitization leads to an exaggerated pain response that has both advantageous and unfortunate consequences. On the plus side, heightened levels of pain ensure that an injured body part is not used. On the regrettable side, pain is not an enjoyable experience. Overall, the neurogenic reactions to tissue damage are physiologically advantageous, albeit psychologically unpleasant, in the face of acute injury because they speed healing and prevent further damage.

In an example of natural parsimony, the efferent functionality of nociceptors serves a protective role in the *absence* of an injury. Under normal, everyday conditions, peptidergic nociceptors promote the health of innervated tissues. Thus, nociceptors that may never signal tissue damage, even over the course of a human lifetime, are responsible for exerting *trophic* effects that maintain the well-being of innervated tissues. In fact, *most nociceptors, most of the time, are more active as trophic influences on target tissues than as sensors of pain-producing stimuli.* Body tissues as diverse as skin, hair follicles, tooth pulp, tympanic membrane, dura, vertebral column, joints, and viscera all receive nociceptor innervation. In the absence of nociceptors, obvious changes in hair and nail growth, skin, bone, and cartilage abound.

As a consequence of nociceptors' important trophic roles, loss of nociceptor innervation greatly retards wound healing, the response of tissue to injury. Such a deficit contributes to the pathology of skin ulcerations observed in some patients with various types of neuropathies: diabetic, hereditary, or traumatic. Without trophic influences from nociceptors, target tissues become less healthy and less resilient in the face of injury. Damage to sympathetic efferents also contributes to deficits in peripheral tissue health. As a result, individuals with peripheral nerve damage often have thickened skin and nails, and wound healing can be very slow. For example, diabetic individuals who have a reduced density of cutaneous nerve terminals exhibit decreased neurogenic inflammation and are prone to ulceration. Furthermore, without nociceptors to recruit immune cells to damaged tissue, an ulcer that develops in a diabetic individual is more easily infected and less easily healed.

CHRONIC INFLAMMATION ACTIVATES A CLASS OF SILENT NOCICEPTORS

Although unpleasant to experience, acute pain and inflammation in response to an injury can be beneficial insomuch as they promote healing and tissue recovery. In contrast, chronic inflammation has negative consequences for the innervated tissue and can exacerbate damage to the target tissue. Several factors contribute to the hyperalgesia and tissue damage that accompany chronic inflammation. Although inactive and unresponsive in healthy tissue, silent nociceptors become spontaneously active and responsive to stimulation once triggered by damage. Inflammation renders these afferents responsive to even innocuous stimulation of the innervated tissue. Silent nociceptors are classified as nociceptors because, when active, their activity boosts nociceptive transmission (not tactile or thermal) in central transmission pathways. Thus, silent nociceptors provide an avenue through which innocuous stimuli gain entrance to nociceptive pathways with the ultimate result that a perception of pain is elicited by innocuous and noxious stimuli alike. Activity in silent nociceptors bump up the pain experienced from damaged tissue, feeding both allodynic and hyperalgesic sensations.

The inflammatory response is most beneficial when it operates as a quick fix, a response that peaks and subsides rapidly. When inflammation persists, tissue damage can be exacerbated. The mechanisms by which chronic inflammation damages tissue are not well worked out. However, it appears that, whereas many components of inflammatory soup protect and maintain tissue health, some are harmful to tissue health, at least when present over an extended period of time.

The mechanisms by which chronic inflammation such as arthritis degrades tissue and the neuronal contribution to this degradation are surely varied. Common to inflamed tissue is an elevation in endogenous proteases that comprise part of the inflammatory soup. By breaking down proteins within a joint (or elsewhere), proteases directly contribute to the degradation of the inflamed tissue. Proteases also act upon *proteinase-activated receptors (PARs)*, G protein-coupled metabotropic receptors (see Chapter 13) present on the terminals of nociceptors. PARs are activated by an unusual mechanism. The extracellular proteases cleave the terminal end of the extracellular domain of a PAR, releasing a still tethered moiety that acts as an agonist on the very same receptor complex (Fig. 17-8).

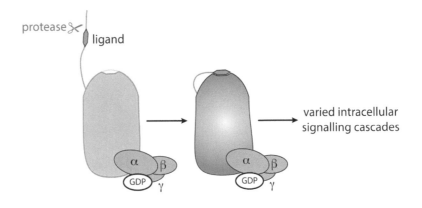

Figure 17-8 Protease-activated receptors (PARs) are G protein-coupled receptors with an extracellular domain containing the same receptor's own ligand. Proteases present in inflamed tissue can cut the N-terminus of the extracellular domain, leaving the tethered ligand free to bind to the PAR binding site. Once activated, PARs can activate a number of downstream signaling cascades.

Signaling mediated by different isoforms of PARs exerts both pro- and anti-inflammatory effects, with the latter predominating. Furthermore, exposure to PAR agonists leads somatosensory afferents to fire action potentials spontaneously and also to respond to innocuous stimulation. Excitement is building over the therapeutic possibilities of small molecules that can interrupt the protease-to-PAR connection.

A common example of the harm incurred by chronic inflammation is *arthritis*, a heterogeneous group of conditions involving joint damage. Arthritic conditions are prevalent, affecting more than a fifth of American adults. Arthritis is more prevalent among women during their reproductive years than among men. This sexual difference appears to depend at least in part upon gonadal hormonal differences because rheumatoid arthritis is ameliorated during pregnancy and in women taking contraceptive pills. Tissue destruction of a joint through inflammatory mechanisms can be aggravated by an increase in synovial volume and by changes in joint usage and mechanics due to pain.

Experimental studies have dramatically illustrated the role of silent nociceptors in signaling arthritic pain. Normally, silent nociceptors that innervate a joint are not activated by physiological stimuli. However, after introduction of inflammatory soup into the joint, silent nociceptors respond to simple joint flexion and extension. This stunning experimental finding explains the severe pain suffered by some individuals with arthritis while making even the simplest movements. Although rheumatoid arthritis is uniformly painful, not all osteoarthritis is associated with pain all the time; the reason for variation across individuals and time is unknown.

MULTIPLE SOMATOSENSORY INPUTS CONVERGE ON NOCICEPTIVE DORSAL HORN CELLS

Each nociceptive dorsal horn cell receives input from many nociceptors. The convergence of numerous individual nociceptors of one type, such as Aδ high-threshold mechanoreceptors, is the basis of a central neuron's receptive field that is smoother and larger than the receptive field of a primary afferent. Furthermore, multiple types of primary afferents converge on single dorsal horn cells. Many nociceptive cells receive input from thermoreceptive and pruriceptive afferents. Some dorsal horn cells that respond to noxious stimulation even receive input from Aβ mechanoreceptors. The extent and significance of the convergence of nociceptive and non-nociceptive input onto some dorsal horn cells are not entirely clear. Yet one outcome of the arrangement is the possibility of facile modulation of dorsal horn neurons. For example, a dorsal horn neuron that receives inputs from multiple afferent types may respond preferentially to one type of input normally and to a different type of input under different conditions, such as after injury.

A BARRAGE OF NOCICEPTOR INPUT CHANGES THE PHYSIOLOGICAL PROPERTIES OF NOCICEPTIVE DORSAL HORN CELLS

Tissue damage has long-lasting effects on nociceptive dorsal horn neurons through a process termed *central sensitization*. Central sensitization leads to an increase in spontaneous activity and to greatly augmented responses to all afferent input, non-nociceptive and nociceptive alike. The behavioral correlates of these changes are familiar by now: spontaneous pain, hyperalgesia, and allodynia. This trio is termed *secondary hyperalgesia* to distinguish it from primary hyperalgesia, which depends on peripheral mechanisms explained earlier. Secondary hyperalgesia involves a large region of heightened sensitivity to somatosensory stimulation expanding well beyond the region of peripheral damage (Fig. 17-6E).

Central sensitization can be initiated by a barrage of nociceptor activity, the type of activity that normally occurs in response to severe tissue damage. Central sensitization also occurs after nerve injury or persistent inflammation. The high-intensity afferent input depolarizes dorsal horn cells enough to relieve the magnesium block of postsynaptic N-methyl-d-aspartic acid (NMDA) receptors (see Chapter 13). Changes similar to those involved in long-term potentiation then occur within dorsal horn cells. However, there is an important difference. Whereas long-term potentiation occurs locally in the synapse receiving strong input, central sensitization affects all synapses in the postsynaptic cell. The result of these universal changes is an enhanced response to all afferent input (Fig. 17-9). This is the mechanism by which central sensitization results in an augmented response to both innocuous and noxious inputs. After central sensitization, inputs that were ineffective at eliciting a response in a dorsal horn cell become effective. Since these subthreshold inputs arise from regions at the margins of the receptive field, the receptive fields of dorsal horn neurons are expanded after central sensitization.

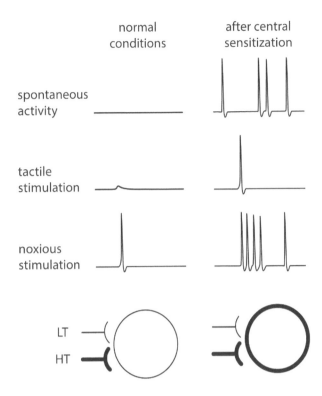

normal conditions   after central sensitization

spontaneous activity

tactile stimulation

noxious stimulation

LT

HT

Figure 17-9 Under normal conditions, high-threshold nociceptive dorsal horn neurons are not spontaneously active and only fire an action potential in response to noxious stimulation. Low-threshold tactile stimulation evokes an excitatory postsynaptic potential (EPSP) but not an action potential. After central sensitization, spontaneous activity and the responses to innocuous or low-threshold (*LT*) and nociceptive or high-threshold (*HT*) inputs are greater.

REFERRED PAIN DEPENDS ON CONVERGENCE FROM SUPERFICIAL AND DEEP INPUTS

Just as we learn to interpret points of light and dark as visual images and auditory tones as meaningful communication, we learn to interpret input from somatosensory pathways as stimulation of our body. A baby learns to associate one particular neural pattern with touch of the right thumb pad and a different neural pattern with heat on the lip and so on. Such associations can be learned for superficial structures because there are data to interpret. Falling and scraping a knee produces activity in visual, auditory, and multiple somatosensory pathways. And the inputs from multiple systems vary systematically according to the site of a stimulus. Using such information, the cerebral cortex learns to correctly assign activity patterns to stimuli of a given nature at a given location. In essence, we learn to *project* activation within somatosensory areas of cerebral cortex as touch or pressure, heat, cold, pricking, and so on.

In contrast to superficial stimulation, stimulation of deep structures produces only a somatosensory feeling with

no other sensory information to anchor that feeling. As a result, we cannot learn the characteristics or the location of stimuli arising from deep structures. Moreover, afferents from deep structures and afferents from cutaneous structures converge onto the same dorsal horn cells (Fig. 17-10). For example, a single spinothalamic tract cell in the thoracic spinal cord may receive input from a visceral afferent that innervates the stomach and from a cutaneous afferent innervating the skin of the upper abdomen. Activity in that spinothalamic tract cell is interpreted as stimulation of the abdominal surface, not of the stomach. Convergent excitation from visceral and superficial afferents of sensory neurons in the dorsal horn and spinal trigeminal nucleus produces a *referral* of deep pain to the body surface. This is the basis for referred pain.

Deep afferents converge with cutaneous afferents onto dorsal horn cells that receive input from nociceptors but not onto dorsal horn cells that receive input exclusively from innocuous mechanoreceptors. As a result, we experience deep stimulation as pain rather than as vibration or light touch, for example. Nonetheless, the complement of somatosensory activity elicited by deep stimuli differs from the complement of somatosensory activity activated by a normal cutaneous stimulus. For example, no innocuous

A. normal conditions

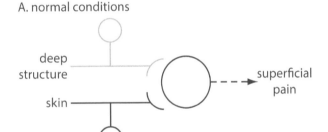

deep structure

skin

superficial pain

B. during conditions of deep pain

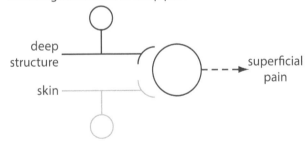

deep structure

skin

superficial pain

Figure 17-10 Referred pain arises from a convergence of deep and superficial input onto single dorsal horn cells. Under normal conditions (A), the superficial input is sometimes active, but the deep input is never active. Therefore, higher structures learn to interpret activity in the dorsal horn cell as arising from the superficial structure. Activity in deep nociceptors (B), when it occurs, excites a dorsal horn cell whose activity is associated with superficial pain. As a consequence, noxious stimulation of a deep structure is interpreted as arising from superficial structures.

mechanoreceptive input arises from regions at the margin of the central skin region. Because the sensation elicited is unlike anything caused by a normal cutaneous stimulus, we are often aware that the stimulus arises from "inside."

THE BRIDGE TO PERSISTENT PAIN IS PAVED BY PERIPHERAL AND CENTRAL CHANGES

Persistent pain is not simply acute pain of long duration. Persistent pain has different characteristics than acute pain because important properties of the nociceptors, peripheral tissue, and central pain pathways are significantly altered. When acute pain turns into a chronic state, the nervous system is changed—often permanently—so that even if any peripheral damage present were rectified, the pain would continue. In other words, persistent pain occurs independently of any stimulus; this is the meaning of the term *neuropathic*. A particularly poignant example of neuropathic pain is phantom limb pain, in which the perceived source of the painful sensation does not even exist. As phantom limb pain exemplifies, nociceptive transmission is uncoupled from any physical stimulus in conditions of neuropathic pain. Neuropathic pain usually involves the three positive signs of allodynia, hyperalgesia, and spontaneous pain.

Most commonly, the triggers for neuropathic pain are one of the following:

- Inflammation

- Nerve injury

- Deafferentation

When inflammation, a normal accompaniment to trauma, infection, or disease, fails to resolve over time, changes in somatosensory pathways script the transition from acute (and often treatable) to chronic (and difficult to treat) pain. Similarly, peripheral nerve lesions can initiate a transformation from healthy to neuropathic. Deafferentation refers to the interruption of somatosensory pathways, either peripherally or centrally. Over time, deafferentation leads to neuropathic pain that co-exists with anesthesia in the affected area. Examples of deafferentation pain include amputation pain and central pain secondary to a stroke that interrupts the ascending somatosensory radiation.

Perhaps the most common form of deafferentation pain can occur after resolution of a herpes zoster (commonly called *shingles*) infection. Recall from Chapter 4 that herpes zoster produces an exquisitely painful rash caused by an awakening of latent *varicella zoster virus*, the causative agent for chicken pox, present in sensory neurons of a dorsal root or trigeminal ganglion. The pain of herpes zoster represents a good example of acute somatic pain. Treatment with antiviral drugs can shorten the duration of a herpes zoster outbreak and analgesics may relieve the pain experienced.

Unfortunately, the story does not always end once an outbreak of herpes zoster resolves. In up to a quarter of patients, a neuropathic pain condition called *postherpetic neuralgia (PHN)* develops. PHN is a potentially devastating, life-altering disease. Common risk factors for the development of PHN are an older age at onset of herpes zoster, severity of the zoster rash, and pain severity at the time of the initial zoster infection. Postherpetic neuralgia is characterized by allodynia and spontaneous pain that can be either deep and aching or sharp and lancinating, or both. In cases where postherpetic pain is accompanied by local anesthesia, the implication is that infected dorsal root ganglion cells have died, setting up a deafferentation-type pain classically termed *anesthesia dolorosa*.

A recently developed and approved vaccine, Zostavax, reduces the incidence of herpes zoster by half and that of PHN by nearly 70%. Although expensive, this vaccine is now being provided to the at-risk populations of immunocompromised and elderly individuals.

Inflammation, nerve injury, and deafferentation produce pathological changes through both shared and unique mechanisms. For example, changes in the excitability of central neurons in the nociceptive pathway contribute to all forms of neuropathic pain. On the other hand, changes in the peripheral chemical environment are critical to persistent inflammatory pain but contribute not at all to deafferentation pain. The mechanisms involved in initiating persistent pain operate at three essential levels:

- The chemical environment of peripheral tissue

- The nociceptor

- Central pathways

Changes at each of these levels work together to produce the symptoms of persistent pain that may co-exist with anesthesia. Invariably, individuals with somatosensory dysfunction are more bothered by *paresthesias* and their unpleasant "cousins," *dysesthesias*, than by an absence of feeling. An example of a paresthesia is a sensation of numbness, whereas sensations of pins and needles or of being impaled by a hot poker are examples of dysesthesias.

Several voltage-gated sodium channel isoforms, most notably Nav1.7, are present either exclusively or are at particularly high levels in nociceptors. Because Nav1.7, a channel found exclusively in nociceptors, only opens at depolarized potentials, nociceptors have an elevated threshold for activation, more depolarized than is the case with other cells. Thus, a given synaptic input is less likely to activate a nociceptor than another type of afferent. Moreover, since Nav1.7 channels inactivate slowly, the maximal rate at which nociceptors can fire action potentials is low. Once activated, nociceptors fire only one or a few action potentials because each action potential inactivates slowly and therefore lasts a long time.

Mutations in Nav1.7, the sodium channel isoform important in action potential generation in nociceptors, cause a congenital insensitivity to pain. Individuals with nonsense mutations in Nav1.7 feel no pain and thus present in a manner similar to that of children with hereditary autonomic and sensory neuropathy. However, these children appear to have fewer symptoms of sympathetic dysfunction, such as anhidrosis.

The importance of an elevated threshold and slow inactivation to nociceptor function is revealed when these firing characteristics are altered by injury. During conditions of persistent pain such as inflammation, nerve injury, or a burn injury, nociceptors change. The threshold for activation is lowered, and inactivation occurs more rapidly. Therefore, in persistent pain conditions, less intense stimuli, often in the innocuous range, activate nociceptors and elicit bursts of action potentials rather than single spikes. Furthermore, the number of sodium channels is elevated. All of these changes mean that nociceptors show bursting discharge under pathological conditions. This firing pattern leads to the *paroxysmal* (i.e., electric and shooting) pain experienced by some individuals in chronic pain.

ULTIMATELY THE BRAIN CONTROLS WHAT WE FEEL THROUGH SOMATOSENSORY PATHWAYS

An intriguing aspect of somatosensory perception is its lability. During self-generated movements, anticipated sensory inputs are suppressed. We saw an example of this in Chapter 16 with the activation of the tensor tympani accompanying chewing. In the context of the somatosensory system, every self-generated movement creates changes that are sensed by cutaneous afferents. Yet, as long as these reafferent changes are those that are expected to occur, they are suppressed. This makes it impossible to tickle oneself. Movement-accompanying sensory suppression is accomplished by projections from somatosensory cortex to the dorsal column nuclei and the dorsal horn. Suppression of anticipated sensory inputs allows us to register surprises or unexpected events and to ignore mundane and uninformative inputs.

Local spinal circuits support modulation through interactions between tactile and nociceptive pathways. One example of this is the inhibition of nociceptive transmission by activity in local Aβ mechanoreceptors. This type of interaction may be the reason that shaking an injured finger, blowing on a burn, or sucking on a paper cut may alleviate the pain of the injury. Local inhibition of nociceptive transmission by Aβ activity is also the basis for the most efficacious, nonpharmacological therapeutic treatment for pain: *transcutaneous electrical nerve stimulation (TENS)*. As Aβ afferents enter the spinal cord and course rostrally within the ipsilateral dorsal column, they give off axonal collaterals that enter the dorsal horn. These collaterals are the source of tactile input to dorsal horn cells. Activity in Aβ afferents has an inhibitory effect on nociceptive transmission. This circuitry may explain why TENS is effective in alleviating pain in many patients. Since Aβ afferents have a lower electrical threshold than do other nerve fibers, it is straightforward to adjust the stimulation intensity to a level that only stimulates Aβ afferents. Because TENS units provide great relief to many patients and carry few risks, they are often worth trying if the funds are available. Unfortunately, for many, the pain relief provided by TENS units is not permanent.

Pharmacological drugs are often the first line of therapy for patients in pain. Opioids mimic endogenous substances and are superb at modifying pain perception. The opioids, such as fentanyl and morphine, represent the prototypical analgesic in clinical use today. They are used to treat postoperative pain and also a number of acute conditions such as a wound, pulled tooth, broken bone, or back pain. The reason that opioids are so effective at alleviating pain is that opioid receptors are present throughout nociceptive transmission circuits. The distribution of opioid receptors throughout pain pathways allows opioids to act at multiple levels. Actions of μ-opioid receptor agonists within the spinal cord are effective in blocking the transmission of nociceptive transmission. This is the basis for epidural administration of opioids. Recall from Chapter 8 that, within the spinal cord, there is a space between the bone and the dura. Epidural injections are given into this space. Drugs introduced into the epidural space cross the blood–brain barrier and reach the spinal cord in relatively high concentrations. Epidurally administered opioids are used to relieve acute pain during childbirth, surgery, and postsurgical recovery and for the treatment of chronic pain, often in terminally ill patients with intractable pain.

Opioids also act supraspinally (in the brain) to modulate pain transmission through engaging a descending pain modulatory pathway. Neurons in the periaqueductal gray (see Chapter 6) and a midline nucleus in the medulla, the *raphe magnus*, respond to opioids by suppressing nociceptive transmission within the spinal cord and the spinal trigeminal nucleus. The suppression of nociceptive transmission initiated by brainstem neurons is termed *descending pain modulation* because it is carried by brainstem neurons that send axons into the spinal cord. Of great relevance to clinical practice, the analgesic effects of opioid actions in the brainstem and spinal cord are synergistic. Thus, opioids administered systemically (orally or by injection) produce a more powerful analgesia than when administered only epidurally or only in the brainstem. Descending pain modulatory pathways not only suppress nociceptive transmission but can also enhance nociceptive transmission. Through such bidirectional effects on ascending nociceptive transmission within the dorsal horn, descending pain modulatory pathways play important roles in both opioid analgesia and the generation of some forms of neuropathic pain.

Opioid drugs have several drawbacks. They cause a myriad of side effects, several of which are both poorly tolerated and difficult to prevent. The most threatening side effect is respiratory depression, which can lead to death. Second, people develop tolerance to opioids, touching off the need for escalating doses in order to achieve an analgesic effect. Third, patients exposed to opioids in the context of appropriate pain management may develop a drug dependency and even debilitating addiction. Indeed, a steep increase in prescriptions for hydrocodone (known in the United States as Vicodin), oxycodone (sold as OxyContin or as Percocet when mixed with acetaminophen), and hydromorphone (Dilaudid) fueled a precipitous rise in prescription opioid abuse during the early 21st century. In the past few years, this trend has begun to reverse with the number of opioid prescriptions dropping for each of the past 3 years. This trend is good news for combatting drug abuse, but it is accompanied by unfortunate caveats. First, the drop in prescriptions has not led to a drop in cases of opioid overdoses. Second, some patients frustrated in attempts to obtain prescription opioids have turned to illegal sources of narcotics. This is reflected in a rise in heroin abuse. Finally, as opioid drugs become more difficult to obtain, some patients are left untreated for severe pain. A failure to treat those in pain runs counter to the physician's commitment to help patients in need. Finding the delicate balance between appropriately treating pain and minimizing prescription opioid abuse is a major challenge for the future.

ADDITIONAL READING

Argyriou AA, Koltzenburg M, Polychonopoulos P, Papapetropulos S, Kalofonos HP. Peripheral nerve damage associated with administration of taxanes in patients with cancer. *Crit Rev Oncol Hematol.* 66: 218–228, 2008.

Basbaum AI, Bautista DM, Scherrer G, Julius D. Cellular and molecular mechanisms of pain. *Cell.* 139: 267–284, 2009.

Berthier M, Starkstein S, Leiguarda R. Asymbolia for pain: A sensory-limbic disconnection syndrome. *Ann Neurol.* 24: 41–49, 1988.

Bessac BF, Jordt SE. Breathtaking TRP channels: TRPA1 and TRPV$_1$ in airway chemosensation and reflex control. *Physiology.* 23: 360–370, 2008.

Cervero F, Janig W. Visceral nociceptors: A new world order? *Trends Neurosci.* 15: 374–378, 1992.

Craig AD. Interoception: The sense of the physiological condition of the body. *Curr Opin Neurobiol.* 13: 500–505, 2003.

Fields HL, Rowbotham M, Baron R. Postherpetic neuralgia: Irritable nociceptors and deafferentation. *Neurobiol Dis.* 5: 209–227, 1998.

Fields HL. *Pain.* New York: McGraw Hill, 1987.

Fischer TZ, Waxman SG. Familial pain syndromes from mutations of the Na V 1.7 sodium channel. *Ann NY Acad Sci.* 1184: 196–207, 2010.

Gawande A. The itch. *The New Yorker*, June 30, 2008.

Holzer P. Neurogenic vasodilatation and plasma leakage in the skin. *Gen Pharmacol.* 30: 5–11, 1998.

Hunter DJ, McDougall JJ, Keefe FJ. The symptoms of osteoarthritis and the genesis of pain. *Rheum Dis Clin N Am.* 34: 623–643, 2008.

Latremoliere A, Woolf CJ. Central sensitization: A generator of pain hypersensitivity by central neural plasticity. *J Pain.* 10: 895–926, 2009.

Lawson SN. Phenotype and function of somatic primary afferent nociceptive neurons with C-, Adelta- or Aalpha/beta-fibres. *Exp Physiol.* 87: 239–244, 2002.

Levine JD, Khasar SG, Green PG. Neurogenic inflammation and arthritis. *Ann NY Acad Sci.* 1069: 155–167, 2006.

Liljencrantz J, Olausson H. Tactile C fibers and their contributions to pleasant sensations and to tactile allodynia. *Front Behav Neurosci.* 8: 37, 2014.

Linden DJ. *Touch: The Science of Hand, Heart, and Mind.* New York: Penguin Books, 2015.

Lumb BM. Hypothalamic and midbrain circuitry that distinguishes between escapable and inescapable pain. *News Physiol Sci.* 19: 22–26, 2004.

Lumpkin EA, Caterina MJ. Mechanisms of sensory transduction in the skin. *Nature.* 445: 858–865, 2007.

McDougall JJ. Arthritis and pain: Neurogenic origin of joint pain. *Arthritis Res Ther.* 8: 220, 2006.

Miller R, Bartolo DCC, Cervero F, Mortensen NJ. Anorectal sampling: A comparison of normal and incontinent patients. *Br J Surg.* 75: 44–47, 1988.

Miller R, Bartolo DCC, Cervero F, Mortensen NJ. Anorectal temperature sensation: A comparison of normal and incontinent patients. *Br J Surg.* 74: 511–515, 1987.

Ramachandran R, Noorbakhsh F, Defea K, Hollenberg MD. Targeting proteinase-activated receptors: therapeutic potential and challenges. *Nat Rev Drug Discov.* 11: 69–86, 2012.

Singer T, Seymour B, O'Doherty J, Kaube H, Dolan RJ, Frith CD. Empathy for pain involves the affective but not sensory components of pain. *Science.* 303: 1157–1162, 2004.

Sweitzer SM, Fann SA, Borg TK, Baynes J, Yost MJ. What is the future of diabetic wound care? *Diabetes Educator.* 32: 197–210, 2006.

Waxman SG. A channel sets the gain on pain. *Nature.* 444: 831–832. 2006.

Woolf CJ, Ma Q. Nociceptors: Noxious stimulus detectors. *Neuron.* 55: 353–364. 2007.

Windebank AJ, Grisold W. Chemotherapy-induced neuropathy. *J Peripheral Nerv Syst.* 13: 27–46, 2008.

18.

THE VESTIBULAR SENSE

THE VESTIBULAR SENSE

BALANCE AND EQUILIBRIUM

Airplanes, ships, and rockets have a set of gyroscopes that detect orientation with respect to gravity. We have an even more sophisticated and far more economical (free for vertebrates) set of *force* sensors within the vestibular apparatus inside our head. Recall that force is the product of acceleration and mass. Accordingly, the vestibular system detects *any* accelerating forces that act on the head. This includes but is not limited to gravity; external forces such as being pushed by another and self-generated forces such as occur during voluntary movements are also detected.

Acceleration is key to vestibular stimulation. We can tell when an elevator starts or stops but we do not sense the steady ascent or descent that occurs in between. Similarly, an ornament hanging from the rear view mirror of a car only swings backward and forward during accelerations and decelerations. When the car is either in constant motion or stopped, the ornament is steady *with respect to the car* even as the ornament careens forward, along with the car, at so many miles or kilometers per hour. The principle that objects maintain a constant velocity unless a force acts upon them is referred to as *inertia* and is also known as *Newton's first law*.

The peripheral vestibular system provides the brain with sensory information about head orientation only because of the ever-present force of gravity. Weighty masses, called *otoconial masses*, are used to sense gravity and other *linear forces*. Just as an ornament hangs from the car mirror, the otoconial masses hang in response to gravity. In other words, car ornaments and otoconial masses are acted upon by the force of gravity even as they maintain a constant position and do not move. The position of the otoconial masses is then translated into the sensory information from which we derive a sense of head position. Sensing gravity

is a phylogenetically ancient function among invertebrate and vertebrate animals. Even plants have a mechanism to detect the direction of gravitational forces, one that is used to direct root growth downward, toward the center of the Earth, rather than perpendicular to the ground. The ubiquity of gravitational sensory systems in both the plant and animal kingdoms speaks to the fundamental importance of adjusting growth and position to Earth's gravity.

Primary afferents with their cell bodies in *Scarpa's ganglion* carry information from the vestibulum to the hindbrain. The central nervous system (CNS) uses information from vestibular afferents to build up a picture of the position and movement of the head. This picture is the starting material for a variety of reflexes that function to stabilize gaze, stabilize the head with respect to the body, and stabilize the trunk and limbs with respect to gravity. The close links between the vestibular sense, vision, and the motor system serve to keep the body in balance or equilibrium. The influence of the vestibular system on motor control is so automatic—and necessarily so—that we take balance, equilibrium, and a steady visual image entirely for granted.

In contrast to the close relationship between vestibular sensation and motor control, the connection between vestibular sensation and perception in a healthy individual is quite weak. Under normal conditions, we are not conscious of the fact that we are upright in the same sense that we are conscious that the sky is blue, the birds are singing, or a cool breeze is in the air. It appears that our perception of equilibrium adapts extraordinarily quickly, vanishing from our consciousness even more rapidly than does awareness of the touch of our clothes. We also do not think anything of the steady visual image that we see from moment to moment. Yet, under pathological conditions, including alcohol intoxication, vestibular dysfunction creates disturbing perceptions that, when present, dominate our conscious experience and imperiously grab our attention.

Two different types of head movements are signaled by vestibular end organs in two different compartments (Fig. 18-1):

- Rotational movements, involving *angular acceleration*, are sensed within the *semicircular canals*.

- Linear accelerating forces, including but not limited to gravity, are sensed by the *otoconial organs*.

The functional division between the canals and otoconial organs is of great clinical importance. The peripheral vestibular system processes information from the two types of end organs separately and differently. Therefore, peripheral vestibular lesions of the otoconial organs or canals can give rise to problems that are restricted to either *disequilibrium* or *vertigo*, respectively, as well as to a combination of the two. To understand the two prominent vestibular

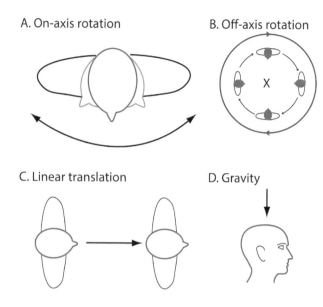

Figure 18-2 Schematic view of angular (A–B) and linear head accelerations are illustrated. A: Shaking your head to indicate "*No*" represents an angular rotation in the yaw plane. The center of the angular rotation is the midpoint of the head, and this is therefore an on-axis rotation. B: The semicircular canals also respond to off-axis angular rotations, such as riding a merry-go-round, in which the center of the rotation is not located at the center of the head. C: Linear motion, or translation, follows a simple linear path. D: Gravity is a constant linear acceleration of about 10 m/s².

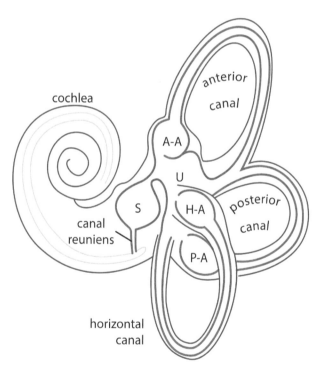

Figure 18-1 The membranous labyrinth, outlined in red, sits within the bony labyrinth (*blue*). The three semicircular canals form the most posterior portion of the inner ear. All three semicircular canals open up into the utriculus (*U*). The sensory epithelium for each canal is contained in a swelling called an ampulla. The ampullae of the anterior (*A-A*), posterior (*P-A*), and horizontal (*H-A*) semicircular canals are labeled. Anterior to the utriculus is the second otoconial organ, the sacculus (*S*). The entire membranous labyrinth is bathed in endolymph.

symptoms, let us back up and look at the two types of accelerating forces.

Angular head acceleration is the acceleration produced by any rotational motion of the head such as occurs on a merry-go-round or when shaking the head to indicate "no" (Fig. 18-2A, B). Linear head acceleration is acceleration of the head along any linear path of motion. Running forward, jumping up, falling down, and moving on an escalator all involve linear motion (Fig. 18-2C). Gravity, an acceleration of roughly 10 m/s², operates on us even when we stand still or lie down (Fig. 18-2D). Because of gravity, static head tilt, which is simply the position of the head with respect to gravity, continuously stimulates the otoconial end organs of the vestibulum (more on this later).

Pathological conditions of the peripheral vestibular system, such as alcohol intoxication, create disturbing perceptions of disequilibrium or vertigo. Disequilibrium refers to an impaired postural stability that stems from dysfunction of sensations arising from the otoconial masses. It represents disordered processing of linear forces. An individual with disequilibrium does not feel in balance, even when standing, sitting, or even lying down. Disequilibrium produces postural instability and often results in injurious falls. Fear of falling and the uncertainty associated with feeling unbalanced lead some individuals with disequilibrium to retreat from the world and social interactions.

Vertigo refers to a perception of spinning, either that the world is moving around a stationary individual or that the self is spinning within a stationary environment. Vertigo results from semicircular canal dysfunction. On the other hand, *dizziness* is a term that people use to refer to an uncomfortable sensation of lightheadedness, the feeling that one is about to faint, *or to vertigo*. But dizziness is not always vertigo. In fact, dizziness is frequently caused by problems outside of the vestibular system, particularly problems with the cardiovascular system such as hypovolemia. Simply getting up quickly can sometimes produce a completely benign lightheadedness that patients may report as feeling "dizzy." Thus, dizziness is by no means an automatic sign of vestibular dysfunction. Despite the distinct definitions of dizziness and vertigo, lay people often use these terms interchangeably. It is important therefore to clarify what an individual means to convey by the terms used. Lightheaded patients should probably see a cardiologist, whereas recurring episodes of vertigo may indicate a problem with the vestibular system.

Along with sensory disturbances, vestibular dysfunction is also tightly associated with autonomic and motor problems. One familiar example is the feeling of nausea that accompanies a perception of vertigo. As discussed later, the vestibular-to-autonomic connection is key to *motion sickness*. A common motor companion to vestibular dysfunction is *nystagmus*, an oscillatory eye movement that occurs normally under certain conditions but also frequently accompanies peripheral or central vestibular pathologies (see much more in Chapter 19). This involuntary and abnormal movement of the eyes in turn alters visual perception, producing *oscillopsia*. Recall from Chapter 5 that oscillopsia is a failure of gaze control in which the visual scene moves continuously with every eye movement. This is akin to watching the world through a hand-held video camera. Movies that intentionally use this device for effect make many viewers feel nauseated. In oscillopsia, the moving visual image persists far longer than the 90–120 minutes of a film; the effect is not only disturbing but also debilitating.

THE VESTIBULAR LABYRINTH AND COCHLEA SHARE THE INNER EAR AND THE EIGHTH CRANIAL NERVE

The inner ear houses the sensory end organs involved in both hearing and vestibular function (Fig. 18-1). Both systems depend on hair cells, and information from cochlear and vestibular afferents travels within the eighth cranial nerve.

The commonalities between cochlear and vestibular end organs are reflected in conditions that are best thought of as *inner ear disorders*. The best example of this is *Ménière's disease*, a disabling and distressing condition that involves recurring cochlear (hearing loss and tinnitus) and vestibular (vertigo and nausea) symptoms and a sensation of fullness in the ear. Ménière's disease can be associated with an increase in endolymphatic pressure, termed *endolymphatic hydrops*, which can result from either overproduction or insufficient absorption of endolymph. Treatment with diet restrictions and steroids designed to reduce endolymphatic pressure can ameliorate the vestibular symptoms of Ménière's disease. Unfortunately, even after such treatment, disabling vertigo continues to afflict about 10% of patients with Ménière's disease. Such patients sometimes elect to undergo either a surgical ablation of the vestibular apparatus or injections of the ototoxic antibiotic gentamicin into the affected labyrinth in order to rid themselves of the vertigo. The willingness of patients to undergo these procedures, which cause permanent vestibular impairment, speaks to the extreme distress of the vertiginous episodes experienced by patients with Ménière's disease.

Ménière's disease is not the only disorder that affects both hearing and vestibular function. Many congenital forms of deafness also involve at least some degree of vestibular impairment. Inflammation of the inner ear, termed *labyrinthitis*, or of the vestibular branch of the vestibulocochlear nerve, *vestibular neuritis*, causes a rapid onset of vestibular symptoms such as vertigo, disequilibrium, and nausea and may also involve hearing loss and tinnitus. Labyrinthitis and vestibular neuritis are thought to be caused by viral infections in most cases, with symptoms typically subsiding in days to weeks.

THE VESTIBULAR LABYRINTH AND COCHLEA OPERATE WITHIN DIFFERENT FREQUENCY RANGES

Despite similarities between vestibular and cochlear transduction, the stimuli involved—airborne sound in the case of the cochlea and accelerating forces acting on the head in the case of the vestibular labyrinth—are quite different. The starts, stops, and changes in the direction of head movements produce accelerations and decelerations that vestibular hair cells respond to. To describe head movements, we use Hertz (Hz), or cycles/s, as was the case for airborne sound. In the case of a force acting on the head, a 2 Hz head movement would be one in which your head moves back and forth twice within a second, returning to the starting position every half second. In humans, the dominant frequencies of head motion are below 10 Hz, about 2–3 Hz during normal walking, a glacial frequency range compared to that of human cochlear hair cells (20 Hz–16 kHz in a young adult). Think about this from the hair cell's perspective. Whereas a cochlear hair cell bundle may have less than 50 microseconds to respond, a 10 Hz head movement moves a vestibular hair bundle in one direction for 50 ms, an ionotropic ion channel "eternity."

Associated with its relatively easy task of transduction, the vestibulum lacks several biochemical and biophysical features that permit the cochlea to respond to high-frequency stimuli. First, vestibular hair cells retain a *kinocilium*, a tall cilium that polarizes the stereocilia bundle during development. In the cochlea, the kinocilium is only present transiently before regressing over the course of normal development. Loss of the kinocilium may serve to increase bundle stiffness and therefore enable responses to the high-frequency displacements that occur in the cochlea. In contrast, vestibular hair bundles are not as stiff and cannot move as fast as cochlear ones. Second, there is only a small endolymphatic potential in the vestibulum (about +10 mV) as compared to the endocochlear potential of +90–100 mV. Thus, the driving force in vestibular hair cells is only about 50–60 mV. Corresponding to this, *abolition of the endocochlear potential does not impair vestibular function even as it causes deafness.* Finally, vestibular hair cells do not express the molecular motor protein prestin; no stimulus amplification occurs in the vestibulum.

Because of the differences between the inner ear's two residents, some disorders affect vestibular or cochlear function, either exclusively or primarily. For example, because prestin is present in the cochlea but not the vestibulum, deafness caused by mutations in prestin occurs without any vestibular dysfunction. Noise-related loss of hearing does not harm vestibular hair cells. Although both types of hair cells are susceptible to damage from ototoxic drugs, some drugs such as the aminoglycoside antibiotic gentamicin affect vestibular hair cells more than cochlear hair cells. Therefore, gentamicin is the drug of choice for intentionally killing vestibular hair cells in conditions such as intractable Ménière's disease.

HAIR CELLS TRANSFORM HAIR BUNDLE DEFLECTION INTO A GRADED MEMBRANE POTENTIAL

Deflection of hair cell bundles leads to a neural response through an intricate transduction mechanism that is largely the same in the cochlea and vestibulum. We examine that mechanism here with a focus on vestibular hair cells. The stereocilia of vestibular hair cells emerge from a hexagonal area at the apical surface of the hair cell; they are arranged from shortest to longest (Fig. 18-3). Tip links connect shorter stereocilia to neighboring longer stereocilia. Recall that the kinocilium is a tall cilium located at the tall end of the hair bundle. When the stereocilia of vestibular hair cells are displaced toward the kinocilium, the tip links pull open the mechanoelectrical transduction (MET) channel, which in turn results in cell depolarization (Fig. 18-3). Thus, movement of the stereocilia toward the kinocilium constitutes the hair cell's preferred (depolarizing) direction. Conversely, when the hair bundle is bent away from the kinocilium (the nonpreferred direction), hair cells hyperpolarize due to closing MET channels. Bending the hair bundle orthogonal to

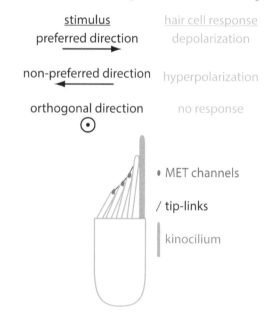

Figure 18-3 Vestibular hair cell stereocilia are arranged from shortest to tallest, with the kinocilium located at the tall end of the bundle. Deflection of the stereocilia toward the kinocilium is the preferred direction of stimulation and results in hair cell depolarization. Deflection of the bundle away from the kinocilium is the nonpreferred direction of stimulation and results in hyperpolarization. Hair cells do not respond to deflection of the stereocilia in the orthogonal direction (into or out of the page). Hair bundle deflection is transformed into a change in membrane potential by tip-links between stereocilia that pull open MET channels, allowing cations in the endolymph to flow into the hair cell.

the preferred-to-nonpreferred axis has no effect on the tip links and therefore does not elicit a hair cell response.

THE UTRICULUS AND SACCULUS SENSE LINEAR MOTION IN ALL DIRECTIONS

Two open bony chambers located posterior to the cochlea and anterior to the three canals, the *utriculus* and the *sacculus*, house the two otoconial end organs that respond to linear accelerations (Fig. 18-1). The utriculus and sacculus each contain a patch of hair cells called the *macula*. Stereocilia of the macular hair cells are embedded in the otoconial mass that is displaced by gravity or other linear forces (Fig. 18-4).

Recall that the otoconial mass serves as a weight, or load, that can be displaced by linear forces. To understand the importance of the otoconial mass's mass, consider a stone and a Styrofoam peanut of the same volume and shape. These two objects, differing only in mass, will fall at very different rates. Compared to the plummeting stone, the Styrofoam peanut's downward trajectory is a slow and lazy meandering. This comparison illustrates the importance of having a heavy object to sense linear acceleration. Essentially, vestibular function requires that the otoconial masses have sufficient mass upon which gravitational and other forces can act.

Each otoconial mass contains about 200,000 tiny weights called *otoconia* (Greek for "ear dust") that consist of calcium carbonate within a matrix of glycosylated proteins called *otoconins*. The otoconia amass together into an otoconial mass that is held together by fibrils and a dense gelatinous matrix that functions as glue (Fig. 18-5). Critically, most otoconins are only made during fetal development, and the mature otoconial masses form at that time. Since no replacements for the primary otoconins are available after birth, the loss of otoconia is irreversible. Unfortunately, the supply of otoconia does not always last for a human lifetime as the otoconial masses degenerate with age. Decalcification of the otoconia and loss of fibrils leads to a progressive degeneration of the otoconial masses that starts by the sixth decade. First pits appear in the otoconial masses. Over time, the pits expand until small pieces of the otoconial masses form, break loose, and eventually float off. Because the degeneration of otoconia occurs preferentially in the sacculus, the sacculus eventually may lack sufficient otoconia to sense gravity in affected individuals. In essence, when an

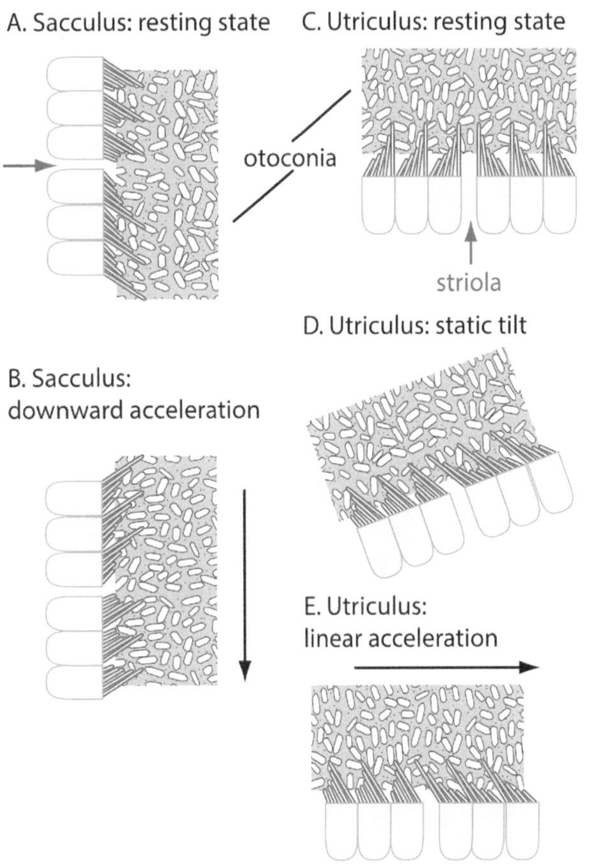

Figure 18-4 A: In an upright person at rest, the otoconial mass of the sacculus is displaced downward due to the force of gravity. During linear accelerations in the vertical plane, the sacculus is displaced either farther downward during upward acceleration or upward during downward acceleration (B). When the sacculus floats up, as occurs during a downward acceleration, the resting effect of gravity on the sacculus is relieved momentarily, resulting in a feeling of "weightlessness." C: The resting state of the utricular otoconial mass in an upright individual involves no displacement of stereocilia. However, during static tilt (D) or linear accelerations (E), the otoconial mass shifts, and the stereocilia are deflected. The deflection of the utricular stereocilia can be the same during a static tilt and a linear acceleration, as is the case in the examples illustrated in D and E. Additional input from the semicircular canals, somatosensory afferents, and motor centers are used by central vestibular neurons to disambiguate these signals. In both the sacculus and utriculus, there is a dividing line called the striola (*red arrows* in A and C).

otoconial mass resembles a feather more than a stone, accurately sensing gravity is no longer a possibility.

Mild to moderate loss of otoconia from the otoconial masses may have little effect on equilibrium. However, a total or near-total loss of the otoconial masses adversely affects balance and contributes to disequilibrium. Because of the finite supply of otoconia, degeneration of the otoconial masses is a progressive problem. As discussed earlier, disequilibrium is a debilitating state that can lead both to

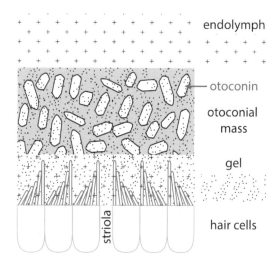

endolymph

otoconin

otoconial mass

gel

striola

hair cells

Figure 18-5 The otoconial mass consists of protein (otoconin), fibrils, and a gelatinous matrix (gel) into which the hair cell bundles extend. Endolymph, present throughout the lumen of the membranous labyrinth, bathes the hair cell bundles and surrounds the otoconial mass. With age or trauma, pieces of the otoconial mass can break off, irreversibly diminishing the otoconial mass. In both otoconial end organs, there is a dividing line called the striola.

falls and to social isolation born of the fear of falling. It may be that impairment in balance secondary to otoconial mass degeneration is as inevitable or likely as other age-related changes, such as presbyopia and presbyacusis. If it were not for the bulkiness of the term, we might talk of "presbyequilibrium" as we do of presbyopia and presbyacusis.

Many refer to the otoconial masses as *otoliths*. In fact, otoliths are inner ear masses that are found in finned fish. They are made of calcium carbonate within a proteinaceous matrix, and they continue to grow, accreting more mass throughout the lifetime of a fish. Thus, even though the mammalian otoconial mass and fish otolith both serve as a load that enables the detection of gravitational force, the difference between the single-edition otoconial mass and the ever-growing otoliths is substantial and of great clinical significance in aging humans.

DISLODGED OTOCONIA FLOAT INTO THE SEMICIRCULAR CANALS AND PRODUCE BENIGN PAROXYSMAL POSITIONAL VERTIGO

Benign paroxysmal positional vertigo (BPPV) is perhaps the most common vestibular condition that brings an individual to seek medical care. BPPV is thought to result when some part of an otoconial mass dislodges and floats into the canals. The displacement of endolymph stimulates canal hair cells, resulting in a perception of head rotation. Since the posterior

canal is the lowest part of the labyrinth when the head is in an upright position (see Fig. 18-8), the dislodged fragments from an otoconial mass tend to move there and stimulate hair cells, resulting in a sudden (paroxysmal) feeling of vertigo that is often accompanied by nausea. Hair cell stimulation occurs preferentially during particular head movements that bring the dislodged mass in contact with vestibular hair cells and is thus dependent on head position.

BPPV can be caused by head trauma or even by riding a roller coaster but tends to occur more frequently with age and often without an identifiable triggering event. Treatment is aimed at maneuvering the head in specific trajectories so that the otoconial mass fragments move from the canals to the vestibule containing the utriculus and sacculus. Since the macular hair cells are embedded in the otoconial mass, they do not respond to free-floating otoconia. With time, BPPV typically subsides, presumably as the free-floating otoconia are resorbed.

THE SACCULUS AND UTRICULUS RESPOND TO LINEAR FORCES

In an upright person, the utricular macula is oriented horizontally and the saccular macula is oriented vertically. Since the stereocilia of the saccular hair cells are embedded in an otoconial mass, they are displaced downward toward the center of the Earth (Fig. 18-4A). This displacement is a response to gravity. In the same stationary and upright individual, the stereocilia in the utricular macula are not displaced (Fig. 18-4C). Now consider the consequences of tilting the head to the side. The otoconial mass in the utricular macula is displaced by gravity downward, toward the side of the tilt (Fig. 18-4D), whereas the downward displacement of the saccular otoconial mass is lessened. Thus, thanks to the constant of the gravitational force, otoconial end organs respond to the static position of the head, whether it be upright or tilted.

The sacculus and utriculus also respond to linear accelerations of the head caused by self-motion, falling, or vehicular movement. During linear accelerations, the heavy otoconial mass lags behind the macula (think of a car ornament lagging behind as the car accelerates forward), so that the hair cell stereocilia are displaced. For example, accelerating forward will cause the utricular otoconial mass to lag backward, bending the stereocilia backward as well (Fig. 18-4E). In the upright person, utricular hair cells are arranged in such a way that they respond to linear acceleration in any horizontal direction, meaning accelerations to either side as well as accelerations forward and backward.

Saccular hair cells, in contrast, respond to accelerations up and down. During an upward acceleration, as occurs during the upward phase of a jump, the otoconial mass lags behind, displaced even more than normal by gravity alone. Conversely, on the downside of a jump, the otoconial mass lags behind at a position that is *above* the macula (Fig. 18-4B). By sensing the displacement of the otoconial mass induced by gravity and other linear accelerations, hair cells in the utriculus and sacculus signal both the static position of the head and linear accelerations of the head.

ANGULAR ACCELERATION PRODUCES ENDOLYMPH MOVEMENT IN SPECIFIC CANALS

There are three semicircular canals on each side. The canals are fluid-filled *tori* (*torus* is the singular form), meaning shapes that resemble inner tubes. The three canals, oriented orthogonal to one another in three planes of space, are:

- The anterior, or superior, semicircular canal

- The posterior, or inferior, semicircular canal

- The horizontal semicircular canal

Each semicircular canal begins and ends in the utriculus. At one end of each semicircular canal is a swelling called the *ampulla*. Within the ampulla, a transverse ridge of sensory epithelium protrudes into the canal (Fig. 18-6). This sensory epithelium is the *crista ampullaris*, or simply the *crista*, where the hair cells are situated, the canal equivalent to the macula.

Accelerations in three different planes of rotation are the stimuli for hair cells in each of the semicircular canals. To understand which rotations stimulate which semicircular canals, we need names for three planes of head rotation. The plane names that we use are those used originally by farmers for plows and seafarers for boats and more recently by aviators for airplanes. The yaw or horizontal plane of movement is described by moving one's head back and forth in the universal signal for "no" (Fig. 18-2A). The pitch plane is that in which the head moves when nodding; imagine a plow or a boat pitching forward (Fig. 18-7A). The third plane of head movement, the roll plane, is used when you lay your head to either side (e.g., on your shoulders; Fig. 18-7B). The nautical or aeronautic analogies, particularly for pitch and roll, are useful in imagining and remembering the three planes of rotational head motion.

The key to inner ear function is transformation of the adequate stimulus into a stimulus of mechanical displacement that stimulates well-positioned hair cells. For semicircular canals, the transformation is accomplished within the fluid-filled tori of the canals. For our purposes, a fluid-filled torus attached to a rotating surface such as a "Lazy Susan" approximates a semicircular canal. Now, imagine that the

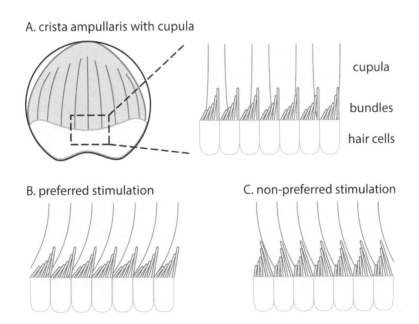

Figure 18-6 Within the ampulla of each semicircular canal, the sensory epithelium, termed a crista ampullaris (*blue*), is located on top of the ridge of the crista. The stereocilia of the hair cells within the crista are embedded in a gelatinous structure called a cupula. B: When the cupula is displaced in the preferred direction, all the hair cells depolarize. When the cupula is displaced in the nonpreferred direction, the hair cells hyperpolarize. Only accelerations in the plane of the canal lead to displacement of the cupula and therefore hair cell responses.

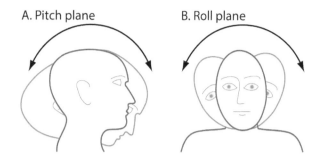

A. Pitch plane **B. Roll plane**

Figure 18-7 A: Rotations moving the head forward and backward as when nodding yes, or nodding off, are contained in the pitch plane. The center of rotation in the pitch illustrated is within the head. An example of an off-axis pitch would be the rotation involved in doing a handstand or flip. B: Side-to-side rotations of the head are contained in the roll plane, with the center of rotation located within the head. A cartwheel is an example of an off-axis roll rotation. The yaw plane of rotation is illustrated in Figure 18-2A, B.

torus is rotated clockwise. The fluid in the torus has inertia and stays stationary. Thus, the fluid moves in a counterclockwise direction *relative* to the torus walls. Moreover, the fluid moves the *cupula*, a gelatinous structure that stretches across the lumen of the canal (Fig. 18-6). The stereocilia of hair cells in the crista are embedded in the cupula so that deflection of the cupula deflects the hair cell bundles of the canal ampullae.

In the inner ear, instead of a torus attached to a rotating tray, the membranous labyrinth is fixed within the bony labyrinth, which is fixed within the rotating head. The cristae and resident hair cells are all located at one end of the canal where the labyrinth meets the utriculus. For each of the canals, there is a specific end that houses the crista and overlying cupula: the rostral end of the horizontal canal, the

posterior end of the posterior canal, and the anterior end of the anterior canal (Fig. 18-8).

CANAL HAIR CELLS RESPOND TO RELATIVE ENDOLYMPH MOVEMENT

As simple as it sounds, the arrangement of a fluid-filled torus provides all that is necessary to transform angular motion into fluid movement. Rotation of the head leads to relative endolymph flow, which deflects the cupula and thus the hair cell bundles. The conversion of endolymph movement into a consistent hair cell response is then accomplished by the specific arrangement of hair cells in the canal cristae. *Within each semicircular canal crista, all hair cells are oriented in the same direction* (Fig. 18-6A). As illustrated in Fig. 18-8, the preferred direction of the hair cells is toward the utriculus for the horizontal canals and *away* from the utriculus in the cases of the anterior and posterior canals.

With this last piece of the puzzle in place, we can now understand how a clockwise rotation leads to the depolarization of hair cells in the right horizontal canal and hyperpolarization of the hair cells in the left horizontal canal (Fig. 18-9). Recall that a clockwise rotation leads to counterclockwise (relative) endolymph movement and therefore counterclockwise deflection of the cupula. Since the preferred direction of the horizontal canal hair cells is toward the utriculus, the horizontal canal hair cells on the right are deflected in the preferred direction and depolarize. On the left, horizontal canal hair cell bundles are deflected away from the utriculus, leading to hair cell hyperpolarization.

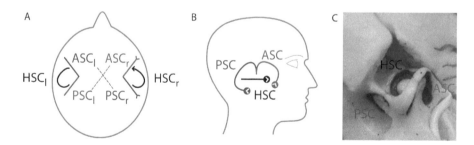

Figure 18-8 The canal orientations are illustrated. A: The horizontal semicircular canals on the left and right side (*HSC*ₗ and *HSC*ᵣ) form a pair. This means that any rotation with a component in the yaw plane will have opposing effects on the two horizontal canals. The other two canal pairs are (1) the right anterior semicircular canal (*ASC*ᵣ) and the left posterior semicircular canal (*PSC*ₗ) shown in red and (2) the left anterior semicircular canal (*ASC*ₗ) and the right posterior semicircular canal (*PSC*ᵣ) shown in blue. The arrowheads on the right side of the head indicate the location and orientation of the hair cells in the ampulla of each canal. The hair cells in the horizontal ampulla are oriented toward the utriculus, whereas the preferred direction of hair cells in the anterior and posterior canals is away from the utriculus. B: The location of the ampullae (*filled circles*) and the preferred direction of hair cells in each semicircular canal (*arrowheads*) are illustrated on a side view of the right canals. From this perspective, it is clear that the lowest point in the vestibular apparatus is the ampulla of the posterior canal. Because of this topography, debris within the membranous labyrinth is thought to preferentially accumulate in the posterior ampulla. B: This view of the three semicircular canals (*green and labeled*) makes clear that the lowest point in the vestibular apparatus is the ampulla of the posterior canal (*asterisk*).

A. Clockwise head rotation

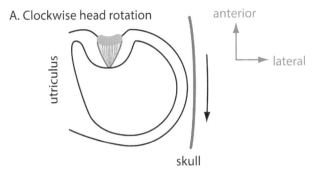

B. Counter clockwise endolymph rotation

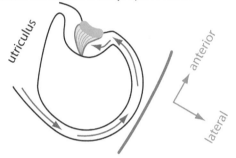

Figure 18-9 The right horizontal semicircular canal, viewed in isolation from above, is diagrammed before (A) and after (B) a clockwise head acceleration. During a clockwise head acceleration, the bony and membranous labyrinths rotate clockwise while the endolymph stays stationary. Because the crista and ampulla are anchored to the membranous labyrinth, endolymph moves relative to these structures (B). The relative motion (*brown arrows*) of the endolymph with respect to the crista and cupula deflects the cupula, which leads in turn to the deflection of hair bundles (not shown). In the rotation illustrated, the stereocilia are deflected *toward* the utriculus, which is the preferred direction of hair cells in the horizontal canals. Thus, a clockwise or rightward acceleration results in the depolarization of right horizontal hair cells. The same logic used here can be employed to deduce the effect of any rotational acceleration.

The preceding example shows how a rotation in the yaw plane produces fluid movement in opposing directions in the two horizontal canals. This same yaw rotation does not elicit fluid movement in either the anterior or the posterior canal. Thus, the horizontal canals form a pair; they are contained in a single plane and respond in opposing fashion to stimulation. Just as the horizontal canals form a pair, so do the right anterior and left posterior canals (Fig. 18-8A). The same goes for the left anterior and right posterior canals. Each canal pair shares a single plane of orientation. The right anterior canal and left posterior canal are contained in the vertical plane that runs from a point that is midway between a rightward roll and a forward pitch to a point midway between a leftward roll and a backward pitch. Similarly, the left anterior canal and right posterior canal form a pair that is oriented in the orthogonal vertical plane. Thus, the posterior and anterior canals do not sit within any one of the three planes described

Table 18-1 THE EFFECT OF ROTATIONS ON HAIR CELLS IN EACH CANAL IS LISTED

ROTATION	L-HOR	R-HOR	L-ANT	R-POST	R-ANT	L-POST
CW yaw	Hyper	Depol	–	–	–	–
CCW yaw	Depol	Hyper	–	–	–	–
FW + R	–	–	–	–	Depol	Hyper
BW + L	–	–	–	–	Hyper	Depol
FW + L	–	–	Depol	Hyper	–	–
BW + R	–	–	Hyper	Depol	–	–

For six rotations, the effect of movement in each direction on hair cell membrane potential is listed. For example, a rotation that is equal parts backward pitch (BW) and left roll (L) causes hyperpolarization (Hyper) of the right anterior canal (R-Ant) hair cells and depolarization (Depol) of left posterior canal (L-Post) hair cells. CCW: counterclockwise, CW: clockwise, Depol: depolarization, FW: forward pitch, R: right roll.

earlier: yaw, pitch, or roll. Instead, their orientations are about equal parts pitch and roll, at 45-degree angles to the pitch and roll planes. An easy way to visualize the orientations of the two vertical canal pairs is to view each pair as one stroke of an "X" through the center of the head when viewed from above.

By knowing the location of the crista and the orientation of the hair cells in each canal, the effect of any head rotation on the hair cells in any of the canals can be deduced. Alternatively, there is an easy shortcut to knowing the effect of any head rotation on any given semicircular canal. As it turns out, head rotations toward a canal's *outer edge* depolarize hair cells in that canal (see Table 18-1). For example, a rotation that is half-pitch forward and half-roll right depolarizes right anterior canal hair cells. The opposite rotation, half-pitch backward and half-roll left, hyperpolarizes the same hair cells of the right anterior canal.

Now that we understand hair cell orientation, we can take a brief look back at the otoconial end organs. The preferred direction of hair cells in the utriculus and sacculus is complicated by the *striola,* a dividing line about which hair cell orientations change (Figs. 18-4, 18-5). In the sacculus, the preferred direction of hair cells is always away from the striola, and, in the utriculus, the preferred direction is toward the striola. The hair cells in the saccular macula are oriented vertically, responding to a vertical displacement of the stereocilia with either a depolarization or a hyperpolarization (Fig. 18-4B). The orientations of hair cells in the utricular macula are radially organized to cover all horizontal directions. Consequently, displacement of the utricular stereocilia in any horizontal direction depolarizes a population of utricular hair cells, hyperpolarizes another population (Fig. 18-6C), and has no effect on utricular hair cells with an orthogonal orientation.

ALCOHOL INTOXICATION CAUSES VERTIGO BY CHANGING THE SPECIFIC GRAVITY OF THE CUPULA

Normally, the cupula is neither heavier nor lighter than the endolymph. However, drinking alcohol dilutes the blood so that it has a lower specific gravity than usual. If enough alcohol is consumed and the specific gravity of the cupula sufficiently decreased, the cupula will float up within the denser endolymph. Movement of the cupula then deflects the stereocilia of hair cells. The pattern of hair cells that are stimulated depends on the position of the crista with respect to gravity, which in turn depends on head position. In any case, the pattern of hair cell responses is unlike any naturally occurring pattern. For example, in a stationary prone position, alcohol intoxication would stimulate both left and right horizontal canals, a pattern that never occurs normally. Moreover, the activation of both horizontal canals at the same time that both vision and otoconial end organs signal a steady environment is a further sign that all is not well. The CNS interprets this odd conglomeration of vestibular and visual input as a spinning motion, leading to a sense of vertigo. A similar vertiginous perception occurs in BPPV due to the excitatory signal from one canal without a concurrent inhibitory signal from the canal's contralateral partner.

The morning after alcohol intoxication, dehydration has set in and the specific gravity of blood is higher than normal. The endolymph, however, is a little less dense than usual, reflecting the state of the dilute blood when it was made several hours earlier. So, now the cupula sinks in the endolymph, and vertigo returns until blood and endolymph equilibrate to their normal specific gravities. Of course, one way to quickly achieve equilibration is colloquially referred to as "the hair of the dog": viz drink more alcohol, thereby lowering the specific gravity of blood and, in turn, of the cupula.

THE VESTIBULAR SYSTEM IS NOT SENSITIVE TO MOVEMENT AT CONSTANT VELOCITY

Vestibular hair cells only respond to acceleration and not to movement at a constant velocity. In the canals, the requirement for acceleration is accomplished because the cupula is only deflected by movement of the endolymph, and endolymph only moves during angular acceleration of the head. However, movement of the endolymph in the canals is opposed by frictional forces arising from the viscosity of the endolymph and the elasticity of the cupula. These opposing forces cause the movement of the endolymph

and cupula to lag head acceleration and to approximate the velocity of the head. Thus, *vestibular hair cells require head acceleration to detect movement of the cupula but code for head velocity.* Another way to view this is that the lag of the endolymph and cupula integrate the acceleration stimulus into a velocity signal. Similarly, macular hair cells in the otoconial organs only respond to linear accelerations but have responses that are proportional to velocity.

That hair cells only respond to acceleration is evident by the lack of any vestibular sensation during constant velocity motion, such as occurs in a car or a plane cruising at a constant speed. In contrast, during takeoff and landing of a plane and during car accelerations and decelerations, a clear sensation of slowing down or speeding up is perceived.

NATURAL HEAD MOVEMENTS ELICIT COMBINED CANAL AND OTOCONIAL ORGAN RESPONSES

Under normal circumstances, head movements rarely adhere neatly to single planes of either angular or linear acceleration. For example, a pitch forward is equal parts forward movement in the plane of the left anterior–right posterior canal pair and in the plane of the right anterior–left posterior canal pair (Fig. 18-10A). As another example, a roll right is equal

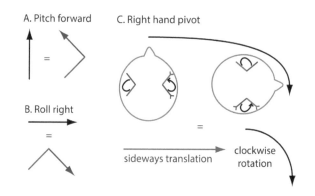

Figure 18-10 The vestibular system operates by decomposing every movement into the components contained within the planes of the canal pairs, the utriculi and the sacculi. Three examples are illustrated. A: A pitch forward (*black arrow*) is equal parts forward movement in the right anterior semicircular canal–left posterior semicircular canal plane (*red*) and forward movement in the left anterior semicircular canal–right posterior semicircular canal plane (*blue*). B: A roll right (*black arrow*) is equal parts forward movement in the right anterior semicircular canal–left posterior semicircular canal plane (*red*) and backward movement in the left anterior semicircular canal–right posterior semicircular canal plane (*blue*). C: Natural head movements typically involve both angular and linear acceleration. The same principle of decomposition applies here. The rightward pivot illustrated is composed of a rightward translation and a clockwise rotation. These movements evoke responses in hair cells in the utriculi and the horizontal semicircular canals.

parts forward movement in the right anterior–left posterior canal pair plane and backward movement in the left anterior–right posterior canal pair (Fig. 18-10B). Application of this type of movement decomposition into component vectors can be extended from exclusively rotational movements to truly natural head movements, which typically include both linear and angular acceleration. For example, a pivot to the right involves both a rightward translation and a clockwise rotation (Fig. 18-10C). In this way, vestibular end organs respond separately to the individual vector components, angular and linear, that make up natural movements.

VESTIBULAR AFFERENTS CARRY INFORMATION FROM THE INNER EAR TO THE BRAINSTEM

As you know, the hair cells in the vestibulum, like their cousins in the cochlea, are non-neural sensory cells derived from the otic placodes. The first *neurons* in the vestibular pathway are the primary afferents in Scarpa's ganglion that synapse on vestibular hair cells and also send a central process into the hindbrain. It is these primary vestibular afferents that take information from the inner ear to the brain.

The hair cell to afferent synapse is heavily trafficked. In both the cochlea and vestibulum, MET channels are slightly open even when the hair cell bundle is in a neutral position and not moving. Therefore, hair cells are depolarized to roughly −50 mV at rest. This depolarization results in constitutive release of glutamate, the hair cell neurotransmitter, which in turn activates primary vestibular afferents.

Thus, vestibular afferents discharge at fairly high rates, in the range of 50–100 spikes per second, even when the head is not moving and even in the canals that do not respond to the ever-present gravity.

The elevated resting potential that is found in inner ear hair cells allows for bidirectional sensory coding. Accelerations in the nonpreferred direction hyperpolarize hair cells and result in less glutamate release from the hair cell. Consequently, the firing rate of the postsynaptic vestibular afferents decreases below the resting rate of 50–100 spikes per second (Fig. 18-11). Of course, hair cell depolarization, as occurs with accelerations in the preferred direction, increases the rate of glutamate release and therefore elicits an increased discharge rate in the vestibular afferents. In this way, *vestibular afferents respond bidirectionally to head acceleration*. This is useful particularly since the preferred and nonpreferred directions are equally meaningful. Bidirectional sensory responses are also present in vision, where dark and light are both informative. Resting discharge and therefore bidirectional responses are notably absent from the somatosensory system, which in turn accentuates deviations from the background quiet as notable.

Vestibular afferents project to neurons in four vestibular nuclei within the hindbrain. A small number of vestibular afferents also project directly to the cerebellum, the only sensory afferents to enjoy such privileged access to the cerebellum. The hindbrain targets of vestibular afferents serve several functions that revolve almost exclusively around motor control. As we see in the next section, the transition from sensory (inner ear, Scarpa's ganglion, and vestibular portion of CN VIII) to motor occurs within the vestibular nuclei.

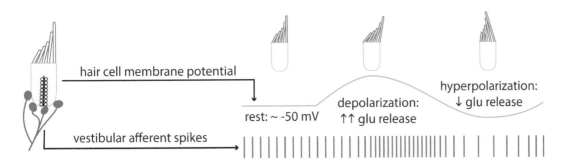

Figure 18-11 The hair cell to primary afferent synapse. As with cochlear hair cells, vestibular hair cells respond to stimulation with graded potentials (*blue line*). They do not fire action potentials. As diagrammed on the left, hair cells release glutamate from a specialized type of active zone called a ribbon synapse (*black*) onto postsynaptic vestibular afferents (*red*). When the hair bundle is in the neutral position (*top row*), the hair cell membrane potential is about −50 mV (*middle row*), and vestibular afferents have a resting discharge of roughly 50–100 spikes per second (*bottom row*). In response to a stimulus that deflects the stereocilia in the preferred direction, the hair cell depolarizes and releases more glutamate. Consequently, the vestibular afferent fires more rapidly. In contrast, in response to a stimulus that deflects the stereocilia in the nonpreferred direction, the hair cell hyperpolarizes and releases less glutamate than at rest. Consequently, the vestibular afferent fires less rapidly. The depolarized rest potential in the hair cell and the resting discharge of the vestibular afferent enable the vestibular system to respond to stimulation in opposing directions.

VESTIBULAR NUCLEI DIRECTLY CONTROL MOTOR OUTPUT

When all is well, vestibular perception plays very little role in our daily life. We normally operate without awareness of our vestibular status. We may notice a warm sunny day or a beautiful bird singing a melodic song, but gravity and rotational forces are not prominent in our conscious life. Reflecting this reality, vestibular pathways to neocortex exist but are dwarfed by vestibular pathways to motor control centers and motoneurons.

In contrast to its miniscule role in perception, the vestibular system plays a central and absolutely essential role in everyday motor control. As terrestrial animals, we battle gravity constantly in order to stay upright and keep the horizon horizontal. Furthermore, gaze can be kept steady even as the body and head move about. As will be elaborated in the next chapter, our mechanism for keeping gaze steady depends on *vestibular* rather than visual input. The vestibular–motor connection is even built into our language. The words that best describe vestibular sensory functions (balance, equilibrium, steady) are all borrowed from the motor side. It is impossible to describe the feeling of falling in the same way that you could describe the color of a visual object, timbre of a musical note, or texture of cloth. Thus, despite the sensory system-style connections from the inner ear to the brainstem, the vestibular system serves a primarily motor function, guiding and modifying all movements in a healthy individual.

Direct connections from vestibular nuclear neurons to specific groups of motoneurons are a primary architectural mechanism that allows for the vestibular system's integral role in motor control. The best example of the vestibular system's importance to motor control is the *vestibuloocular reflex* (*VOR*), which maintains an image on the fovea even as the body and head move about. Essentially, this reflex allows us to read as we walk, ride public transit, or sit in a moving train. In fact, since we are never perfectly still, the VOR also permits us to read or see any image stably as we stand, sway, or sit. Through the VOR, every head movement—to the side, up, or down—elicits an opposing eye movement (see Chapter 19).

OPTIC FLOW INFORMATION INFORMS THE BRAINSTEM OF VERY SLOW ACCELERATIONS

We sense accelerations that are so slow that they do not excite hair cells. How can this be? As it turns out, central vestibular neurons get information about slow accelerations from the *visual system* rather than the inner ear. Midbrain neurons that receive retinal input respond to the overall movement of the entire visual field, or *optic flow*. For example, as you look out the window of a slowly moving vehicle, the world is not stationary but rather flows by, opposite to the direction of travel. Importantly, central vestibular neurons sum inner ear and optic flow inputs *without distinguishing between them*. Because of this free-for-all mixing, a slow (vestibular) acceleration of the self is simply no different (to a vestibular nuclear neuron) from a slow (optical) acceleration in the world. A common example of this is experienced when sitting in a train at a station; we are often fooled into thinking that our own train has begun to move and is accelerating ever so slightly when, in fact, the train on the next track is slowly moving.

The confusion between movement of one's own train and of another train is a strictly modern predicament born of vehicles. Throughout past evolutionary time, adult terrestrial animals traveled only when self-propelled. This situation has changed with the inventions of boats, trains, automobiles, and planes. However, the vestibular system has not evolved to catch up with the recent development of passenger vehicles. Consequently we are prone to suffer the affliction of *motion sickness*, which only occurs when one is moved through space rather than propelling oneself through space. The difference comes from the involvement of the brain's motor control circuits in self-propelled movement but not in passive movement through space. Essentially, each motor command is accompanied by a message to the vestibular system to ignore the vestibular consequences of the intended movement. For example, consider a twirl to the right. Along with the signal that initiates the twirling movement, motor control centers also send a message to suppress the excitation of vestibular nuclear neurons arising from the right horizontal canal. In other words, the predictable sensory consequences of an intentional action are suppressed.

In the absence of a motor signal cancelling anticipated sensory inputs, head movements elicit responses in central vestibular neurons. For example, consider traveling through urban streets, replete with potholes, during the stop-and-start traffic of rush hour. The vestibular stimulation inherent in traveling this course would be canceled in a person walking or running through the streets. However, when a person traverses this same terrain as a vehicular passenger, innumerable accelerations and decelerations in vertical and horizontal planes gain access to central vestibular neurons. Consequently, the overall message from the vestibular system is one of head motion, and lots of it. Now, consider that a bus passenger is reading a book while sitting on the bus. The image of the book type remains steady because gaze is kept constant thanks to the VOR. This creates a mismatch between information from the vestibular system—lots of movement—and information from the visual system—the world is steady.

Sensory mismatch is thought to cause the autonomic symptoms of motion sickness. When traveling on Earth, the mismatch involved is primarily between visual and vestibular signals, as just described. In space, mismatch between the various vestibular end organs occurs because of the microgravity environment. Additionally, somatosensory inputs, such as those along your back as you lie down, are altered in gravity-free space. The *toxin detector hypothesis* holds that, across evolutionary time, vestibular input has always gone haywire in response to the osmotic changes caused by ingested neurotoxins. For example, afferents from the left and right horizontal canals may discharge together after food poisoning. Accompanying the unpleasant and unnatural feeling of vertigo, there is an evolutionarily adaptive reaction of nausea and emesis (vomiting). Although everyone can experience motion sickness given severe enough conditions, some are more susceptible than others; the reason for the individual variation in susceptibility is not known.

The nonpharmacological strategy to avoid motion sickness focuses on avoiding near fixation during passenger travel. This approach yields a moving visual image that is more in line with the vestibular input of motion. The most common pharmacological treatment for motion sickness is directed at the guts rather than at the brain or vestibulum. *Scopolamine*, a muscarinic receptor antagonist, reduces gastrointestinal motility while also blocking accommodation, nasal and oral secretions, and causing some degree of drowsiness.

The lessons regarding sensory mismatch gained from thinking about motion sickness can inform our understanding and even treatment of vestibular disorders. Consider an older individual who experiences episodes in which she feels that objects rotate around her when she is still and even when her eyes are closed. Nausea and vomiting may accompany these episodes. Walking feels unsteady, as though the ground has been transformed into clouds that give way with every step. One simple way to ameliorate these symptoms is to provide a sensory input, beyond vision, that the world is steady. The easy one to use is the somatosensory system. Thus, a person suffering from feeling unsteady can gain a perceptual advantage, beyond any physically stabilizing benefit, by touching a fixed object such as a wall. A great advantage of such treatment is that it comes at no cost.

THE VESTIBULAR NUCLEI ARE NOT SIMPLE RELAYS OF VESTIBULAR AFFERENTS INPUT

Under many conditions, the responses of vestibular nucleus neurons to head movements reflect the responses of vestibular nerve afferents. However, there are exceptions to this general rule. We have already looked at two exceptions. Slow accelerations do not excite vestibular afferent but are conveyed by midbrain neurons responsive to optic flow into the vestibular nuclei. And input arising from motor control centers during self-generated movements cancels the message from predictable vestibular inputs.

Another difference between vestibular afferents and vestibular nucleus neurons is that only the latter can integrate input from more than one end organ. This is useful because the input from only one vestibular end organ or even from an end organ pair can be ambiguous. For example, a backward tilt of the head and a forward acceleration both stimulate the utriculus identically (Fig. 18-4D–E). In this situation, vestibular nucleus neurons cannot use input from both the utriculi alone, but combined input from the sacculi and utriculi are informative and can be used to distinguish between the two stimuli. Somatosensory afferents, particularly from the neck, can also aid in distinguishing between ambiguous vestibular signals. In our example, neck proprioceptive input to the vestibular nuclei differs when the head is tilted versus being upright.

Vestibular ambiguities can have deadly consequences for pilots. A deceleration at constant altitude has virtually the same effect on vestibular afferents as does an upward climb; this ambiguity is just one of a myriad that can occur in an airplane. When the horizon is not visible, pilots can fall victim to *spatial disorientation*, and each year a number of pilots of small planes crash for this reason. This tells us several things. First, visual perception is far more reliable than vestibular perception; without the former, we are at a disadvantage. Second, somatosensory inputs are normally too weak to counteract a vestibular illusion. And yet, despite its ambiguity, vestibular perception powerfully drives reactions, which can transform a minor confusion into a major and uncorrectable crisis within seconds. The only defenses against disorientation are flying during clear conditions or expertise at reading and using instruments to fly.

VESTIBULAR PATHWAYS REACH MOTOR AND HOMEOSTATIC TARGETS

As emphasized earlier, outputs from the vestibular nuclei target motor-related regions that are critical to controlling eye movements and postural balance. Direct projections to oculomotor, trochlear, and abducens motoneurons, which control the extraocular muscles (see Chapter 5), serve the reflexive eye movements of the VOR. Projections to the cervical ventral horn are important in coordinating head and shoulder movements needed for large shifts in gaze. Projections to the spinal ventral horn at all levels are critical to maintaining postural balance. In sum, the motoneuron types targeted by neurons in the vestibular nuclei include:

- *Extraocular motoneurons*: These connections support the VOR that moves the eyes to keep gaze steady during head movements (see Chapter 19).

- *Neck motoneurons*: These connections support the *vestibulocollic reflex* (*VCR*), which serves as another strategy to keep gaze steady during head movements (see Chapter 19). Although humans have a serviceable VCR, the VCR of birds is superb and highly entertaining as multiple online videos demonstrate.

- *Postural extensors*: These connections support the postural reflexes that activate extensors in response to downward acceleration (see Chapter 23).

Thus, the vestibular system's integral role in motor control is built into the architecture of the vestibular nuclear neurons through direct projections to motoneurons. Moreover, vestibular projections to the cerebellum also contribute to the motor coordination of postural balance and eye movements with head position and body movement. This architecture is remarkable, especially compared to the visual system. The secondary sensory neuron in the visual system that corresponds to a vestibular nucleus neuron is in the retina. Of course, no retinal (or geniculate or visual cortex) neuron projects to a motoneuron or even to a motor control center. The contrast between visual and vestibular pathways highlights the extreme motor emphasis of the vestibular system.

Under normal, all-is-well conditions, the output of the vestibular system is entirely motor in character. However, when vestibular well-being is challenged, vestibular perception comes to the fore, along with autonomic distress. Putting on glasses with a poor prescription, spinning, or diving from a high board all can elicit an unpleasant perception of vertigo or disequilibrium. The pathway serving vestibular perception travels through the ventral postero-medial (VPM) nucleus of the thalamus, the same region that receives trigeminal somatosensory information from the face and oral cavity. From thalamus, vestibular information reaches regions near the head representation in somatosensory cortex. Stimulation within "vestibular" cortical areas most frequently produces a sense of movement, imbalance, or vertigo, more evidence that vestibular perception is restricted to impaired conditions.

Vestibular pathways also reach brainstem and cortical regions involved in homeostasis. Connections between vestibular and brainstem regions such as the nucleus of the solitary tract may support the uncomfortable bodily feeling that accompanies falling. Within the forebrain, vestibular information serves two primary purposes. First, vestibular information is critical to spatial orientation and the sense of self in space. Second, vestibular information appears key to a sense of bodily well-being. The comorbidity, or coincidence, of anxiety disorders and symptoms reflective of vestibular dysfunction—dizziness, vertigo, disequilibrium, and nausea—may result from the strong influence of vestibular inputs on emotional and homeostatic systems.

ADDITIONAL READING

Angelaki DE, Cullen KE. Vestibular system: The many facets of a multimodal sense. *Annu Rev Neurosci.* 31: 125–150, 2008.

Balaban CD, Thayer JF. Neurological bases for balance–anxiety links. *Anxiety Dis.* 15: 53–79, 2001.

Berthoz A, Viaud-Delmon I. Multisensory integration in spatial orientation. *Curr Opin Neurobiol.* 9: 708–712, 1999.

Dieterich M. Central vestibular disorders. *J Neurol.* 254: 559–568, 2007.

Fernandez C, Goldberg JM, Abend WK. Response to static tilts of peripheral neurons innervating otolith organs of the squirrel monkey. *J Neurophysiol.* 35: 978–987, 1972.

Freedman EG. Coordination of the eyes and head during visual orienting. *Exp Brain Res.* 190: 369–387, 2008.

Goldberg JM, Fernandez C. Physiology of peripheral neurons innervating semicircular canals of the squirrel monkey. I. Resting discharge and response to constant angular accelerations. *J Neurophysiol.* 34: 635–660, 1971.

Golding JF. Motion sickness susceptibility. *Autonom Neurosci.* 129: 67–76, 2006.

Minor LB, Schessel DA, Carey JP. Ménière's disease. *Curr Opin Neurol.* 17: 9–16, 2004.

Thalmann R, Ignatova E, Kachar B, Ornitz DM, Thalmann I. Development and maintenance of otoconia. *Ann NY Acad Sci.* 942: 162–178, 2001.

19.

GAZE CONTROL

We tightly control the direction of gaze. The large amount of neural territory devoted to gaze control reflects the unique importance of maintaining a steady gaze when so desired or, alternatively, of changing the direction of gaze when needed. Brain circuits exert exquisite control over the position and orientation of the *visual axis* between the pupil and the fovea. We effortlessly keep our gaze steady, never even thinking about this as a task or an accomplishment. In contrast, we cannot keep other important body parts, such as the hands, in a steady position even when we try really hard to do so. To illustrate the difference to yourself, compare how you fare trying to either read or write while walking. Reading is no problem because gaze control circuits keep our point of fixation under tight control so that we do not see text jumping around. However, writing performed while one's body is moving doesn't look pretty; we have no neural system dedicated to keeping our hands steady. Even if the writing surface is stationary, as when walking on a treadmill, we cannot finely maintain a hand position in space. In sum, the control system that governs gaze is unique.

PATTERNS OF GAZE ARE IMPORTANT FOR SOCIAL COGNITION

Gaze is a powerful social signal and, in fact, the original mode of social communication. Mothers bond with their children through mutual gaze, which elicits oxytocin release in the mother, which in turn facilitates attachment and nurturing behavior. This loop between gaze, hormone release, and attachment circling back to gaze is critical to establishing the mother–child bond. Gaze may also facilitate bonds between other individuals, including between people and their pet dogs.

Gaze control is also revealing of temperament and personality. Shifty eyes effectively communicate "person with something to hide." A steady gaze suggests to us that someone is honest, open, and trustworthy. Although these judgments may not always be warranted, they certainly stem from a fundamental truth that eye movements, as with facial expressions and posture, are an expression of self and mood.

Our visual judgments depend utterly and entirely on eye movements. We evaluate the emotional content of a person or situation based on the visual information that we take in (Fig. 19-1). Most people fixate primarily on the eyes and mouth of a face and determine, with high accuracy, the emotion expressed therein. Abnormal face-scanning patterns are associated with damage to the amygdala (see Chapter 7) and with psychiatric diseases such as schizophrenia and autism spectrum disorder. Individuals who fail to scan faces normally often fail at making emotional judgments that are simple for most of us (Fig. 19-1A).

Eye movements dictate our perceptual reality even when we gaze steadily at an object. This is because images that are completely stable on the retina fade from view. Such *visual fading* occurs in a completely immobile person, a person without any head or eye movements. Small eye movements, less than a degree in size, called *microsaccades*, circumvent this problem and prevent images from fading. During fixation, we unconsciously make one to two microsaccades each second, and this is sufficient to prevent visual fading. Thus, although still images disappear, small eye movements are enough to restore image perception, thus providing a clear demonstration of the importance of changes in luminance across time and space as the critical stimuli for vision (see Chapter 15).

Eye movements are easy to elicit even in young children and can be quantitatively measured. Consequently, attention has focused recently on the use of eye movement abnormalities as diagnostic tools for schizophrenia and other developmental psychiatric disorders. One hope is that eye movement abnormalities can serve as biomarkers of psychiatric disease, allowing for early detection, diagnosis, and the evaluation of potential therapeutic interventions. Another possibility exists, which is that eye movement

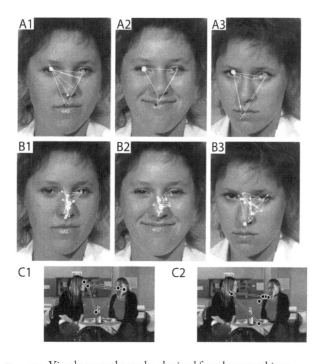

Figure 19-1 Visual scan paths can be obtained from human subjects by videotaping the eyes at high resolution. The resulting scanpaths map both points of fixation (*dots*) and saccades (*lines*) between points of fixation. The scanpaths of control (A) and schizophrenic (B) individuals are shown as the subjects look at a neutral face (*A1, B1*), a happy face (*A2, B2*), and a sad or somber face (*A3, B3*). As illustrated by these representative scanpaths, schizophrenic subjects spend far less time fixating on the eyes and mouth, the most emotionally salient features of a human face, than do control subjects. In contrast to control subjects who showed similar scanpaths regardless of the target expression (*A1–A3*), schizophrenic subjects followed more normal scanpaths when looking at a sad face (*B3*) than at neutral (*B1*) or happy (*B2*) faces. Associated with the different scanpaths, schizophrenic subjects judged sad faces as accurately as did controls, but were worse at detecting neutral and happy faces. C: Control teenagers, teenagers with autism spectrum disorder and impaired language development (*C1*), and teenagers with autism spectrum disorder and normal language development (*C2*) were shown a video of two young women in a restaurant talking about whether to send back disgusting food. Control teenagers (not shown) and teenagers with autism spectrum disorder and language impairment fixated primarily on the eyes of the two faces in the video. In contrast, teenagers with autism spectrum disorder and normal language skills fixated on eyes far less. Furthermore, the amount of time spent fixating on the mouth was directly correlated and the amount of time fixating on the eyes indirectly correlated to language skills among subjects with autism spectrum disorder. Panels A and B are modified from Loughland CM, Williams LM, Gordon E. Visual scanpaths to positive and negative facial emotions in an outpatient schizophrenia sample. *Schizophrenia Res* 55: 159–70, 2002, where a full discussion of these interesting results can be found, with permission of the publisher, Elsevier. Panel C is modified from Norbury CF, Brock J, Cragg L, Einav S, Griffiths H, Nation K. Eye-movement patterns are associated with communicative competence in autistic spectrum disorders. *J Child Psychol Psychiatry* 50: 834-42, 2009, where these intriguing results are discussed fully, with permission from the publisher, John Wiley & Son.

abnormalities may contribute to the pathophysiology of psychiatric disease. The patient with bilateral amygdala damage described in Chapter 7 supports this idea. Recall that the patient could not detect fearful expressions until she was told to look at the eyes of a face. When she looked at the eyes, she performed normally in detecting fearful expressions. Determining the extent to which abnormal eye movements *cause* psychiatric dysfunction, beyond simply serving as potential biomarkers of disease, remains an intriguing question for the future.

EYE MOVEMENTS SERVE TO EITHER STABILIZE GAZE OR CHANGE DIRECTION OF GAZE

As we know by now, gaze depends on both eye and head position. Yet head and eye position are unequal partners because eye movements contribute more than do head movements to gaze shifts, small and large alike. *Saccades*, fast ballistic eye movements, are faster and require less preparatory time than the most rapid head movements. It is the saccade that brings gaze to its new position; gaze remains steady from the point at which the *eyes* reach the target onward (Fig. 19-2). Since gaze stabilization and gaze shifts depend principally on eye movements, we focus our examination of gaze control on the *oculomotor system*, the pathways involved in controlling extraocular muscles. The oculomotor system should not be mistaken for the cranial nerve and nucleus of the same name; the system is inclusive of all brain regions involved in moving the eyes.

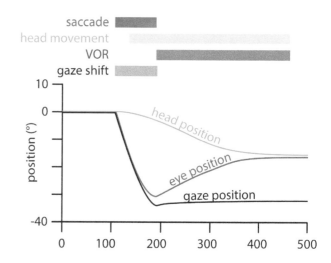

Figure 19-2 During large gaze shifts, both the eyes and head move in the direction of the target. The eyes start moving before the head and bring gaze most of the way to the final target position before the head moves by any appreciable amount. The saccade is very short, providing a fast eye movement that brings gaze to the new target. Then, as the head movement proceeds, the vestibuloocular reflex (VOR) keeps gaze steady by moving the eyes in opposition to the head movement. The result is that gaze stays steady once the target has been reached. Modified from Freedman EG. Coordination of the eyes and head during visual orienting. *Exp Brain Res* 190: 369–87, 2008, with permission of the publisher, Springer.

Progressive external ophthalmoplegia is a disorder that results in progressive weakness and eventual failure of all extraocular muscles and the levators palpebrae superioris. Sporadic mutations in any of a number of mitochondrial genes coding for enzymes in the respiratory chain cause this muscular disease. Initially, weakness is bilaterally symmetric, and head movements compensate for the loss in extraocular mobility. However, eventually it becomes obvious to the patient, or to those around the patient in pediatric cases, that the eyes are not moving and that head movements are producing all gaze shifts. Over time, facial muscles and the long muscles of the legs may also become weak. Surgery is typically used to treat the ptosis resulting from levator palpebrae superioris involvement, but no therapy currently exists for the ophthalmoplegia or other motor weakness. Note that as with the muscular dystrophies, the problem in progressive external ophthalmoplegia is in the muscle and not in the nervous system. Nonetheless, patients are unlikely to know this and may seek care from a general practitioner, ophthalmologist, or neurologist.

Recall from Chapter 5 that passive forces place the eye in the neutral position, looking straight ahead. In a healthy individual, only active eye movements produced by extraocular muscle contractions can move the eyes from the neutral position to an eccentric, or off-center, position. Eye movements fall into two fundamental categories: (1) those that serve to stabilize an image on the fovea at an eccentric position, and (2) those that serve to shift the point of fixation.

Three types of eye movements serve to stabilize eye position:

- *Fixation* is an active process that maintains gaze in a given position.

- The *vestibuloocular reflex* (*VOR*), introduced in Chapter 18, stabilizes gaze during head movements.

- The *optokinetic response* stabilizes gaze when viewing repeating visual patterns. This is what occurs when one looks out of a moving vehicle at a picket fence or grove of trees.

Four types of eye movements serve to change the direction of gaze:

- *Cancellation of the VOR* during head movements allows gaze to shift from one location to another.

- *Saccades* are rapid, sometimes reaching speeds of more than 300 degrees per second, ballistic movements that move the eyes to a new position in minimal time without the possibility of mid-course corrections or adjustments.

- In *smooth pursuit*, gaze stays fixed on a target, such as a bird flying, that moves at speeds of roughly 20–50 degrees per second.

- *Vergence*, the eye movement component of the near triad (see Chapter 5), shifts the fixation target from a far location to a near location.

After a brief foray into extraocular muscles and motoneurons, we examine each of these types of eye movements in turn.

EXTRAOCULAR MUSCLES AND NEUROMUSCULAR JUNCTIONS HAVE SPECIAL PROPERTIES ADAPTIVE TO THEIR FUNCTION

Extraocular muscles and motoneurons have a few peculiar properties that make them different from other skeletal muscles and motoneurons (see Chapter 21). The differences yield differences in susceptibility to disease. For example, both extraocular motoneurons and the motor control cells (in frontal eye fields) that innervate them are spared in amyotrophic lateral sclerosis, which lays waste to virtually all other skeletal motoneurons and motor control neurons. On the other hand, extraocular muscles are particularly vulnerable to damage from autoimmune conditions such as myasthenia gravis (see Chapter 13).

Myasthenia gravis and *Grave's ophthalmopathy* are two diseases that target ocular tissues and result in slow or weak eye movements. Myasthenia gravis is an autoimmune disease that results in failure of the neuromuscular junction, often starting in the eye (see Chapter 13). Patients typically present with ptosis due to reduced levator palpebrae superioris contraction and diplopia secondary to extraocular muscle weakness (Fig. 19-3). Grave's ophthalmopathy is an inflammation of the orbit typically associated with hyperthyroidism. Antibodies against antigens present in the orbit drive an inflammatory reaction that produces extreme swelling of the orbital contents, including the muscles. Consequences include *proptosis*, or bulging of the eye, that is usually accompanied by pain, restriction of eye movements, and, in extreme cases, compression of the optic nerve resulting in blindness. The vulnerability of the extraocular muscles to these two autoimmune diseases may reflect a unique immunological milieu within the orbit.

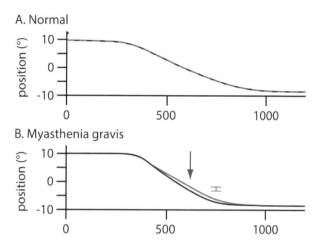

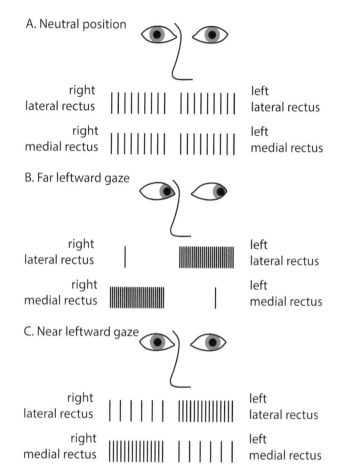

Figure 19-3 Precisely aligned eye movements are necessary for normal vision. A: In healthy individuals with normal eye movements, the vertical positions of the right (*red*) and left (*black*) eyes are the same at every moment in time as a person shifts gaze from up to down. Therefore, traces of the two eye positions overlap completely. The traces are alternately dashed in order to illustrate the overlap. B: In a patient with mild myasthenia gravis, a neuromuscular disease that typically affects eye muscles first, the two eyes are misaligned (*arrow*). Even a small misalignment of only a degree or two is enough displacement to produce diplopia. The distance between the eye positions at the time of the arrow is illustrated by the lines to th right.   Modified from Kaminski HJ, Li Z, Richmonds C, Ruff RL, Kusner, L. Susceptibility of ocular tissues to autoimmune diseases. *Ann NY Acad Sci* 998: 362–374, 2003, with permission of the publisher, John Wiley & Sons.

FIXATION AT AN ECCENTRIC POSITION REQUIRES SUSTAINED MUSCULAR FORCE

Eye position depends on the tonic discharge rate of the six extraocular motoneurons. In the neutral position, eye position is not biased in the pulling direction of any muscle, and extraocular motoneurons have a balanced resting discharge (Fig. 19-4A). Increases in the firing rate of extraocular motoneurons rotate the eye away from the neutral position in the pulling direction of the muscle involved. As the firing rate increases, the eye is increasingly rotated in the pulling direction of the innervated muscle. For example, maximal activation of the motoneurons innervating the left lateral rectus leads to an abduction of the eye all the way to the left. More moderate firing rates have less extreme consequences on eye position (Fig. 19-4B). Thus, a moderate elevation in the discharge rate of left lateral rectus motoneurons may only partially abduct the eye to the left.

A decrease in the firing rate of extraocular motoneurons allows the eye to be pulled but does not, in and of itself, result in eye movement. Thus, neither contraction alone nor relaxation alone predicts eye position; rather, *the balance of activity in muscles with opposing pulling directions determines eye position*. Consider that the right lateral rectus

Figure 19-4 The dependence of eye position on discharge (action potentials represented by vertical lines) in medial and lateral rectus motoneurons. The tonic firing rate of extraocular motoneurons is related to the distance the eye is rotated from the neutral position in the pulling direction of the innervated muscle. A: In the neutral position, all extraocular muscles are at rest, and the resting discharge of all extraocular motoneurons is balanced. B: During fixation to the far left, the left lateral rectus and right medial rectus motoneurons have an elevated discharge rate, whereas the right lateral rectus and left medial rectus motoneurons do not fire or fire very infrequently. C: During fixation to the near left, the left lateral rectus and right medial rectus motoneurons fire at a rate intermediate between the rates during the above two conditions. Similarly, the right lateral rectus and left medial rectus motoneurons fire at a rate below that of resting levels but above the level when the muscles are fully relaxed.

and left medial rectus motoneurons stop firing. If there is still activity in the opposing muscles (left lateral rectus and right medial rectus), then the eye will move to the left. However, if the opposing muscles are also quiet, then the eye will stay where it is. This principle is the basis for understanding the pathophysiology behind deviations from the neutral position. For example, we can now understand why a down and out eye results from an oculomotor nerve lesion (see Chapter 5). In the face of no medial rectus contraction (due to the lesion), the normal resting activity in lateral rectus motoneurons pulls the eye laterally while unopposed activity in the superior oblique pulls the eye down. By similar logic, the eye is adducted by an abducens palsy and elevated in an individual with a trochlear lesion.

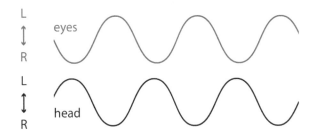

Figure 19-5 The vestibuloocular reflex (VOR) keeps gaze stable during head movements. When the head (*black*) rotates back and forth in the yaw plane, the eyes move in the opposing direction due to the VOR. L: left, R: right.

VERTICAL GAZE IS CONTROLLED IN THE MIDBRAIN AND HORIZONTAL GAZE IN THE PONS

As with the vestibular system, the oculomotor system is a vector-based system. This means that the horizontal and vertical components of every eye movement are processed and organized separately by the horizontal and vertical gaze centers, respectively. The horizontal gaze center is located in the pons, whereas control over vertical and torsional gaze depends on neurons in the midbrain. The midbrain also contains another group of neurons that control vergence. This separation of gaze control makes sense in light of the location of cranial nerve nuclei containing motoneurons innervating the different extraocular muscles. Horizontal gaze depends critically on the abducens nucleus located in the pons, whereas vertical, torsional, and vergence movements all require the oculomotor and trochlear nuclei located in the midbrain.

The division of gaze control labor between the pons and midbrain cuts across all types of eye movements. For example, there are two brainstem saccade generators—one for the horizontal component and one for the vertical and torsional components of every saccade. The pontine horizontal gaze center produces the horizontal component of saccades and smooth pursuit movements. Vertical and torsional components of saccades and smooth pursuit movements are organized in the midbrain. Distinct regions in the pons and midbrain also control the horizontal and vertical components of fixation, respectively.

As we move up from extraocular muscles and motoneurons to motor control circuits, we consider horizontal movements almost exclusively. The principles are the same for vertical and torsional eye movements but the specifics are far more difficult to envisage.

THE VESTIBULOOCULAR REFLEX ENSURES A STEADY FIXATION TARGET DURING HEAD AND BODY MOVEMENTS

As was introduced in Chapter 18, the VOR keeps the image on the fovea stable even as the head and body move about (Fig. 19-5). When active, the VOR counteracts head movement to keep gaze rock steady. Then, when the VOR is suppressed, head movements can be used to help accomplish gaze shifts, typically large ones.

To appreciate the advantages accrued by using *vestibular* input rather than *visual* input to keep gaze steady, do the following experiment. Fixate on your finger in front of your face. Now, turn your head back and forth in the yaw plane. Start slowly and increase the speed of your head movement until your finger gets blurry. You have to move your head fairly fast in order to blur the image of your finger. Now, keep your head steady and move your finger, at first slowly and then more rapidly. Hopefully, you realize that you are much better at stabilizing gaze during head movements than during movements of the visual target (your finger in this case).

There are many reasons why a vestibular initiated reflex is faster than a visually initiated one, starting with the respective transduction mechanisms. Vestibular transduction depends on ionotropic channels, whereas visual transduction depends on metabotropic receptors. Processing of a visual stimulus is still in the retina by the time that a vestibular input has already reached the brainstem. Moreover, in order to use visual input to stabilize gaze, a complex visual signal called *retinal slip* needs to be detected. Retinal slip refers to the change in an image's position on the retina. For example, consider that you are standing still and light from a fixation target is hitting your fovea. Now, as you start to move, your head moves, shifting your gaze (= head + eyes) so that light from the desired fixation target is no longer hitting your fovea. Instead, light from the erstwhile fixation target hits a peripheral spot on the retina. Thus, the place on the retina where the image of the target is represented has slipped. Any such shift in image position is retinal slip. Neural detection of retinal slip requires extrastriate cortex and takes oodles of processing time. Accordingly, movements such as smooth pursuit that require a calculation of retinal slip cannot start any earlier than about 200 milliseconds. In contrast, the latency to the VOR is about 10 milliseconds!!

THE VOR IS A DISYNAPTIC REFLEX

The VOR is a disynaptic reflex that requires a minimum of three neuronal types (Fig. 19-6A):

- Primary vestibular afferent
- Vestibular nuclear neuron
- Extraocular motoneuron

Although head movements in all directions elicit a VOR, we look in detail at the VOR that is simplest to understand, which is, of course, that elicited by a rotation in the yaw plane (see Chapter 18).

We start with a clockwise head rotation (rightward head turn as viewed from above) that excites afferents innervating the right horizontal semicircular canal (Fig. 19-6B). Vestibular afferents from the right horizontal canal excite neurons in the ipsilateral vestibular nuclei. Vestibular nuclear neurons in turn directly excite ipsilateral medial rectus motoneurons and contralateral lateral rectus motoneurons (Fig. 19-6B). The result is a rapid contraction of the left lateral rectus and right medial rectus and therefore a leftward or counterclockwise eye movement that opposes the initiating head movement.

As mentioned earlier, the VOR produces a very rapid eye movement that opposes the effects of a head rotation in any plane, not just the horizontal plane. The correspondence between head rotation and evoked eye movement arises from the connectivity of vestibular nuclear neurons that connect afferents from one canal pair to a specific pair of extraocular motoneuron pools. As we saw earlier, a head movement that excites a horizontal canal excites the ipsilateral medial rectus and contralateral lateral rectus to produce a contralateral eye movement. The other two extraocular muscle pairs (see Chapter 5) pair with specific anterior or posterior canal activation (see Table 19-1). A backward pitch that excites a posterior canal elicits a downward VOR, which is accomplished by the inferior rectus and superior oblique (Fig. 19-7C, D). Similarly, a forward pitch of the head excites an anterior canal and elicits an upward VOR, requiring the superior rectus and inferior oblique (Fig. 19-7A, B).

To step through one example, consider a half pitch forward and half roll left head rotation that excites afferents to the left anterior canal (Fig. 19-7A). The resulting VOR brings the eyes up and to the right, a movement that involves contraction of the left superior rectus and right inferior oblique. Thus, vestibular nuclear neurons that receive input from afferents from a given canal are

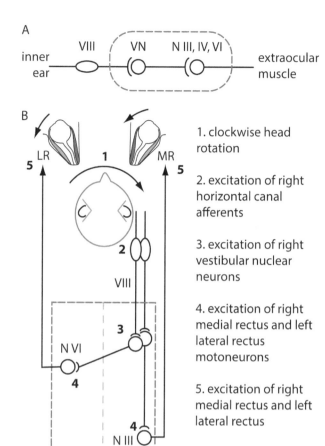

Figure 19-6 **A:** The vestibuloocular reflex (VOR) is a disynaptic, three-neuron reflex. Vestibular afferents (*VIII*) enter the central nervous system (*dashed green line*) and synapse on neurons in the vestibular nuclei (*VN*). Vestibular nuclear neurons project to extraocular motoneurons in cranial nerve nuclei (*N III, IV, VI*) and spinal motoneurons that innervate neck muscles (not shown). **B:** The circuit of a horizontal VOR evoked by clockwise head rotation (*1*) is diagrammed. Clockwise head rotation excites right horizontal canal afferents (*VIII, 2*), which then excite vestibular nuclear neurons (*3*). Vestibular nuclear neurons in turn excite contralateral abducens motoneurons and ipsilateral medial rectus motoneurons (*4*). The result is contraction of the contralateral lateral rectus and ipsilateral medial rectus (*5*), producing a contralateral, in this case counterclockwise, eye movement. Thus, a head rotation elicits a compensatory eye movement in the opposite direction.

Table 19-1 **EXTRAOCULAR MUSCLE PAIRS PARTNER WITH ONE SEMICIRCULAR CANAL**

HEAD MOVEMENT	SEMICIRCULAR CANAL	EXTRAOCULAR MUSCLE PAIR
Yaw (CW or CCW)	Horizontal	Ipsilateral medial rectus Contralateral lateral rectus
Downward pitch	Anterior	Ipsilateral superior rectus Contralateral inferior oblique
Backward pitch	Posterior	Ipsilateral superior oblique Contralateral inferior rectus

The following labels appear in Figure 19-6:

A
inner ear — VIII — VN — N III, IV, VI — extraocular muscle

B
1. clockwise head rotation
2. excitation of right horizontal canal afferents
3. excitation of right vestibular nuclear neurons
4. excitation of right medial rectus and left lateral rectus motoneurons
5. excitation of right medial rectus and left lateral rectus

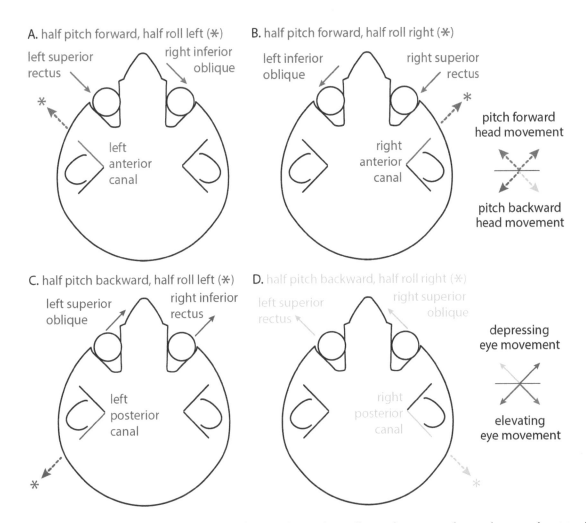

A. half pitch forward, half roll left (✱)

left superior rectus

right inferior oblique

left anterior canal

B. half pitch forward, half roll right (✱)

left inferior oblique

right superior rectus

right anterior canal

pitch forward head movement

pitch backward head movement

C. half pitch backward, half roll left (✱)

left superior oblique

right inferior rectus

left posterior canal

D. half pitch backward, half roll right (✱)

left superior rectus

right superior oblique

right posterior canal

depressing eye movement

elevating eye movement

Figure 19-7 The pairings of each semicircular canal with a pair of extraocular muscles are illustrated in cartoons showing the eyes and semicircular canals as viewed from above. Only head movements involving a pitch forward (*upward dashed arrows*; A–B) or backward (*downward dashed arrows*; C–D) are diagrammed; yaw movements are not illustrated. Excitation of the left (A) or right (B) anterior canal excites the ipsilateral superior rectus and contralateral inferior oblique, whereas excitation of the left (C) or right (D) posterior canal excites the ipsilateral superior oblique and contralateral inferior rectus. In this way, the vestibuloocular reflex (VOR) produces an eye movement (*inset at bottom right*) that opposes head movement (*inset at top right*).

connected to a specific pair of extraocular motoneuron pools, one ipsilateral and one contralateral. In this way, head movement that stimulates a canal elicits eye movement in the opposing direction.

Relaxation of antagonist muscles accompanies the contraction of a pair of extraocular muscles. The easiest example to understand is, of course, a horizontal eye movement. In the case of a leftward eye movement, the left medial rectus and right lateral rectus muscles relax. This allows contraction of the opposing muscles to rotate the eyes leftward. Muscle relaxation comes about through a process of reducing excitatory input, known as *disfacilitation*. Every canal excitation is paired with a canal inhibition (see Chapter 18) so that, along with exciting afferents to the ipsilateral horizontal canal, any acceleration in the yaw plane also *inhibits* afferents from the contralateral

horizontal canal. As you recall, vestibular afferents are active at rest. Therefore, inhibition of canal afferents leads to less excitation—rather than to inhibition—of vestibular nuclear neurons. The disfacilitated vestibular nuclear neurons in turn provide less excitatory drive to target motoneurons, which are, in turn, also disfacilitated. In the example of a rightward head rotation, the discharge of left medial rectus motoneurons and right lateral rectus motoneurons decreases due to disfacilitation, and the innervated muscles relax allowing the eyes to be pulled to the left.

In sum, VOR circuitry uses synaptic connectivity to automatically link any given head movement to the motoneurons that will lead to an opposing eye movement. The circuitry requires a minimum of neural processing and therefore is complete within a very short time. A head movement elicits an opposing eye movement that begins within 10 milliseconds!

Linear head accelerations also elicit a compensatory VOR, in this case a translational one. In addition, the vestibulocollic reflex produces head movements that oppose head rotations. The vestibulocollic reflex depends on circuitry that closely parallels that of the VOR except that the targeted motoneurons innervate neck muscles. The latency of the vestibulocollic reflex is a little longer than that of the VOR. Nonetheless, the vestibulocollic reflex can compensate, at least partially, for the VOR in individuals with extraocular muscle or motoneuron impairment.

NYSTAGMUS CAN RESULT FROM UNBALANCED PERIPHERAL VESTIBULAR INPUT

Ordinarily, afferents from the paired semicircular canals provide a balanced signal to the left and right vestibular nuclei (Fig. 19-8A). Pathological conditions can produce an imbalance in the left and right vestibular nerve inputs (Fig. 19-8B, C). For example, imagine that the left semicircular canals are damaged by surgery, trauma, or infection so that the afferents on that side fall silent. Yet the contralateral inner ear functions normally so that there is normal resting discharge in vestibular afferents on the healthy side. Centrally, the imbalance in vestibular afferent input (Fig. 19-8C), in this case more activity on the side of the healthy inner ear, is interpreted by the vestibular nuclei as a rotational head movement toward the healthy side (Fig. 19-8B). The nervous system reacts to the imbalanced inputs as it would to a rotational head movement, resulting in a VOR toward the damaged side (VOR in Fig. 19-8D). Once the eye reaches the edge of the orbit, a quick saccade to the healthy side is made (saccade in Fig. 19-8D). At this point, the imbalanced afferent input still exists, and so another compensatory VOR to the damaged side is made, setting off another saccade, and so on and on. This repeated cycle of a slow eye movement (VOR) in one direction followed by a fast reset (saccade) in the opposite direction is a form of *nystagmus* (Fig. 19-8D).

Jerk nystagmus is any form of nystagmus with alternating fast and slow movement. In the nystagmus just described due to peripheral damage, the pathology involved produces the slow eye movement, the VOR. However, when observing nystagmus, it is the saccade that stands out and not the VOR. Therefore, the direction of a jerk nystagmus is named for the direction of the fast (saccade) movement.

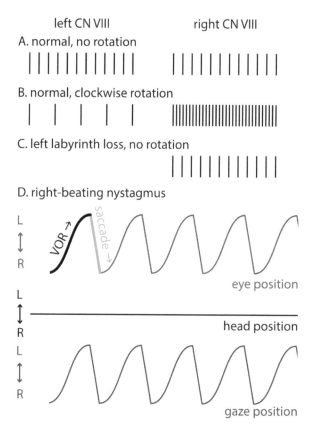

Figure 19-8 A: At rest and in the absence of any head rotation, activity in the left and right horizontal canal afferents is balanced. B: During clockwise head acceleration, left horizontal canal afferent activity decreases while activity in the right horizontal canal afferents increases over rest levels. C: When one labyrinth is injured or surgically removed, there is no more input from vestibular afferents on that side. The afferents contralateral to the damage continue to fire, leading to an imbalance in the vestibular input from the two sides. Thus, in a person with unilateral vestibular damage, the vestibular input resembles the input arising during head rotation, even when the individual is at rest and the head is not rotating. D: Unilateral vestibular damage leads to nystagmus that *beats* away from the direction of the damage. This nystagmus consists of a vestibuloocular reflex (*VOR*) toward the side of the damage followed by a fast reset (*saccade*) in the direction away from the side of the damage. In this example, gaze position (*blue line*) is determined entirely (*red line*) by eye position since head position (*black line*) is steady.

Caloric testing is a way to test for peripheral vestibular health by intentionally eliciting nystagmus. Caloric testing uses hot and cold water to artificially evoke nystagmus to test peripheral vestibular function. A person is laid in a supine position, which places the horizontal canal in the vertical plane. Recall that the hair cells in the ampullae of the horizontal semicircular canals are at the anterior end of the canals and are oriented toward the utriculus (see Chapter 18). In a supine individual, then, the hair cells are at the upper end of the horizontal canal and, importantly, are above the level of the external auditory meatus. Warm or cold water is then introduced into the external auditory meatus. When warm water is placed in the ear, endolymph flows up—as the warmed fluid rises—which results in excitation of the hair cells in the horizontal canal ampulla. Although the head has not moved, the brain receives a signal that the head is rotating toward the ipsilateral side. This evokes a VOR toward the contralateral side. The eye comes to the end of the orbit and quickly resets to the ipsilateral side. Still receiving the message that the head is rotating toward the ipsilateral side, another VOR toward the contralateral side occurs and so on. In this way, warm water evokes an ipsilateral-beating nystagmus (remember that nystagmus is named for the direction of the quick reset). By similar reasoning, please convince yourself that cold water elicits a nystagmus to the opposite side. Thus, the best mnemonic in neurobiology is born: COWS—cold opposite, warm same—referring to the direction of the nystagmus (not the direction of the VOR) elicited by irrigating cold or warm water into the ear.

Caloric testing is used in unconscious patients. It has two advantages over simply turning the head of an unconscious patient. First, it is a very strong stimulus and will elicit a VOR if a VOR is possible. The strength of the vestibular stimulus is also the reason that caloric testing would not be tolerated in awake patients, in whom it would cause nausea and discomfort. Second, patients with some forebrain lesions do not maintain fixation. In these patients, caloric testing is one way to determine if VOR pathways are intact. This is critical in determining if a patient is brain dead, a designation that requires that all brainstem reflexes, including the VOR, are absent.

NYSTAGMUS IS VARIED IN APPEARANCE AND CAUSE

Nystagmus comes in many different forms. Jerk nystagmus, with its slow and fast phases, is common. *Pendular nystagmus* involves the eyes moving back and forth like a pendulum, oscillating back and forth in a pattern that resembles the eye movements used to watch a tennis volley. Pendular nystagmus often occurs in individuals suffering from multiple sclerosis. Nystagmus can also be named for the direction of movement involved. For example, a downbeat nystagmus has a slow upward phase followed by a fast downward resetting saccade. Torsional nystagmus, almost always due to a central lesion, involves a slow torsional rotation in one direction followed by a fast torsional movement in the opposite direction.

In the most common form of jerk nystagmus, *gaze-evoked nystagmus*, visual fixation at an eccentric position

Table 19-2 **PERIPHERAL AND CENTRAL LESIONS CAN BOTH LEAD TO NYSTAGMUS**

PERIPHERAL LESION	CENTRAL LESION
Unidirectional	Uni- or bidirectional
Typically horizontal; rarely torsional	May be horizontal, vertical, or torsional
Tinnitus or hearing loss often present as well	Tinnitus or hearing loss not present
Usually associated with a sense of vertigo	May occur without vertigo

cannot be maintained. Therefore, the eye relaxes back to the neutral position. There is then a saccade back to the desired point of fixation followed by relaxation back to the neutral position, and so on. Understanding the mechanisms of gaze-evoked nystagmus requires knowledge of saccade-generating circuits, and this is discussed later.

Nystagmus can result from damage in a large diversity of sites, central as well as peripheral. Lesions of the extraocular muscles, cranial nerves, labyrinths, vestibular nuclei, horizontal and vertical gaze centers, and cerebellum can all produce nystagmus. Determining the underlying cause of nystagmus is definitely a task for a specialist. Nonetheless, there are a few key differences between nystagmus that arises from a peripheral lesion and that which arises from a central lesion (Table 19-2).

Finally, we consider the *sensory* consequences of nystagmus. As one or both eyes oscillate back and forth, the visual scene also oscillates. This can produce *oscillopsia* (i.e., the perceived visual image moves unintentionally; see Chapter 5). To get a sense of oscillopsia, watch a video taken with a hand-held camera that is moved about; the result is nauseating. Note that when both eyes move together, oscillopsia occurs *without diplopia*. Luckily, the perception of oscillopsia can be suppressed. Individuals born with congenital nystagmus, including patients with albinism or Down syndrome, learn from an early age to suppress visual motion and therefore rarely report oscillopsia. In fact, if the retinal image of individuals with congenital nystagmus is artificially stabilized, the *patients then report oscillopsia*. This indicates that such patients effectively suppress visual motion all the time. Adjustment of the visual image continues when the visual image is artificially stabilized so that this adjustment then is perceived as visual motion! Adults who acquire a form of nystagmus learn to suppress visual motion and thus eventually can largely ameliorate the visual effects of nystagmus (Fig. 19-9).

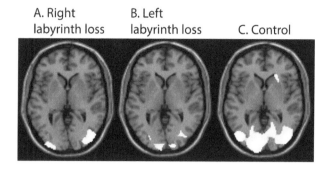

A. Right   B. Left
labyrinth loss   labyrinth loss   C. Control

Figure 19-9 Patients with unilateral vestibular loss learn to suppress visual motion. Functional magnetic resonance images from patients with failure of the right (A) or left (B) vestibular apparatus and from controls (C) were obtained during optokinetic nystagmus, a physiological form of nystagmus that can be elicited by a repeating visual pattern. The scans are horizontal sections with the occipital cortex at the bottom. Patients showed less activation of visual areas of cortex than did control patients. This was interpreted as evidence that patients were effectively suppressing visual motion stimulation and thus had smaller responses to the oscillopsia accompanying optokinetic nystagmus.   Reprinted from Deutschlander A et al. Unilateral vestibular failure suppresses cortical visual motion processing. *Brain* 131: 1025–1034, 2008, with permission of the publisher, Oxford University Press.

THE VESTIBULOOCULAR REFLEX IS CONSTANTLY MODULATED BY THE CEREBELLAR FLOCCULUS

We change the gain of our VOR (= eye movement / head movement) all the time, and we do this without any conscious involvement. Sometimes, the gain may be greater than 1, meaning that the eye moves more (in degrees) than the head does. At other times, the VOR gain is less than 1; the VOR may even be *turned off*, meaning that the gain is zero. *Cancellation of the VOR* occurs during voluntary shifts in gaze that are accompanied by head movements. For example, when making large gaze shifts, such as from one side of an auditorium to the other, the head may move while the eyes stay stationary within the head.

A frequent use of VOR gain modulation occurs when switching between near and far viewing. To see this, ask a friend to fixate on a near target, a finger, or on a far target, a tree at the horizon, and move her head back and forth in the yaw plane. You will see that your friend's eyes move far more when fixating on a near target than on a far target (this is a simple consequence of the optics involved). In other words, the gain of the VOR is greater during near viewing than far viewing. The reason that we are able to effectively fixate near and far targets during head movements is because the cerebellar *flocculus* seamlessly modulates the VOR gain. The flocculus also adjusts the gain and timing of the VOR as conditions change, such as during adaptation to a new pair of glasses or after damage to the inner ear.

Purkinje cells in the flocculus adjust the gain of the VOR by modulating the synapse between presynaptic vestibular afferents and postsynaptic vestibular nucleus neurons (Fig. 19-10A). The Purkinje cells receive information about eye and head movements and also information about retinal slip. When retinal slip is detected, output from the flocculus adjusts the vestibular nuclear synapse to minimize retinal slip during ensuing head movements. In this way, the flocculus mediates short-term motor learning. In an individual with floccular damage, the VOR will have a fixed gain of 1.

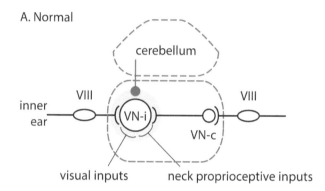

A. Normal

cerebellum

VIII   VIII
inner
ear   VN-i
                    VN-c

visual inputs   neck proprioceptive inputs

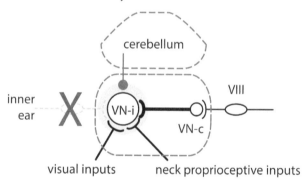

B. After unilateral labyrinth lesion

cerebellum

                                    VIII
inner
ear   VN-i
                    VN-c

visual inputs   neck proprioceptive inputs

Figure 19-10 The cerebellum, principally the posterior vermis, uvula, nodulus, and flocculus, modulates the inputs to vestibular nuclear neurons (*VN*). In a healthy individual with the eyes open, the predominant input to the vestibular nucleus arises from afferents of the vestibular nerve (*VIII*). Ipsilateral vestibular afferents synapse directly on vestibular nuclear neurons (*VN-i*), whereas commissural pathways bring input from the contralateral vestibular nucleus (*VN-c*). There are also visual and neck proprioceptive inputs to vestibular nuclear neurons. By modulating the synapses onto vestibular nuclear neurons, the cerebellum can change the gain of the vestibuloocular reflex (VOR) as conditions warrant. The red shading encircles the neural elements that are most heavily influenced by cerebellar output. B: After unilateral labyrinth loss (*red X*), the cerebellum modifies the synaptic strength of inputs to vestibular nuclear neurons. As a result, synapses bringing in commissural, visual, and proprioceptive information are strengthened. Consequently, individuals rapidly compensate for the damaged ear and have a normal or near normal VOR after a short period of learning. Since visual inputs are far more important after vestibular damage, the VOR functions far better in the light than in the dark in affected individuals.

The flocculus can induce long-term changes in the synaptic weights of a variety of inputs to vestibular nuclear neurons. This comes into play when, for example, there is damage to a vestibular end organ. The flocculus can modify the weight given to incoming signals from the unaffected ear, from neck proprioceptors, and from visual pathways (Fig. 19-10B). In essence, the flocculus can turn down or turn off the influence of afferents from the injured ear and increase the weight given to inputs from other sources. After vestibular injury, visual input dominates the VOR so that, after a period of adjustment, the VOR is fine when performed in the light but works poorly, if at all, in the dark. In sum, the VOR can be modified to function after many types of injury. However, after floccular damage, VOR gain is fixed and the VOR's usefulness is severely compromised.

VOR cancellation occurs all the time during voluntary gaze shifts in awake people, but an unconscious person does not cancel or otherwise modify the gain of the VOR. Thus, a physician can expect to see a VOR with a gain of 1 in an individual with compromised consciousness. As the physician turns the unconscious patient's head to the right or the left, the eyes continue to look straight up using the VOR; this is termed *doll's eyes*. This outcome is (relatively) good news as it indicates that the patient has intact VOR pathways. If, however, the physician observes that the patient's eyes stay fixed in the head so that gaze changes with the imposed head movement, then the patient's VOR circuits are damaged. Caloric testing (described earlier) can also be used to check VOR function in the unconscious patient.

OPTOKINETIC RESPONSES GIVE RISE TO PHYSIOLOGICAL NYSTAGMUS

As mentioned in Chapter 18, vestibular hair cells do not respond to head movements that are at a constant velocity or to very slow head movements. Since constant velocity and very slowly accelerating head movements do not engage the vestibular system, the VOR does not occur in response to either of these stimuli. Yet we are able to stabilize moving images in these conditions, and we do so by using the *optokinetic response*. The stimulus that elicits the optokinetic response is a *visual* stimulus, movement of the whole visual field, which elicits an eye movement in the opposite direction so that images stay steady on the retina.

Whole-field visual movement occurs with either self-motion or visual field motion. An example of the former (you are moving, the object is still) occurs when looking out of a moving train. The latter, visual field motion (you are still, the object is moving in the world) can be accomplished

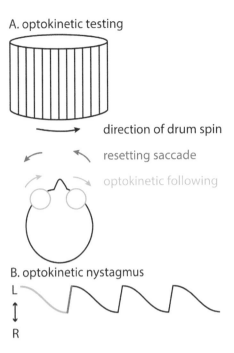

Figure 19-11 In optokinetic testing (A), a striped drum is rotated in front of a person. The repeating visual pattern, in this case moving to the right, elicits an eye movement that follows the whole field movement rightward (*blue arrows*). Upon reaching the edge of the orbit, a quick saccade (*red arrows*) brings the eye back to the central position, from where optokinetic following begins again. B: Optokinetic nystagmus, a healthy form of nystagmus, is elicited by a horizontally rotating drum as in A. Optokinetic following (*blue*) moves the eyes far more slowly than do saccades (*red*). Optokinetic testing and responses can occur in vertical as well as horizontal orientations.

by passing a repeating visual pattern in front of a stationary individual. Physicians typically use a rotating black-and-white striped drum to elicit an optokinetic response (Fig. 19-11). The eyes track the image until the eyes are at the edges of the orbits at which point a quick saccade in the opposite direction is made. This slow eye movement in one direction and fast reset in the other direction constitutes *optokinetic nystagmus*. This form of nystagmus is entirely normal and is in fact a sign of health.

SACCADES ARE BALLISTIC MOVEMENTS

As you know by now, saccades are ballistic eye movements that change the direction of gaze, placing a new visual field target on the fovea. Saccades can be voluntarily initiated by areas in cortex or can occur more automatically, as happens with orienting saccades to an unexpected sound or sight. After the saccade is initiated, its direction and magnitude cannot be changed even if the target position changes. Thus, saccades are ballistic (see Chapter 20). The eyes move very quickly during saccades, with eye speeds that can monentarily reach 600 degrees per second. The saccade itself takes about 200—250 milliseconds to initiate and 50–100 milliseconds to complete (Fig. 19-12A). The size or amplitude of the saccade is the distance in degrees between the starting and ending positions. As saccade size increases, the duration and peak velocity of the saccade increase as well.

A saccadic eye movement has two components: pulse and step. The pulse is the ballistic movement, and the step is the maintenance of the eye in the new desired position (Fig. 19-12A). Although images move across the retina during the pulse portion of a saccade, visual input is suppressed during the pulse so that no blur is perceived as the eye moves.

As you know, the horizontal and vertical gaze centers are located in distinct regions, the former in the pons and the latter in the midbrain. The horizontal gaze center is located in the *pontine paramedian reticular formation* (*PPRF*; see Chapter 6) that surrounds the abducens nucleus (Fig. 19-12B). The vertical gaze center is located in the midbrain just rostral and lateral to the oculomotor complex. Upstream areas, the superior colliculus and frontal eye fields, provide separate input to the two gaze centers. Thus, information about the horizontal component of an intended saccade is sent to the horizontal gaze center, and information about the vertical component of an intended saccade is sent to the vertical gaze center. Ultimately, horizontal and vertical components of a saccade are added together again at the level of the muscles.

THE CIRCUIT FOR HORIZONTAL SACCADES INVOLVES PREMOTOR NEURONS IN THE HORIZONTAL GAZE CENTER

Saccades are controlled by multiple premotor neurons that sit within the gaze centers (Fig. 19-12B). The first neurons to foretell an imminent saccade are omnipause neurons. *Omnipause neurons* fire tonically and then stop firing just before the pulse portion of a saccade. Omnipause neurons are GABAergic and therefore are inhibitory. When they pause, the target neurons, *saccade burst neurons* that are also located in the gaze center, are disinhibited and fire a burst of activity. Between saccades, omnipause neurons fire continuously, and burst neurons are silent because they are being inhibited by the omnipause neurons. In order for a saccade to occur, the inhibition of saccade burst neurons must be briefly interrupted, allowing the burst neurons to fire a burst.

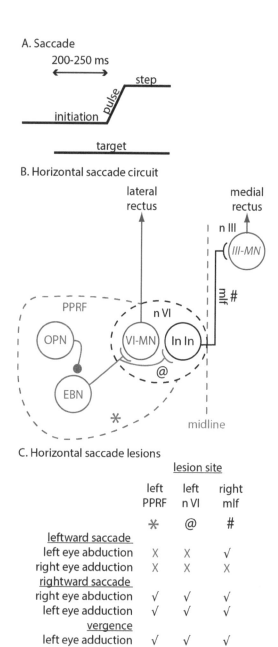

A. Saccade

B. Horizontal saccade circuit

C. Horizontal saccade lesions

	lesion site		
	left PPRF	left n VI	right mlf
	*	@	#
leftward saccade			
left eye abduction	X	X	√
right eye adduction	X	X	X
rightward saccade			
right eye abduction	√	√	√
left eye adduction	√	√	√
vergence			
left eye adduction	√	√	√
right eye adduction	√	√	√

Figure 19-12 A: A saccade requires 200–250 ms to initiate after a target appears. The actual movement, or pulse, is very rapid after which the eye must be actively maintained at an eccentric position (step). B: The generation of a horizontal saccade is organized by premotor neurons in the horizontal gaze center (*PPRF, red dashed line*), abducens nucleus (*n VI, black dashed line*), medial longitudinal fasciculus (*mlf*), and oculomotor nucleus (*n III*). Premotor neurons in the PPRF include omnipause neurons (*OPN*) and excitatory burst neurons (*EBN*). Upon being released from inhibition by the omnipause neurons, excitatory burst neurons (*EBN*) excite two types of neurons in the ipsilateral abducens nucleus. Excitation of abducens motoneurons (*VI-MN*) leads directly to contraction of the ipsilateral lateral rectus while excitation of the internuclear interneurons (*In In*) excites contralateral medial rectus motoneurons (*III-MN*), which in turn produce contraction of the medial rectus muscle. The internuclear interneuron sends an axon across the midline (*dashed green line*) at the level of the abducens nucleus. This axon travels through the medial longitudinal fasciculus to reach the oculomotor nucleus. C: The effects of lesions in the PPRF (*), abducens nucleus (@), or medial longitudinal fasciculus (#) on saccades and vergence are listed.

There are two types of burst neurons in the horizontal gaze center: excitatory and inhibitory. *Excitatory burst neurons* excite motoneurons in the ipsilateral abducens nucleus, and *inhibitory burst neurons* inhibit motoneurons in the contralateral abducens nucleus (Fig. 19-12B). In response to a pause in omnipause firing, excitatory burst neurons burst, which in turn results in excitation of the abducens motoneurons and contraction of the lateral rectus. Thus, the eye is pulled laterally. The duration and peak discharge of the burst determine the duration and velocity—and therefore the size—of the saccade. In response to a burst in an inhibitory burst neuron, contralateral abducens motoneurons slow their firing (disfacilitation), allowing the eye to be pulled medially.

INTERNUCLEAR INTERNEURONS YOKE MEDIAL RECTUS MOTONEURONS TO LATERAL RECTUS MOTONEURONS

To ensure that the appropriate medial and lateral rectus motoneurons are activated together during saccades and smooth pursuit movements, there is a special neuron type called the *internuclear interneuron*. Internuclear interneurons are located in the abducens nucleus and receive the same input as do their neighbors, the abducens motoneurons. However, *internuclear interneurons do not contact muscle*. Instead, *they carry a copy of the message received by abducens motoneurons to contralateral medial rectus motoneurons* (Figs. 19-12B, 19-13A). Because of this pathway, the medial and lateral rectus muscles on opposite sides receive the same message. Consequently, the two eyes move together during horizontal gaze shifts.

As you recall from Chapter 5, the vertically oriented extraocular muscles are also paired. One input has to reach two different pools of motoneurons that control muscles on opposite sides of the midline. As illustrated in Figure 19-13, bilateral routing of vertical and torsional motor command messages is accomplished by motoneuron axons that cross the midline:

- *Superior oblique-inferior rectus*: Axons innervating the superior oblique muscle cross along the dorsum of the midbrain (see Chapter 5).

- *Inferior oblique-superior rectus*: Motoneurons innervating the superior rectus muscle send their axon out of the oculomotor nucleus and then directly across the midline within the brainstem.

Thus, for the two extraocular muscle pairs involved in vertical gaze, one muscle in each pair is located contralateral to the innervating motoneurons. As a result, motoneurons innervating each of the rectus-oblique muscle pairs are located on the same side. This arrangement allows an eye movement command from an upstream region to project unilaterally while ultimately controlling muscles on opposite sides.

DAMAGE TO INTERNUCLEAR INTERNEURON AXONS IS THE PATHOLOGICAL BASIS OF INTERNUCLEAR OPHTHALMOPLEGIA

Internuclear interneuron axons follow a stereotyped trajectory from the abducens nucleus to the medial rectus motoneuron pool in the contralateral oculomotor nucleus. These axons cross the midline immediately upon exiting the abducens nucleus and then make a 90-degree turn to course rostrally in the contralateral medial longitudinal fasciculus, eventually terminating in the oculomotor nucleus (Figs. 19-12B, 19-13A). Medial longitudinal fasciculus axons are heavily myelinated, which allows for rapid action potential conduction from the abducens to the oculomotor nucleus. The heavy myelination also makes medial longitudinal fasciculus axons vulnerable to demyelinating diseases such as multiple sclerosis. A common symptom of multiple sclerosis, which as you recall causes central demyelination, is *internuclear ophthalmoplegia*.

In internuclear ophthalmoplegia, the eye ipsilateral to the lesion (remember that the internuclear axon travels on the side of the medial rectus motoneuron that it innervates) does not adduct during a contralateral saccade (Fig. 19-14A). For example, a person with a right internuclear ophthalmoplegia would be able to saccade to the right normally. However, when looking to the left, the left eye would abduct, while the right eye would stay in the neutral position (Fig. 19-14A). Bilateral lesions of the medial longitudinal fasciculus result in the inability to adduct either eye during lateral gaze (Fig. 19-14B). The perceptual result of internuclear ophthalmoplegia of the eyes is horizontal gaze diplopia. In other words, when gaze is shifted laterally, the images hitting the two retinas are different.

Internuclear interneurons only receive inputs related to horizontal saccades and smooth pursuit. Inputs related to the VOR contact abducens motoneurons but not internuclear interneurons. Vergence movements are coordinated by midbrain neurons that contact medial rectus motoneurons;

A. lateral rectus - medial rectus: internuclear interneuron crosses inside pons

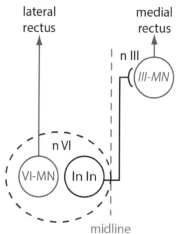

lateral rectus

medial rectus

n III
(III-MN)

n VI
(VI-MN) In In

midline

B. superior oblique - inferior rectus: CN IV crosses outside midbrain

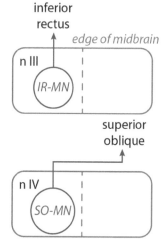

inferior rectus

edge of midbrain

n III
(IR-MN)

superior oblique

n IV
(SO-MN)

C. superior rectus - inferior oblique: SR motoneuron crosses inside midbrain

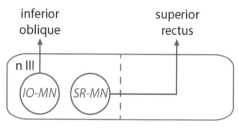

inferior oblique

superior rectus

n III
(IO-MN)   *(SR-MN)*

Figure 19-13 Premotor commands to pairs of extraocular muscles involved in conjugate eye movements contact neurons on the same side although the pairs include a muscle on each side of the midline. A: Internuclear interneurons (*In In*) take the same message that lateral rectus motoneurons (*LR-MN*) receive to medial rectus motoneurons (*MR-MN*) on the other side. B: Motoneurons innervating the superior oblique muscle (*SO-MN*) cross the midline after exiting from the dorsal side of the midbrain. C: Motoneurons innervating the superior rectus (*SR-MN*) travel medially and cross the midline within the midbrain.

internuclear interneurons and lateral rectus motoneurons are not involved. For these reasons, internuclear ophthalmoplegia

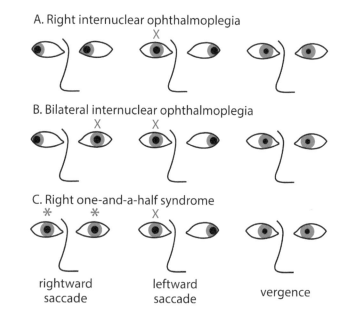

A. Right internuclear ophthalmoplegia

B. Bilateral internuclear ophthalmoplegia

C. Right one-and-a-half syndrome

rightward saccade   leftward saccade   vergence

Figure 19-14 Internuclear ophthalmoplegia results from damage to the axons of internuclear interneurons as they travel in the medial longitudinal fasciculus. A: An individual with right internuclear ophthalmoplegia will be able to look to the right normally (*left column*) but will not adduct the right eye (*red X*) when looking to the left (*middle column*). Vergence (*right column*) is not affected. B: An individual with bilateral internuclear ophthalmoplegia cannot adduct either eye (*red X*) when looking to either side (*left and middle columns*). Vergence in this individual is normal (*right column*). C: In one-and-a-half syndrome, the medial longitudinal fasciculus and abducens nucleus on the same side are damaged, usually by small strokes. Because of damage to the abducens nucleus, the ipsilateral (in this case right) eye does not abduct (*red asterisk*) nor does the contralateral eye adduct (*red asterisk*) during ipsilateral saccades (*left column*). Damage to the medial longitudinal fasciculus prevents the ipsilateral eye from adducting (*red X*) during contralateral saccades (*middle column*). Thus, of the two possible horizontal saccades (two eye movements involved in looking left and two needed to look right), one and a half are impaired; only contralateral abduction is unaffected. Vergence movements depend on midbrain circuits and not upon connections between the pons and midbrain. Therefore, vergence movements (*right column*) are normal in all of the conditions of pontine damage illustrated.

impairs adduction accompanying saccades and smooth pursuit, whereas adduction involved in VOR and vergence are normal.

Beyond multiple sclerosis, small ischemic strokes in the dorsal pons may also cause internuclear ophthalmoplegia. When this happens, the abducens nucleus is often affected along with the adjacent medial longitudinal fasciculus. When both the abducens nucleus and the medial longitudinal fasciculus are lesioned, a *one-and-a-half syndrome* occurs (Fig. 19-14C). This syndrome is not particularly common, but it serves as a good litmus test of your understanding of saccade circuits. Individuals with one-and-a-half syndrome cannot look ipsilaterally with either eye; this is due to the lesion of the abducens nucleus. They also cannot adduct the ipsilateral eye when looking contralaterally. Thus, one and a half of the two possible lateral gaze movements are impaired. The only working movement among horizontal gaze shifts is contralateral abduction. Because vergence depends on midbrain inputs to medial rectus motoneurons located in the oculomotor nucleus, vergence movements remain normal.

SACCADES MOVE EYES TO A NEW POSITION AND THEN MAINTAIN THAT POSITION

As you recall, saccades include two different phases that move (pulse) and then maintain (step) the eye at an eccentric position. We considered the pulse phase earlier. The step component of a saccade produces fixation at a new eye position, which is maintained by discharge in extraocular motoneurons. The horizontal and vertical/torsional components of the fixation position are calculated separately in the hindbrain and midbrain, respectively. The *nucleus prepositus hypoglossi* serves as the eye movement integrator for horizontal eye position, and the *interstitial nucleus of Cajal* codes for vertical and torsional eye position. The nucleus prepositus hypoglossi is located in the dorsal medullary midline, just anterior to the hypoglossal nucleus, and the interstitial nucleus of Cajal is located just rostral to the oculomotor complex. Neurons in these nuclei provide continuously updated information about eye position that is used to maintain eccentric fixation.

Here, we take horizontal fixation as an example. Neurons in nucleus prepositus hypoglossi receive input from saccadic burst neurons (Fig. 19-15A). The activity of these neurons then drives the tonic firing rate of abducens motoneurons, which is needed to maintain an eccentric eye position (Fig. 19-15B). Via the internuclear interneuron, prepositus hypoglossi neurons also excite contralateral medial rectus motoneurons.

A lesion of either integrator results in gaze-evoked nystagmus in which the pulse phase of a saccade works fine, bringing the eye to an eccentric position. However, the saccade step phase does not work (see Fig. 19-15C), and the eye relaxes back to the neutral position. Lesions in a number of locations can produce gaze-evoked nystagmus. For example, individuals with a weakness in the abducens nerve may be able to make a saccade to a lateral position but cannot maintain that position. This would result in a gaze-evoked nystagmus upon trying to maintain a lateral fixation point.

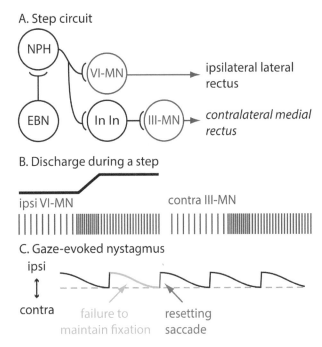

A. Step circuit

B. Discharge during a step

ipsi VI-MN   contra III-MN

C. Gaze-evoked nystagmus

ipsi

contra   failure to maintain fixation   resetting saccade

Figure 19-15 At the end of the pulse phase of a saccade, fixation is maintained by discharge in extraocular motoneurons that is proportional to the component of eye position that is in the pulling direction of the innervated muscle. A: Nucleus prepositus hypoglossi neurons (*NPH*) receive and integrate input from burst neurons (*EBN*) to produce the step component of a saccade. Nucleus prepositus hypoglossi neurons send an eye position signal to motoneurons (*VI-MN*) and internuclear interneurons (*In In*) of the ipsilateral abducens neurons. Internuclear interneurons contact contralateral oculomotor motoneurons that innervate the medial rectus (*III-MN*). B: This circuit results in ipsilateral abducens motoneurons and contralateral medial rectus motoneurons increasing their tonic discharge. C: The most common form of nystagmus stems from a failure of the step phase of a saccade. In gaze-evoked nystagmus, there is insufficient tonic discharge to maintain an eccentric eye position. As a result, the eye relaxes back to the neutral position. The saccade is made again because there is nothing wrong with the pulse component of the saccade. Once again, the eye cannot be maintained at an eccentric eye position, and an oscillatory eye movement occurs. The case illustrated is termed *ipsilateral-beating* since nystagmus is always named for the direction of the saccade.

SPECIFIC REGIONS IN THE MIDBRAIN AND CEREBRAL CORTEX INITIATE SACCADES

Activity in several regions can lead to the initiation of saccades. An important presaccadic signal arises from the *superior colliculus*, which contributes to both reflexive orienting saccades and voluntary saccades. The superior colliculus transforms sensory information into a *motor map*, where activity produces a gaze shift to a particular location regardless of the current eye or head position. To support gaze shifts, the superior colliculus projects through the *tectospinal tract* to the spinal cord to contact motoneurons that move the neck, shoulders, and body in support of gaze shifts. The superior colliculus selects a target but does not dictate a motor strategy to reach that target. For example, the superior colliculus fires regardless of whether the eyes alone or the eyes and the head are used to shift gaze to a given target. Axons leaving the superior colliculus cross the midline. Thus, the superior colliculus on one side projects to the contralateral horizontal gaze center to generate saccades that move the eyes toward the contralateral side.

The superior colliculus can initiate reflexive or automatic orienting movements that occur in response to sensory input signaling an unexpected sound or flash of light. The participation of the superior colliculus in voluntary saccades stems from input that the colliculus receives from a number of cortical regions. The *frontal eye fields*, essentially the primary motor cortex for eye movements, are particularly important as a source of the motor command for volitional saccades. The frontal eye fields contact the contralateral brainstem gaze centers directly and also indirectly via the ipsilateral superior colliculus. Thus, activity in the frontal eye fields engages contralateral gaze centers to produce saccades that are ipsilateral to the gaze center, which is contralateral to the cortex.

A lesion in any of the gaze control areas of cortex results in impairment of *voluntary* contralateral gaze shifts, including resting gaze. For example, a stroke in the frontal eye field prevents gaze shifts to the contralateral side. In addition, the eyes deviate to the side of the lesion at rest. Without excitatory drive from the damaged frontal eye field, contralateral eye saccades and fixation do not happen.

SMOOTH PURSUIT CIRCUITS STABILIZE A SLOWLY MOVING TARGET ON THE FOVEA

Smooth pursuit movements are voluntary eye movements that shift the direction of gaze to match a moving target. The velocity of pursuit movements is quite a bit slower than that of saccades. Pursuit movements typically achieve velocities of 50 degrees per second or less and do not exceed 100 degrees per second. During pursuit movements, visual perception is maintained. Intriguingly, smooth pursuit movements cannot be "imitated" in the absence of a moving target. In other words, we cannot pretend we are watching a bird fly across the sky. When we try to do this, we make a series of small saccades. Pursuit movements *require* the presence of a slowly moving target, and, when such a target is present, the velocity of the pursuit movement matches the velocity of the target.

Smooth pursuit movements are initiated by cortical neurons in several regions including the frontal eye fields, the lateral intraparietal area, and regions in the dorsal visual stream. Smooth pursuit movements are complex in that they must integrate processing of visual motion in extrastriate cortex with processing of motor error in the cerebellar vermis to ensure that eye velocity matches target velocity. Changes in head position, signaled through the VOR, also are necessary to successful smooth pursuit. The same brainstem gaze centers in the pons and midbrain that support saccades also produce smooth pursuit.

This organization of funneling motor commands from a number of areas (frontal eye fields, lateral intraparietal area, superior colliculus, vestibular nuclei) through a limited number of lower motor control centers (horizontal and vertical gaze centers, vergence control center) and then through the final common pathway of motoneurons is familiar. It represents the motor hierarchy for eye movements just as primary motor cortex, ventral horn interneurons, and spinal motoneurons comprise the motor hierarchy for actions involving the arms and legs.

OCULOMOTOR PATHWAYS ARE MODULATED BY BOTH CEREBELLUM AND BASAL GANGLIA

Gaze control, like all other motor systems, is modulated by the cerebellum and basal ganglia, the two great loops of the brain. As is true for other movements, the cerebellum compares actual eye movements to intended eye movements. When movements are off target, the cerebellum provides the fine adjustment needed so that subsequent eye movements are corrected. The flocculus also coordinates eye movements with visual feedback and thus plays critical roles in the adjustment of the VOR to changing circumstances, to eccentric fixation, and to smooth pursuit movements.

The oculomotor loop of the basal ganglia runs through the caudate and the substantia nigra pars reticulata (see Chapter 25). Nigral cells *must pause* in their discharge in order for saccades to occur. In parkinsonian patients, nigral neurons are hyperactive, and saccades are slow. In contrast, in patients with hyperkinetic disorders, nigral neurons are hypoactive, resulting in excess saccades and an inability to maintain an eccentric gaze.

ADDITIONAL READING

Deutschländer A, Hüfner K, Kalla R, et al. Unilateral vestibular failure suppresses cortical visual motion processing. *Brain.* 131: 1025–1034, 2008.

Freedman EG. Coordination of the eyes and head during visual orienting. *Exp Brain Res.* 190: 369–387, 2008.

Gittis AH, du Lac S. Intrinsic and synaptic plasticity in the vestibular system. *Curr Opin Neurobiol.* 16: 385–390, 2006.

Kaminski HJ, Li Z, Richmonds C, Ruff RL, Kusner L. Susceptibility of ocular tissues to autoimmune diseases. *Ann NY Acad Sci.* 998: 362–374, 2003.

Keller EL, Missal M. Shared brainstem pathways for saccades and smooth-pursuit eye movements. *Ann NY Acad Sci.* 1004: 29–39, 2003.

Nagasawa M, Mitsui S, En S, et al. Social evolution. Oxytocin-gaze positive loop and the coevolution of human-dog bonds. *Science.* 348: 333–336, 2015.

Krauzlis RJ. The control of voluntary eye movements: New perspectives. *Neuroscientist.* 11: 124–137, 2005.

Leigh RJ, Dell'Osso LF, Yaniglos SS, Thurston SE. Oscillopsia, retinal image stabilization and congenital nystagmus. *Invest Ophthalmol Visual Sci.* 29: 27–82, 1988.

Loughland CM, Williams LM, Gordon E. Visual scanpaths to positive and negative facial emotions in an outpatient schizophrenia sample. *Schizophrenia Res.* 55: 159–170, 2002.

Martinez-Conde S, Otero-Millan J, Macknik SL. The impact of microsaccades on vision: Towards a unified theory of saccadic function. *Nat Rev Neurosci.* 14: 83–96, 2013.

Norbury CF, Brock J, Cragg L, Einav S, Griffiths H, Nation K. Eye-movement patterns are associated with communicative competence in autistic spectrum disorders. *J Child Psychol Psychiatry.* 50: 834–842, 2009.

Poletti M, Rucci M. Eye movements under various conditions of image fading. *J Vision.* 10: 1–18, 2010.

Rucker JC. Oculomotor disorders. *Semin Neurol.* 27: 244–256, 2007.

Rucker JC. Overview of anatomy and physiology of the ocular motor system. In Eggers SDZ, Zee D, eds. *Vertigo and Imbalance. Clinical Neurophysiology of the Vestibular System. Handbook of Clinical Neurophysiology.* Vol. 9. New York: Elsevier, 2010.

Sweeney JA, Takarae Y, Macmillan C, Luna B, Minshew NJ. Eye movements in neurodevelopmental disorders. *Curr Opin Neurol.* 17: 37–42, 2004.

Wilson VJ, Schor RH. The neural substrate of the vestibulocollic reflex. *Exp Brain Res.* 129: 483–493, 1999.

SECTION 5

MOTOR CONTROL

In Section 4, a consideration of the vestibular system, clearly a sensory pathway, naturally transitioned into a final chapter on gaze control, a topic that fits squarely within the motor domain. In point of fact, the transition to motor control could have been made just as easily from somatosensation and with only marginally more sleight of hand from vision or hearing. This sensory-to-motor connection is no coincidence, for while we humans greatly revel in our perceptual experiences, evolution acts on actions and behaviors. In other words, evolution only "sees" perception insomuch as those perceptions drive actions and behaviors. Ultimately, we are here today because the human nervous system has been adequate to allow for the survival and reproductive continuation of our ancestors through the ages.

In this section, we turn our attention to the nervous system's ultimate function of driving skeletomotor behavior. The brain directs cognitive actions that form expressions of inner affect and deliberative thought while also influencing the most basic reflexive and semi-automatic movements. The result is a unified motor expression of self, from spoken words to gait to facial expression. Thus, although we discuss the motor system in heuristically convenient chunks, the biological reality is one of integrated function and coherent output. Let us begin.

20.

VOLUNTARY MOTOR CONTROL

THE MOTOR SYSTEM WORKS
WITH SENSATION, HOMEOSTASIS, AND
COGNITION TO PRODUCE UNIFIED
AND COHESIVE BEHAVIOR

Before embarking on our journey from skeletal muscle contraction to action, we explicitly recognize that *movement is interdependent with sensory, homeostatic, and cognitive brain function*. A few examples should suffice to convince you of the necessary interactions between motor control and sensory, homeostatic, and cognitive function.

As we will explore in Chapter 22, voluntary movements require somatosensory feedback, a fact that is placed in dramatic relief by the experiences of Ian Waterman, a young man who lost all proprioception and touch input from his body due to a viral infection. Without proprioception or tactile sensation, Waterman had to painstakingly teach himself to deliberately perform even the most common of movements such as standing. His complete dependence on visual feedback replacing somatosensory feedback in maintaining posture is evident from his collapse when the lights went out. Simple acts such as lighting a match are not possible when a local anesthetic is injected into the fingertips. In sum, we do not stand, walk, speak, chew, write, or pick berries without sensory feedback that, in the vast majority of us, is somatosensory. Afferents from skeletal muscles and skin are so critical to the skeletal motor system that we include them as part of the motor system even though they are somatosensory afferents—embryologically, anatomically, and physiologically—rather than motoneurons.

The connections between homeostasis and voluntary movement are myriad. When walking, and even more so when running, autonomic changes in cardiac output and blood supply to skeletal muscles are critical to permitting one to continue without fainting. Cutaneous vasodilation, another autonomic function that occurs automatically during motor activity, increases thermal exchange between skin and the environment. This enables the active body to dissipate heat and continue without overheating. When vasodilation is insufficient to reduce core temperature, sweating is elicited. These examples make clear that *skeletal muscles alone cannot accomplish our goals as we move through the world*. Similarly, autonomic control of smooth and cardiac muscle cannot keep the body in homeostasis without the participation of skeletal muscles that support breathing, thermoregulation, and other necessary functions. Accommodation, micturition, and mating all require both skeletal and smooth muscle participation, revealing the somewhat artificial divide between somatomotor and autonomic movements.

All movements proceed upon a platform that depends entirely on motivation, mood, and thought. Most fundamentally, without motivation—either conscious or unconscious—we simply do not make voluntary movements. The converse also holds: communicating motivation, mood, and thought depends absolutely on the final common currency of skeletal muscle excitation. This statement is essentially a tautology because we derive all that we know about cognitive function from the contraction of skeletal muscles. The manner in which a person walks, stands, writes, and speaks depend on skeletal muscle excitation. *Movements inform us of who a person is and are in fact the only clues we have as to the nature of a person's inner self.* We instantly recognize a stranger as uptight, relaxed, or depressed, words which, although they describe abstract traits of personality and affect, derive from and readily conjure up physical images. Because of the interdependence of self and movement, we feel that we know public figures and have a sense whether we would like them or not simply after watching their *movements* in films or on television, all without ever exchanging words or coming face to face.

Despite the extensive interdependence of motor, sensory, homeostatic, and cognitive systems, we identify neural circuits that are particularly central to movement and action and prone to malfunctions of great clinical importance. In the chapters of this section, we focus on these key motor circuits.

The brain faces an incredible challenge in creating the full range of motion that humans are capable of and producing movements at the appropriate and desired times. The muscles that are involved in even a simple motion—for example, turning the palm upward—are numerous and act at several joints (digits, wrist, and elbow). Motor command must be further adjusted to account for muscle fatigue, balance, and weight, or *load*. The specific forces and muscles required to turn the palm upward will be different in the water or in the air; when supine, prone, or upright; when carrying a heavy bag versus being load-free. An unanticipated protruding tree root across the path or a bee sting requires adjustments to keep planned movements "on track" while avoiding injury and maintaining balance. Yet, in most cases, the motor system is able to anticipate and avoid impediments to reaching motor goals rather than correcting an action only after a motor blunder. Visual, auditory, tactile, and vestibular information, together with past experiences, are used by the brain to coordinate complex motor strategies that have the best chance of achieving the intended goal.

VOLUNTARY ACTION DEPENDS ON A SUBSET OF ALL MUSCLES, THE SKELETAL MUSCLES

The body contains *smooth* and *striated* muscles. Smooth muscle has a histologically smooth appearance and is controlled automatically rather than voluntarily. Two types of muscle contain visible striations of actin and myosin: *cardiac* and *skeletal*. Cardiac muscle resembles smooth muscle in that it cannot be controlled consciously but differs from smooth muscle in its lightly striped appearance. *Skeletal muscle can, in general, be controlled purposively* and is the subject of this section.

Although skeletal muscle supports purposeful movement, we are incapable of willfully contracting most skeletal muscles *in isolation*. Instead, we contract most skeletal muscles as part of a group. For instance, when pulling a door open, our biceps muscle contracts along with a number of other muscles in the arm, shoulder, trunk, and even legs. In another example, we have exquisite control over laryngeal muscles, allowing us the power of vocalization, but we cannot willfully contract or relax a single laryngeal muscle, such as the left oblique arytenoid muscle. Some skeletal muscles, such as the two middle ear muscles are simply not available for voluntary control, even as part of a group.

Many muscles that can be controlled voluntarily are also controlled unconsciously. For example, the diaphragm, the skeletal muscle critical to breathing, continues to contract rhythmically during sleep or general anesthesia and, alternatively, can be willfully controlled when we intentionally take a deep breath.

The term *skeletal muscle* is used because most noncardiac striated muscle attaches, at least at one end, to a bone. Of course, there are exceptions to this rule, just as there are exceptions to the "skeletal-muscle-is-voluntarily-controlled" rule. Exceptions include muscles of facial expression that attach only to skin and intrinsic laryngeal muscles that attach to cartilage, as well as muscles that surround or attach to the trachea, esophagus, and urethra. Nonetheless, throughout this book, I employ the imperfect shorthand of referring to all noncardiac striated muscle as skeletal.

MOVEMENT CAN BE VERY FAST BUT INFLEXIBLE OR SLOWER AND CONTROLLED

Movements are characterized as either *ballistic* or controlled. Ballistic movements are projectile in the old-fashioned, pre- "smart bomb" sense. After movement initiation in a particular direction and with a given force, no additional steering or guidance of a ballistic movement occurs. Common examples include saccades, swinging a bat, or throwing a punch. In contrast, smooth, controlled movements may start with one trajectory but that trajectory may be altered during the course of the movement, just as a "smart bomb" changes heading to hit an evasive target. Examples of controlled movements include watching a bird fly across the sky, threading a needle, peeling an apple, and caressing a loved one.

In general, ballistic movements utilize axial and proximal limb muscles and can be initiated reflexively, automatically, or voluntarily. Most controlled movements use proximal and distal limb muscles and are controlled through a constant dialogue with the brainstem and cerebral cortex. Many muscles, such as the extraocular muscles, support both ballistic and controlled movements. Even axial movements can be controlled as well as ballistic; examples of controlled axial movements abound in dance.

Ballistic movements offer the major advantage of being very fast. However, speed comes at the cost of flexibility and accuracy: if the expected target location changes after the aim–fire sequence initiates, the movement will end up off target. Even when a target remains stationary, ballistic movements are often less accurate than controlled ones. Although controlled movements are far more flexible and often more accurate than ballistic movements, they are also far slower. Supporting flexible behavior is neurally more complicated than supporting fixed behavior. Therefore, the brainstem and cerebral cortex generate controlled movements, whereas simpler circuits in the brainstem and spinal cord can generate ballistic movements.

THE MOTOR HIERARCHY MAKES ACTIONS OUT OF MUSCLE CONTRACTIONS

As introduced in Chapter 1, skeletal muscles cannot contract independently, without input from the central nervous system. They only contract in response to action potentials fired by innervating motoneurons. Even when a motoneuron fires an action potential and a muscle contracts, the result is a *twitch*, the simplest of movements. Although a twitch is a physical movement, it is certainly not a useful or natural one.

The motor hierarchy uses twitches as building blocks and organizes the timing, strength, and distribution of muscle contractions to produce *movements* ranging from simple to complex (Fig. 20-1). The lowest elements of the motor hierarchy, local circuits in the ventral horn involving motoneurons and motor interneurons, support the simplest movements, such as flexions or extensions of a single limb. Activity in sensory afferents from both muscle and skin reaches these local circuits to elicit quick reflexive adjustments. Within the spinal cord and brainstem, *central pattern generators* produce the basic motor sequences involved in far more complex movements such as standing upright, breathing, chewing, or walking. *Central pattern generators are circuits of neurons that create a patterned progression of motor activity and can do so in the absence of peripheral feedback* (see more in Chapter 22).

Brainstem motor control centers, such as the red nucleus (see Chapter 6), employ circuits in lower parts of the motor hierarchy to produce fairly complex movements, such as ingestion or locomotion. However, these movements have no meaning. They resemble the movements that result from motor cortex stimulation in awake neurosurgical patients. Recall that in response to electrical stimulation of the motor cortex, patients report that a body part moved or "could not move" or that the body part "wanted" to move (see Chapter 14). In these reports, the body part rather than the person is the *actor*: patients do not report "I moved my hand." This distinction is

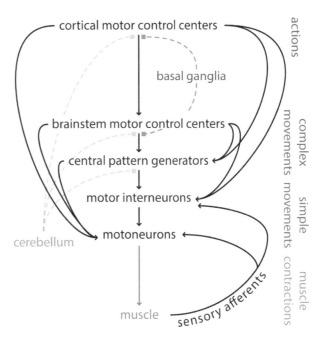

Figure 20-1 The motor hierarchy (*black*) consists of one-way connections from higher motor centers to lower motor centers. Ultimately, a motor message is delivered to motoneurons, the final common pathway controlling skeletal muscle. Motoneurons are capable of producing muscle contractions. Simple circuits involving motor interneurons can produce simple movements, whereas central pattern generators and brainstem motor control centers produce complex movements such as chewing, walking, and the like. Cortical circuits imbue movements with meaning and thus produce actions. Feedback from primary somatosensory afferents that innervate the muscles and joints reaches motoneurons and motor interneurons directly. All other sensory input to motor areas is indirect (not shown). The two major motor modulatory regions—the cerebellum and the basal ganglia—modulate higher motor centers but do not directly connect to motoneurons.

key to the contribution of the cerebral cortex. The cerebral cortex is required to make movement personal, to transform physical movement into a physical expression of the self. Movement so imbued with personal meaning and motivation is termed *action*. We are so accustomed to being responsible for our own movements that we take conscious credit for automatic movements where such credit may not be warranted, as in "I stumbled but just caught myself in time."

Since the brain adds meaning to movements, two different actions can share the same component movements. For example, a smile of enjoyment, a smile used as a greeting, and a smile in response to a command during a game of Simon Says all share a similar up-turning of the mouth. Yet, these three smiles are three different actions, each occurring in a different context. The context depends on the brain. Nerves and other peripheral structures do not "do" context. Therefore, *context-specific* impairment is pathognomonic or diagnostic of a central nervous system lesion.

TWO MODULATORY LOOPS ARE CRITICAL TO SMOOTH, RECOGNIZABLE MOVEMENTS

The motor hierarchy does not and cannot produce recognizable human motion without running its motor plan through two brain loops that provide indirect and modulatory input back to the motor hierarchy (Fig. 20-1). These two regions serve critical motor functions:

- The *cerebellum* smoothes, coordinates, and sequences movements and is required for motor learning

- The *basal ganglia* suppress most movement most of the time and also select which movements to make when, often chaining together several actions into one seemingly unitary action

Both modulatory regions modulate motor centers in the brainstem and forebrain rather than exerting effects directly on either motoneurons or motor interneurons. The importance of the cerebellum and basal ganglia in generating the smooth movements that humans make, movements that involve multiple muscles, joints, and limbs and take place over the course of minutes or even hours, cannot be overestimated. Indeed, several of the most common motor disorders are those of the cerebellum or basal ganglia.

DIFFERENT TYPES OF MOVEMENT INDEPENDENTLY OPERATE OR FAIL TO FUNCTION

Consider the consequences of damage to a cerebral motor control center. We use a simple example: the frontal eye fields, which organize gaze to the contralateral side so that an individual with damage to the right frontal eye field cannot make a willful saccade to the left. Does this mean that this person cannot abduct the left eye under any circumstances? Absolutely not: this person still makes reflexive movements to the left and still orients to a rapidly moving stimulus streaking to the left. In contrast, a person with an injury to the right abducens nerve cannot abduct the right eye under any circumstances. As this example illustrates, *different actions employ overlapping but not identical motor pathways, all of which funnel through the common pathway of the motoneuron.* Therefore, dysfunction of any central motor region above the level of the motoneuron affects one or more, but not all, types of movements.

The movement types that we recognize are:

- *Passive movement* occurs without any neural input, as, for example, when a physician bends the arm about the elbow or during a stretch produced by active contraction of an antagonist muscle. A deficit in passive movement is commonly felt by the physician as a resistance against imposed movement. Deficits in passive movement are termed *rigidity*. Rigidity is caused by central rather than peripheral nervous system lesions. One common example, *cogwheel rigidity*, accompanies Parkinson's disease, a basal ganglia disorder.

- *Reflexes* are very simple movements, such as flexion withdrawals from a painful stimulus. Reflexes can occur without voluntary control. An absence of reflexive movement, termed *areflexia*, is caused by impairment of motoneurons or the connection of motoneurons to muscles. A condition of *exuberant* reflexes, termed *hyperreflexia*, typically results from lesions of descending motor tracts (discussed in Chapter 23).

- *Stereotyped, semiautomatic movements* include rhythmic behaviors, such as chewing, walking, and swimming, as well as nonrhythmic ones such as vomiting, micturition, and even postural control, which depend on central pattern generator circuits. Central pattern generator circuits and their component neurons are critical to producing the basic pattern of stereotyped movements.

- *Self-generated actions* include a large variety of motions that we initiate. Self-generated actions may occur in response to a stimulus—gazing at a beautiful painting or gasping at a story told by a friend. Yet, unlike a reflex, a self-generated action is far removed from sensory input in terms of both time and neural distance traveled. Self-generated movements are heterogeneous but fall primarily into two motivational categories:
  - A subset of self-generated actions are *volitional* or *voluntary actions*, also called *willful, purposeful*, or *deliberate* actions. Volitional actions require the participation of the cerebral cortex. Moving in response to a command, as occurs during a game of Simon Says, is an example of a voluntary and conscious movement. Yet, voluntary actions account for a minority of our skeletal muscle contractions. An absence of voluntary movement is commonly called *paralysis* but *volitional paresis* is a more accurate term, referring to a selective impairment of voluntary movement with sparing of nonvolitional self-generated actions (Fig. 20-2).

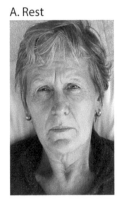 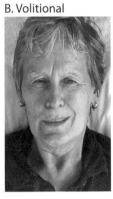 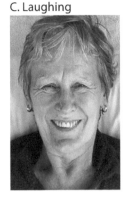 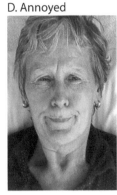

A. Rest B. Volitional C. Laughing D. Annoyed

Figure 20-2 The facial expressions of a patient with a lesion in the left supplementary motor area, a cortical motor control center, at rest (A), in response to a verbal command (B), and during natural emotional states (C–D) are shown. A: The facial expression at rest is symmetrical and normal. The nasolabial folds are symmetrically apparent in this patient in contrast to patients with Bell's palsy. B: In response to a request to show her teeth, the left side of the patient's face moves normally, but there is little change in the right side of the face. C–D: During feelings of enjoyment and annoyance, the patient makes symmetrically normal facial expressions of emotion. Impairment of volitional facial expressions coupled with intact emotional facial expressions is termed *volitional facial paresis*. Note that, in this patient, impairment of movement is *context-specific*, accompanying volitional but not emotional facial expressions. Context-specificity is pathognomonic for a central nervous system lesion. In contrast, Bell's palsy, due to a peripheral lesion, impairs all movements of the ipsilateral face, regardless of context.   Photographs kindly provided by Adrian Danek. Additional information about this patient's case is available in Jox et al., 2004.

• Most self-generated movements are *emotional actions* initiated for reasons that often do not reach consciousness. We may assign a post hoc reason, often inaccurate, to the occurrence of emotional actions. Pathways from the cerebral cortex to motoneurons that are critical to producing emotional actions are distinct from the pathway required for voluntary actions. *Our emotional actions reflect our emotions far more accurately than do our verbal explanations, underscoring the inherent honesty of the emotional motor system.* Some patients show an impairment of emotional actions with relatively preserved volitional action; this condition has been termed *emotional paresis* or *amimia* (Fig. 20-3).

Paralysis and the suffix *-plegia* refer to an inability to move, whereas *-paresis* refers to weakness. *Palsy* is a term that is ambiguous and thus is inclusive of paralysis, weakness, or an indeterminate level of immobility.

Paralysis can be either *flaccid* in the case of a complete paralysis or *spastic* in the instance of a voluntary paralysis. As an example of a flaccid paralysis, consider a lesion or complete dysfunction in the motoneuron, neuromuscular junction, or muscle. The affected muscle cannot contract under any context. This type of paralysis is complete; the muscles never contract and, therefore, over time, they lose their tone and become *flaccid*. In contrast, paralysis caused by a lesion in the corticospinal pathway only disrupts the ability to move in response to a verbal command. Patients with this type of paralysis, which is typically termed *spastic paralysis*, have hyperreflexia (see Chapter 23). These patients may

A. Smile in response to a command

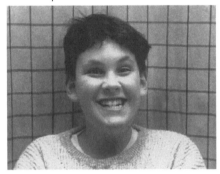

B. Smile in response to a funny joke

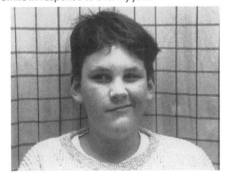

Figure 20-3 This young patient with *emotional facial paresis* smiles normally in response to a command but fails to smile symmetrically in response to a funny joke. This patient has essentially the reverse condition from that of the patient illustrated in Figure 20-2. Yet, like the patient illustrated in Figure 20-2, this patient has a context-specific impairment, automatically implicating a lesion *within* the central nervous system. Lesions that give rise to emotional facial paresis are varied in location. In this patient, the lesion is in the striatum and anterior internal capsule on the left side, contralateral to the side of impaired emotional movement.   Reprinted from Trosch RM et al. Emotional facial paresis with striatocapsular infarction. *J Neurol Sci* 98: 195–201, 1990, where more information about this case is available, with permission of the publisher, Elsevier.

even be able to generate emotional movements, as is true of the patient illustrated in Figure 20-2. Thus, it is important to understand that despite sharing a common moniker, the two forms of paralysis are not equivalent. Stereotyped and emotional actions are relatively spared, and reflexes are actually enhanced after lesions of the corticospinal pathway that cause spastic paralysis. In contrast, all muscle contractions are obliterated by motoneuron lesions that produce a flaccid paralysis.

The terminology used to describe patients who do not move is further complicated by *akinesia*, a symptom resulting from damage to basal ganglia circuits. Akinesia is a prominent symptom in patients with severe Parkinson's disease. Akinetic patients do not move much at all either for internal motivational reasons or in response to a voluntary command. However, they *can* move because *there is absolutely nothing wrong with the motor hierarchy and cerebellum*. Reflective of a healthy motor hierarchy, akinetic patients make relatively normal visually guided and reflexive movements.

No skeletal muscles contract in isolation; all skeletal muscle activity requires input from motoneurons of the central nervous system. Yet there is a valuable distinction to be made between movements that stem from the forebrain and those that do not. Throughout this book, I use the term *self-generated* to refer to actions that emerge from forebrain motor control centers. These include semiautomatic, emotional, and voluntary movements but do not include spinal or brainstem reflexes.

In the next several chapters, we explore the function of the motor system with an eye to understanding clinical presentations such as those illustrated in Figures 20-2 and 20-3. We start at the lowest level of the motor hierarchy—the muscles and motoneurons—before working our way up to the motor control centers and then to the motor modulatory regions.

ADDITIONAL READING

Cole J. *Pride and a Daily Marathon*. Cambridge, MA: MIT Press, 1995.

Holstege G. Emotional innervation of facial musculature. *Move Dis.* 17 (Suppl 2): S12–16, 2002.

Jox R, Bruning R, Hamann G, Danek A. Volitional facial palsy after a vascular lesion of the supplementary motor area. *Neurology.* 63: 756–757, 2004.

Trosch RM, Sze G, Brass LM, Waxman SG. Emotional facial paresis with striatocapsular infarction. *J Neurol Sci.* 98: 195–201, 1990.

21.

THE MOTOR UNIT AND ORDERLY RECRUITMENT

MUSCLES VARY IN FORCE, SIZE, SPEED, AND ENDURANCE

Different movements require different physical feats, and, to accommodate this variety, the basic physiological features of different muscles vary. In other words, one muscle type does not fit all movements. The physical requirements of elevating the eyelid for the better part of a day differ from those of yanking open a door. Hand muscles used to hold and direct a pencil for writing differ from the diaphragm, which supports breathing, whispering, singing, and shouting. *Fine and coarse movements with different requirements for maximal force, speed of contraction, and resistance to fatigue are controlled differently by the brain and also utilize muscles that differ in their basic properties.*

MUSCLE FIBERS DIFFER IN THEIR CONTRACTILE PROPERTIES

Our bodies' skeletal muscles support varied movements ranging from the steady opposition to gravity required to stand to the fast push-off needed for track and field competition and the meticulous fine movements needed to articulate a tongue twister or pick a raspberry without crushing it. *Different types of muscle fibers are mixed in proportions appropriate to the common usages of each muscle.*

Skeletal muscle comes in two basic varieties that we will call *slow-twitch* and *fast-twitch* fibers. In scientific literature, these fiber types are referred to by the uninformative names of *type I* and *type II* fibers:

- Slow-twitch fibers (type I fibers) generate forces slowly and maintain these forces for a long time.

- Fast-twitch fibers (type II fibers) generate large forces rapidly but tire quickly.

Slow-twitch fibers require oxygen to function and are supplied amply with capillaries carrying oxygenated blood.

They derive their red appearance from myoglobin, a heme-containing protein that transports oxygen to muscle mitochondria that support aerobic metabolism. Because slow-twitch fibers depend on diffusion of oxygen from nearby capillaries, there is an upper limit to their physical size.

Fast-twitch fibers differ from slow-twitch fibers in almost all respects. Fast-twitch fibers function either partially or entirely by anaerobic glycolysis. Fast-twitch fibers that can function both aerobically and anaerobically using glycolysis are called *oxidative glycolytic fast-twitch fibers* (or *type IIa*), whereas fast-twitch fibers that function exclusively by anaerobic glycolysis are called *glycolytic fast-twitch fibers* (or *type IIb*). Muscle fibers that rely progressively more upon glycolysis are progressively paler in color and less vascularized, which leads to the culinary distinction between dark (red) and light (white) meat (*ex vivo* skeletal muscle). Most flying birds have exclusively or nearly exclusively slow-twitch muscles to maintain muscle contractions for long-duration flights; thus, game birds yield mostly dark meat. However, domesticated chickens do not fly much. Only their leg muscles are slow-twitch whereas the chicken's breast muscles, that would normally serve flying, are composed of fast-twitch muscle (white meat).

Because fast fibers depend either in part or wholly on glycogen stores that are distributed throughout the cell, fast fibers *can* be large in size. However, they are not always large. For example, the size of fast-twitch fiber-dominated muscles in the hand, face, or orbit is far smaller than in the legs and arms. In general, the size of a fast muscle increases as the natural load on that muscle increases—a lot less force is needed to move a finger or an eyeball than a leg. The force exerted by a contracted muscle fiber depends on its cross-sectional area. Therefore, the maximal contractile force is greater in the largest fast-twitch fibers than it is in slow fibers.

Slow- and fast-twitch muscle fibers differ in two main *contractile* features:

- Speed of force generation

- Endurance or ability to maintain force over time

Table 21-1 THE CHARACTERISTICS OF THE THREE TYPES OF MUSCLE FIBERS ARE SUMMARIZED

CHARACTERISTIC	SLOW-TWITCH FIBERS	OXIDATIVE GLYCOLYTIC FAST-TWITCH FIBERS	GLYCOLYTIC FAST-TWITCH FIBERS
Energy source	Aerobic only	Aerobic and anaerobic glycolysis	Anaerobic glycolysis only
Speed of contraction	Slow	Intermediate	Fast
Maximal duration of continuous activation	Hours	≤30 minutes	2–3 minutes
Upper size limit	Small	Intermediate	Large
Upper limit for twitch tension	Low	Intermediate	High

The upper size limit refers to the largest physical dimensions of a fiber of each type. Slow-twitch fibers depend on oxygen for their operation and thus have the smallest upper limit in fiber diameter of the three types. The fiber size is the major determinant of the maximal amount of tension produced by a twitch. Therefore, the upper limit of twitch tension largely reflects the upper limit on fiber size. Note that there are muscle fibers of each type that are smaller in diameter and produce less tension than the upper limits possible.

The difference in contractile speed stems from variations in contractile molecules and their regulation by calcium. Fast-twitch muscle fibers contract two to three times more rapidly than do slow-twitch muscle fibers. Yet slow fibers can contract for longer periods of time. In slow fibers, oxygen keeps coming, but in fast fibers, glycogen stores last for only a limited amount of time before depletion. After glycogen depletion, fast glycolytic fibers cannot contract again until the glycogen stores are replenished, a process that can take hours. Fast oxidative glycolytic fibers, on the other hand, function aerobically after their glycogen supply is exhausted so that these fibers can operate for a longer time than can fast glycolytic fibers although still not as long as slow fibers.

In sum, we recognize three types of skeletal muscle fibers (see Table 21-1):

- Oxidative slow-twitch muscle fibers generate forces slowly and are highly resistant to fatigue. They are active during small, steady contractions that last for hours.

- Oxidative glycolytic fast-twitch muscle fibers generate forces at an intermediate speed and fatigue within 5–30 minutes.

- Glycolytic fast-twitch muscle fibers generate forces very rapidly. Yet they cannot sustain contractions for more than a few minutes and after exhaustion may require hours to recover.

In muscles that are active for long periods, such as those that maintain posture, close off the urethra during hours of urine storage, or grip a briefcase while walking to work, slow-twitch fibers, which can provide long-lasting, tonic contractions, predominate. One can think of cardiac muscle, which can only operate aerobically and does so for a lifetime (by definition), as the epitome of a slow-twitch muscle. In contrast, muscles with a large proportion of fast-twitch fibers support ballistic movements such as jumping and blinking.

The proportions of slow-, oxidative glycolytic fast-, and glycolytic fast-twitch muscle fibers in a muscle match the functions of that muscle (Fig. 21-1). Here, it is useful to introduce the

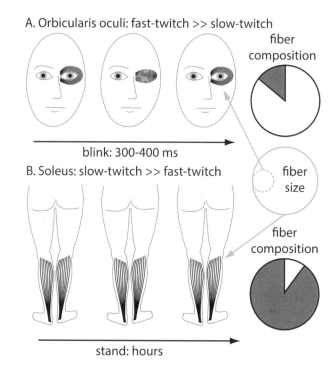

Figure 21-1 A: One major use of the orbicularis oculi is for blinking, a ballistic movement, that is initiated and completed in less than a half second. The orbicularis oculi consists mostly of fast-twitch fibers (*white area in pie graph*) and has only a small proportion of slow-twitch fibers (*red area in pie graph*). B: The soleus muscle flexes the ankle, keeping the body from falling backward. The soleus is the primary muscle employed in standing and can continue to contract for hours. Befitting its long duration use, the soleus muscle contains mostly slow-twitch fibers. The average fiber size of orbicularis oculi muscle fibers (*dashed blue circle*) is far smaller than the average fiber size of soleus muscle fibers (*solid blue circle*). Data obtained from Johnson MA, Polgar J, Weightman D, Appleton D. Data on the distribution of fibre types in thirty-six human muscles: An autopsy study. *J Neurol Sci* 18: 111–129, 1973; and Polgar J, Johnson MA, Weightman D, Appleton D. Data on fibre size types in thirty-six human muscles: An autopsy study. *J Neurol Sci* 19: 307–328, 1973.

terms *tonic* and *phasic*, which refer to prolonged and transient time courses, respectively. Tonic muscle activity, such as that in paraspinous muscles during prolonged sitting or standing, is ongoing for a relatively long period of time. In contrast, phasic muscle activity refers to a burst of activity that starts and ends within a short period of time, a pattern that is used for sprinting, gasping, plucking, and so on. Exemplary of a tonic muscle, the soleus muscle is an ankle extensor that is nearly maximally contracted during standing and maintains close to the same level of tension during locomotion. Thus, the soleus, like other postural extensors, shows tonic contraction for long periods of time as it opposes the force of gravity; correspondingly, the soleus muscle contains predominantly slow-twitch fibers. The small force and long endurance provided by slow-twitch fibers exactly match the requirements for optimal soleus function. On the other hand, the orbicularis oculi is active almost exclusively during eye blinks—rapidly initiated, phasic, ballistic movements—and appropriately contains mostly fast-twitch muscle fibers.

The size of muscle fibers in any given muscle is appropriate to the force requirements of movements made by that muscle and does *not* only depend on fiber type. For example, fast-twitch fibers in the orbicularis oculi are used for eye blinks, whereas limb and axial muscles operate on much heavier objects, including the body itself. In addition to the orbicularis oculi having fewer fibers than a limb muscle such as the biceps, the average diameter of fast-twitch fibers in the orbicularis oculi is less than half that of fast-twitch fibers in limb and axial musculature (Fig. 21-1).

Most muscles are "mixed," containing both slow- and fast-twitch fibers, and therefore can participate in both tonic and phasic activities. For example, the gastrocnemius (the superficial calf muscle) is minimally contracted during standing, but activated increasingly during walking, jogging, running, and sprinting. Appropriately, the gastrocnemius contains both slow- and fast-twitch fibers with more fast oxidative glycolytic than fast glycolytic fibers, allowing for long-lasting engagement in locomotion.

THE MOTOR UNIT IS THE SMALLEST DIVISION OF MOVEMENT

As emphasized throughout this book, the motoneuron is the only conduit from the central nervous system to skeletal muscle. I use the term *motoneuron* in order to underscore the unique role as well as distinctive properties of the neurons that innervate skeletal muscle. *Motor neuron*, a term

that is common elsewhere, is not used here because it does not differentiate between somatic and autonomic neurons.

Regardless of the author's commitment to the word "motoneuron," the medical student must be aware that motoneurons are termed *lower motor neurons* within clinical circles. The "lower" implies an "upper" and, indeed, clinical vernacular recognizes cells in motor cortex as *upper motor neurons*. The idea behind the upper and lower motor neuron terminology is that cortical motor control cells influence motoneurons so strongly that activity in the former inevitably leads to activity in the latter. However, this is absolutely not the case. Motoneurons directly contact muscle fibers and control motor contraction absolutely, whereas cells of motor control centers are only one of many sources of influence upon motoneurons. As we shall see, loss of cortical motor control neurons can lead to more movement, whereas loss of motoneurons *always* diminishes or abolishes movement.

Each motoneuron innervates a number of muscle fibers at a single site, termed the *endplate*. Yet any single muscle fiber is innervated by only one motoneuron in the adult. *The smallest functional unit of the motor system is one motoneuron and the muscle fibers that it innervates.* This is the *motor unit*. When a motoneuron fires, all muscle fibers innervated by that motoneuron contract. The converse is also true; in the absence of input from a motoneuron, none of the innervated muscle fibers contracts. This one-to-one connection between motoneuron activity and contraction of the innervated muscle fibers means that *the motor unit is the quantum of the motor system, the smallest operating unit that can be engaged.*

Muscles used for finely graded movements contain motor units with fewer fibers than do muscles used for more forceful and less carefully controlled movements. Some motoneurons innervating muscles that produce coarse movements (e.g., gastrocnemius and quadriceps muscles) innervate hundreds or thousands of muscle fibers in the human. In contrast, motoneurons innervating muscles that produce finely controlled movements (e.g., hand muscles) innervate far fewer muscle fibers, typically less than 100, whereas motoneurons innervating muscles that allow for extremely precise movements, such as extraocular muscles, innervate fewer than 10 muscle fibers.

All muscle fibers innervated by any one motoneuron are of one type—either slow-twitch, oxidative glycolytic fast-twitch, or glycolytic fast-twitch (Fig. 21-2). Luckily, the muscle fibers innervated by each motoneuron, although of the same type, are dispersed throughout the muscle. Consequently, injury to one region of a muscle does not preferentially affect one muscle fiber type over another.

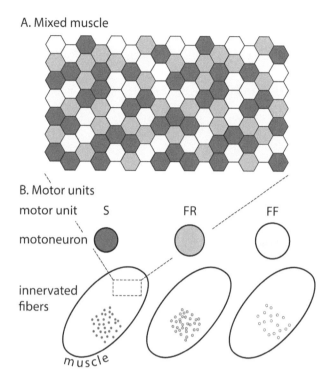

A. Mixed muscle

B. Motor units

motor unit   S   FR   FF

motoneuron

innervated
fibers

muscle

Figure 21-2   A: In mixed muscles, different fiber types are interspersed rather than segregated in one portion of the muscle. This cartoon diagrams the muscle fibers (*hexagons*) in a cross-section through a mixed muscle such as the gastrocnemius. Slow-twitch (*red*), oxidative glycolytic fast-twitch (*pink*), and glycolytic fast-twitch (*light gray*) muscle fibers are interspersed in an apparently random fashion.
B: Motor units consist of a motoneuron and the muscle fibers that that single motoneuron innervates. Motor units are the quanta of the motor system. S motor units innervate slow-twitch muscle fibers. Fast fatigue-resistant (*FR*) motor units innervate oxidative glycolytic fast-twitch muscle fibers. Fast fatigable (*FF*) motor units innervate glycolytic fast-twitch muscle fibers. The muscle fibers of a single motor unit, of any type, are scattered through a region of muscle and are rarely contiguous.   Modified from Burke RE, Tsairis P. Anatomy and innervation ratios in motor units of cat gastrocnemius. *J Physiol* 234(3): 749–165, 1973, with permission of the publisher, Wiley.

Reflecting the one-to-one relationship between motor units and fiber type innervated, there are three types of motor units and associated motoneurons (Fig. 21-2). Slow or *S* motoneurons innervate slow-twitch muscle fibers. Activation of S motor units produces slowly building muscle tension that can be sustained for hours. Fast fatigue-resistant or *FR* motoneurons innervate oxidative glycolytic fast-twitch muscle fibers. Activity in FR motor units produces rapid increases in muscle fibers that use both aerobic and anaerobic metabolism to sustain contractions for tens of minutes. The final type of *motoneuron* is the fast fatigable or *FF* motor unit. Activity in FF units leads to very rapid increases in muscle tension. However, the glycolytic fast-twitch fibers excited by FF units can only maintain a contraction for a few minutes at most. In this way, *the characteristics of each motor unit type reflect the properties of the innervated muscle fibers.*

MAXIMAL FORCE PRODUCED BY A MOTOR UNIT DEPENDS PRIMARILY ON THE NUMBER OF MUSCLE FIBERS INNERVATED

The maximal force produced by a motor unit depends mainly on the number of muscle fibers innervated; this number is called the *innervation ratio*. In general, the innervation ratio is lowest in S units, greatest in FF units, and intermediate in FR units. Thus, one S motor unit innervates a small number of muscle fibers and produces a small total force, whereas one FF motor unit innervates a large number of muscle fibers and produces a relatively large force.

Because of the small force exerted by each S motor unit, a large number of S motor units make a disproportionately small contribution to the maximal contractile force of a muscle (Fig. 21-3). Similarly, because of the large force exerted by each FF motor unit, FF motor units contribute disproportionately more than their numbers to the maximal contractile force of a muscle. In other words, S motor units contribute much less and FF units more to the total force of a muscle than would be predicted by their representation within the motoneuron population.

The profiles of different motor unit types allow us to predict the consequences of injury to selected motor unit populations. *Loss of just a few FF or FR motor units will drastically compromise maximal muscle contraction.* In contrast, many S motor units must be injured before a serious reduction in contractile force would be observed. However, *the loss of even a few S motor units may negatively impact the endurance capacity of a muscle without significantly weakening it.*

People vary in the proportions of fast- and slow-twitch muscle fibers that they possess. Although these proportions are set genetically, exercise can change the relative force

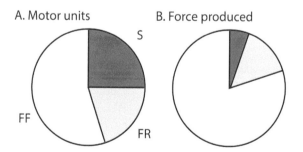

A. Motor units   B. Force produced

S

FF

FR

Figure 21-3   In the case of the gastrocnemius muscle, a typical mixed-limb muscle, S motor units (*red*) make up 25% of the total motor units (A) but contribute less than 5% of the force (B). In contrast, FF motor units (*white*) make up 55% of the motoneuron pool (A) and contribute 80% of the force (B). The number and contribution of FR motor units (*pink*) are intermediate.

contributions of the different muscle fiber types to overall motor performance through changes in metabolism, contractility, and muscle fiber diameter. As an example of the influence of exercise on muscle fiber size, strength training leads to a selective increase in the diameter of fast-twitch muscle fibers whereas endurance training has the opposite effect. Thus, an average individual genetically endowed with a roughly even split of fast- and slow-twitch muscle fibers can selectively augment the force contributed by one or the other type of fiber through a targeted exercise regimen. The lability of muscle force is a two-way street. Inactivity rapidly leads muscle fibers to return to their initial size prior to any exercise regimen. For clinicians, it is important to recognize that inactivity due to either a sedentary lifestyle, injury, or illness may diminish motor performance below levels needed for ordinary activities such as standing, walking, and lifting.

MOTONEURON FIRING RATE AND PATTERN ARE CRITICAL TO SETTING MUSCLE TENSION

The relationship between motoneuronal firing and muscle tension depends on two factors:

- The immediate (tens of milliseconds) history of activity in the innervating motoneuron

- The "warm-up" (minutes) history of the innervating motoneuron

The immediate influence of motoneuron firing on muscle fiber tension is fairly simple: the more frequently a motoneuron fires, the greater the muscle tension that develops. This positive correlation between motoneuron firing rate and muscle tension operates until the maximal tension possible is produced. This maximal tension is termed *tetanus*, which is discussed in more detail later. Warm-up exerts its effect on muscle tension only after a delay by amplifying the effect of subsequent action potentials. Thus, a warmed-up muscle produces greater tension in response to a train of action potentials than does a cold muscle.

To understand how these processes work together, we first look at the muscle tension or twitch produced by a single action potential. Regardless of muscle fiber type, increases in muscle tension persist for a far longer time than the duration of the motoneuron action potential (Fig. 21-4). Slow-twitch fibers produce the longest lasting twitches (up to 100 ms), fast glycolytic fibers the shortest lasting ones (as short as 3 ms but typically closer to 20–30 ms), and fast

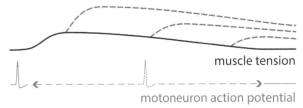

A. Slow-twitch muscle fiber

muscle tension

motoneuron action potential

B. Fast-twitch muscle fiber

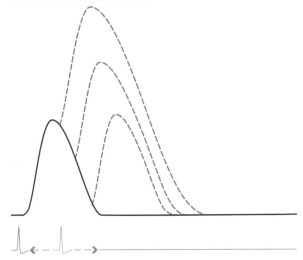

Figure 21-4 Action potentials are short (~1 ms), but produce long-lasting changes in muscle tension. A: A single action potential (*lower trace in green*) produces a slowly developing, long-lasting, small increase in the tension of a slow-twitch motor unit (*black*). A second action potential (*dotted green*) following the initial action potential within about 100 ms (*period encompassed by green arrows*) produces an additive effect on muscle tension (*dashed red traces*); this effect decreases with increasing intervals. B: A single action potential (*lower trace in green*) produces a rapidly developing and large magnitude, but short-lived increase in the tension of a glycolytic fast-twitch muscle fiber (*black*). A second action potential (*dotted green*) must follow the initial action potential within about 40 ms (*period encompassed by green arrows*) to produce an additive effect on muscle tension (*dashed red traces*), an effect that, as in the case with a slow-twitch muscle fiber, decreases at longer intervals.   Modified from Burke RE, Rudomin P, Zajac FE 3rd. The effect of activation history on tension production by individual muscle units. *Brain Res* 109: 515–529, 1976 with permission of the publisher, Elsevier.

oxidative glycolytic fibers produce twitches of intermediate duration (30–50 ms). Because of the long-lasting muscle twitches, muscle tension summates with the arrival of every subsequent action potential that occurs during an ongoing twitch for as long as muscle tension is elevated.

When a train of action potentials occurs in a motoneuron, the forces generated in the innervated muscle fibers resulting from each successive action potential sum until contraction reaches a maximal level, representative of the maximal contraction possible for that muscle (Fig. 21-5A). At moderate rates of motoneuron discharge, the individual contractions due to each action potential are still distinguishable in a recording of muscle force; this is termed an *unfused tetanus*. At higher rates, however, the individual contractions evoked by single action potentials are no longer

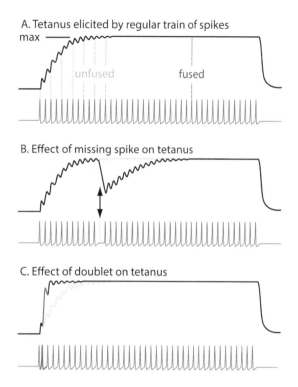

A. Tetanus elicited by regular train of spikes

max unfused   fused

B. Effect of missing spike on tetanus

C. Effect of doublet on tetanus

Figure 21-5 **A:** A train of regularly timed action potentials in a motoneuron produces regularly timed and summating increases in muscle tension. When the maximal muscle tension (*max*) is initially reached, the effect of each action potential is still apparent. This is termed *unfused tetanus*. Fused tetanus occurs when action potentials have no additional effect on muscle tension. **B:** Omission of a single action potential (*pale green*) greatly decreases muscle tension and prolongs the latency to fused tetanus. **C:** Two action potentials occurring at a short interval are termed a *doublet*. The effect of a doublet (*red*) is a large increase in muscle tension (*red*) and an augmentation of the effect of each subsequent action potential. As a result, both unfused and fused tetanus occur at earlier latencies. In B and C, the original tetanus shown in A is drawn in gray. Modified from Burke RE, Rudomin P, Zajac FE 3rd. The effect of activation history on tension production by individual muscle units. *Brain Res* 109: 515–529, 1976 with permission of the publisher, Elsevier.

distinguishable. Instead, the tension generated during a *fused tetanus* reaches and maintains a smooth plateau level. *Fused tetanus represents the maximal force that a muscle can*

generate; *increasing the motoneuron firing rate beyond that which produces fused tetanus produces no additional force.*

If one action potential is missed from a regular train of action potentials, the result is a disproportionately large drop in muscle tension (Fig. 21-5B). Conversely, if an extra action potential sneaks into an otherwise regular train of action potentials, muscle tension is abruptly and inordinately increased (Fig. 21-5C). The sensitivity of muscle tension to the pattern of action potentials is important because alterations to the timing of action potentials, such as occur in *demyelinating* diseases, profoundly alter the profile of muscle contraction.

Just as the occurrence of an action potential alone or within a train influences the magnitude of the resulting muscle tension, past usage of the muscle also influences the tension evoked by a single spike. *Excitation of a previously tetanized muscle fiber results in a far larger output than does excitation of a previously inactive fiber.* Full tetanus maximally facilitates muscle tension per action potential, but even a few isolated twitches augment the ensuing level of muscle tension produced by a single action potential. In sum, "warming-up" multiplies the muscle tension produced by every subsequent action potential occurring over the course of the next several minutes. Maximal warm-up, achieved by reaching tetanus minutes prior, maximally facilitates the effect of subsequent action potentials.

ORDERLY RECRUITMENT PRODUCES MOVEMENTS THAT INCREASE IN FORCE SMOOTHLY

Motoneurons belonging to the three types of motor units differ in physiological properties, most importantly input resistance. The input resistance of S motoneurons is greatest and that of FF motoneurons lowest (see Table 21-2). Recall

Table 21-2 **THE CHARACTERISTICS OF THE THREE CATEGORIES OF MOTOR UNITS ARE SUMMARIZED**

PHYSIOLOGICAL PROPERTY	S MOTOR UNITS	FR MOTOR UNITS	FF MOTOR UNITS
Type of muscle fiber	Slow-twitch fibers	Oxidative glycolytic fast-twitch fibers	Glycolytic fast-twitch fibers
Rise time	Slow (50–100 ms)	Intermediate (30–50 ms)	Fast (3–30 ms)
Maximal duration of continuous activation	Hours	≤ 30 minutes	≤5 minutes
Innervation ratio	Lowest	Low	Highest
Upper limit for tetanic tension	Low	Intermediate	High
Input resistance	High	Intermediate	Low
Current threshold for activation	Low	Intermediate	High

The kinetic properties of motor unit types reflect the properties of the muscle fiber types innervated. The innervation ratio, input resistance, and current threshold of activation are all characteristics of the motoneuron. The upper limit for tetanic tension produced is primarily a consequence of the innervation ratio but is also influenced by fiber type.

from Chapter 9 that, because of Ohm's Law ($V = I * R$), a cell with a high input resistance requires a lower synaptic current to reach the action potential threshold than does a cell with a lower input resistance. As a result, cells provided with the *same synaptic current* are activated in the order of decreasing input resistance. This means that S motoneurons are activated before FR motoneurons, which are activated before FF motoneurons, so that *if provided with a common input, motor units are activated in a sequence of increasing force*. S motor units are activated first, FR units second, and FF units last (Fig. 21-6). The sequential engagement of S, FR, and FF motor units is termed *orderly recruitment*.

Orderly recruitment matches output to demand. To understand this concept, consider three activities: standing, walking, and jumping. Of the three activities, standing requires the smallest force but lasts the longest amount of time. The attributes of S motor units match the low force and long endurance requirements of postural muscles. Walking depends on greater muscular forces, but these forces are needed for less time than in the case of standing. Thus, FR motor units, working with still-engaged S motor units, are suited to support walking. Finally, jumping requires a large contractile force for a very short time, needs met by adding activation of FF motor units to the already-activated S and FR units. Even when not exercising, we continually engage S motor units to exert small forces that maintain our body position, whether we are prone, sitting, or standing. Only upon this background do we start to move about, engaging FR units to walk or jog. Similarly, we typically run before leaping, a brief action that requires activation of FF units in the context of still-contracted S and FR units.

The sequential engagement of motor units in the S → FR → FF order combines with a progressive increase in the number of innervated muscle fibers in each successively activated motor unit. Thus, the first S motor units activated innervate fewer muscle fibers than do subsequently activated S motor units and so on. *The progressive increase in force produced by successively activated motor units ensures that muscle tension increases smoothly, devoid of sudden jerks or failures.* Derecruitment (i.e., relaxing a muscle) happens in the reverse order from recruitment. So, FF motor units "drop out" first followed by FR motor units, whereas S motor units remain contracted for hours. As discussed later, minimally invasive electromyography, which allows a glimpse into the recruitment and drop-out of motor units in accessible human muscles, is used to diagnose myopathies and motoneuron diseases.

Advantages derive from the sequential activation of S, FR, and FF motor units and the reverse order drop-out of motor unit types. First, *failure due to fatigue is minimized* because S motor units are activated first and for the longest time during long-lasting activities. Second, *the increment of force produced by the recruitment of each additional motor unit is proportional to the existing force in the muscle*. This is a sort of motor equivalent to Weber's sensory law (see Chapter 14) that enables a person to both exert finely graded pressure on a foot pedal and kick a ball. Thus, small increments of force add up on a background of low force to enable finely controlled movements, whereas large increments of force add up on a background of great force for ballistic movements.

Orderly recruitment depends on a common input to all of the motor units innervating a muscle. However, not all inputs are distributed evenly to motoneurons of all three types. For example, cutaneous nociceptors excite FF and FR motor units but not S motor units. This advantageous organization

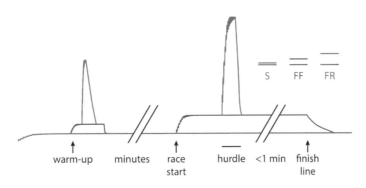

Figure 21-6 A cartoon showing the recruitment and derecruitment of motor units in a leg muscle before and during a 400 m hurdle race. S motor units (*brown*) are recruited first to support standing and walking. In a brief warm-up, FR motor units (*blue*) are recruited followed by FF motor units (*red*). Even tetanic muscle activation during the warm-up does not produce maximal muscle tension but permits production of maximal force in the ensuing minutes. When the race starts, FR motor units are rapidly recruited and stay active for the duration of the approximately 1-minute race. At each hurdle (only one is shown), FF motor units are rapidly recruited and then de-recruited. At the end of the race, as the racer warms down by walking, FR motor units are derecruited while activation of S motor units continues. The right-hand inset shows the relative increment of muscle tension produced by one motor unit of each type.

allows a noxious input to elicit a rapid and ballistic movement without a slow build-up in muscle tension. Beyond cutaneous afferents, few additional inputs that may utilize this "shortcut" to FF and FR motor units have been identified.

In sum, the tension generated by a muscle fiber depends on a combination of warm-up history and immediate input from the innervating motoneuron. In turn, the force produced by the entire muscle depends on the number, type, and size of the motor units recruited and on the number and frequency of action potentials fired by the recruited motoneurons in the immediate and recent past. By ensuring that each increase in contractile force is proportional to the existing level of muscle activation, orderly recruitment prevents both an inappropriately large and therefore jerky contraction during standing and an inappropriately small, and therefore inconsequential and potentially disastrous, contraction during actions requiring great force.

WEIGHT-BEARING EXERCISE ALTERS MOTOR UNIT RECRUITMENT

S motor units are used daily, but FF and FR motor units are used much less often. In sedentary individuals, engagement of FF motor units is rare, particularly in muscles that are not used in everyday activities. When asked to make a maximal contraction, sedentary adults produce no more than 95% of the maximal force that their muscle can produce. The unactivated fibers, those with the highest threshold for activation, are FF motor units. An immediate effect of exercise, an effect that is sustained for weeks after a single workout of strength training, is the facilitation of FF motor unit recruitment. This enables the voluntary contraction of more FF motor units and the capacity to reach 100 % of a muscle's contractile strength.

A pair of action potentials that occurs in rapid succession, termed a *doublet*, evokes a very large and abrupt increase in muscle force (Fig. 21-5C). Doublets increase the force of muscle contraction more than would the same pair of action potentials separated by a longer interval. Exercise may increase the incidence of doublets in motoneurons. It is also possible that strength training increases the synchrony of motor unit recruitment so that more motor units are recruited together at one time.

EXTRAOCULAR MUSCLES AND THEIR INNERVATION DIFFER

Extraocular muscles are qualitatively different from skeletal muscles found in the rest of the body and head.

They are heterogeneous, comprising multiple anatomical subtypes split between (1) *global fibers* that insert on the sclera of the globe and provide the force that rotates the eye and (2) *orbital fibers* that form pulleys and insert onto the global muscle fibers themselves. It appears that contraction of orbital muscle fibers alters the effect of the global muscle fibers, for example, maintaining an eccentric gaze even after global muscle fibers have relaxed.

Extraocular muscles have contractile and innervation properties distinct from those of other muscles. For example, most orbital muscle fibers contract rapidly and are also highly fatigue-resistant, demonstrating a blend of slow- and fast-twitch muscle fiber properties. This combination of features make extraocular muscle fibers ideally suited for quickly reaching an eccentric eye position and then sustaining that position for a long period of time. In contrast to most skeletal muscles that are innervated by one motoneuron at a single endplate, many extraocular muscle fibers receive innervation from multiple motoneurons, resulting in up to 10 endplates. The effect of an action potential at one endplate is a regional and graded contraction. The rapid, localized, fatigue-resistant graded contractions of selected extraocular muscles are ideal for fine adjustments to eye position.

There is a lower safety factor at extraocular neuromuscular junctions than in skeletal muscles elsewhere in the body. This is due to smaller endplates and to an acetylcholine receptor isoform retained from embryonic development. The lower safety factor is in part compensated for by the high, ongoing discharge of extraocular motoneurons. The peak-firing rate of extraocular motoneurons is around 600 Hz, far higher than observed in motoneurons innervating limb skeletal muscles. Because of this, extraocular muscles can rapidly reach a steady level of contraction and then stay contracted. The steady contraction is akin to the fused tetanus observed in limb skeletal muscles except that further increases in motoneuron discharge rate can still generate larger forces. Thus, as the discharge rate of extraocular motoneurons increases up to maximal rates, muscle tension continues to smoothly increase.

As mentioned in Chapter 19, extraocular muscles have vulnerabilities to disease that differ from those of other skeletal muscles. Of particular note, extraocular muscles are particularly susceptible to certain autoimmune diseases such as myasthenia gravis and *Grave's ophthalmopathy* but are spared in other diseases such as *amyotrophic lateral sclerosis* and *Duchenne muscular dystrophy*.

ELECTROMYOGRAPHY IS A MINIMALLY INVASIVE CLINICAL TEST THAT CAN MEASURE MOTOR UNIT FUNCTION

The motor unit is one of the most accessible physiological processes in the nervous system. Thin needles placed in muscles allow physicians to make *electromyographic (EMG)* recordings of muscle activity. These EMG tests help distinguish between problems in muscle (termed *myopathies*), motoneuron diseases, and dysfunction of higher motor centers, such as can occur with multiple sclerosis or stroke.

Electromyography, typically called *EMG testing*, involves inserting a metal recording electrode through the skin into the belly of a muscle. The electrode records extracellular action potentials in surrounding muscle fibers. The nearer the electrode is to the muscle fiber, the larger the recorded action potential. Since the muscle fibers innervated by each motoneuron are scattered throughout the muscle, activity in any motor unit is likely to include at least some fibers within the range of the recording electrodes. However, remember that either all or none of the fibers in a motor unit contract at one time. Therefore, activity in each motor unit will cause a particular size and shape of voltage deflection so that the waveform serves as that motor unit's signature.

Let us begin by considering how EMG testing should appear in a healthy individual. At rest, there should be no activity, meaning no action potentials, in a muscle (Fig. 21-7A). As the patient voluntarily contracts the muscle being studied, one or a few S motor units are recruited; this appears as repeated action potentials (Fig. 21-7B). Once a motor unit fires at about 10 Hz, another motor unit is recruited. When the second one also fires at a rate of at least 10 Hz, additional motor units are recruited, and so on. With increasing strength of voluntary contraction, more and more motor units become active. Eventually, when a person is voluntarily contracting at maximal strength, many motor units are all firing together, giving rise to a noisy and large-amplitude recording in which single motor units are no longer discernible (Fig. 21-7C).

Now, let us consider what to expect in patients with motoneuron disease such as spinal poliomyelitis, colloquially known as polio. The poliovirus kills motoneurons, resulting in muscle weakness or paralysis. As more and more motoneurons die, there are fewer motor units available. So, when the first motor unit reaches 10 Hz, another motor unit may not be available. If another motor unit is not available—because the motoneuron has died—the first motor unit fires faster, without a second motor unit being recruited. This is termed *reduced recruitment*. Reduced recruitment occurs in *neuropathic* conditions that reduce the number of motoneurons (Fig. 21-7D). Since muscle fibers that lose their innervation—are denervated—waste away and atrophy with time, there is an eventual loss of

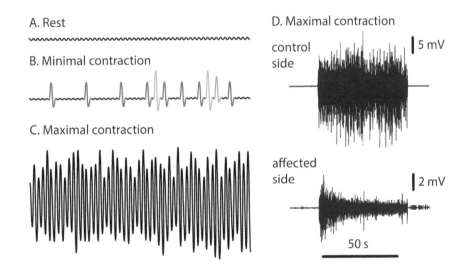

Figure 21-7 Electromyographic (EMG) testing can be used to identify neuropathic or myopathic motor disorders. A–C: Schematic cartoons illustrate the principles of a normal EMG recording. A: At rest, no motor units are active. B: During minimal contraction, distinct motor units (different colors), characterized by particular waveforms or electrical signatures, appear. Of the three units illustrated, the red unit is most active, and with time, the blue and orange units are recruited. C: During maximal contractions, individual units are no longer detectable. The activity during maximal contractions is continuous and larger in amplitude than the activity during minimal contractions. The large amplitude of EMG recordings during maximal contractions reflects (1) the recruitment of glycolytic fast-twitch fibers, which have larger amplitude waveforms; and (2) the addition of waveforms from simultaneously active motor units. D: Recordings from a patient with a motor neuropathy taken from the unaffected side (*top*) and the affected side (*bottom*). Reduced recruitment is evident along with rapid fatigue. Note the different vertical scales for the two traces. Panel D is modified from Kaji R et al. Activity-dependent conduction block in multifocal motor neuropathy. *Brain* 123: 1602–1611, 2000, with permission of the publisher, Oxford University Press.

muscle fibers in neuropathic conditions. In the presence of denervated muscle fibers, the existing motoneuron axons sprout new endings that innervate the denervated muscle fibers. Thus, the remaining motoneurons innervate extra muscle fibers, resulting in motor unit potentials that are larger than normal. Abnormally large motor units combined with reduced recruitment are signs of a neuropathic condition.

In *myopathic* conditions, muscle fibers waste away and become atrophied due to a defect in the muscle itself. For example, in patients with a primary muscle disease such as Duchenne muscular dystrophy, the potentials recorded from muscle are small in amplitude and are relatively few, even at maximal contraction. The distinct characteristics of EMG recordings in neuropathic and myopathic conditions make EMG testing a valuable diagnostic tool.

Fasciculations are visible twitches that result from activation of an entire motor unit. In patients with motoneuron disease, fasciculations can be quite large because the surviving motoneurons innervate extra muscle fibers, as just explained. Before a large portion of you panics that you have motoneuron disease—as much as 50–60% of the population experiences fasciculations—and most fasciculations are benign. Furthermore, people with benign fasciculations are not more likely than others to develop motoneuron disease.

In contrast to fasciculations, *fibrillations* represent single muscle fiber contractions that are not visible. Thus, fibrillations are an "electrical sign"—a sign only seen with EMG recording methods—rather than an observable symptom. Fibrillations arise in denervated muscle, which has supersensitive acetylcholine receptors that respond to acetylcholine circulating in the blood. Note that, in contrast to fasciculations (i.e., visible twitches resulting from activation of an entire motor unit), fibrillations involve the contraction of lone muscle fibers rather than all of the muscle fibers in a motor unit. Fibrillations are the only type of muscle contraction involving a muscle division smaller than the motor unit. Fibrillations are associated with any condition that involves muscle denervation, including amyotrophic lateral sclerosis, polio, neuropathy, or traumatic nerve injury.

ADDITIONAL READING

Burke RE. Motor units: Anatomy, physiology, and functional organization. In: *Handbook of Physiology*. Vol. II. Bethesda, MD: American Physiological Society, 1981: 345–422.

Burke RE. Some unresolved issues in motor unit research. *Adv Exp Med Biology.* 508: 171–178, 2002.

Burke RE. Revisiting the notion of 'motor unit types'. *Prog Brain Research.* 123: 167–175, 1999.

Burke RE, Levine DN, Tsairis P, Zajac FE, 3rd. Physiological types and histochemical profiles in motor units of the cat gastrocnemius. *J Physiol.* 234: 723–748, 1973.

Burke RE, Rudomin P, Zajac FE, 3rd. The effect of activation history on tension production by individual muscle units. *Brain Res.* 109: 515–529, 1976.

Burke RE, Rudomin P, Zajac FE, 3rd. Catch property in single mammalian motor units. *Science.* 168: 122–124, 1970.

Burke RE, Tsairis P. Anatomy and innervation ratios in motor units of cat gastrocnemius. *J Physiol.* 234: 749–765, 1973.

Enoka RM, Fuglevand AJ. Motor unit physiology: Some unresolved issues. *Muscle Nerve.* 24: 4–17, 2001.

Gabriel DA, Kamen G, Frost G. Neural adaptations to resistive exercise: Mechanisms and recommendations for training practices. *Sports Med.* 36: 133–149, 2006.

Karpati G, Hilton-Jones D, Bushby K, Griggs RC. (Eds.). *Disorders of Voluntary Muscle.* 8th ed. Cambridge: Cambridge University Press, 2010.

Moritani T, Stegeman D, Merletti R. Basic physiology and biophysics of EMG signal generation. In Merletti R, Parker P, eds. *Electromyography.* New York: Wiley InterScience, 2005.

22.

REFLEXES AND GAIT

otoneurons are executors, not planners. Just as muscles require instructions from motoneurons for contraction, motoneurons require inputs in order to compose those instructions. Then the motoneurons simply act out whatever they are told. Instructions from primary motor cortex are the flashiest and most celebrated inputs to motoneurons, but they are clearly not the most important. Sensory inputs from muscles, joints, and skin are the most critical inputs to motoneurons needed for movement. Without the reflexes elicited by these sensory inputs, movement as we all know it is impossible.

The critical importance of reflexes to movement is stunningly illustrated by the experience of Ian Waterman as described in Jonathan Cole's book, *Pride and a Daily Marathon*. Waterman permanently lost function in all proprioceptive and tactile spinal afferents at the age of 19 (see Chapter 20). This singular condition manifested itself as a severe motor disability for all movements involving muscles below the neck. Initially, Waterman was unable to walk, stand, or even sit. Early in the course of the illness, he was propped up in the corner of an ambulance, on the way to a neurological treatment center. Since he received no proprioceptive input, Waterman fell over at the first curve in the road, saved from injury only because of an attentive attendant.

Waterman worked assiduously to teach himself to move using visual feedback. In a staggeringly impressive feat, he taught himself to sit, stand, and even walk. Yet he continued to rely on visual feedback to guide his movements. His dependence on vision was so complete that when the lights went out, he collapsed on to the floor. Moreover, at no time did movement of any type become automatic. He had to deliberately perform each part of each action, every heel strike and toe-off in a walk across a room. The thousandth repetition of a movement was as effortful and deliberate as the first. He was unable to take notes while sitting in a meeting because just sitting alone used too much of his cognitive reserve.

Without reflexes, unexpected changes in the environment were dangerous. Tall buildings were difficult since "high winds . . . altered his postural relation to the horizon"

in an unpredictable way that could not be counteracted through conscious anticipation. Cole writes of Waterman being patted on the back from behind. In response, "he all but collapsed." Without proprioceptive feedback, Waterman could only react after visual cues told him he was already falling.

Ian Waterman's condition is dramatic proof that voluntary movement requires a full partnership between motor and sensory neurons. Reflexes are the marriage that binds sensory afferents to the motor hierarchy, allowing us to react to unexpected obstacles and to effectively produce repetitive movements by rote despite ever-changing conditions.

In this chapter, we consider inputs to motoneurons from sensory afferents and local motor interneurons that are critical in producing reflexive and semiautomatic movements. Motor interneurons within the spinal cord and brainstem organize reflexive movements such as the quick adjustments made to ongoing movements when a change in load occurs. *Central pattern generator* circuits comprised of local motor interneurons produce semiautomatic movements that constitute most of the human movement repertoire, including walking, running, and chewing. We then look at how sensory inputs and reflexes modify central pattern generator–supported movements. For example, reflexes allow a person to stumble and catch herself before falling over an unanticipated tree root or to adjust her gait when the ground turns unexpectedly soft.

THE STRETCH REFLEX CORRECTS FOR UNEXPECTED LOADS

Thus far, we have described how action potentials in motoneurons produce contractions in selected muscle fibers. Now, what happens when something unexpected occurs? Consider walking along and encountering a tree root in the path. As your foot hits the immovable root, a reflex to recover from stumbling takes over, preventing a fall. You do not have to plan this motion, prepare for it, think about it, or practice it daily. Instead, you recover from a stumble *reflexively*, without practice or forethought. The automatic engagement of the stumbling corrective reflex is rooted in spinal circuits and happens very quickly, within 10–50 ms of encountering the obstacle, thus allowing people to recover from stumbles before actually falling to the ground.

The spinal cord and brainstem mediate a number of stereotyped, behavioral responses called *reflexes*. The stumbling corrective reflex is a highly intricate reflex; at the opposite end of the complexity spectrum, the *stretch reflex*, also known as the *myotactic reflex*, is the simplest vertebrate reflex. Clinicians typically refer to the stretch reflex as *deep tendon reflexes*. The precipitating stimulus for the stretch reflex is a stretch, also termed a *load*, an added and unexpected force that stretches a muscle. The stretch reflex involves only one synapse within the central nervous system and therefore is termed *monosynaptic*. In counting synapses involved in a circuit, we count only those between two neurons; the synapse from motoneuron to muscle is not counted. *The only monosynaptic reflex in the human is the stretch reflex.* Although operating in many skeletal muscles, *the stretch reflex is most easily viewed as the knee-jerk or patellar reflex* of doctor's office fame. Stretch reflexes are absent in muscles that do not attach to bone and do not contain stretch sensors; this group includes the muscles of facial expression and circular sphincter muscles, such as the external urethral sphincter.

Muscle contraction refers to the tension produced by sliding molecules of actin and myosin. However, muscle shortening does not always accompany the tension produced by the biochemical process of muscle contraction. In *isometric* muscle contractions, muscle does not change length while exerting force. For example, the biceps exerts force to hold a baby while maintaining a constant length. Perhaps less widely appreciated are muscle contractions associated with muscle-lengthening, termed *eccentric*. Eccentric muscle contractions occur commonly. For example, to lift a baby in the air, the biceps contracts but also lengthens. When the load on a muscle exceeds the muscle's *maximal contractile force*, all contractions are eccentric. Thus, you can carry (isometric) and put down (eccentric) a weight that you may not be able to lift (muscle-shortening). Interestingly, eccentric exercise strengthens muscles more effectively than isometric or muscle-shortening exercises. Eccentric contraction also creates tiny muscle tears. These tears appear to be largely responsible for the muscle soreness that occurs on the days following a new or particularly strenuous workout. With time, these small tears and the associated soreness resolve.

The stretch reflex is elicited by passive stretch or load and acts to oppose that stretch or load. Consider using the biceps to hold an empty mug when all of a sudden, tea is poured into the mug. The weight of the tea increases the load on the biceps, stretching the muscle. The stretch reflex automatically and rapidly leads to a small contraction of the biceps that opposes that stretch. All is well, and tea does not spill from the mug. Minute stretches engage sensory afferents, permitting us to maintain our posture on a moving train, carry a squirming child, and catch a softball.

To sense muscle stretch, a special group of sensory afferents—*Ia afferents*—innervate a peripheral structure called a *muscle spindle*. A muscle spindle is a capsule containing a group of *intrafusal muscle fibers* that are stretched passively when the whole muscle stretches (Fig. 22-1).

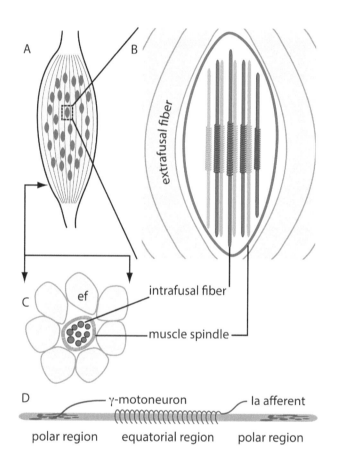

Figure 22-1 Intrafusal fibers are modified skeletal muscle fibers that do not stretch the length of the muscle, as extrafusal fibers (*ef*) do. Intrafusal fibers do not contribute to the force produced by skeletal muscle contraction but rather house muscle stretch receptors. Groups of intrafusal fibers are contained in a capsule called the muscle spindle. A: Muscle spindles (*green oblongs*) are scattered throughout skeletal muscle. B: A tangential view of a muscle spindle surrounded by extrafusal fibers is shown. C: A cross-section through a muscle spindle shows that the diameters of intrafusal fibers are much smaller than those of extrafusal fibers. D: Each intrafusal fiber contains an equatorial region surrounded on either side by polar regions. A mechanoreceptive sensory afferent called the Ia afferent weaves around the equatorial region of an intrafusal fiber. Stretch of this middle portion of the intrafusal fiber excites the Ia afferent. The polar regions of intrafusal fibers are contractile and contract in response to input from a γ-motoneuron.

Implied in the fact that there are intrafusal muscle fibers is the existence of a category of *extrafusal muscle fibers*, which are the fibers that we have been calling simply muscle fibers. Extrafusal muscle fibers produce visible muscle contractions. In contrast, intrafusal fibers:

- Are very thin and short

- Do not contribute to the force of contraction

- Are fewer in number than extrafusal muscle fibers

Intrafusal fibers are oriented parallel to extrafusal fibers. Each intrafusal fiber receives sensory innervation from a stretch-sensitive Ia afferent. Ia afferents that sense the stretch of intrafusal fibers have myelinated axons that conduct action potentials *rapidly*, at 70 m/s or more in humans, allowing for the quick transmission of information regarding unexpected loads. *Spindle afferents weave around the central region of an intrafusal fiber to sense the amount and rate of stretch in the fiber.* This central or equatorial portion of the intrafusal fiber is passively stretched by load-elicited changes in muscle length (Fig. 22-1D).

Despite serving a sensory function, intrafusal fibers are true motor fibers and are therefore contractile. However, they are only contractile at their polar ends (Fig. 22-1D). A special type of motoneuron, termed the *γ-motoneuron*, provides the motor innervation of intrafusal muscle fibers. The motoneuron that we have discussed heretofore is called an *α-motoneuron*. Note that the unqualified term *motoneuron* always refers to the α-motoneuron rather than the γ-motoneuron.

The γ-motoneuron contacts the intrafusal fiber at its *polar* ends where contraction is possible (Fig. 22-1D). Although contraction of the polar ends of the intrafusal fibers stretches the *equatorial* portion, it does not generate sufficient force to contribute to movement or load-bearing.

Ia afferents enter the spinal cord through the dorsal root and course ventrally to synapse directly onto all of the α-motoneurons of the same or *homonymous* muscle and onto many of the motoneurons that innervate its *synergists*, meaning muscles that act at the same joint and pull in the same direction (Fig. 22-2A). When a load stretches a muscle, muscle spindles and the intrafusal fibers within are stretched, eliciting a barrage of impulses that travel up Ia afferent fibers. Ia afferent activity, in turn, directly excites motoneurons that innervate the homonymous muscle and motoneurons that innervate synergists. The resulting contraction of homonymous and synergist muscles opposes the original stretch.

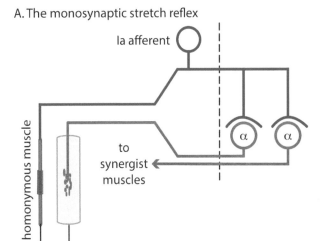

A. The monosynaptic stretch reflex

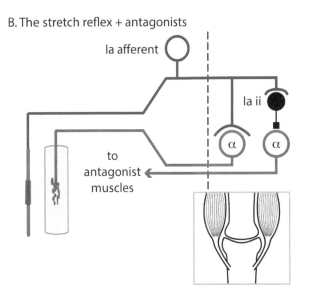

B. The stretch reflex + antagonists

Figure 22-2 The essential circuits of the stretch reflex. A minimum of anatomical details are illustrated in order to most clearly convey the essential circuitry. More anatomical detail on the spinal cord is included in Chapter 4. A: Two types of neurons form the fundamental stretch reflex circuit. The endings of Ia afferents wrap around intrafusal fibers (*if*) and are activated by stretch. Ia afferents cross from the periphery into the central nervous system (*dotted line*) and directly contact α-motoneurons (*α*) that project into the periphery to innervate extrafusal fibers (*ef*) in the same or homonymous muscle, as well as in synergist muscles. Synergist muscles are those that work in concert to produce the same action. The fundamental stretch reflex circuit contains one central synapse, the synapse from the Ia afferent to an α-motoneuron. B: Muscle stretch also results in the inhibition of antagonist muscles. The inhibition of antagonist muscles is accomplished through activation of the glycinergic Ia inhibitory interneuron (*Ia ii*). The inset (*blue box*) shows an agonist–antagonist pair of muscles. The members of an agonist–antagonist muscle pair move a joint in opposing directions.

When a muscle is stretched and the homonymous muscle contracted, activity in muscles that oppose contraction of the homonymous muscle is inhibited. Inhibition occurs via a synapse from the Ia afferent onto an inhibitory interneuron that in turn inhibits motoneurons innervating the *antagonist muscle* (Fig. 22-2B). The Ia afferent-to-inhibitory interneuron-to-antagonist motoneuron circuit is the basis for reciprocal inhibition. This pathway is *disynaptic* since it involves two synapses—the first between the Ia afferent and the inhibitory interneuron and the second between the inhibitory interneuron and the motoneuron. The inhibitory interneuron in this case is such an important cell that it has its own name: the *Ia inhibitory interneuron*. The Ia inhibitory interneuron contains *glycine*, the second most prevalent fast inhibitory neurotransmitter behind γ-aminobutyric acid (GABA) and the most prevalent one in the spinal cord.

In general, the stretch reflex is strongest in muscles that oppose gravity, termed *physiological extensors*, thus helping to maintain postural control. The term *physiological extensor* refers to muscles that, when contracted, oppose gravity, whereas the term *physiological flexor* denotes a muscle that works in concert with gravity. According to this classification scheme, the quadriceps is a physiological extensor. Similarly, jaw-closing muscles, such as the masseter or temporalis, elevate the jaw against gravity and thus are also physiological extensors, even though their activation decreases joint angle. The terms of physiological extensors and flexors are robust in that they are invariant across different joints: the quadriceps, whether extending the knee or flexing the hip, opposes gravity. Furthermore, these terms are useful because motor circuits are organized around physiological extensors and flexors rather than around joint extensors and flexors. To stay upright and to avoid a permanently slack-jawed appearance, brainstem motor centers project to the spinal cord and tonically excite physiological extensors—not joint extensors (see Chapter 23). Thus, motor circuits respect a classification of muscles according to their work with respect to gravity.

γ-MOTONEURONS ENSURE THAT THE STRETCH REFLEX IS ONLINE DURING ACTIVE MUSCLE CONTRACTION

The stretch reflex is not only interesting because it is a monosynaptic reflex but also because it illustrates an important element in motor control—the role of peripheral feedback. In order to make movements correctly, motoneurons need to receive input on the *current* state of the muscles: their length, rate of lengthening or shortening, and whether they are contracting or relaxing. The Ia afferent innervation of muscle spindles provides some of this information.

As explained earlier, activity in α-motoneurons leads to contraction of extrafusal fibers but not intrafusal fibers. This presents an immediate problem: if a muscle contracts and the extrafusal fibers shorten but the intrafusal fibers do not contract, then the intrafusal fibers will become slack (Fig. 22-3A, B). In a slack configuration, no change in muscle length can be signaled by the spindle receptors. It is therefore crucial that intra- and extrafusal fibers are the same length at all times. γ-Motoneurons serve to ensure this by synapsing on the polar regions of intrafusal muscle fibers. When a γ-motoneuron fires, the polar ends of the innervated intrafusal muscle fiber contract, which in turn stretches the equatorial region of the fiber.

During most reflex and voluntary movements, α- and γ-motoneurons are coactivated. This *α-γ coactivation* mandates that the intrafusal and extrafusal muscle fibers are maintained at similar lengths (Fig. 22-3C). α-Motoneurons lie in the same motoneuron pools with γ-motoneurons innervating the same muscle. In the case of the stretch reflex, Ia afferents synapse on both α- and γ-motoneurons. Similarly, axons descending from brainstem or cortex, important for self-generated movements, typically synapse on γ-motoneurons as well as on α-motoneurons. This circuitry ensures that muscle spindles are ready to signal any changes in muscle length due to unexpected stretches or loads that may occur during reflexive or voluntary movements.

ACTIVATION OF γ-MOTONEURONS ALONE CAN LEAD TO MUSCLE CONTRACTION

One result of the stretch reflex circuitry is that *by activating γ-motoneurons alone, one can indirectly excite α-motoneurons: this is called the γ-loop* (Fig. 22-3D). We go through this step by step:

1. γ-Motoneuron activity contracts intrafusal fibers at the polar regions.

2. Contraction of the intrafusal fibers at the poles stretches the equatorial region of the intrafusal fiber.

3. Stretch of the equatorial portion of the intrafusal fiber excites Ia afferents.

4. Activity in Ia afferents excites α-motoneurons innervating the homonymous muscle.

In sum, the γ-loop starts with excitation of a γ-motoneuron and ultimately results in a force-producing muscle contraction (Fig. 22-3D).

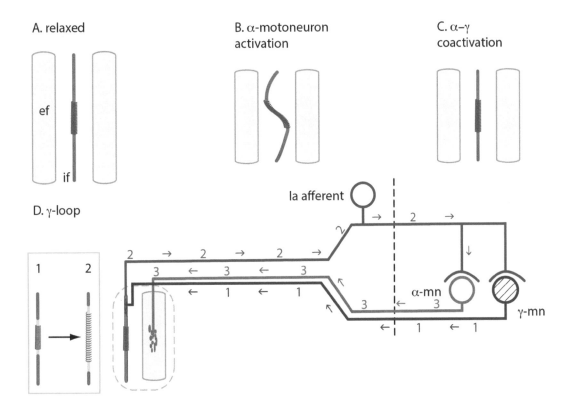

A. relaxed

B. α-motoneuron activation

C. α–γ coactivation

D. γ-loop

Ia afferent

α-mn

γ-mn

Figure 22-3 A: In the relaxed state, intrafusal fibers (*if*) are taut and sensitive to stretch. However, if an α-motoneuron were to be activated alone (B), the extrafusal fibers (*ef*) would contract but the intrafusal fibers would go slack. In this situation, a load would have no effect on an intrafusal fiber. Consequently, Ia afferents would go "off-line" as they could no longer sense stretch. C: α-γ coactivation resolves this problem by maintaining the intra- and extrafusal fibers at matching lengths. D: The γ loop starts with γ-motoneuron (*γ-mn*) activation (*brown arrows marked 1*). The effect of γ-motoneuron activation is contraction of the polar ends of the intrafusal fibers (*see inset in blue box*). Contraction of the polar ends of the intrafusal fibers stretches the equatorial region of the intrafusal fibers, resulting in Ia afferent activation (*blue arrows marked 2*). Ia afferent activation leads to excitation of α-motoneurons (*α-mn*). Activity in α-motoneurons (*red arrows marked 3*) leads to extrafusal fiber contraction and muscle tension. Thus, the γ-loop starts with γ-motoneuron activation and culminates in muscle tension that is dependent on sensory activity in Ia afferents.

The γ-loop is conceptually important. Despite the rule of α-γ coactivation, motor control centers in the brainstem preferentially excite γ-motoneurons over γ-motoneurons under particular conditions. Upon selective or preferential activation of γ-motoneurons, tension of the intrafusal fiber increases, thereby increasing the sensitivity of the Ia afferents and the gain of the stretch reflex.

Gain is the ratio of output to input. In the case of the stretch reflex, gain refers to the amount of homonymous muscle shortening per stretch of that muscle. For example, if a muscle is stretched by 5 mm, and the stretch reflex contracts the muscle by 3 mm, the gain of this reflex would be 3/5 or 0.6. When the gain of a reflex equals 0, the reflex is fully suppressed. When the gain of a reflex is 1, the reflex acts as a perfect *servomechanism*, meaning that the reflex responds to a stretch with an opposing contraction of equal magnitude.

Let's return to selective activation of γ-motoneurons by descending motor control axons. When γ-motoneurons are activated, subsequent muscle stretches will elicit larger contractions, reflecting a higher stretch reflex gain. *An increase*

in the gain of the stretch reflex may be particularly useful when delicate movements are being performed in unpredictable environments. For instance, when walking on ice, extreme sensitivity to even the minutest slippage—which inevitably stretches physiological extensors—may prevent a serious fall and resulting injury. The gain of the stretch reflex varies across conditions such as sleep, wake, exercise, walking, and so on. In addition, some motor disorders are associated with either an increase or decrease in reflex gain.

REFLEX TESTING IS A MINIMALLY INVASIVE PROCEDURE THAT TESTS THE INTEGRITY OF THE STRETCH REFLEX CIRCUIT

In *reflex testing*, an electromyographic (EMG) recording electrode is placed in a muscle and a stimulating electrode is inserted transcutaneously into the nerve leading to that muscle (Fig. 22-4A). Within the nerve, the axons with

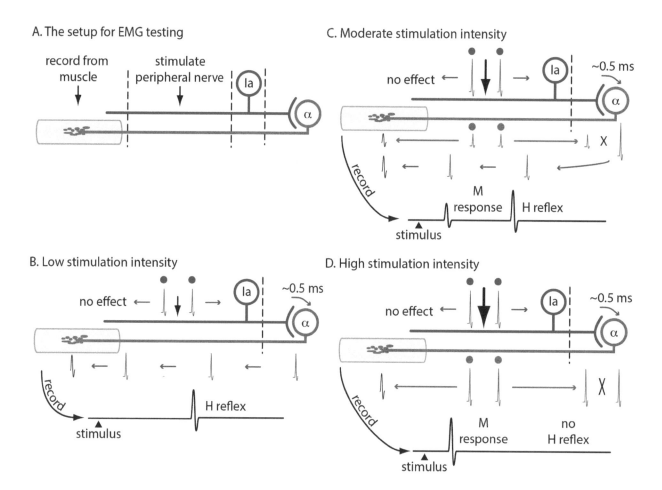

Figure 22-4 The basic setup and ideal results of electromyography (EMG) testing are illustrated. A: Electrical stimulation of a peripheral nerve has the potential to excite the axons of Ia afferents (*blue*) and motoneurons (*red*). The effect of nerve stimulation on muscle activity is measured using EMG recording from the muscle. B–D: The height of the action potentials is proportional to the number of axons excited. B: At the lowest stimulation intensities (*small black arrow*), only Ia afferents are excited (*filled blue circles*), producing action potentials in Ia afferents that travel away from the stimulation electrode toward either side. The action potentials in Ia afferents that travel toward the muscle have no effect. The Ia afferent action potentials that travel orthodromically toward the spinal cord synapse on and excite α-motoneurons, leading to a muscle contraction after a delay of several milliseconds, depending on conduction distance to the muscle. This muscle contraction is termed the *H reflex*. C: At moderate stimulation intensities (*medium black arrow*), more Ia afferent axons along with some motoneuron axons are excited. Action potentials are color coded according to whether they occur within Ia afferent axons (*blue*) or motoneuron axons (*red*). Electrical stimulation produces action potentials that travel away from the stimulation electrode on either side of both Ia and motoneuron axons. The orthodromically traveling action potentials in motoneuron axons reach the muscle and elicit a muscle contraction. This is termed the *M response*. The M response occurs much earlier than the H reflex because: (1) there is no synaptic delay; and (2) the conduction distance and time are far less. There are also action potentials that travel antidromically in the motoneuron axon. These action potentials collide with action potentials arising from the synaptic responses in motoneurons to Ia afferent input. Since action potentials that collide (*small x*) do not continue on, only a portion of the action potentials continue to travel orthodromically in the motoneuron axons. The result is a small M response followed by an H reflex. C: At the highest stimulation intensities (*large black arrow*), all Ia afferent and motoneuron axons are excited. Therefore, *all* of the action potentials arising from synaptic responses in motoneurons to Ia afferent input collide with action potentials traveling antidromically in the motoneuron axon (*large x*). Consequently, there is a large M response and no H reflex.

the lowest electrical activation thresholds are Ia afferents. Therefore, at low stimulating intensities, only Ia afferents are activated (Fig. 22-4B). After a delay of 5–30 ms (depending on how far the stimulating electrode is from the muscle), a muscle contraction occurs. The pathway taken is Ia activation → α-motoneuron excitation → muscle activation recorded by the EMG electrode. This is the *H reflex*.

When the stimulation intensity is increased, *motor axons are directly activated*, and a muscle action potential

occurs at very short latency (<5 ms)—this is called the *M response* (Fig. 22-4C). After the M response, an H reflex still occurs. Note that this sequence occurs only after increasing the stimulation intensity because motoneuron axons have a greater electrical threshold for activation than do Ia afferent axons. When the stimulation intensity increases even further, the M response grows but the H reflex shrinks. At the highest intensities, only an M response occurs. Try to work your way through why this happens before reading on.

Hint: Remember that when you stimulate an axon, action potentials travel in both directions.

To understand the spoiler, we need to define two terms regarding how action potentials travel. *Antidromic* refers to the wrong direction or the direction that is counter to the normal direction of action potential traffic. *Orthodromic* is the right direction, the direction of normal action potential traffic.

Now, here is the spoiler. As the stimulation intensity increases above the threshold for activating motoneuron axons, more and more motoneuron axons are activated along with the full complement of Ia afferents. An action potential in a motoneuron axon travels both orthodromically to the muscle, producing the M response, and antidromically to invade the cell bodies of motoneurons in the spinal cord (Fig. 22-4D). Meanwhile, action potentials in Ia afferents travel orthodromically to the spinal cord to synapse on homonymous motoneurons. By the time that the Ia afferent action potential excites the motoneuron, the motoneuron is still in the absolute refractory period from the action potential that arrived antidromically from the motoneuron axon. Consequently, the motoneuron cannot fire an action potential in response to excitatory synaptic input from the Ia afferent. Thus, action potentials that travel antidromically *occlude* or *collide with* action potentials arriving orthodromically. When *all* the motor axons are activated, the maximal M response occurs, and the action potentials in the motor axons traveling centrally invade all of the motoneurons, thereby blocking the H reflex from occurring at all.

ACTIVATION OF TENDON RECEPTORS DISYNAPTICALLY INHIBITS CONTRACTION

A second muscle reflex, the *inverse stretch reflex* or *inverse myotactic reflex*, is a disynaptic reflex (i.e., it involves two synapses and three neurons). The inverse stretch reflex is engaged during active contraction and acts to oppose the contraction itself! Although this may appear counterproductive at first glance, this reflex serves a number of purposes, including protecting muscle injury from overcontraction during very forceful movements. *Opisthatonos*, a symptom of *tetanus* (see Chapter 11), dramatically illustrates the damage wreaked by unchecked, excessive muscle contraction.

The inverse stretch reflex depends on the *Ib afferent*, another fast-conducting proprioceptive receptor like the Ia afferent (Fig. 22-5). The endings of the Ib afferent weave in and among the *Golgi tendon organs* formed by a tendon's collagen fibers located at the junction between tendon and extrafusal fiber. *Ib afferents are excited by tension generated by muscle*

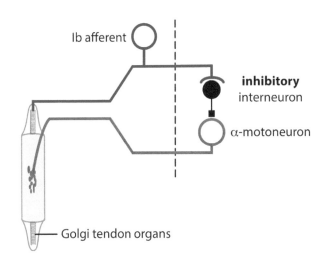

Figure 22-5 Ib afferents weave in and out through the Golgi tendon organs located at the junction of tendon and muscle. During active contraction, but not during passive stretch, the Golgi tendon organs are stretched and Ib afferents are excited. Ib afferents excite inhibitory interneurons, which in turn inhibit homonymous α-motoneurons.

contraction rather than by passive stretch. Inhibitory interneurons in the ventral horn are activated by Ib afferents and, in turn, inhibit homonymous α-motoneurons (Fig. 22-5). The inhibitory interneurons involved in the Ib reflex are among those targeted by tetanus toxin.

Ib afferent–mediated inhibition of α-motoneurons serves to increase stiffness by dampening changes in muscle tension. The strength of the Ib afferent–mediated reflex is regulated by input from local interneurons and supraspinal sources. Thus, when a great deal of force is required, Ib afferent–mediated inhibition can be turned down, turned off, or even reversed, allowing large increases in muscle tension to occur without feedback inhibition. For instance, when trying to hit a home run, the Ib reflex is suppressed. In contrast, when a highly controlled touch is required, as during threading a needle, the strength of the Ib reflex can be increased.

Ia and Ib afferents are both excited by changes in muscle, but their response characteristics are distinct. Ia afferents respond to *passive stretch* of the muscle spindles, such as occurs when a load is added to a muscle, but they do not respond to active contraction. In contrast, Ib afferents respond to stimulation of the Golgi tendon organs during active muscle contraction but do not respond to passive stretch.

THE NOCICEPTIVE WITHDRAWAL REFLEX REQUIRES LEARNING

The stretch, inverse stretch, and vestibuloocular reflexes (VOR; see Chapter 19) are just a few of many reflexes in the human and other mammals. The *nociceptive withdrawal reflex* is representative of most reflexes in its complexity. Additionally, the nociceptive withdrawal reflex is of great clinical importance. We therefore examine it here.

The nociceptive withdrawal reflex serves an important protective function because it automatically removes a body part, such as a hand, from harm's way, such as a flame. Consider that you step on a thorn with your heel, with the ball of your foot, or with your little toe. A withdrawal occurs, not because of a cognitive decision but automatically. Moreover, the withdrawal is *tailored* to the location of the stimulus. Thus, the heel is removed from the ground in the case of a thorn in the heel, the toe is withdrawn in the case of a thorn in the toe, and so on. For example, stimulation on the ball of the foot leads to reflex activation of the soleus muscle, and activation of the soleus muscle then *removes* the ball of the foot from the ground. Similarly, heel stimulation leads to reflex activation of the tibialis anterior muscle, which in turn leads to the heel being lifted from the ground. In this way, the area of stimulation matches the area of withdrawal. Put in other terms, the *withdrawal* field of the nociceptive withdrawal reflex overlaps the receptive field.

The nociceptive withdrawal reflex is a polysynaptic circuit that involves a minimum of two central neurons. One of the necessary central neurons is, of course, a motoneuron. The other neuron required for the nociceptive withdrawal reflex is an interneuron that we will call a *reflex encoder*. Reflex encoding neurons are sensorimotor and are present in the deep dorsal horn, close to the ventral horn. They receive input from a variety of sensory afferents, both nociceptors and Aβ mechanoreceptors, and they target motoneurons to specific muscles. In the adult, the sensory input to reflex encoders is weighted proportionally to the withdrawal or unloading action of the targeted muscles. For example, a reflex encoder that targets soleus motoneurons weights sensory input from the ball of the foot far more than input from the heel, *and* the withdrawal field produced by soleus muscle activation is centered over the ball of the foot (Fig. 22-6). In sum, the nociceptive withdrawal reflex transforms sensory input into a muscle-centric signal. Consequently, reflex encoders within the dorsal horn are organized topographically by muscle, termed *musculotopic*, rather than *somatotopically* by skin area. Ultimately, the musculotopic organization is functionally advantageous because it best aligns the reflex's effect to the triggering stimulus.

Aligning the withdrawal field to the point of injurious input means that sensory input and motor output do not necessarily arrive and emerge from the same spinal segment. For example, sensory input from the ball of the foot arrives

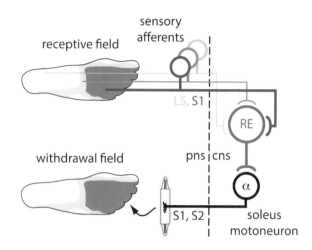

Figure 22-6 Sensory afferents from the foot synapse on reflex encoder neurons (*RE*) in the deep dorsal horn. Sensory input arrives into L5 and S1 segments, and motor outflow emerges from the upper two sacral segments (*S1, S2*). Sensory inputs from different areas of the foot have different levels of influence on the RE neuron through synapses of differing weights (proportional to the width of the line). The most heavily weighted inputs to reflex encoders are from areas of skin that are withdrawn by the contraction of the motoneurons targeted by those reflex encoder neurons. In this way, the receptive field of a reflex encoder neuron maps onto the withdrawal field produced by activation of the same reflex encoder neuron.   Modified from Schouenborg J. Action-based sensory encoding in spinal sensorimotor circuits. *Brain Res Rev* 57: 111–117, 2008 with permission of the publisher, Elsevier; and from Sonnenborg FA, Andersen OK, Arendt-Nielsen F. Modular organization of excitatory and inhibitory reflex receptive fields elicited by electrical stimulation of the foot sole in man. *Clin Neurophysiol* 111: 2160–2169, 2000, with permission of the publisher, Elsevier.

into L5 and S1 segments, whereas the motor innervation of the soleus emerges from the S1 and S2 segments. As another example, input from fingers innervated by dorsal roots from C7 and C8 elicits a withdrawal that depends largely on muscles innervated by ventral roots from C5 and C6. The functional hookup of sensory input to motor output critical to the withdrawal reflex differs substantially from the anatomically simpler connections involved in the homonymous stretch reflex. Indeed, it now appears that circuits for the nociceptive withdrawal reflex are forged during development through a learning process that has been termed *somatosensory imprinting*.

MODULATION OF REFLEXES OCCURS ACROSS MULTIPLE TIME SCALES

Modulation is common to all reflexes. At one extreme, reflexes can be turned off, their gain set to zero. This occurs with the VOR during intentional gaze shift or with the Ib reflex during an emphatic arm swing. Even the stretch reflex can be "turned off" through willful suppression. Of enormous importance, reflexive movements are continually modulated to optimally accommodate the circumstances. The VOR gain is increased or decreased for near or far vision, whereas modulation of Ia and Ib reflexes serves fine, delicate movements.

Beyond the moment-by-moment modulation of reflexes, quite a few reflexes only occur during the early postnatal period (see Table 22-1). These developmentally regulated reflexes are sometimes termed *primitive reflexes*; indeed, many are shared across mammals. For example, the *suck reflex* is automatically elicited by a touch of the hard palate in babies. The *root reflex*, elicited by a touch near the mouth, leads to a baby "rooting around" with its mouth open. As may be obvious, the suck and root reflexes serve to aide newborns in getting started with their very first job, which is sucking milk from the mother's nipple.

Primitive reflexes are transient in that they are not observed after some number of months. For example, the root, suck, and other reflexes that aid feeding are not observed after about 6 months of age, even though the baby may still be suckling. Importantly, although the reflexes are not observed, they are still present. They have not vanished even though they are not apparent in healthy adults. *Past the early postnatal period, primitive reflexes are suppressed by descending signals from the brain.* Any interruption of this descending suppression *releases* the reflexes, thereby serving as a useful sign of brain damage. The presence of such *release signs* is clinically important because it indicates damage of normal descending suppression. After damage to the corticospinal tract, the *plantar reflex* appears; this is known as the *Babinski sign* (see Chapter 23). Damage to

the prefrontal cortex through stroke or neurodegeneration (e.g., *frontotemporal dementia* or *FTD*) releases the *grasp reflex* from suppression. Severely affected patients are even unable to deliberately stop a reflex grasp, vividly illustrating that release signs represent reflexes in an unmodulated state (i.e., without potential suppression).

CENTRAL CIRCUITS CAN GENERATE PATTERNED MOVEMENT SEQUENCES

Most of our actions are repeats. The specifics of how we say "good morning" change little from day to day. Whenever we walk, whether across a carpet or an icy and uneven field, the core fundamentals of our walk remain the same. The confident walk on carpet and the tentative one on ice share a single basic gait of alternating leg steps of swing and stance. What neural mechanisms generate this and other fundamental movement patterns? Walking is too complicated to be a reflex, or even a chain of reflexes, and too simple and repetitive to require deliberate or volitional control at every step. Indeed, the basic gait pattern and other movement fundamentals comprise a category of *semiautomatic* movement patterns that depend on central networks of neurons.

As a neural compromise, circuits within the spinal cord and brainstem, termed *central pattern generators*, generate the core element of rhythmic and repeated movements such as walking, chewing, and micturition. *Central pattern generators create a patterned activation and relaxation of specific muscles through selective central connections and can do so in the absence of peripheral feedback or supraspinal input.* For example, a brainstem central pattern generator rhythmically activates jaw closer motoneurons to produce a chewing motion.

Central pattern generators *do not depend on sensory feedback from the periphery* and therefore do not require contributions from reflexes. Yet, central pattern generators cannot produce fully elaborated versions of rhythmic and repeated movements without input from the periphery *and* the participation of reflexes. For example, the force of jaw closure is stronger and perhaps slower when chewing a hard candy than gum.

The actual neuronal elements that comprise a central pattern generator are interconnected neurons that form a circuit. Our understanding of central pattern generator function stems in large part from experiments in invertebrates and also from experiments in early vertebrates such as the lamprey. These basic investigations have demonstrated that *a single circuit can be reconfigured to produce multiple related movements*. In the mammal, this means that a single

Table 22-1 REFLEXES DEVELOPMENTALLY RESTRICTED TO INFANCY

REFLEX NAME	DESCRIPTION	AGE
Grasp	Stroking palm elicits a grasp	<6 months
Moro	Unexpected sound elicits extension of neck and all four limbs and cry, followed by flexion of the limbs	<6 months
Plantar	Firm stroke to the sole elicits dorsiflexion of large toe and fanning of the remaining toes	<2 years
Root	Stroke to corner of the mouth elicits a turn toward the stimulus and mouth-opening, useful for suckling	<4 months
Snout	Tapping the lips elicits pursing of the lips so that they resemble a snout	<1 year
Suck	Touch to the roof of the mouth elicits sucking	<4 months
Tonic neck	Head turn to one side elicits ipsilateral arm extension along with contralateral flexion at the elbow	<7 months

circuit serves walking and running or chewing and sucking. An important limitation to the central pattern generator concept as it is applied to humans is that we do not know the exact boundaries of human central pattern generator circuits, nor can we enumerate the neuronal elements that comprise central pattern generator circuits. Thus, central pattern generator circuits, particularly those in humans, are better established as conceptual framework than as specific anatomical reality.

To better understand the control of semiautomatic movements, we examine walking in some depth because it is both exemplary and important:

- All parts of the motor system participate, in characteristic ways, in producing walking. Examining each region's contribution to walking will illuminate that region's general mode of operation.

- Locomotion is an integral human function, which, when impaired, leads to a severe compromise of a person's quality of life. In other words, people are fairly unhappy if they lose their ability to get around.

HUMAN LOCOMOTION REQUIRES FORWARD PROPULSION WHILE REMAINING BALANCED ON TWO LIMBS

Locomotion in humans is different from locomotion in other animals because we face the dual challenge of (1) staying upright and (2) advancing forward. Thus, successful locomotion requires postural stability or balance, provided by the brainstem, as well as some form of propulsion, typically termed *gait*, that employs contributions from both spinal and brainstem circuits. In the following section, we examine gait, and, in the next chapter, postural control is discussed.

Normal human gait involves stepping movements controlled by central pattern generators in the spinal cord. Coordination of the two legs' stepping movements with each other and with the arms, shoulders, and head also involve a central pattern generator in the midbrain. Thus, there are at least two central pattern generators involved in producing the walking gait. Here, we focus on the stepping central pattern generator present in the spinal cord.

To best understand gait, we examine the gait cycle from its most elemental component—the movements of one leg—to its most integrative—coordination of the two legs with trunk and arm movements. Each leg cycles between swing and support during locomotion (Fig. 22-7):

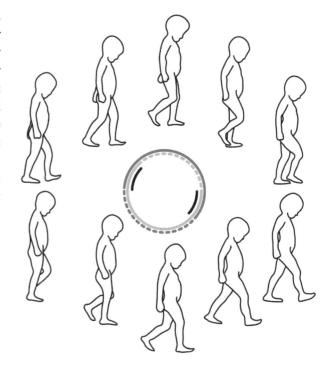

Figure 22-7 The walking cycle of a young infant. The cycle proceeds in a clockwise direction. This child's gait is not fully mature, but shows the essential features of human locomotion. Each leg alternates between support (*solid blue and red lines in the circle*) and swing (*dotted lines*). Support starts at heel strike and swing starts with lift off. For example, the left leg (*red*) begins the support phase with a heel strike as the right leg (*blue*) is still in contact with the ground. Weight transfers to the left leg as the body is propelled forward. As the left leg assumes the weight of the body, the right leg begins the swing phase and so on. Between the left and right legs' swings, both legs are in contact with the ground, a period of double support (*black arcs*). The immaturity of the gait is evident in the minimal arm swing, the downward head posture, and less ankle flexion than is typically present in a healthy adult.   Modified from Muybridge E. The human figure in motion: An electro-photographic investigation of consecutive phases of muscular actions. London: Chapman & Hall, 1904.

- In the *swing phase*, the foot is not in contact with the ground.

- To initiate the swing, the hip and knee flex, lifting the toes off the ground. This is termed *toe-off*.

- The leg advances forward to a point ahead of the body.

- During the *support phase*, the foot is in contact with the ground, providing support to the body.

- To begin the stance, the leg extends and the heel lands on the ground, termed *heel strike*.

- Weight is loaded onto the extended leg, which when flexed at the knee, acts as a spring, accepting the load.

- At mid-stance, the knee straightens and the leg, positioned directly below the body with a flat foot, supports the entire weight of the body.

- The leg is extended backward, propelling the body forward. The foot rolls forward on to the toes, ready for lift-off, as the other leg touches down to begin a period of double support.

Each leg cycles repetitively through stance and swing phases. The movements of the two legs are coordinated so that after one leg contacts the ground, the other leg lifts off. In the moments intervening between heel strike on one side and lift-off on the contralateral side, both feet are in contact with the ground. During two periods of *double support*—each accounting for about 10% of the walking cycle—the weight of the body shifts from the leg that is about to lift off to the leg that has just landed. As the leg that is about to lift off swings forward, the contralateral leg moves to a position directly underneath the body. Trunk, arm, and head movements are coordinated with alternating leg movements during locomotion.

LOCOMOTOR CENTRAL PATTERN GENERATORS IN SPINAL CORD AND MIDBRAIN

The central pattern generator in the lumbar spinal cord generates a rudimentary version of gait. A circuit on each side produces the fundamental pattern of a leg stride, and commissural connections between the sides provide basic coordination between the two legs. By alternating the strength of synaptic connections within the central pattern generator, the same spinal circuit that produces a walking gait, differently configured, can give rise to related movements such as crawling, skating, the kicking component of swimming, and, of course, running. Thus, by modulating the connectivity and level of excitation within one basic, step-producing circuit, not one, but a multitude of gaits becomes possible. One weird-but-true consequence of this organization is that the cerebellum (a primary source of motor modulation) can engage circuits on either side of the cord such that the two legs walk at different speeds *or even in different directions* when on a treadmill with two independently controlled half-belts (more about this in Chapter 24).

Running represents a variant of the walking pattern. During running, the support phase decreases in duration so that one leg lifts off while the other is still swinging. This results in the body being airborne for a time. With increasing speed, the support period progressively shortens, the length of time airborne increases, and greater muscle force is used to propel the body forward.

The spinal central pattern generator for gait does not operate solo and indeed needs an external trigger to be initiated. A central pattern generator in the midbrain, the *mesencephalic locomotor region*, provides the start signal to gait-producing circuits in the spinal cord. *As the output of the mesencephalic locomotor region increases, the locomotion generated increases in speed, from a slow to a faster and faster walk and eventually to a jog, a run, and a sprint.* Using this flexible arrangement, the midbrain and lumbosacral cord work together to produce locomotion at different speeds by adjusting the strength of the intervening signal.

PERIPHERAL FEEDBACK REINFORCES GAIT AND ADJUSTS LOCOMOTION TO EXTERNAL CONDITIONS

Remember that central pattern generators produce a baseline movement and do not require any peripheral, sensory feedback or reflex participation to do so. Although true, this principle is a somewhat artificial construct because the movement produced by a deafferented central pattern generator will only work under ideal circumstances (i.e., when a person in the peak of health walks load-free across a flat, hard surface). Even in these idealized circumstances, the movement provided by a central pattern generator alone would be clearly "off," not quite normal. On the other hand, when a middle-aged professor with the beginnings of arthritis, carrying a briefcase in one hand and a gym bag in the other, cuts across a rain-slick football field, sensory feedback is absolutely critical to reinforce and modify the core movements involved in gait and thereby prevent stumbling.

An example of sensory feedback occurs when the leg is extended behind the body and about to lift off. The leg is extended behind the body through the activation of hip extensors, which produces a passive stretch of the hip flexors. In this case, passive stretch does not result from an external load but instead from the active contraction of antagonist muscles. Thus, just prior to toe-off, backward leg extension stretches hip flexor muscles. Ia afferents that innervate hip flexors such as the iliopsoas and quadriceps muscles are excited, which in turn leads to contraction of the homonymous muscles. Iliopsoas and quadriceps contraction facilitates hip flexion and lifting the leg off the ground. In sum, *extending the leg backward passively stretches the relaxed hip flexors, triggering a stretch reflex that in turn helps lift the leg to start the swing phase* (Fig. 22-8A, B).

In a second example of sensory feedback, activity in Ib afferents reinforces the fundamentals of gait and ensures that muscle strength matches load. Consider a person

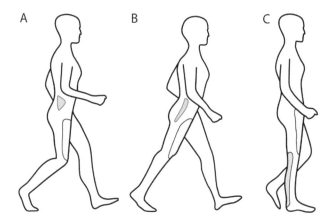

Figure 22-8 A–B: Feedback from Ia afferents innervating the iliopsoas (*red*) and quadriceps (*blue*) muscles signals the stretch caused by hip extensors and excites homonymous muscles contributing to the hip flexion needed for lift off. In A, both muscles are short and neither is stretched. When the leg extends back (B), extending the hip joint, both muscles are stretched. Stretching these muscles facilitates hip flexor motoneurons through the stretch reflex. C: During stance, the quadriceps (*blue*) and gastrocnemius (*tan*) muscles contract to bear the weight of the body and load. The stronger the contraction, the more excitation of Ib afferents occurs. During locomotion, Ib activation leads to *excitation* of the homonymous muscles. Note that the excitatory effect of Ib afferents on the homonymous muscle only occurs during locomotion and is exactly opposite to the effect mediated by the Ib reflex at other times.

carrying a toddler in one arm and groceries in the other. The combined weight of the loads is opposed by strong contractions of leg extensors acting at the knee and ankle, the quadriceps and gastrocnemius muscles, respectively. Recall that the quadriceps serves as both a hip flexor, as in the first example, and a knee extensor, as in this example. The strong contractions of the quadriceps and gastrocnemius muscles excite Ib afferents—and here a funny thing happens. Instead of inhibiting the homonymous muscles, the effect of Ib afferents is reversed—*during locomotion*—to excite them (Fig. 22-8C). The *excitation of leg extensors prolongs the stance, ensuring that the leg does not take off until the other leg has accepted enough weight.* Thus, this reflex guarantees that a person's leg will not buckle while walking with a heavy load. In people with weakened muscles, the body itself may be sufficiently heavy to elicit a prolongation of the stance phase, resulting in a delay in lift off and a general slowing of gait.

Unexpected external objects elicit rapid reflex reactions, rapid enough to allow people to recover from a stumble or slip without actually falling and to do so with time to spare. In fact, *healthy people rarely trip or fall, largely because the stumbling correction reaction is excessively fast and highly redundant.* Many things have to go wrong before the system fails, a feature commonly referred to as a large "safety factor."

Although the core movements involved in walking are stereotyped, walking varies with speed, walking surface, and body condition. At a distance of a block, we recognize friends and can even tell something about their mood. We discern this information by recognizing a friend's individual and distinctive gait rather than by making out the details of that friend's face. As another example of gait changing with circumstances such as mood, fatigue, injury, and motivation, compare a teenager's gait when walking to the principal's office after being caught passing notes in class, shoulders slumped and rotating minimally, with the same individual's gait when walking up to deliver a valedictorian speech, shoulders back and torso rotating in full swagger.

Walking is a learned motor pattern that continues to change with age. When children learn to walk, they begin with a characteristically different gait, and, as age takes its toll on joints, muscles, and vim, we alter our gait again. The riddle of the Sphinx asks, "Which creature in the morning goes on four feet, at noon on two, and in the evening upon three?" The answer, provided according to mythological legend by Oedipus who interpreted time of day as a metaphor for time in life cycle, is a human. A baby crawls on four feet before learning to walk on two and until needing a third leg, or cane, to ambulate. That is to say that walking proceeds through a series of predictable changes as a person develops and then ages.

When babies, top heavy with their disproportionately large heads, first begin to walk while holding on to objects to provide balance, they walk in a side-to-side waddle with little forward motion. The arms are held up, used entirely for balance, and do not swing. The legs are held fairly rigidly, particularly at the ankle, and the initial touch down is on either the toes or a flat foot. An infant's walk involves no true swing phase but rather consists mainly of double support, briefly interrupted by lifting of alternating legs. Each leg leaves the ground, raised from the hip en masse, and "plops" down shortly thereafter. As an infant's ability to maintain balance matures, the ability to walk independently is gained. By 3 years of age, a relatively mature walk is in place, complete with heel strike upon touch down and alternating arm motions.

Walking is learned, and that is very important. Apparently by instinct, babies get the itch to move themselves about in the world. However, they have to learn how to ambulate. What advantages emerge from a baby's learning to walk rather than simply being born with the innate ability to walk? One advantage is that babies born with a physical anomaly can learn an effective, albeit different, method for ambulating. Think of conjoined twins. If at all possible, conjoined twins will find a way to get around, something that would be impossible with a rigid, inborn program for walking wholly inappropriate to the twins' anatomy. A second, probably more important advantage stems from the fact that one must lead either a very short or a very charmed life to avoid any injury that impacts walking. Whether it be a pulled muscle, a broken bone, or a central nervous system disease, things happen in a typical life. Yet, for the most part, people learn, probably using similar learning circuits to those used in infancy, to adjust their locomotor pattern to achieve their ambulatory goals.

For infants, practice plays a critical role in learning to walk. Infants walk for hours each day, apparently by biological mandate. If their strides were of average adult length, infants would cover an average of more than 8 miles (13 km) in a day. Given the intensity with which infants practice walking, one may wonder whether intense practice rather than immobility would better serve people trying to recover after injury.

An unfortunate exception to the generalization that people compensate for injuries and continue to move about is spinal cord injury. One of the first questions that a patient with spinal cord injury typically asks is, "Will I ever walk again?" Right now, the answer, for someone with a complete or nearly complete transection, is typically no, at least not in the same way as before the injury. For one, bipedal walking requires balance that, as discussed in the next chapter, requires a connection from the brainstem to the spinal cord. This connection is interrupted by many spinal cord injuries.

It is reasonable to ask whether gait would be possible if balance and an upright posture were assured in a spinal cord injured patient. Consistent with the presence of a central pattern generator for gait in the lumbar spinal cord, this is possible in cats with a transected thoracic cord. Such an injured cat will step if supported upon a moving treadmill and given drugs, such as dopamine receptor agonists, that facilitate motor excitability. However, this same approach does not work in humans. People with spinal cord injuries who lose the ability to walk do not recover spontaneous ambulation. Although innovative prosthetic interventions have allowed a limited number of experimental subjects to recover limited motor function, such treatments cannot be scaled up to serve even a fraction of the population paralyzed by spinal cord injury.

As people age, muscle strength decreases. In addition, older people have a compromised sense of balance, in part due to age-related otoconial degeneration. The resulting impairment in maintaining balance is largely responsible for older people adopting a conservative gait characterized by:

- More time spent in double support
- Reduction in stride length
- Reduction in speed

Even in athletic people of advanced age, the amount of walking time in double support increases, and the amount of running time spent airborne decreases. Older people tend to walk with less agility, bending their ankles less, extending their hips less, and swinging their arms less. In general, the safety factor for walking decreases in the elderly. An older person runs a high risk of tripping and falling because the clearance between the foot and ground during the swing phase decreases. Deterioration in vision further exacerbates the risks of walking. Finally, the psychological impact of fear should not be underestimated because the elderly may have either fallen themselves or watched a loved one fall, learning first-hand the difficult struggle required to recover from such an event. Along with physical and neurological deterioration, fear of falling leads people to overcompensate by, for example, widening their stance, which unfortunately increases, rather than decreases the chance of falling.

ADDITIONAL READING

Cole J. *Pride and a Daily Marathon*. Cambridge, MA: MIT Press, 1995.

Hultborn H, Nielsen JB. Spinal control of locomotion—from cat to man. *Acta Physiol (Oxf)*. 189: 111–121, 2007.

Nilsson J, Thorstensson A, Halbertsma J. Changes in leg movements and muscle activity with speed of locomotion and mode of progression in humans. *Acta Physiol Scand*. 123: 457–475, 1985.

Pierrot-Deseilligny E, Burke D. *The Circuitry of the Human Spinal Cord*. Cambridge: Cambridge University Press, 2005.

Rose J, Gamble JG. *Human Walking*. 3rd ed. Philadelphia: Lippincott Williams & Wilkins, 2006.

Schouenborg J. Action-based sensory encoding in spinal sensorimotor circuits. *Brain Res Rev*. 57: 111–117, 2008.

Sonnenborg FA, Andersen OK, Arendt-Nielsen J. Modular organization of excitatory and inhibitory reflex receptive fields elicited by electrical stimulation of the foot sole in man. *Clin Neurophysiol*. 111: 2160–2169, 2000.

23.

FROM MOVEMENT TO ACTION

POSTURAL STABILITY, ORIENTING, AND PRAXIS

solated from the brain, the spinal cord does not generate recognizable movements. Even the knee jerk reflex looks very different in a person with a complete spinal transection than in a healthy individual. How could this be if the stretch reflex only requires intact Ia afferents and motoneurons, neither of which is damaged by a spinal transection? The reason is simple: all spinal functions degrade when the spinal cord operates in isolation. Although the absolutely essential circuit for the stretch reflex consists of only two neurons, the reflex circuit is influenced by thousands of synaptic inputs from other neurons and does not work normally without these myriad inputs. In this chapter, we examine how motor control centers in the brainstem and forebrain influence the activity of motoneurons in the spinal cord and brainstem, taking us one step closer to a more integrated and realistic picture of how we move.

MOTOR CONTROL CENTERS MAINTAIN POSTURE AND GENERATE PURPOSEFUL MOVEMENTS

When all motor control centers that influence motoneurons are in working order, we move as normally as the condition of our bones, muscles, and other body parts permits. The failure of one motor control center will severely impact some movements, slightly impact others, and only subtly or not change still others. In this chapter, we concentrate on the core functions of the most important motor control centers and their tracts. Thus, the role of the vestibulospinal tract in postural control is emphasized even though the vestibulospinal tract also contributes to orienting, reaching, and many other types of movements. The student should understand that this teaching strategy hits the highlights of motor control function without being either complete or free of oversimplifications.

Regions in the brainstem and forebrain comprise the highest levels of the motor hierarchy that direct

motoneuronal activity, participating in the full complement of movements that humans and other mammals can make. This chapter focuses on how neurons in motor control centers initiate movements that fall into two categories:

- *Postural stability* means maintaining the position of the body, or *posture*, during self-generated movements and against unexpected perturbations.

- Volitional and emotional actions include speech, facial expressions, reaching, grasping, playing the piano, and so on. I will refer to these forebrain-initiated actions by the umbrella term of *praxis* (meaning "action" or "practice" in ancient Greek).

In focusing on the high clinical yield topics of praxis and posture, we leave out a full consideration of orienting movements. *Orienting movements* work with eye movements to enable gaze shifts to any location in order to fixate on an unexpected stimulus, a moving target, or a remembered place in space (see Chapter 19).

Neurons in *motor control centers* located in the brainstem and cerebral cortex influence movement through descending tracts of axons. Descending axons target the spinal ventral horn and brainstem motor cranial nerve nuclei, where they contact motoneurons and motor interneurons. As you recall from Chapter 4, motoneurons located in the medial portion of the ventral horn innervate axial muscles, and more laterally located motoneurons innervate progressively more distal limb muscles. Thus, *the major descending tracts that influence motoneuron activity can be divided into medial tracts that control posture through effects on the axial and proximal limb musculature and lateral tracts that mostly control the movements of the hands, feet, and face* (Fig. 23-1):

- Medial tracts for posture:
  - Lateral vestibulospinal tract

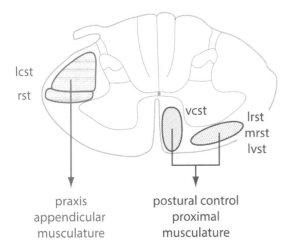

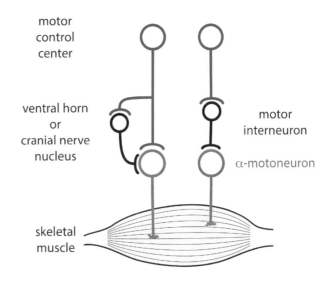

Figure 23-1 The tracts that mediate postural control lie medial to those responsible for praxis. The corticobulbar tract terminates in the caudal medulla and therefore is not present in this section of the cervical enlargement. The lateral corticospinal (*lcst*) and rubrospinal (*rst*) tracts are the primary tracts used for voluntary praxis using appendicular or limb muscles. The corticobulbar tract (not present here) is used for voluntary praxis using facial, oral and upper airway musculature. The ventral corticospinal (*vcst*), reticulospinal (lateral, *lrst*; and medial, *mrst*), and lateral vestibulospinal (*lvst*), tracts are the primary tracts used for ensuring postural stability. Proximal musculature in limbs along with trunk muscles are used for most postural adjustments.

Figure 23-2 Neurons in motor control centers (*blue*) project to motor interneurons (*black*), motoneurons (*red*), or both. Pathways with at least some direct projections to motoneurons support fine fractionated movements of the distal limbs and lower face. Projections from motor control centers to interneurons, including neurons that participate in central pattern generator circuits, support axial, proximal, and bilaterally symmetrical movements.

- Reticulospinal tracts
- Ventral corticospinal tract

- Lateral tracts for control of appendicular and face musculature:
  - Lateral corticospinal tract
  - Corticobulbar tract
  - Rubrospinal tract

The nervous system makes a further distinction between simple, often bilaterally symmetric, movements that employ axial and proximal muscles—standing up from a chair, waving hello, taking a bow—and complex, fractionated movements that require distal muscles—opening a latch, playing the piano, writing, playing a game of paper-rock-scissors. Although axial and appendicular are not useful terms with respect to facial, tongue, and upper airway musculature, distinct brain circuits support simple movements—raising both eyebrows, frowning, opening one's mouth, sticking out one's tongue, humming—and more complex movements such as dislodging a piece of food from between two teeth, raising one eyebrow to convey disbelief, or articulating "She sells seashells by the seashore."

All descending motor tracts, medial and lateral, contribute to simple movements, but only the corticospinal and corticobulbar tracts support complex, fractionated movements. Indirect projections from motor control centers to motoneurons, via motor interneurons, are sufficient to produce simple, bilaterally symmetric movements (Fig. 23-2). In contrast, complex, fractionated movements arise from direct projections from corticospinal and corticobulbar neurons to motoneurons.

Beyond the medial and lateral tracts listed here, there are additional pathways that are collectively called *extrapyramidal*. Extrapyramidal pathways travel separately from the pyramidal tracts (lateral corticospinal and corticobulbar tracts) and support nondeliberate, emotional actions. Of clinical importance, one descending motor pathway can be lesioned and therefore not working while others remain intact and functional, leading to a selective motor impairment. As seen in Chapter 20, patients can fail to smile on command while still smiling in response to a joke. As another example, a patient with a lateral corticospinal injury that prevents them from dancing the jig may still be able to walk, albeit differently than was the case pre-injury.

THE GOAL OF POSTURAL CONTROL IS TO KEEP THE CENTER OF FORCE DIRECTLY ABOVE THE SUPPORT SURFACE

Humans adopt a number of *postures* or body positions and maintain them against gravity and other forces by the neural process of *postural control* or *balance*. The difficulty of holding a given posture depends on two factors:

- The location of the *center of mass*: This is relatively high for an upright human (of normal weight), located at a spot just below the belly button (Fig. 23-3). In the sagittal plane, the center of mass is just behind the hip joint and in front of the knee.

- *Support surface*: Points where the body contacts the ground define the outer edge of the support surface (Fig. 23-3). For a standing human, the support surface includes the area of the feet and the space between, a relatively small area compared to a quadruped such as the cat. The size of the support surface depends on posture, being smaller when the feet are placed

together and even smaller when a person stands on tip-toes.

The point where the gravitational force vector passing through the center of mass intersects with the ground is called the *center of pressure* (Fig. 23-3A). Before we move on to the multijointed human body, let us consider an inert body or object. As long as the center of pressure is centrally located in the support surface, the inert body will stand upright without any external force required. However, an object with a high center of mass and a center of pressure peripherally located within the support surface, or one that is outside the support surface, will fall.

Bipedal humans deviate from the inert body scenario in important ways. The force vector passing through the

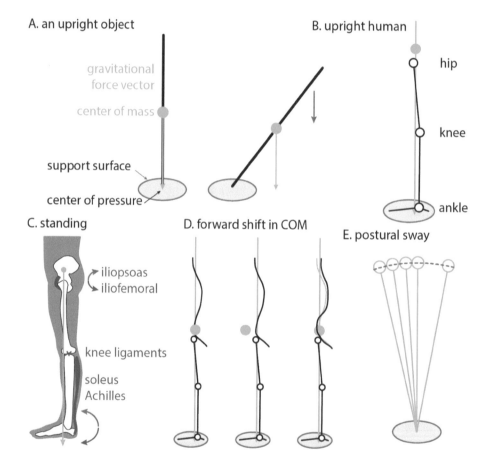

Figure 23-3 A: An inert object with a high center of mass (*green dot*) will stay upright as long as the center of pressure is centrally located within the support surface. If the gravitational force vector (*green arrow*) passing through the center of mass hits a spot that is located outside the support surface, the object will fall (*red arrow*). B: In the upright human, the gravitational force vector passing through the center of mass passes just behind the hip joint and in front of the knee and ankle joints. C: During standing, the gravitational force vector produces a dorsiflexion torque at the ankle and extension torque at the hip (*red arrows*) and knee (*not shown*). Dorsiflexion at the ankle is opposed by muscle activity (*blue arrows*) in the soleus muscle through its connection to the Achilles tendon, rendering both muscle contraction and tendon integrity required for standing. The ligaments of the knee prevent hyperextension of the knee without muscular contribution. The iliofemoral ligament and iliopsoas muscle oppose hip extension through passive and active (muscle contraction) mechanisms, respectively. D: The sway of the back is shown for a woman of normal weight (*left*). If the same posture were adopted during pregnancy, the center of mass would be shifted forward. However, pregnant woman adopt a lordotic posture that extends the back (*right*), bringing the center of mass back to its normal position relative to the sacrum. E: Postural sway can be viewed as the motion of an inverted pendulum. The magnitude of sway is greatly exaggerated here for illustrative purposes.

center of mass does not pass through the center of any of the three joints—hip, knee, or ankle (Fig. 23-3B). Thus, gravitational force exerts a torque on all three joints of the leg. Additionally, a human is far from inert; small movements, even those associated with breathing, constantly alter the location of the center of mass. Seen in this light, postural stability is a marvel. It is in fact unparalleled by any existing artificial circuit. Given a comparable physical starting point to that of humans (similarly high center of mass and small support surface area), no robot, no matter how advanced, could remain upright while riding a city bus or exploring Mars (see Box 23-1).

The ease of maintaining balance increases as the size of the support surface increases. This is because the area over which the center of mass can be passively supported increases as the support surface area gets larger. Of course, the support surface depends on posture in a straightforward way:

- When *lying prone*, the support surface is at a maximum, and postural control is relatively easy.

- When *sitting*, the support surface is intermediate in area, and postural control is of intermediate difficulty.

- The *bipedal upright* position utilizes a limited support surface and, consequently, is challenging to maintain, even more so with a narrow than with a broad stance.

As we saw earlier, the center of pressure of a *passive* body must lie near the center of the support surface, the area within which the body contacts the ground (Fig. 23-3A). Recall from Newtonian physics that:

FORCE = MASS * ACCELERATION

From this equation, we realize that *for an active, moving body, it is the center of force that must lie over the support surface.* Two basic types of disturbances can impact the center of force:

- *Mass*: Imagine picking up an infant at arm's length. Without postural adjustments, the body falls forward.

- *Acceleration*: Imagine throwing a punch or being punched. Without compensatory postural adjustments, the body topples in the direction of the acceleration or, in other words, with the punch.

To oppose disturbances of mass or acceleration and move the center of force back to a spot overlying the support surface, we use muscular force. A myriad of abdominal muscle-strengthening exercises use exactly this principle by requiring force from the abdominal musculature to maintain balance when the body's center of mass does not lie above the support surface.

Box 23-1 BALANCE ON TWO LEGS WITH A HIGH CENTER OF GRAVITY IS DIFFICULT

Since the landing of the Mars *Pathfinder* in 1997, a series of robotic, all-terrain vehicles have roamed, for increasingly long journeys, over the surface of Mars. Designers of these Mars rovers were so concerned about balance that they gave the rovers six wheels and placed the center of mass very low, allowing the vehicles to remain upright even at tilts of up to 45 degrees. Thus, Mars rovers are built for postural stability, not speed. The *Curiosity*, which landed on Mars in 2012, travels at a *peak* speed of 90 meters (or 98 yards) per hour. The average human walking speed is 5 kilometers per hour (about 3 mph), more than 150 times faster than *Curiosity's* average speed of 30 meters per hour. Along with speed, flexibility is another casualty of the Mars rover design. One of *Curiosity's* predecessors, the *Opportunity*, spun its wheels forward and backward for nearly 5 weeks, trying to step over a 20-centimeter (8-inch) high "hill." In 2014, *Curiosity* could not gain purchase on the slippery Martian sands, leading a NASA employee to quip, "we need to gain a better understanding of the interaction between the wheels and Martian sand ripples and Hidden Valley [on Mars] is not a good location for experimenting." The rover was programmed to give up and alter course.

Upright humans, with their high center of mass and small support surface, are able to achieve much faster speeds than those achieved by the bottom-heavy, "sextupedal" Mars rovers. Moreover, humans have neural circuits that utilize sensory input to maintain balance. These brain circuits are neither easy nor cheap to imitate. Engineers working in the field of robotics have steadily made progress, producing more and more biologically inspired robots over the years. Boston Dynamics has produced one such robot, named PETMAN, that walks bipedally, can match its walking speed to treadmill speed, and remains upright even when pushed off balance. This extraordinary achievement was made possible by programming gait, proprioceptive, and vestibular systems that resemble those present in us into the robot. So, with a great deal of money and the efforts of many talented engineers and scientists, it is has been possible to inch closer to the performance of the human brain and body that we are all born with.

Everyday tasks such as holding an infant at arms' length or carrying a bag of groceries requires isometric contractions of the gastrocnemius and paraspinous muscles that provide a force in the backward direction to oppose the forward shift in center of force that would occur in the absence of any muscular effort. The farther that the center of mass shifts from the support surface, the more force is required to oppose the shift and maintain balance. Only very strong, well-practiced gymnasts, dancers, and body contortionists can keep a steady posture in which the center of pressure lies far outside the center of pressure (Fig. 23-4).

Bipedal human standing relies on both passive biomechanics and active muscular force (Fig. 23-3C). The elastic properties and stability of the ankle, as well as ligaments that limit extension of the knee and hip joints, reduce the need for muscular involvement. Thus, standing depends on activity in relatively few muscles. Chief among these muscles is the soleus. As you know by now, the center of pressure for a standing human's mass lies in front of the ankle; because of this, the body is pulled forward at the ankle. Tonic muscle activity in the soleus muscles opposes this force and keeps the body from falling forward. Similarly, the center of mass is located just behind the hip's center of rotation; this has the effect of slightly extending the hip. The iliofemoral ligament and the iliopsoas muscle oppose hip extension. Thigh muscles, including the quadriceps, are largely relaxed during standing. In healthy people, the low muscular demands involved allow for extended periods of standing at little energetic cost.

The location of the center of mass during standing varies across individuals and across time. If a woman adopted her normal, nonpregnant standing posture in the third trimester of her pregnancy, then her center of mass would be shifted forward by more than 3 centimeters (more than 1 inch; (Fig. 23-3D). However, pregnant women adopt a lordotic posture that increases the concavity of the lower back and extends the upper back. These adjustments bring the center of mass back to its normal position relative to the sacrum, but they also require muscular involvement to maintain. Thus, simply standing while pregnant requires an extra contribution from leg and core muscles. Similarly, central obesity, meaning weight concentrated at the waist, is likely to alter the biomechanical requirements of a standing posture, typically requiring greater active involvement from muscles of the legs and core. From this perspective, centrally located weight associated with either obesity or pregnancy predictably leads to sore muscles and back pain.

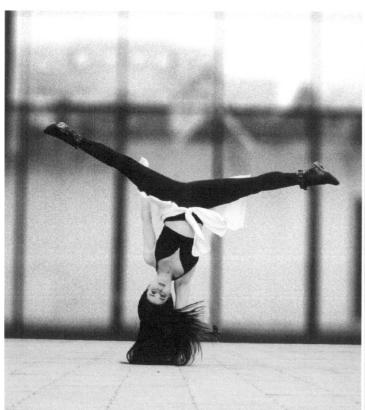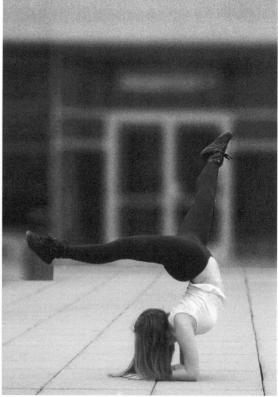

Figure 23-4 Postures in which the center of pressure is far removed from the support surface require great muscle strength. In poses such as these, the position of the body at each joint is maintained through a combination of biomechanical limitations and muscular force. Photographs by Nathan Lee are kindly provided by Jocelyne Muñoz and Brianna Pinder.

Standing still is an illusion. Since the late 19th century, we have known that "standing still" involves continuous adjustments, albeit small ones, that generate an oscillatory *postural sway*. The sway can be imagined as the motion of an inverted pendulum (Fig. 23-3E). Postural sway tends to increase with age.

What is remarkable about reflexes during human standing is that they are primarily *feed-forward* or *anticipatory* rather than feedback in nature. With each activation of the soleus muscle, reflex sensitivities are adjusted to minimize the potential disturbance produced by the ensuing soleus action. In this way, *major perturbations to balance are prevented before they happen rather than being corrected after they have occurred.*

All self-generated actions, not just standing, elicit anticipatory movements that prevent postural instability before it happens. To convince yourself of this, take this textbook in your right hand and raise it to the right. No problem, right? Then stand with your left shoulder and side next to a wall. If you now try to perform the same action, you will fall over, to the right, *toward the location of the shifted center of mass.* This is because the postural shift made "unconsciously" *prior to* lifting the textbook was prevented by your proximity to the wall. As another example, when standing up from a seated position, people visibly move their center of mass forward before propelling themselves upward (Fig. 23-5). More subtle postural adjustments accompany all self-generated movements, even those made from a supine position.

During all self-motion—kneeling down, carrying an infant, running, reaching—the center of mass moves rapidly in varied directions, and anticipatory postural adjustments prevent falling from happening. Postural adjustments, visible or subtle, prevent any loss of balance before it even has a chance to occur. Although postural adjustments can precede a primary movement (the one that is intended), the order of the primary and postural activations is less important than the fact that *postural adjustments occur in the absence of any actual postural perturbation, precluding any disturbance of equilibrium before it happens.* Thus, postural control circuits *anticipate* potential disturbances to equilibrium that our intentional movements would cause if uncorrected and thereby prevent the occurrence of such disturbances.

A great deal of brain power is devoted to postural stability. Postural control circuits contain so many safeguards

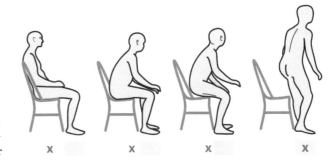

Figure 23-5 In preparation for rising from a sitting position, people lean forward to advance their center of mass before rising. Leaning forward is necessary, as you will learn if you try to rise straight up from a seated position. In this cartoon of a man rising from a chair, the projection of the body's center of mass is marked by a red x. The position of the support surface after standing is marked by a blue rectangle. Note that, in the seated position, the support surface includes the region of contact between the body and the chair. To rise from a sitting position, the center of mass is first advanced by leaning forward. Yet even leaning forward does not place the center of mass within the standing support surface. To move the *center of force* over the support surface, force from the contraction of leg muscles shifts the center of force both forward and up.   Modified from Muybridge E. The human figure in motion: An electro-photographic investigation of consecutive phases of muscular actions. London: Chapman & Hall, 1904.

that quite a bit of damage to the system can be tolerated, enabling humans to stand even in their advanced years and after a lifetime of accumulated insults. Unexpected perturbations, to physiological extensors especially, elicit reflexive adjustments with a high *safety factor*. All measures help to make postural balance fail-safe. In fact, *healthy people do not fall normally, certainly not during everyday activities such as standing and walking.* Therefore, a person falling, in the absence of an obvious cause such as an icy or slick surface, typically signifies a problem.

DESCENDING POSTURAL TRACTS GENERATE ADJUSTMENTS USING A VARIETY OF MECHANISMS

Challenges to balance occur when people stand in unpredictable environments, such as on a boat in stormy seas or on icy ground, and when people balance on a small support surface, such as a narrow beam or tree limb. Somatosensory afferents detect and signal unexpected forces that impact the center of mass and elicit *feedback* corrections from descending postural motor tracts. Basic motor reflexes provide rapid, appropriately sized, and effective adjustments to *unanticipated* perturbations. Visual input—"Gee everything looks tilted"—can also initiate postural adjustments. Finally, vestibular input makes a critical contribution to postural stability. *In terms of postural control, falling rapidly excites lateral vestibulospinal tract neurons that increase physiological extensor activity, opposing gravity and promoting an upright posture.* The lateral vestibulospinal tract descends ipsilaterally from the lateral vestibular nucleus for the entire length of the spinal cord (Fig. 23-1).

The descending motor tracts most closely concerned with posture control—lateral vestibulospinal, reticulospinal, and ventral corticospinal tracts—contribute to both feedback and anticipatory postural adjustments. For anticipatory postural adjustments, the command initiating a primary action is *copied* to one or more of the descending *postural* tracts, which in turn contact motor interneurons. For example, action commands that arise in the motor cortex and travel through the lateral corticospinal tract ensure postural adjustments through signals in the ventral corticospinal tract.

The lateral vestibulospinal and reticulospinal tracts produce postural adjustments through projections onto γ-motoneurons. Recall from Chapter 22 that activation of γ-motoneurons excites α-motoneurons via the γ-loop (excitation of γ-motoneurons → contraction of polar regions of intrafusal fibers → stretch of intrafusal fiber equator → excitation of Ia afferents → excitation of α-motoneurons → muscle contraction). Thus, *descending postural tracts can influence muscle activation at least in part through an indirect mechanism that starts with γ-motoneuron activation and depends on sensory input from Ia afferents.*

Although top-down connections routed through the descending postural tracts are clearly needed for the adjustments that occur in concert with self-generated movements, descending postural tracts also play a role in *feedback* postural reactions by modifying the sensitivity of corrective reflexes. The reversal of the Ib reflex from inhibition to excitation during locomotion is one example of reflex modulation (see Chapter 22). Another example is the increased sensitivity of the Ia reflex during situations of equilibrium instability, such as walking on a narrow beam. Projections from descending tract neurons to γ-motoneurons and motor interneurons modify the sensitivity of basic spinal motor reflexes. In this way, *descending postural tracts provide a central control system that regulates the center of force and also adjusts reflex sensitivities, even reversing the gain of a reflex, to stabilize posture and maintain balance during self-generated movements.*

Lesions in descending postural tracts produce abnormal tonic postures. These postures, typically seen in unresponsive patients, are clinically useful as a quick, noninvasive tool for identifying the level of a brain lesion. With a lesion at or above the rostral midbrain, people lie in a *decorticate* or *flexor posture*, marked by foot and leg extension along with elbow flexion and adduction. More caudal lesions, in the caudal midbrain or hindbrain, cause a *decerebrate* or *extensor posture* in which both arms and legs are fully extended and the head dorsiflexed with teeth clenched. The decerebrate posture is of historic significance because Nobel Prize winner Sir Charles Sherrington studied it intensively. Sherrington showed that in cats, decerebrate posturing involves activity in lateral reticulospinal and lateral vestibulospinal tract cells that is unopposed by damaged medial reticulospinal tract cells that would normally activate flexors. The decerebrate posture in cats is reversed by cutting the dorsal roots, evidence that it depends on the γ-loop. Both decorticate and decerebrate postures signal brainstem damage and thus a medical emergency; neither is associated with a good outcome.

PRAXIS FORMS THE CONNECTION BETWEEN THE BRAIN AND THE OUTSIDE WORLD

The inability to effect one's internal ideas upon the physical world produces great suffering in locked-in patients such as Jean-Dominique Bauby, introduced in Chapter 1. This inability stems from a loss of voluntary praxis. Consciously deliberate actions arise from cognitive processes, including internal thoughts and perceptions of external events. Two pathways connect the internal thoughts and processes of the forebrain to volitional movement-producing circuits in the brainstem and spinal cord:

- Volitional actions of the skeletal muscles in the neck, body, and limbs—particularly fine motor acts—depend on the *lateral corticospinal tract.*

- Volitional movement of the skeletal muscles in the oral cavity, larynx, and face, such as are required for eating, winking, and articulation, depend on the *corticobulbar tract.*

Before considering the pyramidal motor pathways in depth, we briefly look at two other motor pathways: the *rubrospinal tract* and *extrapyramidal pathways.*

Cortical neurons engage neurons of the rubrospinal tract for fundamental movements of the body such as walking or reaching but not for fine movements such as berry-picking, finger-snapping, or foot-tapping to a musical beat. The rubrospinal tract arises from neurons in the red nucleus (see Chapter 6). Axons immediately cross the midline within the midbrain at the level of the red nucleus and travel down into the spinal cord, just ventrolateral to the lateral corticospinal tract (Fig. 23-1). Although its precise function in humans is unclear, the rubrospinal tract is *the* motor command center in vertebrates that lack a well-developed motor cortex. Patients with lesions of the motor cortex who cannot, for example, lift their leg in response to a verbal command can still stand and walk, admittedly awkwardly, probably in large part due to their intact rubrospinal tract. Similarly, *patients with a brain lesion of the lateral corticospinal tract may still stand, walk, and reach under certain circumstances, exhibiting residual functions that likely depend on an intact rubrospinal tract.*

As you recall from Section 2 "Neuroanatomy," the lateral corticospinal tract and parts of the corticobulbar tract travel through the pyramids at the base of the medulla. Additional descending pathways, including the rubrospinal tract, also contribute to motor control but since they travel outside of the pyramids, these additional tracts are called "extrapyramidal." Extrapyramidal pathways arise from diverse cortical and subcortical areas, travel heterogeneous routes, and generate movements that are automatic, subconscious, or emotional rather than deliberate. The term is essentially a term of exclusion and as such refers to a catch-all category of motor pathways. Despite its lack of specificity, the term is useful in referring to pathways that produce nondeliberate, self-generated movements that are typically emotionally motivated. For example, the smile in response to a joke depends on an extrapyramidal pathway. A better understanding of the trajectories traveled by extrapyramidal tracts is an important area for future investigation.

FINE VOLUNTARY MOVEMENTS OF THE BODY, ORAL CAVITY, AND FACE DEPEND ON THE LATERAL CORTICOSPINAL AND CORTICOBULBAR TRACTS

We exert exquisitely fine control over our facial, oral, and distal appendicular muscles using corticobulbar and corticospinal tracts. Consider how many English consonant sounds require that the tip of the tongue touch the anterior pole of the palate: /d/, /l/, /n/, /t/. Although very few of us could describe the fine differences in muscle usage that allow us to say "ta" in place of "da" or vice versa, virtually all who grew up speaking English encounter no difficulty in producing these two sounds when desired. Just as speech and "making a scary face" depend on the corticobulbar tract, shuffling cards, dicing vegetables, and braiding hair depend on the lateral corticospinal tract.

Despite the reader's familiarity with the course traversed by the corticospinal and corticobulbar tracts, these pathways merit further review, with added details regarding somatotopy, due to their importance to human motor function. The corticospinal and corticobulbar tracts arise from neurons in a wide cortical distribution, including primary motor cortex, somatosensory areas of parietal cortex, premotor cortex, and the supplementary motor area. Also recall that the extraocular muscles are not represented in primary motor cortex but are controlled by a separate motor control area—the frontal eye fields. The corticospinal and corticobulbar tracts target primarily interneurons as well as some motoneurons in the spinal cord and cranial nerve nuclei.

Each of the cortical regions contributing to descending motor tracts is somatotopically organized. Primary motor cortex exhibits a striking somatotopy, with very large regions of cortex devoted to certain small parts of the body such as the lips and small areas of cortex concerned with large body sections such as the trunk (see Chapter 7). *The relative cortical area controlling different body parts is related to the precision with which movements of the regulated muscles are controlled.*

Beyond the gross topography from medial (toes) to lateral (face), the topographic organization of the primary motor cortex is rough. It is also fractured, with discrete areas eliciting different movements that nonetheless may involve contraction of the same muscle. For example, activation of one area of the motor cortex may produce an eating motion while stimulation of another region produces sucking movements. The important point here is that the motor cortex is organized around everyday movements rather than by individual muscles. There is no one-to-one correspondence between a cortical region and a single muscle. Instead, multiple regions control multiple movements that involve both overlapping and distinct muscles. In sum, the organization of motor cortex is around ethological movements not specific muscles. Therefore, cortical lesions lead to difficulties with sets of complex movements but do not lead to the inability to use a single muscle, as would result from a nerve injury. The motor deficits affected by brain lesions are context-specific, occurring under one circumstance and not under another. The loss of smiling in response to a command while retaining emotionally motivated smiling exemplifies this type of context-specificity.

Corticospinal and corticobulbar axons descend from cortex through the corona radiata and into the internal capsule, where the face is represented in the genu and the arms, trunk, and leg in progressively more caudal regions of the posterior limb. The internal capsule continues caudally to form the middle third of the midbrain cerebral peduncles. Within the cerebral peduncles, corticobulbar fibers travel medially to corticospinal fibers. Arm-, trunk-, and leg-controlling fibers course in progressively more lateral locations, all within the middle third of the peduncles. The peduncles feed into the base of the pons, where corticospinal and corticobulbar tract axons travel in bundles, interspersed like islands within a sea formed by the pontine nuclei. In the pons, the somatotopy is roughly similar, but far cruder, to that present in the cerebral peduncles, with face represented most medially and legs most laterally. Upon entering the medulla, fibers descending from cortex coalesce within the pyramids, where the somatotopy shifts slightly so that the remaining face-controlling axons lie dorsomedially and leg-controlling axons lie most ventrolaterally.

At the spinomedullary junction, virtually none of the corticobulbar tract remains. The only exception is axons destined for the spinal accessory nucleus within the most rostral cervical spinal segments. At this point, 90% of the corticospinal tract fibers decussate to descend within the dorsal part of the lateral funiculus, contralateral to the motor cortex where they originated, as the lateral corticospinal tract. *Thus, voluntary control of muscles on one side depends on neurons in the motor cortex on the other, contralateral side. Remember that within the forebrain and brainstem, lateral corticospinal tract axons travel contralaterally to the muscles that they ultimately influence. However, within the spinal cord, the lateral corticospinal input courses on the same side as the muscles that it influences.* The 10% of the corticospinal tract that fails to decussate descends ipsilaterally within the ventral corticospinal tract, which serves primarily to stabilize posture during voluntary movements and to voluntarily control axial movements.

THE CORTICOBULBAR INNERVATION OF THE FACIAL NUCLEUS CONTROLS EXPRESSIONS OF THE BOTTOM HALF OF THE CONTRALATERAL FACE

As they descend through the brainstem, corticobulbar tract axons terminate within the cranial nerve motor nuclei. The corticobulbar tract resembles the lateral corticospinal tract *except* that it does not always control motoneurons or movements contralateral to the side of the tract's origin. Furthermore, since innervated structures such as the jaw and tongue are joined across the midline, unilateral lesions in the corticobulbar pathway are often not symptomatic. Table 23-1 lists the *typical* projection pattern of the corticobulbar tract to each cranial nerve motor nucleus and the clinical consequences of damage. However, it should be noted that the clinical effects of lesions vary considerably between individuals, probably due to variation in the underlying anatomy of the corticobulbar tract.

The corticobulbar innervation of the facial nucleus, important for facial expressions, differs from the remainder of the corticobulbar pathway in being relatively conserved across individuals and in its disruption having profound clinical consequences. We therefore discuss facial expressions and their cortical control in some detail here. Ultimately, the physician must recognize the difference between symptoms produced by a facial nerve lesion (see Chapter 5) and those that follow a *supranuclear* lesion. A supranuclear lesion is one that is located above the targeted nucleus, which in this case refers to a lesion of the corticobulbar tract before it has reached the facial nucleus.

There is fine control of muscles in the bottom half of the face compared to those in the top half. This aids humans

Table 23-1 LATERALITY OF CORTICOBULBAR TRACT PROJECTIONS TO CRANIAL NERVE NUCLEI

CRANIAL NERVE NUCLEUS	CORTICOBULBAR TRACT PROJECTION	EFFECT OF CORTICAL LESION (RELATIVE TO SIDE OF LESION)
Motor trigeminal nucleus	Bilateral	Typically asymptomatic
Facial nucleus (to upper face)	Bilateral from supplementary motor area	Typically asymptomatic
Facial nucleus (to lower face)	Contralateral from M1	Contralateral volitional paralysis
Nucleus ambiguus	Mostly bilateral, ipsilateral to palate	Dysarthria, dysphagia
Spinal accessory nucleus—trapezius	Ipsilateral	Ipsilateral shrug is weak
Spinal accessory nucleus—sternocleidomastoid	Decussates in pons and then crosses back in spinal cord	Weakness turning to contralateral side for suprapontine lesions or ipsilateral side for hindbrain lesions
Hypoglossal nucleus	Bilateral with ipsilateral predominance	Transient weakness, tongue points contralaterally, dysarthria

in eating, a function shared with all other animals, and in speech, a function shared with few other mammals. You can easily demonstrate to yourself the difference in the pattern of fine motor control between the lower and upper halves of the face. Simply compare your ability to make a discrete unilateral movement with the top and bottom halves of your face. First, try to pull one side of your mouth up, leaving the other side unmoved; then try the other side (Fig. 23-6A). Next, try to specifically raise one eyebrow without contorting any other facial muscles, and now the other eyebrow (Fig. 23-6B). I am guessing that you were able to raise each side of the mouth. I am also guessing that none of you remember the moment you figured out how to do so or even can imagine having to "figure out" such a movement. There was never a Eureka moment for raising the side of your mouth. In contrast, an informal survey (conducted by the author) of more than 4,000 people showed that only 9% reported being able to raise both left and right eyebrows alone. And these eyebrow-raisers have stories to tell about why, how, and when they started to practice: "I started practicing the first time I saw Spock do it" or "I spent one very foggy Maine vacation learning to raise each one independently" or "I practiced raising my right eyebrow when I was a child because my piano teacher use to do this when I played badly and I thought this was a hilarious thing to do."

These examples of mouth and eyebrow movements exemplify a fundamental difference between the cortical control of upper and lower facial musculature. In humans and other primates, the corticobulbar projection controlling the lower half of the face projects directly to motoneurons and is entirely crossed. In other vertebrates,

motor cortex influences *all* facial motoneurons only indirectly via projections to interneurons and central pattern generators in the brainstem reticular core. *Humans retain a pattern of predominantly indirect motor control in the case of the top half of the face*: forehead and eyebrows (frontalis muscle), eyes (orbicularis oculi), and so on. The corticobulbar tract innervation of facial motoneurons that control upper face muscles is bilateral and arises from the supplementary motor area rather than from primary motor cortex. The direct contralateral pattern of motoneuron control allows for fine control of the muscles of the lower half of the face in everyone. In contrast, the indirect, bilateral pattern of innervation for muscles of the upper half of the face does not support finely controlled movements. Three points are worth explicitly stating:

- Direct projections from motor control centers to motoneurons support the ability to deliberately make fractionated unilateral movements.

- Indirect projections from motor control centers to motoneurons support simple bilateral movements.

- Indirect projections from motor control centers to motoneurons (via interneurons) can support discrete unilateral movements, but successful engagement of this pathway for this purpose does not come automatically and may not be possible in all individuals.

There are parallels between the two corticospinal tracts and the cortical control of facial motoneurons. As with the lateral corticospinal tract, the corticobulbar tract innervation of lower facial motoneurons is directly onto motoneurons and crossed. In contrast, an indirect connection from motor cortex to motoneurons is sufficient to produce coarse, bilateral facial movements just as the ventral corticospinal tract supports coarse, typically bilateral movements of the trunk.

Corticobulbar axons bound for the facial nucleus travel on the side of their origin until reaching the level of the facial nucleus. Within the caudal pons, axons from primary motor cortex cross the midline to innervate facial motoneurons that innervate muscles of the lower half of the face (Fig. 23-7B). Axons from supplementary motor area that target facial motoneurons controlling the upper half of the face either cross or remain on the same side (Fig. 23-7C). Thus, the upper face motoneurons receive cortical innervation from both hemispheres. As a consequence, a unilateral lesion of

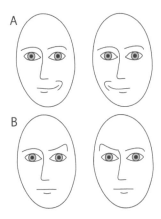

Figure 23-6 Motor control of the upper and lower facial musculature is fundamentally different. This difference is reflected in the ubiquitous ability to pull up the mouth on either side (A) versus the comparatively rare (and always practiced) faculty of raising each eyebrow in isolation (B).

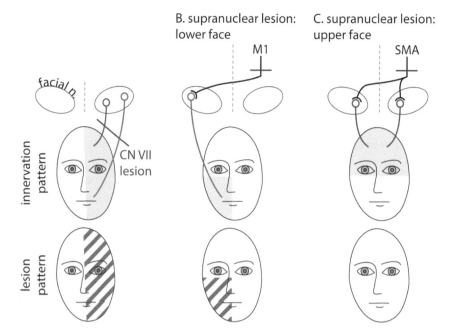

Figure 23-7 The innervation pattern (*beige area in top row of faces*) of motoneurons in the facial nuclei (*facial n.*) that serve upper (*blue*) and lower (*red*) facial musculature is illustrated. Lesions at the sites marked by the brown lines produce deficits in volitionally moving facial areas marked by red stripes (*bottom row of faces*). A: Within the facial nucleus, motoneuron pools that innervate muscles in the top half of the face are located medial to pools that innervate muscles in the lower half of the face. A lesion of the facial nerve (*brown line*), often produced by a viral infection, produces Bell's palsy. The movement component of Bell's palsy is an inability to move the ipsilateral face for any reason, volitional, emotional, or automatic. B: Neurons in the primary motor cortex (*M1*) project directly to motoneuron pools that innervate the contralateral lower face. Therefore, a supranuclear lesion of the corticobulbar tract (*brown line*) produces a volitional paralysis of the lower face contralateral to the damaged hemisphere. This lesion does not alter emotional facial movements, including those that employ the part of the face that is unable to make volitional movements. C: Neurons in the supplementary motor area (*SMA*) project bilaterally to motoneuron pools that innervate the upper face. Even in cases of a complete loss of innervation from one hemisphere, the other hemisphere compensates. Therefore, a supranuclear lesion of the corticobulbar tract (*brown line*) has no detrimental effect on movements of the upper face.

the supranuclear projection to upper face motoneurons has no effect.

As is evident from the anatomy, supranuclear corticobulbar lesions and complete lesions of the facial nerve will produce very different sets of symptoms. Recall from Chapter 5 that a person with a facial nerve lesion cannot move the *entire* face on the side of the lesion *for any reason* (Fig. 23-7A). The most common cause of facial motoneuron paralysis is an infection or inflammation of the facial nerve that produces a transient weakness or paralysis termed Bell's palsy. When Bell's palsy affects all branches of the facial nerve, as often occurs, it also produces:

- Hypersensitivity to loud sounds, termed *hyperacusis*, due to paralysis of the stapedius muscle

- Dry eye and dry mouth, due to lesioning of preganglionic parasympathetic nerves to lacrimal and salivary glands

- Pain radiating from the external ear through effects on the small number of sensory afferents carried in the facial nerve

In contrast to Bell's palsy, difficulty in making *volitional* facial expressions is the only symptom resulting from a supranuclear lesion of corticobulbar fibers destined for the facial nucleus. This follows from the fact that the corticobulbar tract contains axons from motor cortex involved in controlling facial expression but not axons related to the stapedius muscle, the parasympathetic ganglia, or somatosensation. The difference between a supranuclear lesion and a nerve lesion exemplifies the functional variety of cranial nerves and the functional unity of central tracts such as the corticobulbar tract.

The distinction between supranuclear facial paresis and Bell's palsy can easily be discerned by asking a person to smile and frown. Someone with a supranuclear facial paresis cannot lift his mouth on the side opposite to the lesion in a deliberate smile but can frown bilaterally, whereas a patient with a lesion of the facial nerve can neither frown nor smile on the side of the lesion (Fig. 23-8).

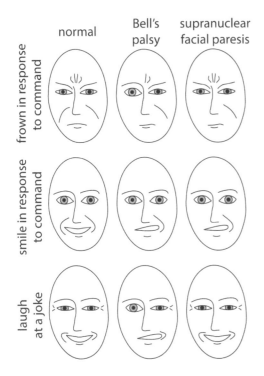

frown in response to command

smile in response to command

laugh at a joke

Figure 23-8 Volitional facial expressions (frown or smile in response to command, *top two rows*) are compared to an emotional facial expression (laugh at a joke, *bottom row*) in a healthy adult (*left*) and in individuals with Bell's palsy (*middle*) or supranuclear facial paresis (*right*). Damage to the facial nerve (Bell's palsy) or facial motoneurons impairs movement of the entire ipsilateral face. A lesion of the corticobulbar tract carrying information from M1 to the facial nucleus impairs volitional movements of the bottom half of the face only. The side affected is ipsilateral to the targeted facial nucleus and contralateral to the hemisphere of origin for the corticobulbar tract involved. Projections from the anterior cingulate gyrus support emotional movements, so that smiling in response to a joke is preserved in people with corticobulbar lesions.

EMOTIONALLY MOTIVATED MOVEMENTS DO NOT DEPEND ON CORTICOSPINAL AND CORTICOBULBAR PATHWAYS

Regions critical to the generation of voluntary actions are distinct from those needed for the production of emotional actions. This concept is best understood and illustrated by comparing the ability of people with different brain lesions to make facial expressions in response to a command or in association with an emotion. For all but the most talented actors, a volitional imitation of an emotional movement differs from the real thing. We easily distinguish a smile of enjoyment from a smile produced in response to a command. A child expertly discerns how angry a parent is by a glance at the parent's facial expression. Patients with lesions

in the corticobulbar tract cannot voluntarily make facial expressions but encounter no problem reacting with their face for emotional reasons (see Figs. 20-2, 20-3, and 23-8).

Some patients make facial expressions in response to a command but not in association with an emotion, a condition termed *amimia*. Patients with amimia can act volitionally—smiling for the camera—but cannot act for emotional reasons—smiling when enjoying a funny story (see Fig. 20-3). Amimia has been reported after lesions in a variety of sites including the frontal cortex, internal capsule, caudate, putamen, and thalamus. This rare condition is worth mentioning because it provides insight into how the cortex divides up different types of movement.

The unanimated face often bears little resemblance to the animated face. Even our resting "neutral" face expresses emotion. See, for example, the normal resting facial expression made by the patient with volitional facial paresis, illustrated in Fig. 20-2. Emotion is so important to one's appearance that a person devoid of expression due to sleep or death can be unrecognizable. In "The Bridge of San Luis Rey," Thornton Wilder wrote, "Camila had a very beautiful face, or rather a face beautiful save in repose. In repose one was startled to discover that the nose was long and thin, the mouth tired and a little childish, the eyes unsatisfied. . . ." This quote eloquently reflects the active nature of the facial expression at so-called rest. The abnormally appearing frozen faces of patients receiving a little too much botulinum toxin supports the conclusion that facial expression is actively maintained during waking hours.

Neurons in the *anterior cingulate gyrus*, a part of the limbic system, control emotional facial expressions. Neurons in the anterior cingulate become active during arousing conditions such as pain or disgust, giving rise to automatic facial expressions that accompany strongly emotional experiences. One example is the involuntary wince that accompanies a sharp pain. The pathway from the anterior cingulate to facial motoneurons does not travel with the corticobulbar tract arising from motor cortex, and thus is extrapyramidal.

LESIONS OF DESCENDING MOTOR TRACTS PRODUCE SYMPTOMS DISTINCT FROM MOTONEURON LESIONS

Descending motor tracts influence but do not completely control the activity of motoneurons. Illustrative of the influence exerted by descending tracts upon motoneurons is a comparison of the effects of lesions to descending motor tracts and motoneuron lesions. As you know, there is no possibility for movement after motoneurons are damaged. Thus, when a motoneuron disease such as poliomyelitis kills motoneurons, no active movements, not even reflexes, are possible using the denervated muscle. In contrast, when the corticospinal tract is lesioned, volitional movements are impaired even as emotional actions and reflexes may remain possible. Reflexes are even enhanced after lesions of descending motor tracts, a condition known as *hyperreflexia*.

The movements spared by central nervous system damage depend on the level and extent of the lesion. For example, after a middle cerebral artery stroke damaging the primary motor cortex, emotional actions typically remain intact. In contrast, spinal cord injuries are rarely surgical and therefore lead to a loss of emotional as well as volitional actions. Subcortical lesions in the cerebral white matter or brainstem have variable effects. In lesions at all levels, hyperreflexia occurs.

The areflexia resulting from motoneuron death and the hyperreflexia that accompanies descending motor tract damage have further consequences (see Table 23-2). Areflexive muscles lose tone and become atrophied from disuse. Muscle fibers that are not innervated by a motoneuron show spontaneous contractions of entire motor units (fasciculations) and of single muscle fibers (fibrillations) (see Chapter 21). In contrast, after damage to the corticospinal tract, stretch reflexes are large in magnitude and occur *briskly*, whereas muscle tone is often elevated, leading to the term *spastic paralysis*. Hyperreflexia and the

consequent increase in muscle tone mitigate the muscle atrophy that would normally result from disuse of a muscle due to an inability to willfully use that muscle.

A lesion of descending tract input to the lumbosacral cord releases the plantar reflex. A release of the plantar reflex is termed the *Babinski sign*. Recall that the plantar reflex is one of the developmentally transient reflexes that neonates show (see Chapter 22). This reflex involves dorsiflexion of the big toe coupled with fanning of the remaining toes in response to a firm stroke along the sole of the foot. In an adult, the presence of the plantar reflex and of brisk stretch reflexes, or hyperreflexia, both stem from a loss of descending inhibition that travels in or with descending motor tracts. It is not clear which of the descending motor tracts is most critical to reflex inhibition; lesions both within and outside of the corticospinal tract appear to contribute.

A person with a cerebral lesion of the corticospinal tract can be recognized readily from his posture and gait (Fig. 23-9). The affected leg is extended and adducted. Weight is shifted away from the affected leg, raising the hip. The affected arm is adducted and flexed at the elbow while the hand is tucked in and held in a fist. With corticobulbar involvement, the head may be turned away from the paralyzed side, a result of lesioned input to the (ipsilateral) spinal accessory nucleus. When the frontal eye fields are affected, gaze is turned toward the unlesioned side. Recall that since the frontal eye fields control contralateral gaze, a lesion produces a resting ipsilateral gaze. In the *hemiparetic gait*, the affected leg does not bend but is swung around in an arc, a pattern known as *circumduction*. It should be noted that lesions of the spinal cord that affect the corticospinal tract almost inevitably involve additional tracts, and patients with any motor involvement are rarely able to either stand or walk.

Many diseases only affect motoneurons or only affect descending motor tracts, but some affect both. The prototypical example of the latter is amyotrophic lateral sclerosis. Patients with amyotrophic lateral sclerosis typically seek medical help because of muscle weakness exhibited as dysarthria, dysphagia, clumsiness, or foot drop. When first seen, these patients present with signs of damage to descending tracts—muscle weakness, hyperreflexia, and increased muscle tone—as well as signs of motoneuron damage—muscle atrophy, fibrillations, and fasciculations. The involvement of both motoneurons and descending tracts reflects the suspected pathophysiology of amyotrophic lateral sclerosis, in which connected pairs of corticospinal tract neurons and motoneurons degenerate. Unfortunately, amyotrophic lateral sclerosis is fatal, usually within a year or two, and

Table 23-2 THE SYMPTOMS ASSOCIATED WITH LESIONS OF MOTONEURONS, THEIR AXONS, OR THE NEUROMUSCULAR JUNCTION ARE DIFFERENT FROM THE SYMPTOMS ASSOCIATED WITH LESIONS IN DESCENDING MOTOR TRACTS

	MOTONEURON LESION	LESION OF CORTICOSPINAL TRACT
Volitional movement	None	None
Reflexive movement	Areflexia	Hyperreflexia
Muscle tone	Absent	Increased
Muscle appearance	Atrophy from disuse	Mild atrophy from disuse mitigated by hyperreflexia
Electromyographic findings suggestive of muscle denervation	Fibrillations, fasciculations	Typically transient if present
Plantar reflex	Unaffected	Released (Babinski sign)

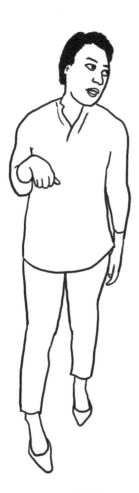

Figure 23-9 The hemiparetic stance involves leg extension and adduction that results in a shift of weight-bearing to the unaffected leg. The arm is held in a flexed and adducted position with the hand in a fist. The posture of the leg and arm resemble that seen in the decorticate posture. The head is twisted toward the unaffected side due to unopposed sternocleidomastoid contraction on the affected side (contralateral to the lesion). The frontal eye fields are often damaged by strokes of the middle cerebral artery that give rise to hemiparesis. In such cases, the working frontal eye fields on the nonlesioned hemisphere shift gaze contralaterally, toward the unaffected side, an effect that is unopposed by the damaged frontal eye fields in the lesioned hemisphere. In the patient illustrated here, nonfluent or Broca's aphasia is likely due to the lesion's location in the left hemisphere.   Drawing kindly provided by Sharon Rosenzweig.

no treatment currently exists. Ultimately, patients with amyotrophic lateral sclerosis lose mobility and become wheelchair-bound. Fatal complications include weakness in swallowing, potentially causing insufficient nutrition or aspiration of food, and weakness in respiratory muscles.

In sum, reduced reflexes indicate a problem at the level of the motoneuron, and brisk reflexes signal damage to descending motor tracts. Only a few specific diseases, such as amyotrophic lateral sclerosis, involve signs of damage to both motoneurons and descending motor tracts. Reflex testing is invaluable in rapidly narrowing down the diagnostic possibilities in a patient with a motor disorder.

NEONATAL LESIONS IN DESCENDING MOTOR TRACTS PRODUCE CEREBRAL PALSY

The immature brain is typically more plastic, adaptive, and less susceptible to permanent damage from injury than is the mature brain. A major exception to this rule involves *cerebral palsy*, a relatively common condition (~2 per 1,000) that results from perinatal damage to cerebral motor regions. Cerebral palsy is a diverse set of permanent, but not progressive, conditions with motor deficits that range in severity from mild to debilitating. In the most common form, impairment is limited to excessive contraction of adducting lower limb muscles; this brings the thighs and knees together, resulting in a *scissors gait*. In its most debilitating form, affected individuals may need use of a wheelchair for mobility as well as assistance with eating and drinking. Altered developmental programs during gestation or early neonatal life set up cerebral palsy. By infancy, these abnormal motor circuits are set, and the underlying pathophysiology does not deteriorate further although the implications for the patient may evolve over time.

It should be noted that since cerebral palsy stems from damage to *motor* regions of the brain, intellectual impairment does not necessarily occur along with the defining motor disabilities. Intellectual impairment only occurs when brain damage extends beyond motor areas.

Most cases of cerebral palsy result from damage to the corticospinal tract, producing *spastic* cerebral palsy, which is discussed here. Damage to the cerebellum produces *ataxic* cerebral palsy, and damage to the basal ganglia produces *athetoid* cerebral palsy. Maternal infections, placental insufficiency, perinatal trauma, and oxygen deprivation are all potential causes of cerebral palsy. Prematurity is associated with a higher risk of cerebral palsy. Regardless of the etiology, cerebral palsy results when damage to a motor control or modulatory region occurs. Many, possibly most, spastic cerebral palsy cases result from lesions of the white matter surrounding the ventricles, where axons of the corticospinal tract pass.

The pathophysiology of cerebral palsy revolves around competition within the spinal cord between corticospinal axons from the left and right hemispheres. In a healthy baby, corticospinal axons from each motor cortex reach both sides of the spinal cord. With time, contralateral axons dominate ipsilateral axons, and the former make permanent synapses. The ipsilateral axons, on the losing end of this competition, retract their axons. Unfortunately, damage to the corticospinal tract on one side prevents the normal competition between descending axons from the two hemispheres. As a result, ipsilateral corticospinal axons do not retreat from the spinal cord, and motoneurons on both sides receive descending input from the same motor cortex. This aberrant descending corticospinal innervation leads to changes in spinal reflex circuits and even in muscle fiber composition. Ultimately, all of these changes cause permanent motor impairment for which no cure and few efficacious treatments currently exist. Nonetheless, many cerebral palsy patients have productive and happy lives and are achieving increasing levels of independence thanks to the advent of adaptive equipment and technology.

HIGHER MOTOR CORTICAL REGIONS DICTATE ACTIONS RATHER THAN MOVEMENTS

Neurosurgeons Wilder Penfield and Theodore Rasmussen reported extensively on their experiences stimulating the cerebral cortex of awake neurosurgical patients (see Chapter 7). Although stimulation of primary motor cortex evokes movements, patients typically say nothing as a part of their body moves. Alternatively they may say, "my _____ wanted to move." Of note, the *patients do not own the movements*. Rather the movements occur *to them*. This reflects the role of the motor cortex as movement executor but not movement organizer or initiator.

Movements evoked by primary motor cortex stimulation range from simple, such as hand-opening or hand-closing, to complex, such as a vocalized cry that requires coordination between the diaphragm, larynx, upper airway, and facial muscles. Both the simple and complex movements are innate in that they are present at birth and do not require learning. Moreover, these movements lack meaning. On the other hand, actions such as the hand gestures for rock-paper-scissors or the utterance of a word are learned. The instructions for learned actions arise from outside the primary motor cortex. Thus, the command for volitional actions does not originate in the motor cortex even as the movements are organized for execution there. Consequently, lesions of the primary motor cortex can prevent the execution of learned movements such as rock-paper-scissors gestures even though stimulation of motor cortex does not produce these movements. Here, we examine the brain regions that send instructions for volitional actions into the primary motor cortex.

Recall that actions are movements imbued with meaning. They advance an individual toward a goal that is independent of any specific movements or muscles. For example,

reaching a cookie jar may mean kneeling down, standing on tip-toes, twisting to the right, or ducking under a shelf on the left. Regardless of which movement is used in the quest for a cookie, reaching for the cookie jar is the meaningful deed that constitutes the action. The myriad of specific reasons that compel people to act—move with meaning—fall into two broad categories: deliberate and emotional. The motor cortex is required for volitional acts but not for emotional ones.

Deliberate actions can occur in response to a verbal request, as when a person passes the saltshaker to a dining companion or a patient touches her finger to her nose during a medical visit. In the clinical vernacular, such movements are said to be in response to a *command* (although a gentle request would surely do). Deliberate actions may also occur as the result of an internal and conscious thought process, as when a person juliennes carrots, texts a friend to say that she is running late, or splits a bar tab. Some actions are tied to external stimuli. A baby who grabs at glasses or dangling earrings, an adolescent who plays a video game, and a sales clerk who looks up when the entry bell rings are all reacting to stimuli in the world.

The *supplementary motor area* and *premotor cortex* are two regions that organize volitional actions. The prefrontal cortex sends motivational and executive function information to the supplementary motor area, which organizes actions made for internal reasons. In contrast, premotor cortex, which receives input from parietal cortex, is critical to movements made in response to external stimuli. The pathways involved in moving in response to a command are not entirely clear but certainly involve input from language comprehension areas.

Emotional actions likely comprise the bulk of our actions. They occur for affective reasons that are typically not well understood on a conscious level even by the person performing the action. Examples range from the "pained" facial expression and cry of "Ow! Ow! Ow!" evoked by a bee sting to the hug shared by good friends, the spry stroll through a park on a beautiful spring day, or the walk to the refrigerator to look for food when hungry. The cingulate gyrus is one place where emotional actions are organized. For example, regions in cingulate gyrus project directly to the facial nucleus and are responsible for facial expressions such as a pain-wince or the smile in response to a joke.

Since the pathways that access the motor cortex differ, lesions may affect one pathway but not others. As a result, actions that occur for one reason may be impaired, whereas actions using the same muscles that occur for a different reason are unaffected. Although rare, this type of disorder, termed *apraxia*, dramatically illustrates the diverse paths leading to praxis or action. There are several types of apraxia, each with heterogeneous presentations. In the most common form of *ideomotor apraxia*, a patient cannot perform an action in response to a command but can make that very same action in the course of everyday life. For example, a patient may be unable to pour water from a pitcher in response to a command, but still be perfectly able to do so when thirsty. As this example demonstrates, there is nothing wrong with the motor hierarchy or with the muscles themselves in a patient with apraxia. Moreover, there is no deficit in language. Instead, the issue in apraxia is in connecting language comprehension to the volitional motor system. Apraxia is commonly thought to result from a lesion in the left hemisphere within the parietal lobe or its connection to frontal motor areas.

ADDITIONAL READING

Brown S, Ngan E, Liotti M. A larynx area in the human motor cortex. *Cereb Cortex.* 18(4): 837–845, 2008.

Clowry GJ. The dependence of spinal cord development on corticospinal input and its significance in understanding and treating spastic cerebral palsy. *Neurosci Biobehav Rev.* 31: 1114–1124, 2007.

Ekman P. Facial expressions of emotion: An old controversy and new findings. *Philos Trans R Soc Lond B Biol Sci.* 335: 63–69, 1992.

Eyre JA. Corticospinal tract development and its plasticity after perinatal injury. *Neurosci Biobehav Rev.* 31: 1136–1149, 2007.

Graziano MS. Ethological action maps: A paradigm shift for the motor cortex. *Trends Cogn Sci.* 20: 121–132, 2016.

Holstege G. Emotional innervation of facial musculature. *Move Dis.* 17 (Suppl 2): S12–16, 2002.

Holstege G, Subramanian HH. Two different motor systems are needed to generate human speech. *J Comp Neurol.* 524: 1558–1577, 2016.

Horak FB, Nashner LM. Central programming of postural movements: Adaptation to altered support-surface configurations. *J Neurophysiol.* 55: 1369–1381, 1986.

Jenny AB, Saper CB. Organization of the facial nucleus and corticofacial projection in the monkey: A reconsideration of the upper motor neuron facial palsy. *Neurology.* 37: 930–939, 1987.

Mastaglia FL, Knezevic W, Thompson PD. Weakness of head turning in hemiplegia: A quantitative study. *J Neurol Neurosurg Psychiatry.* 49: 195–197, 1986.

Morecraft RJ, Louie JL, Herrick JL, Stilwell-Morecraft KS. Cortical innervation of the facial nucleus in the non-human primate: A new interpretation of the effects of stroke and related subtotal brain trauma on the muscles of facial expression. *Brain.* 124: 176–208, 2001.

Morecraft RJ, Stilwell-Morecraft KS, Rossing WR. The motor cortex and facial expression: New insights from neuroscience. *Neurologist.* 10: 235–249, 2004.

Morecraft RJ, Stilwell-Morecraft KS, Solon-Cline KM, Ge J, Darling WG. Cortical innervation of the hypoglossal nucleus in the non-human primate (Macaca mulatta). *J Comp Neurol.* 522: 3456–3484, 2014.

Mori S, Iwakiri H, Homma Y, Yokoyama T, Matsuyama K. Neuroanatomical and neurophysiological bases of postural control. *Adv Neurol.* 67: 289–303, 1995.

Oddsson LI. Control of voluntary trunk movements in man. Mechanisms for postural equilibrium during standing. *Acta Physiol Scand Suppl.* 595: 1–60, 1990.

Penfield W, Rasmussen T. *The Cerebral Cortex of Man: A Clinical Study of Localization of Function.* New York: The Macmillan Company, 1950.

Ross ED, Reddy AL, Nair A, Mikawa K, Prodan CI. Facial expressions are more easily produced on the upper-lower compared to the right-left hemiface. *Percept Mot Skills.* 104: 155–165, 2007.

Staudt M. (Re-)organization of the developing human brain following periventricular white matter lesions. *Neurosci Biobehav Rev.* 31: 1150–1156, 2007.

Van der Fits IB, Klip AW, van Eykern LA, Hadders-Algra M. Postural adjustments accompanying fast pointing movements in standing, sitting and lying adults. *Exp Brain Res.* 120: 202–216, 1998.

Waller BM, Vick SJ, Parr LA, et al. Intramuscular electrical stimulation of facial muscles in humans and chimpanzees: Duchenne revisited and extended. *Emotion.* 6: 367–382, 2006.

Walker HK. Cranial nerve XI: The spinal accessory nerve. In: Walker HK, Hall WD, Hurst JW, eds., *Clinical Methods: The History, Physical, and Laboratory Examinations.* 3rd ed. Boston: Butterworths; 1990.

Waxman SG. Clinical observations on the emotional motor system. *Prog Brain Res.* 107: 595–604, 1996.

Whitcome KK, Shapiro LJ, Lieberman DE. Fetal load and the evolution of lumbar lordosis in bipedal hominins. *Nature.* 450: 1075–1078, 2007.

24.

CEREBELLUM

The cerebellum is a data-hungry computational powerhouse that specializes in associative learning. Its circuitry and connections are perfectly suited to learning from errors. The cerebellum uses what it learns to match outputs to either static or changing conditions and thereby prevent future errors before they happen. The cerebellum makes no assumptions. It is therefore not surprising that the cerebellum does not come "online" until after birth, when the associations between brain activity and the world can first be made from actual evidence.

Judging from the enormous quantity of sensory input it receives, the cerebellum appears to be a *sensory processor*. Yet cerebellar lesions cause few or no deficits in sensation as such. Instead, most animals and patients with cerebellar disease or injury exhibit dramatically uncoordinated movements, providing compelling evidence for a major cerebellar role in motor coordination. As we shall see, the cerebellum coordinates movements through learning to associate appropriate sensory feedback with intended motor output, an approach whereby the cerebellum utilizes its massive sensory input to regulate and smoothen motor function.

The cerebellum lacks direct connections to α-motoneurons. Therefore, it exerts its powerful influence on movement through *modulation* of motor control cells in the cerebral cortex and brainstem. Although motor coordination is most obviously impaired by cerebellar dysfunction, the human cerebellum may also modulate nonmotor functions. Recently, the cerebellum's contributions to the development of typical social behavior has received a great deal of attention. In this chapter, we examine the role of the cerebellum in movement in some detail before briefly considering its potential role in other brain functions.

Our understanding of the pathophysiology and ability to treat cerebellar disorders is only beginning to benefit from the enormous body of basic science information about this well-studied part of the brain. In this chapter, I emphasize aspects of cerebellar biology that offer the greatest clinical payoff. This emphasis comes at the expense of a traditional description of the anatomy and physiology of the cerebellum, a fascinating topic for which a myriad of resources exist; interested students are encouraged to take advantage of these resources.

THE CEREBELLUM OPERATES AS THE CONDUCTOR OF MOVEMENTS

Recall that the cerebellum can be thought of as a conductor of movements. A conductor plays no musical instrument but coordinates dozens of musicians in actualizing the intention of a musical score. Under the conductor's direction, one orchestral section starts up just as another section rests. Similarly, the cerebellum does not contract muscles but tells motor control centers when and how much to activate which muscles in order to achieve the action orchestrated by the cerebral cortex. We can pursue this analogy a bit further. A solo musician has no need for a conductor because no intermusician coordination is required. In the same vein, simple movements restricted to one muscle or even a small group of synergist muscles—extending the index finger—take place without the cerebellum's assistance. However, just as an orchestral conductor cues the entry of one instrument section and the decrescendo of another, the cerebellum coordinates agonist relaxation with antagonist excitation in movements involving multiple muscles.

Timing is integral to the roles of both conductor and cerebellum. The conductor is far more critical to starts, stops, changes in loudness, and so on than to the continued playing of a passage of music. Likewise the coordinated timing of agonist and antagonist muscle contractions is far more difficult to achieve—impossible without the cerebellum—than is a maintained muscle contraction. When contractions of agonist and antagonist muscles occur with just the right timing, a movement will be executed as intended, exactly on target. Otherwise, ataxic or dysmetric movement results.

Finally, the conductor's influence on an orchestra differs during rehearsal and performance. During rehearsal, the conductor may interrupt musicians, correct errors, alter phrasing, and direct the repetition of several bars until satisfied. In contrast, during a performance, the conductor does not interrupt but uses the experience gained through practice to direct the orchestra. She or he ensures that the well-rehearsed orchestra stays on track principally through cueing musicians as discussed earlier. Additionally, a conductor must be responsive to changing conditions, altering the musical interpretation to fit the mood of the audience, the feeling of the occasion, or the acoustics of the venue. The cerebellum also plays distinct roles in the practice and execution of movements. While a movement is being learned, the movement is broken down or *decomposed* and rehearsed in parts. The cerebellum learns from errors made and corrects the ensuing movements. Corrected movements are repeated until learned. Once movements are learned, the cerebellum plays a different role. It correctly times muscle contractions according to what was learned during rehearsal and ensures that a movement occurs as intended. Yet the occasion for every repetition of an action differs in small or large ways, and the cerebellum flexibly adapts movements to changed conditions just as a conductor can change the performance of a musical piece from that which was practiced.

THE CEREBELLUM COORDINATES THE LEARNING AND PERFORMANCE OF MOVEMENTS

Simple movements, involving one or a few synergist muscles acting across only one joint, often proceed without the cerebellum's involvement. In contrast, *the motor circuits of the cerebellum act on movements employing multiple muscles working together across single or multiple joints.* The cerebellum ensures smooth movements through a two-step process:

1. *Motor learning*: After much repetition, at first deliberately executed and then progressively less and less so, movements are learned. Once learned, motor memories endure. A person does not forget how to skip, write her name, or pronounce multisyllabic words.

2. *Motor coordination*: After a movement is learned, the cerebellum makes its ensuing repetition feel automatic, despite the learned movement's actual complexity. The cerebellum also constantly updates previously learned movements, ensuring their smooth completion during changing conditions. Once expertise of a given movement has been achieved, the cerebellum directs the movement, altering the program to account for the condition of the body (e.g., energetic or fatigued) or external world (e.g., walking surface or writing implement) and adding flourishes as an occasion warrants.

For learning movements, the cerebellum develops, through practice, a series of associations between motor intention and motor reality—"when cells in one part of motor cortex fire a particular pattern of action potentials, my arm abducts so many degrees, but if these other cells fire, my arm elevates." After much trial and error during infancy and throughout life, the *cerebellum learns to associate actual movements with intended movements.*

Many of our motor memories are of movements that we have repeated millions or billions of times or more. For example, babies learn to stand and walk and then proceed to stand and walk *a lot.* The repetition of trillions of moments of postural sway or billions of walking steps ensures that the cerebellum has learned the motor expectations associated with standing and walking, and has learned them very well. These memories are difficult, if not impossible to forget, even in one who stops walking for months due to an injury. Yet there are limits. An individual who learns to juggle one afternoon and then practices juggling for an hour will need far more time to "recall" juggling movements after a break of 5 years than will an "over-practiced" expert juggler who takes a 5-year break. Along the same vein, the beginner juggler will pick juggling back up faster after not juggling for 1 day than 5 years. Nonetheless, eventually, after less time than required initially to learn how to juggle, the motor sequence involved in juggling will come back to even the erstwhile juggler.

Motor memories appear to operate best when done without thinking. Imagine a seasoned pianist sitting down in front of a grand piano on a stage in a concert hall full of people. After the lights dim, the audience applauds and the pianist begins to play. The pianist's playing is automatic, an act linked to the sensory setting and internal feelings by the cerebellum. A pianist who "thinks" too much about performing may freeze or perform poorly and haltingly. Similarly, professional athletes often attribute slumps to "over-thinking" and find that they perform optimally when relaxed and "on autopilot."

The cerebellum's involvement does not stop after a movement is learned. Changing conditions, external and internal, demand that our actual movements be continually measured against our intentions. Therefore, *the cerebellum continually checks for a match between intended and actual movements by determining whether the sensory feedback received matches the feedback that it expects to receive.* With a timed sequence of anticipated feedback information secured in memory, the cerebellum "knows" what sensory feedback to expect and when to expect it for each intended movement. When an already-learned movement goes off track, signaled by errant sensory feedback that deviates from the cerebellum's expectation, the cerebellum triggers an adjustment so that the received feedback once again matches the anticipated feedback. In this way, the cerebellum coordinates and ensures the smooth performance of semiautomatic movements that we and other mammals are innately destined to learn—standing, walking, running, reaching for food and bringing it to our mouth, looking around—as well as of movements peculiar to our modern lives—driving a car, writing Chinese script, typing on a keyboard, standing on a moving bus.

DIFFERENT CEREBELLAR PARTS REGULATE DIFFERENT TYPES OF MULTIMUSCLED MOVEMENTS

As you recall from Chapter 6, the cerebellar vermis occupies the midline and is flanked by a thin strip termed the *paravermis* and then by the expanse of the lateral hemispheres (Fig. 24-1A). Perpendicular to this broad sagittally oriented organization is a transverse organization of the cerebellum into anterior, central, posterior, and flocculonodular zones (Fig. 24-1B). The flocculonodular zone, consisting of the *flocculonodular lobe* and uvula and parts of the central vermis coordinate eye and head movements with vestibular and visual inputs. These areas are sometimes termed the *vestibulocerebellum*.

There is a broad somatotopy within the cerebellum. The vermis coordinates midline movements: speech, gait, postural control, and stance. The paravermis regulates the coordination of movements involving more distal musculature: reaching, grasping, and other appendicular movements. Paravermis lesions typically produce appendicular ataxia, similar to that illustrated in Fig. 6-5. In contrast, damage to the vermis, particularly the rostral portion, results in truncal ataxia. Truncal ataxia is characterized by a wide stance and unsteady gait, much like that of an infant or an intoxicated adult. As with an intoxicated adult, an individual with truncal ataxia is not able to walk heel to toe. Midline cerebellar lesions can also cause ataxic speech, which has an irregular pace and volume, similar to the speech of an intoxicated person. The similarities between the movements of patients with cerebellar lesions or disease, young infants, and drunken adults is no coincidence. In all three situations, the cerebellum is not working optimally. In young infants, granule cells are still being born, axons have not yet been myelinated, and cerebellar circuits have not been "calibrated." The mechanisms through which alcohol impairs cerebellar function are not entirely clear and are likely to be varied.

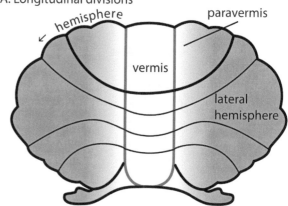

A. Longitudinal divisions

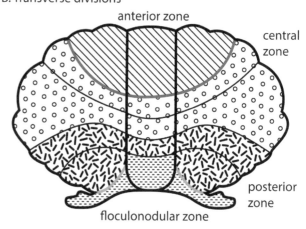

B. Transverse divisions

Figure 24-1 The gross longitudinal (A) and transverse (B) divisions of the cerebellum are diagrammed on a cartoon of a flattened human cerebellum. A: The vermis is an anatomically distinct region separated from the hemispheres by sulci (*red lines*). In contrast, the lateral edge of the paravermis is indistinct (*color gradient*). Lateral to the paravermis is the lateral hemisphere. B: The most anterior transverse division of the cerebellum is the anterior zone, which is separated from the rest of the cerebellum by the primary fissure (*red line*). The most caudal transverse division of the cerebellum is the flocculonodular zone. The hemispheric portion of the flocculonodular zone is separated from the rest of the cerebellum by the posterolateral fissures (*blue lines*). The vermal portion of the flocculonodular zone includes the nodulus and the uvula (unlabeled). The other two transverse divisions are the central and posterior zones. Modified from Apps R, Hawkes R. Cerebellar cortical organization: A one-map hypothesis. *Nature Rev Neurosci* 10: 670–681, 2009, with permission of the publisher, Macmillan Publishers Ltd.

The lateral portions of the cerebellar hemispheres are largest in animals with highly complex movement repertoires. For example, in a human, the lateral cerebellar hemisphere forms the bulk of the cerebellum and dwarfs the vermis, whereas the reverse is true in the rodent.

The entire motor map, including both axial and appendicular muscles, is represented in the lateral hemispheres. The anterior cerebellar hemispheres are reciprocally interconnected with motor areas of the cerebral cortex, primarily in the frontal cortex. The anterior cerebellar hemispheres are essential to complex motor tasks, tasks initiated by

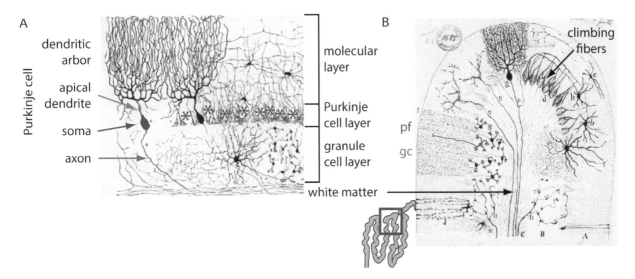

Figure 24-2 The cerebellar cortex is intricately organized, as originally described and drawn by Ramón y Cajal. These modified drawings from Cajal show the basic laminated structure of the cerebellar cortex and illustrate the principal cell and afferent fiber types. A: Cerebellar cortex has a cell-poor molecular layer, a Purkinje cell layer, and a granule cell layer. The Purkinje cell layer contains the somata of Purkinje cells. One such soma is colored in blue. An additional Purkinje cell soma is drawn in black. The climbing fibers innervate Purkinje cells so densely that the afferent fibers outline the location of the Purkinje cell somata. The blue asterisks show the location of Purkinje cells present at the center of concentrations of climbing fibers. The Purkinje cell sends an axon into the white matter below, and this axon eventually terminates in the appropriate deep cerebellar nucleus. The apical dendrite of the Purkinje cell branches extensively to form an elaborate dendritic arbor. B: A drawing of a transverse section through a folium shows a Purkinje cell (*top*), climbing fibers, the underlying white matter, and a number of granule cells. One granule cell (*gc*) is colored red, and its axon, which gives rise to a parallel fiber (*pf*), is colored in blue. The granule cell axon travels into the molecular cell layer, bifurcates, and then extends for up to millimeters in the medial-lateral direction, in and out of the plane of the paper. Drawings are adapted from Sotelo C. Viewing the brain through the master hand of Ramón y Cajal. *Nature Rev Neurosci* 4: 71–77, 2003, with permission of the publisher, Macmillan Publishers Ltd.

prefrontal cortex that often involve synergistic coordination across the body, actions such as painting, dancing, piano-playing, diving, or singing an aria, as well as in visually guided movements. The posterior portion of the hemispheres connects with nonmotor regions of cerebral cortex and may play important, albeit less widely recognized, roles in language, affect, thought, executive function, and social behavior.

PURKINJE CELLS ARE ORGANIZED INTO PARASAGITTAL STRIPES

Recall that the outer rind of the cerebellum is a cortex and that the *Purkinje cell* is a cerebellar cortical neuron with several remarkable anatomical features. Purkinje cells form a layer within the cerebellar cortex that is one cell wide (Fig. 24-2A). In other words, Purkinje somata are lined up like boxcars with absolutely no vertical stacking. The apical dendrite branches exuberantly, and the entire dendritic arbor is covered with spines. The Purkinje cell dendritic tree is oriented so that it is narrow, about the width of the soma (~50–75 microns), in one plane (parallel to the folia) and measures hundreds of microns across in the plane perpendicular to the folia. Since the sagittal plane is perpendicular

to the folia (for most of the cerebellum), Purkinje cell dendrites line up in the orientation of a Mohawk hairdo (Fig. 24-2B). The orientation of Purkinje cell dendrites dictates the organization of the cerebellar cortex. Purkinje cells within parasagittal stripes, oriented from rostral to caudal, form functional groupings or *microdomains*. The stripes occupied by the functional units only extend a short distance in the caudal to rostral direction. Consequently, there are thousands of microdomains in the cerebellum, and each functional grouping contains a few hundred Purkinje cells.

THE DEEP CEREBELLAR NUCLEI ARE THE SOLE CEREBELLAR OUTPUT

Deep to the cerebellar cortex is white matter, and deep within the white matter are bilateral sets of *deep cerebellar nuclei* (Fig. 24-3). Neurons in the deep cerebellar nuclei carry the output of the cerebellum to the brainstem and thalamus. The deep cerebellar nuclei receive input from the cerebellar cortex in a topographical fashion:

- Cerebellar cortex within the vermis projects to a pair of deep cerebellar nuclei, the *fastigial nuclei*, situated just off midline to either side.

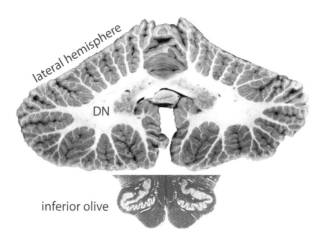

lateral hemisphere

DN

inferior olive

Figure 24-3 An unstained section through the cerebellum (*top*) and a myelin-stained section through the medulla (*bottom*) illustrate the relationship between the outlines of the lateral cerebellar hemisphere, dentate nucleus (*gray matter labeled DN*), and inferior olive. The resemblance between the outside contours of these three structures stem from their anatomical relationships. Cells in the main inferior olivary nucleus project topographically to Purkinje cells in the lateral hemisphere, and Purkinje cells in the lateral hemisphere in turn project topographically to the dentate nucleus. Top photograph reprinted with permission from deArmond S et al., *Structure of the human brain: A photographic atlas.* New York: Oxford University Press, 1989. Bottom photograph reprinted with permission from Bruni JE, Montemurro D. *Human neuroanatomy: A text, brain atlas, and laboratory dissection guide.* New York: Oxford University Press, 2009.

- Each paravermis projects to an interposed nucleus located lateral to the fastigial nucleus. On each side, there are two *interposed nuclei—posterior* and *anterior—* which are often called the *globose* and *emboliform* nuclei in older texts.

- The lateral hemispheres project to the large *dentate nuclei* whose elaborate shape resembles the contour of the hemispheres themselves (Fig. 24-3).

Thus, the gross somatotopy of the cerebellar cortex to deep cerebellar nuclei connection includes ipsilateral projections from vermis to fastigial nucleus, paravermis to interposed nucleus, and lateral hemisphere to dentate nucleus.

On top of the gross somatotopy, there is an extremely fine topography in the cerebellar cortex to deep nucleus projection pattern. Essentially, neighboring Purkinje cells project to neighboring deep cerebellar nuclear neurons. This means that the Purkinje cells in one microdomain project to a patch of neighboring deep cerebellar nuclear neurons. Since neurons in each deep cerebellar nucleus send axons out of the cerebellum to reach specific brainstem and diencephalic targets, Purkinje cells in one microdomain ultimately influence one motor control center. One final important aspect of the microdomains is that neighboring Purkinje cells receive input from neighboring cells in

the *inferior olives.* Because of the fine topography between inferior olives, Purkinje cells, and the deep cerebellar nuclei, the three areas actually resemble each other in appearance although not in scale. This resemblance is most clearly seen by comparing the outlines of the lateral cerebellar hemisphere, the dentate nucleus, and the principal portion of the inferior olive (Fig. 24-3).

In sum, the specific function of cerebellar cortical processing is shared by Purkinje cells in a microdomain. The idea is that Purkinje cells within a single functional unit influence the contribution of a particular motor control center to a particular type of movement via a projection to a restricted region in the deep cerebellar nuclei. For example, one group of microdomains may modulate corticospinal control of wrist movements while another set of microdomains modulates vestibulospinal control of postural sway and so forth. Lesions restricted to a small number of microdomains impair fewer movements than do lesions inclusive of many microdomains.

INFORMATION PASSES THROUGH TWO LOOPS WITHIN THE CEREBELLUM

The number of axons coming into the cerebellum outnumbers the number of axons that leave the cerebellum by a factor of 40 (Fig. 24-4A). The enormous influx of information into the cerebellum targets two regions: the cerebellar cortex and the deep cerebellar nuclei. These two regions are the only two areas where neurons reside. The relatively paltry (in number but not significance) output from the cerebellum leaves from the deep cerebellar nuclei. This extreme degree of convergence reflects the combined processing power of the cerebellar cortex and the deep cerebellar nuclei.

Since neurons of the deep cerebellar nuclei carry the output of the cerebellum to the brainstem and forebrain, the simplest cerebellar loop (Fig. 24-4B) consists of only one cerebellar synapse, the synapse between incoming fibers and a deep cerebellar nuclear neuron. A second pathway loops through the *cerebellar cortex* (Fig. 24-4C), which processes incoming information, transforming it into a *single coherent message* carried by the Purkinje cell, the only cell type in the cerebellar cortex that projects out of the cortex. The Purkinje cell targets neurons in the deep cerebellar nuclei, which then carry the final cerebellar message to the brainstem and forebrain. This second loop includes several synapses within the cerebellar cortex and provides the cerebellum with an enormous amount of additional processing power.

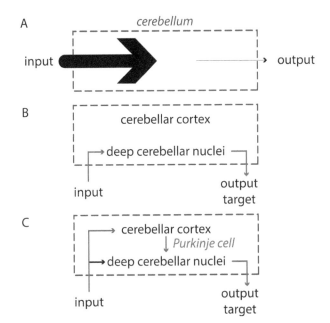

A

B

C

Figure 24-4 The basic inputs and outputs of the cerebellum are diagrammed. A: There are 40 times more afferent axons into the cerebellum (*thick black arrow*) than there are efferent axons from the cerebellum (*thin black arrow*). B: The simplest circuit through the cerebellum involves input to deep cerebellar nuclear neurons, which send axons out of the cerebellum to target structures. C: More processing power is contained in the circuit that includes a loop through the cerebellar cortex than in the simpler circuit diagrammed in B. Afferents to the cerebellum project to the cerebellar cortex. After processing in the cerebellar cortex involving multiple neurons, Purkinje cells within the cerebellar cortex send an axon to the deep cerebellar nuclei. Deep cerebellar nuclear neurons send an axon out of the cerebellum to a target structure in the brainstem or thalamus. Note that the Purkinje cell is the only cell that projects out of the cerebellar cortex.

As one consequence of the dependence on the deep cerebellar nuclei to carry the output of the cerebellum, *injury to the deep cerebellar nuclei or to the output of the deep cerebellar nuclei, principally carried in the superior cerebellar peduncle, will mimic an injury to the cerebellum itself.* A lesion of the decussation of the *brachium conjunctivum*, or superior cerebellar peduncle, will look like a lesion of almost the entire cerebellum. Incomplete lesions of the cerebellar output give rise to symptoms like those caused by lesioning upstream regions. So, for instance, a lesion of the fastigial nucleus has devastating effects on gaze control, equivalent to the consequences of damage in the nodulus, uvula, and central vermis. In contrast, injuries to the cerebellar cortex cause less severe and less permanent symptoms than do those to the deep cerebellar nuclei.

The simple loop through the deep cerebellar nuclei already tells us something about the role of the cerebellum in movement. The inputs to the deep cerebellar nuclei are excitatory, and, in turn, deep cerebellar nuclear neurons

powerfully excite their target neurons in the thalamus and brainstem, which causes excitation of motor control centers including the motor cortex. Thus, *cerebellar output strongly facilitates motor control center activity to such an extent that deep cerebellar nuclear neurons play an important role in the initiation and cessation of movements.* Activity in deep cerebellar nuclear neurons occurs before movements start and leads to movement initiation. Cerebellar dysfunction, therefore, leads to slower movements. When deep cerebellar nuclear neurons stop firing, movement stops, too. In sum, the cerebellum exerts a strong excitatory effect upon motor control centers and ultimately upon *movement*. Lesions or injuries to the cerebellum, particularly to the deep cerebellar nuclei, cause a slowing of movements and poorer performance at rapidly paced movement sequences.

Although neurons in both the cerebellar cortex and the deep cerebellar nuclei transform incoming information, the cerebellar cortex surpasses the deep cerebellar nuclei in processing power. *The cerebellar cortex is particularly important in learning new movement combinations.* All together, the speed and informational throughput of cerebellar processing far surpasses and is in fact in a different galactic realm than that of even the most sophisticated computer chips.

THE CEREBELLUM USES SENSORY REAFFERENCE AND MOTOR EFFERENCE COPY TO COORDINATE MOVEMENTS

The cerebellum anticipates the coordination necessary for smooth movements, ensuring that the movements that we make are those that we intend to make, even as conditions change. For example, when we reach for a cup handle, anything short of reaching the handle is a failure. Yet it would not work to spend our lives practicing all the possible situations that may call for this movement: reaching for differently sized cup handles located above or below you, near or far from you, a cup that is sitting upright or hanging on a hook. Instead, the cerebellum learns a number of different movement basics— arm extension, abduction, wrist pronation, grasp, and so on. Then, to perform a multimuscled, multijointed movement such as reaching for a cup, the cerebellum combines these basic movements together by sending a sequence of signals to motor control centers that cues the appropriate forces in specific muscles, each at the right time.

To compare actual with intended movements, information about both is needed. Information is provided by two types of information that reach the cerebellum (Fig. 24-5):

- *Reafference* is sensory information, coming back into the central nervous system (CNS) from the periphery, about the movement actually occurring.

- *Efference copy*, also called *corollary discharge*, is a neural copy of the intended or desired action.

We term sensory information arising from joints, muscles, and skin as "reafference" because it is sensory (afference) feedback back (re-) from a motor program that we are executing. Think of a pilot's pressing a button to lower the wing flaps and then receiving feedback from sensors signaling that the wing flaps are indeed in the down position; this feedback from sensors is akin to reafference. *In ideal circumstances, we would receive no surprises from reafference. Information coming back from the periphery to the cerebellum would match exactly the expected information, so that the movement would "feel right."* However when an individual does not "do" a movement quite right, the incoming reafference deviates from cerebellar expectations. In these circumstances, the returning sensory input "feels wrong" all of

a sudden. A person typically *senses* the exact moment when he made a wrong move, veering off course. Reafference can also differ from expectations because of unexpected changes, such as an unexpectedly soft spot in the ground or the sudden buckling of a knee.

Clearly, in order to render reafference meaningful, an expected outcome is required. *Information about the expected movement is carried by efference copy signals that serve as the gold standard to which actual movement is compared.* If reafference matches efference copy, all is well. However, when there is a mismatch, the cerebellum dictates appropriate adjustments. As the cerebellum modulates movement in a feed-forward fashion, it corrects *future* iterations of an errant movement. Thus, when stepping off the sandy beach and onto the sidewalk, the first step is too forceful, more appropriate for sand than concrete. The cerebellum quickly adjusts the gait, so that ensuing steps are appropriate.

Reafference and efference copy information to the cerebellum is carried by a heterogeneous group of afferents called *mossy fibers*. Mossy fibers arise from a number of sources but primarily from:

- The periphery via spino- and cuneocerebellar tracts (*reafference*)

- Motoneurons, motor interneurons, and central pattern generators via spino- and cuneocerebellar tracts (*efference copy*)

- Vestibular information, arriving via the vestibular nerve and nuclei (*mixed*)

- Cortex, including motor, premotor, somatosensory, and visual areas, via a synapse in the pontine nuclei (*efference copy*)

Mossy fibers travel primarily in the *middle* and *inferior cerebellar peduncles*. Mossy fiber input is *massive* in number and effect, providing the major excitatory energy that drives the cerebellum. Mossy fibers enter the cerebellum, travel through the white matter, and terminate in two places, reflecting the two cerebellar loops (Fig. 24-4B, C):

- *Deep cerebellar nuclei*: Mossy fibers directly excite neurons that project out of the cerebellum.

- *Cerebellar cortex*: Mossy fibers excite *granule cells* that in turn indirectly excite Purkinje cells.

Because mossy fibers carry both reafference and efference copy, *mossy fiber discharge increases by virtue of sensory input of any modality and from efference copy during self-generated movements.*

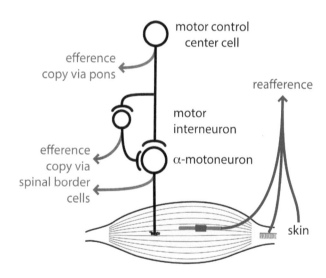

Figure 24-5 The sources of efference copy and reafference are shown on a diagram of the basic motor hierarchy. A motor control cell in the cerebral cortex contacts motoneurons and motor interneurons and sends efference copy information to the cerebellum via the pontine nuclei. Additional efference copy input derived from the discharge of motoneurons and motor interneurons arises from the ventral horn and is carried by spinal border cells into the cerebellum. Reafference information comes primarily from cutaneous mechanoreceptors and also from muscle afferents. Reafference input to the cerebellum is carried by spinal and medullary cells that receive primary afferent input from the dorsal columns. Note that, in all cases, there is an intermediary cell, or a *precerebellar* cell, between the source of the input (motor control center, motor interneuron, motoneuron, primary afferent) and the cerebellum.

THE CEREBELLAR CORTEX PROCESSES INPUTS THROUGH A STEREOTYPED CIRCUIT

Within the cerebellar cortex, the bulk of the input arrives via mossy fibers that synapse onto granule cells. Recall that the granule cells reside in their own layer—the *granule cell layer*—and account for more than half of all the neurons in the brain. Generating all of these neurons from the rhombic lip happens primarily after birth and requires years for completion.

Several mossy fibers converge onto each granule cell, which in turn sends out an axon that travels toward the pial surface, through the Purkinje cell layer, and bifurcates within the molecular layer into two long branches, termed *parallel fibers*, that travel along the long axis of the folia (Fig. 24-6A). Since parallel fibers travel perpendicularly to the orientation of the Purkinje cell dendrites, each parallel fiber contacts the dendrites of a multitude of Purkinje cells spread over many millimeters (Fig. 24-6B). This means that *information from a mossy fiber that contacts a granule cell within one region of the cerebellum is distributed to Purkinje cells in near and distant regions.* So, for example, information that comes into the paravermis may reach the vermis via the

far-reaching parallel fibers. This allows a Purkinje cell in the vermis that controls trunk musculature to "know" at least a little bit about, for example, the state of the elbow joint.

The ultimate destination for all cerebellar cortical circuitry is the Purkinje cell, which provides the only output from the cerebellar cortex. The Purkinje cell's processing of mossy-parallel fiber input represents the computational bottleneck of the cerebellar cortex: *each* Purkinje cell receives input from up to 200,000 parallel fibers and thus indirectly from a million or more mossy fibers (Fig. 24-6B). The effect of discharge in one parallel fiber upon a Purkinje cell is small, either resulting in an excitatory postsynaptic potential (EPSP) or a single action potential, which is termed a *simple spike*. Yet, *Purkinje cells receive such a multitude of synapses from parallel fibers that mossy fiber input constitutes their major excitatory drive.*

Purkinje cell firing reflects activity in mossy fibers as delivered by parallel fibers. On the output side, Purkinje cell axons leave the cerebellar cortex and project to the deep cerebellar nuclei. Since Purkinje cells contain γ-aminobutyric acid (GABA), they are inhibitory. They are also spontaneously active (Fig. 24-7). As one would expect, the next cells

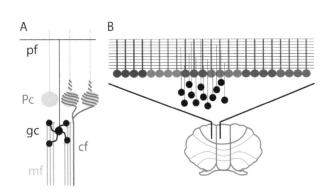

Figure 24-6 Cerebellar circuitry in the coronal plane. In this plane, the dendritic arbor of the Purkinje cells (*Pc*) is narrow and is represented here as simply a line. A: Purkinje cells receive indirect input from mossy fibers (*mf*). Many mossy fibers end on each granule cell (*gc*). Each granule cell sends an axon up into the molecular layer. The granule cell axon bifurcates into a parallel fiber (*pf*), which extends for long distances in the longitudinal plane of the folia. Along the way, a parallel fiber can contact thousands of Purkinje cells, and each Purkinje cell receives hundreds of thousands of synapses from parallel fibers. The second source of afferent input to the Purkinje cell is the climbing fiber (*cf*), which arises from the inferior olive. A climbing fiber innervates a few to several Purkinje cells, but each Purkinje cell receives input from only one climbing fiber. B: Recall that Purkinje cells form functional units or microdomains that are oriented as short sagittal stripes in the rostral to caudal direction. Here, Purkinje cells belonging to distinct microdomains are denoted by different colors. The parallel fibers arising from granule cells extend across many microdomains and can even cross the midline or traverse the divisions of the cerebellum.

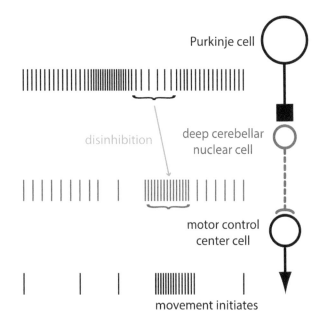

Figure 24-7 The firing patterns of three connected cells. Purkinje cells are GABAergic cells that inhibit deep cerebellar nuclear neurons. Each vertical line represents an action potential. At rest, Purkinje cells fire more rapidly than do either deep cerebellar nuclear neurons or cells in motor control centers. When the discharge rate of the Purkinje cell increases, the deep cerebellar nuclear neuron fires less rapidly, and, when the discharge rate of the Purkinje cell decreases, the deep cerebellar nuclear neuron is disinhibited. Disinhibition results in an increase in the firing rate of the postsynaptic cell and, in this case, in a burst of activity in the motor control center cell. This burst of activity can initiate a movement.

in line, deep cerebellar nuclear neurons, are also spontaneously active. Purkinje cells fire at typical rates of 50 Hz to more than 200 Hz, whereas deep cerebellar nuclear neurons fire at slightly more modest rates, commonly about 20–50 Hz. When Purkinje cells increase their firing rate, deep cerebellar nuclear neurons are inhibited, maybe even pausing. In contrast, when there is a relative lull in Purkinje cell firing, deep cerebellar nuclear neurons are *relieved from inhibition*, a process termed *disinhibition* (Fig. 24-7). Disinhibition involves a decrease in incoming inhibition. The firing rate of the postsynaptic cell—in this case, a deep cerebellar nuclear neuron—then increases. Thus, when Purkinje cell firing slows, the discharge of targeted deep cerebellar nuclear neurons increases. As you already know, more firing in deep cerebellar nuclear neurons results in facilitation of motor control centers and thereby movement initiation.

LEARNING IN THE CEREBELLAR CORTEX DEPENDS ON CLIMBING FIBERS

As you can imagine, correctly anticipating the effects of muscle contractions is the key to proper cerebellar function. Remember that most cerebellar neurons are born, receive afferents, and become myelinated axons postnatally, at a time when a baby can learn to associate motor commands with their consequent physical effects. After the cerebellum has developed and an infant has spent sufficient time playing, babbling, and gesticulating seemingly without purpose, cerebellar neurons have learned enough from past motor experiences to "know" what reafference to expect from a given movement. By anticipating the correct reafference, the cerebellum can prevent errors before they occur. So, movements, at least simple ones, are "spot-on" even when performed for the first time. A child who learns how to take her sippy cup from a parent can also pick the cup up from the floor. Even when physical conditions change—imagine the sippy cup being either nearly empty or completely full—the cerebellum quickly learns how those changes will alter the anticipated feedback and thereby adjusts the movement after minimal disruption.

Climbing fibers, the axons of inferior olive neurons, are key to the learning performed by the cerebellar cortex. Climbing fibers only arise from the inferior olive; all other afferents to the cerebellum are mossy fibers. Climbing fibers arise from the inferior olive, enter the cerebellum through the contralateral restiform body, and excite Purkinje cell dendrites directly. Each climbing fiber wraps itself around the soma and dendrites of a small number of Purkinje cells

that are contained within a single microdomain (Fig. 24-6A). Early in development, multiple climbing fibers synapse onto a single Purkinje cell. However, these multiple inputs are pruned so that in healthy adults each Purkinje cell receives only one climbing fiber.

Climbing fibers do not fire rapidly, discharging irregularly at an average rate of about once per second. Yet the climbing fiber makes up in magnitude what it lacks in quantity. The climbing fiber-to-Purkinje cell synapse is so strong that a single presynaptic potential elicits a large depolarization upon which about five action potentials ride in the postsynaptic Purkinje cell. This response is termed a *complex spike*. Despite the large excitatory response to climbing fiber input, the *net effect of climbing fiber input is actually to suppress Purkinje cell firing*. This decrease in Purkinje cell discharge rate stems from a decrease in the strength of the parallel fiber input through a form of long-term depression (LTD) (see Chapter 13). The molecular mechanisms responsible for LTD in the cerebellum, an area of active investigation by several groups, resemble those responsible for long-term potentiation (LTP) in hippocampus.

The mechanism by which climbing fibers *teach* Purkinje cells is the subject of great and ongoing controversy. Regardless of the specific sequence of events, the upshot is that *climbing fibers provide a teaching signal that tells the Purkinje cell what set of parallel fiber inputs to anticipate and when to anticipate these inputs for any given intended movement*. As mentioned earlier, the learning step occurs when climbing fiber input depresses the strength of parallel fiber synapses active at the same time. In other words, the teaching signal from the climbing fiber depresses Purkinje cell firing in response to reafference and efference copy inputs of the moment. Thereafter, the parallel fiber inputs (both reafference and efference copy) that led to the errant movement will be weakened, and other inputs will gain in relative strength. In this way, Purkinje cells receive stronger inputs from a new set of parallel fiber inputs, a set of inputs that was not associated with the immediately preceding movement error. Through repeated corrections in response to repeated errors, the Purkinje cell input is dominated by inputs that have not been depressed because they were not associated with movement error. This basic learning mechanism supports one of the cardinal features of cerebellar learning: *cerebellar learning requires movement errors*. To reiterate, the cerebellum cannot operate on flawless movements. Luckily, errors come naturally to any animal that moves on earth. Movement begets errors, and errors beget learning.

Through trial and error, repeated rehearsal of a movement trains the cerebellum to associate a set of reafference inputs with a particular efference copy message. Imagine stepping onto a boat for the first time. The feed-forward adjustments that allowed for postural stability and a balanced gait on land will fall short at sea. You will have to use your cerebellum to modify your postural control and gait programs over the course of several days. In other words, you need to "get sea legs." Even as a person learns the sea-legs program, she does not forget how to walk on land. This illustrates the cerebellum's ability to learn and retain multiple, distinct motor programs that operate on the same body parts. These motor programs do not interfere with each other, nor do they degrade over time. Thus, a sailor who returns to land after months at sea can quickly return to normal terrestrial walking and standing. Similarly, after establishing cerebellum programs for walking, marching, running, and cycling, one can seamlessly and perfectly switch between these motor activities without bleed-through of one activity into another.

THE CEREBELLUM PROVIDES FEED-FORWARD MODULATION

Cerebellar coordination of movement operates in anticipation, in a *feed-forward* manner. Thus, in the absence of the cerebellum, mistakes continue to be made and continue to be corrected *after* the fact. This type of error occurs in ataxia. Ataxic movements involve an abnormal sequence of muscle contractions and relaxations, with the error being greatest as the target is neared. Ataxic movements result from the replacement of anticipatory modulation with feedback corrections. Figure 24-8A, B shows the movement trajectories of control subjects and subjects with an inherited form of ataxia on two different tasks. In one task, subjects were asked to move their hands through a target into a soft barrier that stopped their arms' forward movement, whereas, in the other task, subjects were asked to move their hands to a square and stop there. Patients' arm trajectories on the former task, in which a barrier ended the movement, were indistinguishable from those of control subjects. In this situation, arm extension was stopped by arm mechanics. In contrast, patients overshot the target in the latter task and subsequently made a corrective return movement.

Cerebellar dysfunction stems from an inaccurate or unavailable predictive model. As discussed earlier, the cerebellum coordinates movements by anticipating a sequence of appropriate inputs as the movement is carried out. When an error occurs, the inputs received do not match those expected by the cerebellum's *internal model*. A correction

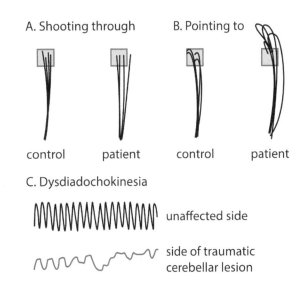

A. Shooting through   B. Pointing to

control   patient   control   patient

C. Dysdiadochokinesia

unaffected side

side of traumatic cerebellar lesion

Figure 24-8 Control subjects and patients with inherited spinocerebellar ataxia were asked to move a joystick on a trajectory that passed through but did not stop in the red square (A) or to move the joystick into the square and stop there (B). The lines indicate the trajectories on four attempts by each subject at this task. Control and patient trajectories were very similar on the "shoot through" task. However, on the pointing task, control subjects' trajectories all ended within the target square, whereas the patients' trajectories all overshot (= hypermetria) and then had to come back to the target. C: In a patient with a gunshot wound in the cerebellum, tracings of the hand trajectory while alternating patting the thigh with the palm and dorsum of the hand. Diadochokinesia is normal on the side contralateral to the lesion but severely impaired on the side of the lesion. Note that performance on the affected side degrades over time, suggestive of fatigue. Panels A and B are adapted from Tseng Y, Diedrichsen J, Krakauer JW, Shadmehr R, Bastian AJ. Sensory prediction errors drive cerebellum-dependent adaptation of reaching. *J Neurophysiol* 98: 54–62, 2007, with permission of the publisher, American Physiological Society. Panel C is adapted from Holmes G. The Croonian lectures on the clinical symptoms of cerebellar disease and their interpretation. *Lancet* 200: 59–65, 1922, with permission of the publisher, Elsevier.

is made that prevents that error from occurring in subsequent movements. However, in patients with cerebellar lesions or disease, often, the internal model itself is off. The result is impaired predictive coordination of movement. In particular, agonist muscle contraction is slow to start and lasts too long. To compound matters, antagonist muscle activation is delayed. Finally, insensitivity to load or other inertial changes during movement prevents adjustments to changing conditions. All of these factors lead to abnormal movements.

Patients with ataxia cannot hit a target with one smooth movement. They find that they need to make movements quite deliberately, "thinking" through each piece of the movement. When agonist–antagonist muscle pairs are not activated in a coordinated fashion, the component movements happen sequentially, producing a *decomposition of movement*. Movement also occurs more slowly. Finally, feedback corrections occur only after mistakes have been made, resulting in a sometimes prolonged series of corrective movements.

CEREBELLAR DAMAGE DISRUPTS THE INTERNAL MODEL

As you now understand, the cerebellum is critical to timing and sequencing the muscle contractions that make up a movement. Let us once again consider the example of reaching for a cup handle. To extend the arm, the triceps needs to be activated, but once the arm nears the cup, the triceps activation needs to be terminated and the biceps activated as a brake. If arm flexion occurs too early or too late, the target will be undershot or overshot, respectively. Likewise, activating the "biceps-brake" at the wrong time or for too short or for too long a time results in a movement that misses the target. Making movements that are too short or too long is termed *dysmetria*. Patients with cerebellar lesions or disease often make *hypermetric* or *hypometric* movements, movements that reach beyond the targeted goal or fall short of it, respectively.

The critical contribution of the cerebellum to starting and stopping movements is particularly evident in the performance of rapidly alternating movements. Joseph Babinski, a French neurologist and student of Jean-Martin Charcot (of Charcot-Marie-Tooth fame), introduced the use of rapid back-and-forth movements, termed *diadochokinesia* (Greek for "succeeding movement"), as a test for cerebellar function One way to test diadochokinesia is to ask a person to move his palm up and down rapidly on his thigh. Such a quickly alternating movement requires tight coordination between supinating and pronating forearm muscles that rotate the palm up and down. As another example, repeated articulation of "pa-ta-ka" tests for cerebellar coordination of lip, tongue, and soft palate movements critical to phonation. Cerebellar patients are able to perform each component movement of a diadochokinesia test but are unable to make the same movements in quick sequence. The difficulty appears to be in the synergy that connects component movements. The slowing of or inability to make rapidly alternating movements is termed *dysdiadochokinesia* and is highly suggestive of a cerebellar problem (Fig. 24-8C).

In individuals with dysdiadochokinesia, agonist muscle contraction continues for an abnormally long time and initiation of antagonist muscle contraction is delayed. As a result, agonist and antagonist muscle contractions overlap. As the number of joints involved increases, the number of movement torques that need to be accounted for also increases, and cerebellar modulation is increasingly critical. Thus, slapping the thigh as just described is more challenging than making the motion that screws in a light bulb. The former requires shoulder in addition to wrist movement whereas the latter relies almost exclusively on wrist

movements. Asking a patient to perform diadochokinesia at a faster pace also increases the difficulty level because the speed of performance limits the availability of reafference information, which requires time to reach the cerebellar cortex.

Clumsiness is frequently associated with cerebellar dysfunction. Objects may fall out of a patient's grasp. Interestingly, grasp issues occur independently of ataxia; they result instead from a failure to match grip force to load. For example, consider a person who pours water from a pitcher held in the left hand into a glass held in the right hand. In a healthy individual, there is no delay between the glass getting heavier and the individual's grasp increasing in strength. This is because the cerebellar cortex anticipates the load change stemming from the self-generated movement of pouring and sends a signal to increase grasp strength. This signal is sent before the load actually changes. Due to having an inaccurate internal model, cerebellar patients are impaired at predictive load matching.

Understanding the role of the internal cerebellar model has led to a clever approach to treating cerebellar patients with dysmetria. Because each patient's internal model is altered in a particular direction, patients are consistently hypermetric or consistently hypometric. For example, hypermetric patients overshoot but do not undershoot movements. As it turns out, hypermetric patients underestimate limb inertia and start movements slowly. As the movement deviates increasingly from the intended course, the hypermetric patient reacts by increasing the force of the movement, leading to an overshoot. On the other hand, hypometric patients overestimate limb inertia and start movements with too much force. They then react to the increasing error by slowing down, resulting in an undershoot. To treat these problems, neuroscientist Amy Bastian and colleagues changed each patient's arm inertia to match their internal model. For example a load was added to the arm of a hypometric patient. This added load meant that the patient's excessively fast and forceful start kept the arm on track. No error occurred, and the patient's dysmetria was corrected.

INPUTS TO THE VERMIS, PARAVERMIS, AND LATERAL LOBES

The entire cerebellum shares the same basic circuit architecture. Mossy fibers provide sensory reafference and efference copy information to the cerebellar cortex. Purkinje cells sum up the deliberations of the cerebellar cortex and deliver the resulting message to deep cerebellar nuclear neurons.

Deep cerebellar nuclear neurons then carry the output from the cerebellum to outside brain regions. Although these general principles hold throughout all divisions of the cerebellum, the particular tracts and brain regions involved differ across the divisions. In this and following sections, the major inputs to and outputs from the vermis, paravermis, and lateral hemispheres are outlined.

The cerebellum receives direct reafference and efference copy about the arms, trunk, and legs from four different tracts that ascend from the spinal cord and caudal medulla (Table 24-1). Two tracts carry direct reafference—one from the legs and trunk and one from the arms—and two carry direct efference copy—again one from the legs and trunk and one from the arms.

Reafference input arises from secondary sensory neurons (i.e., neurons that receive primary afferent input). These secondary sensory neurons are located in the spinal cord in the case of the legs and trunk, and in the caudal medulla in the case of the arms. Leg and trunk proprioceptive input to the cerebellum arises from neurons in *Clarke's nucleus*, located in the thoracic spinal cord, via the *dorsal spinocerebellar tract*. Arm proprioceptive input to the cerebellum arises from the *external* (or *accessory*) *cuneate nucleus* (just lateral to nucleus cuneatus) and travels in the cuneocerebellar tract. Both the dorsal spinocerebellar and cuneocerebellar tracts course through the *restiform body* and enter the cerebellum through the inferior cerebellar peduncle.

Spinal border cells located in the ventral horn receive copies of motoneuron and motor interneuron discharge and give rise to two tracts that carry efference copy into the cerebellum. Spinal border cells in the lumbosacral and cervical cords carrying efference copy information give rise to the *ventral* and *rostral spinocerebellar tracts*, respectively. Like the tracts carrying reafference information, the rostral spinocerebellar tract enters the cerebellum through the

inferior cerebellar peduncle. The ventral spinocerebellar tract is unusual in two ways:

- The ventral spinocerebellar tract enters the cerebellum through the *superior* cerebellar peduncle and is the only afferent tract to do so.

- The ventral spinocerebellar tract crosses within the spinal cord, whereas the other spinocerebellar and cuneocerebellar tracts travel ipsilaterally. The ventral spinocerebellar tract crosses again upon entering the superior cerebellar peduncle, thus terminating ipsilateral to its site of origin.

The cerebellum receives vestibular and visual inputs as well as somatosensory afferents. Because the vermis is most involved in controlling axial musculature including the head, it is not surprising that the vermis also receives auditory information and proprioceptive input from eye, head, neck, and shoulder muscles.

In addition to inputs from the spinal cord and medulla, the cerebellum receives a *massive* amount of input from most areas of the cerebral cortex. Cerebral cortical neurons do not project directly to the cerebellum but rather reach the cerebellum via pontine nuclear neurons. Pontine nuclear neurons receive afferents from the neocortex and in turn send an axon across the midline, through the middle cerebellar peduncle, and into the cerebellum (see Fig. 6-4). The *basis pontis* and middle cerebellar peduncle are entirely utilized by the pathway from cerebral cortex to cerebellum. The enormity of these two structures embodies the scale of the connection from cerebral cortex to cerebellum.

As you understand, the cerebral cortex and cerebellum are not so far apart that one neuron could not traverse the entirety of the distance. Yet cortical neurons only access the

Table 24-1 THE FOUR MAJOR PRECEREBELLAR TRACTS ARISING FROM THE SPINAL CORD AND CAUDAL MEDULLA ARE LISTED

	DORSAL SPINOCEREBELLAR TRACT	VENTRAL SPINOCEREBELLAR TRACT	CUNEOCEREBELLAR TRACT	ROSTRAL SPINOCEREBELLAR TRACT
Type of information	Reafference	Efference Copy	Reafference	Efference Copy
Body parts	Legs and trunk	Legs and trunk	Arms	Arms
Arises from	Clarke's nucleus	Ventral horn	External cuneate nucleus	Ventral horn
Enters through	Restiform body/Inferior cerebellar peduncle	Superior cerebellar peduncle	Restiform body/Inferior cerebellar peduncle	Restiform body/Inferior cerebellar peduncle

Two tracts carry reafference information, and two tracts carry efference copy input. One tract carrying input of each type concerns the legs and trunk, and one tract of each type concerns the arms. The cells of origin for each tract, as well as the cerebellar peduncle through which the tract enters the cerebellum, are also listed. The restiform body is a tract that forms the bulk, but not all, of the inferior cerebellar peduncle. The other tract within the inferior cerebellar peduncle is the juxtarestiform body, which contains the output from the fastigial nucleus bound for reticular and vestibular nuclei.

cerebellum through the *pontine nuclei.* The obvious implication is that pontine neurons contribute to the translation or compilation of cerebral cortical information for the cerebellum. Unfortunately, we know and understand little about pontine nuclear function at present.

Motor-related input from the cerebral cortex destined for the cerebellum arises from somatomotor and prefrontal cortices. There are particularly strong projections from primary motor cortex, supplementary motor area, somatosensory, and parietal association cortices. Much of the input from frontal cortex carries information about movements that are either in progress or are being mentally rehearsed.

THE OUTPUT OF THE VERMIS TARGETS DESCENDING POSTURAL CONTROL AND ORIENTING TRACTS

The output of the vermis reaches motor centers primarily concerned with postural control and orienting movements. Purkinje cells in the vermis project to the fastigial nucleus. Neurons in the fastigial nucleus project out of the cerebellum to four main targets:

- Ventrolateral thalamus, and from there to primary motor cortex to cells that give rise to the ventral corticospinal tract

- Superior colliculus to control tectospinal output

- Reticular nuclei that give rise to reticulospinal tracts

- Vestibular nuclei that give rise to vestibulospinal tracts

The output from the fastigial nucleus to the ventrolateral thalamus and superior colliculus travels through the superior cerebellar peduncle, as do the vast majority of cerebellar efferents (Fig. 24-9A). However, cerebellar outputs to reticular and vestibular nuclei travel through the *juxtarestiform body,* which joins with the restiform body to form the inferior cerebellar peduncle (Fig. 24-9B).

The vermis modulates postural control and axial movements, as well as orienting movements including gaze (see Chapter 19). Of great clinical importance, the vermis modulates gait. As you recall from Chapter 22, central pattern generators in the lumbar spinal cord support the basic stepping cycle or gait. Yet, even in our modern world, stepping needs to be adjusted to the task at hand and to the environment. Slowing down to walk with a child, speeding up to get to class on time, turning, and walking up a rocky incline all require modifications of gait. The cerebellum coordinates the needed modifications, and recent evidence shows that the cerebellum contributes to the coordination of the left and right legs' step cycles. The belt on a treadmill can be split so that the left and right halves of the treadmill are controlled independently. A person walking on a split-belt treadmill matches each leg's gait to its half belt so that, for example, the right leg may be going at a faster speed than the left leg. People are even able to walk in different directions with their two legs—stepping forward with one leg and backward with the other. A healthy person's ability to perform this "cerebellar task" depends on performing it without thinking about it directly, in an automatic-like fashion. Individuals with cerebellar disease or lesions cannot walk on a split-belt treadmill, evidence that this type of gait modulation depends on a working cerebellum.

Patients with lesions of the anterior vermis often have an impairment of gait. Affected patients walk at a slow pace with a wide stance and longer lasting stance and double support phases. Yet it appears that most of these gait alterations are compensatory adjustments rather than primary effects of the lesion or disease. The primary issue may be a lack of coordination between the two legs, between legs and trunk, and so on. The "cerebellar gait" is highly variable from one step to the next and this unpredictability only serves to increase the chance of error and ultimately instability.

THE OUTPUT OF THE PARAVERMIS TARGETS THE LATERAL CORTICOSPINAL AND RUBROSPINAL TRACTS

The output of the paravermis targets rubro- and corticospinal pathways necessary for reaching, grasping, and other movements using appendicular muscles. Purkinje cells in the cerebellar cortex of the paravermis project to the interposed nucleus, which in turn sends efferents through the superior cerebellar peduncle to synapse in:

- Ventrolateral thalamus, and from there to primary motor cortex and other cortical regions where cells give rise to the lateral corticospinal tract

- Magnocellular portion of the red nucleus, which gives rise to the rubrospinal tract

Through these connections, the paravermis is particularly important to reaching and grasping movements (Fig. 24-9C).

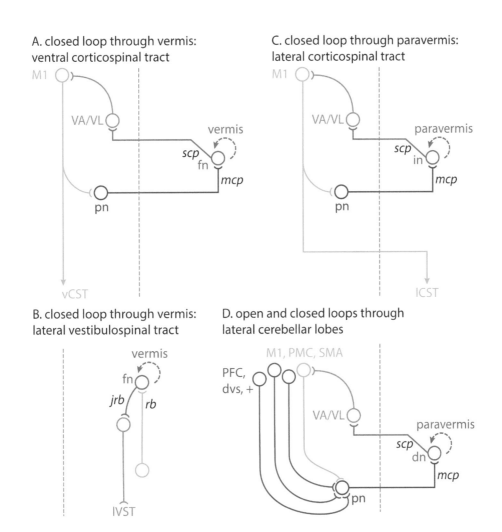

A. closed loop through vermis:
ventral corticospinal tract

C. closed loop through paravermis:
lateral corticospinal tract

B. closed loop through vermis:
lateral vestibulospinal tract

D. open and closed loops through
lateral cerebellar lobes

Figure 24-9 Exemplary loops through each cerebellar division are illustrated. A: Neurons in motor cortex (*M1*) that give rise to the ventral corticospinal tract (*vCST*) send a collateral to the pontine nuclei (*pn*). Pontine nuclear neurons project across the midline (*dashed gray line*) and enter the vermis through the middle cerebellar peduncle (*mcp*). Neurons in the fastigial nucleus (*fn*) carry a signal that is modulated by the output from cerebellar cortical circuits (*dashed red line*). They project through the superior cerebellar peduncle (*scp*) and across the midline to the thalamus (*VA/VL*). Neurons in VA/VL thalamus project back to M1. B: The connections of the vermis with the vestibulospinal and reticulospinal tracts are entirely ipsilateral. Afferent input to the vermis comes in through the restiform body (*rb*) and superior cerebellar peduncle (not shown). Efferents from the fastigial nucleus travel through the juxtarestiform body (*jrb*) to hindbrain targets including the vestibular nuclei that give rise to the lateral vestibulospinal tract (*lVST*). C: The closed loop through the paravermis differs from the circuit of the ventral corticospinal tract through the vermis in two ways. The motor cortex cells involved give rise to the lateral corticospinal tract (*lCST*) and the participating deep cerebellar nucleus tract is the interposed nucleus (*in*). D: The lateral lobes of the cerebellum receive an enormous influx of afferents from most areas of cerebral cortex, especially from motor areas, prefrontal cortex (*PFC*) and parietal cortex of the dorsal visual stream (*dvs*). Projections from the dentate primarily target neurons in somatomotor cortex. Abbreviations: PMC: premotor cortex; SMA, supplementary motor area.

CEREBELLAR LOOPS THROUGH THE VERMIS AND PARAVERMIS CONTINUALLY CHECK MOVEMENTS

Pathways through the vermis and paravermis start and end in the same place, forming a closed loop. For instance, when a postural adjustment arises from lateral vestibulospinal tract neurons or when cells in motor cortex initiate a reach and grasp movement, the output of the cerebellum reaches the vestibulospinal or motor cortical cells either directly in the former case or indirectly via the thalamus in the latter case.

When the motor cortex, red nucleus, or reticulospinal or vestibulospinal neurons initiate a movement, efference copy from the spinal cord border cells reaches the cerebellum via mossy fibers from the spinocerebellar tracts (Fig. 24-9A, C). The Purkinje cells compare the planned movement with reafference received from mossy fibers from the dorsal spinocerebellar or cuneocerebellar tracts. When the end of a movement is reached and position equals intended target, the Purkinje cell is strongly activated, which in turn essentially stops all activity in the deep cerebellar neuron, thereby reducing the excitatory drive on the motor center targeted by the cerebellum so that the movement ends. This loop through the cerebellum takes about 20 ms to complete and is happening all the time. Essentially, this loop keeps our movements smooth and coordinated.

LOOPS THROUGH THE LATERAL CEREBELLAR HEMISPHERES ARE USED TO LEARN FANCY NEW MOVEMENTS

Movements that involve the lateral lobes of the cerebellum are typically fancy or skilled movements rather than the movements such as walking and postural balance that we are innately destined to learn. They often require coordination between multiple limbs or between vision and movement, so-called *eye–hand coordination*. They include skilled movements, such as a fancy dance step, or motions used to play a new musical instrument or sport. As an example, consider teaching a child how to serve a tennis ball. To do this, the eventually fluid motion is initially broken up into segments: stance, toss the ball, knee bend, upswing, hit the ball, follow through. At first, each motion is practiced separately and then combined in a deliberate fashion. Practice utilizes the lateral cerebellum to recognize the proper feel of each serve component and eventually to sequence them together seamlessly. When learning is complete, the entire serve is performed without thought: it is a motor memory, and the cerebellum then simply oversees its future repetition by rote execution.

The input to the lateral lobes comes from a wide swath of neocortex dominated by afferents from somatomotor and prefrontal cortex. In addition, parietal cortex involved in visual processing, primarily the dorsal visual stream, sends information to the lateral lobes (Fig. 24-9D). Purkinje cells in the lateral cerebellar hemispheres project to neurons of the dentate nucleus, which in turn send efferents through the superior cerebellar peduncle to terminate in:

- Ventrolateral thalamus, and from there to cells primarily located in primary motor cortex, premotor cortex, and supplementary motor area
- Parvocellular portion of the red nucleus, which in turn projects to the inferior olivary nuclei, the source of climbing fibers

Loops through the lateral lobes are either closed, starting and ending in the same cortical region, or open, starting and ending in different cortical regions. In the case of open loops, input to the cerebellum arrives from a far wider swath of cerebral cortex than is targeted by the output pathway. In this way, language, vision, emotions, motivations, and memories can all be brought to bear on the way in which the cerebellum coordinates a given movement.

The lateral hemispheres are critically involved in coordinating movements under visual or other mental guidance. Yet, curiously, individuals can withstand large lesions of the lateral cerebellar hemispheres with little motor dysfunction. Ataxia is not typically seen after damage to the lateral hemispheres. Thus, it may be that the lateral hemispheres contribute more to learning new skilled movements than to correctly making previously learned ones. The lateral lobes are also critical to visually guided actions and to nonmotor functions as well.

THE CEREBELLUM MAY ALSO MODULATE NONMOTOR FUNCTIONS INCLUDING COGNITION, AFFECT, AND HOMEOSTASIS

Language, cognition, affect, and visceral function may rely on contributions from cerebellar circuits. This idea has been controversial but is gaining wider acceptance. Major support for nonmotor cerebellar functions comes from neuroanatomy: most parts of the cerebral cortex, including nonmotor areas, project into the cerebellar cortex, via the pontine nuclei. Although nonmotor problems resulting from cerebellar injury or disease are typically overshadowed by obvious ataxic and dysmetric movements, deficits in language, cognition, affect, and visceral function are documented in patients with cerebellar lesions. Some of the nonmotor roles that have been proposed for the cerebellum include:

- Input from the temporal lobe of the dominant hemisphere, critical to language, reaches the contralateral posterolateral cerebellum, a region within the territory of the posterior inferior cerebellar artery (PICA; see Chapter 8). During language tasks, this part of the cerebellum is active. Furthermore, lesions of this area, typically due to a PICA stroke, produce difficulties in language that are well beyond those expected by motor difficulties in speech and articulation.

- Prefrontal cortex, critical to so many functions that make us "human," forms a loop with the posterior lateral lobes and the dentate nucleus. This loop may be important for people to match their behavior and affect to the appropriate situation, meaning that, in the absence of this function, people act inappropriately—being overly familiar with strangers, flat with loved ones, swearing in a formal situation, or joking when faced with a serious situation.

- The vermis contributes to normal visceral function. Through connections with the hypothalamus, the vermis influences cardiorespiratory adjustments to postural changes, exercise, and stimuli that elicit fear.

Since the microarchitecture of the entire cerebellum is the same, the processing transform imposed on nonmotor inputs is likely to be the same as that imposed on motor inputs. If you imagine cerebellar processing as a set of gears (would it be so simple), then motor and nonmotor information alike are changed or transformed by similar sets of gears. While we do not yet enjoy a deep understanding of the "cognitive transform" or the "cerebellar transform," the deficits suffered by patients with cerebellar lesions suggests that the cerebellum may process virtually every brain function. This idea is further supported by modern imaging studies showing activation of cerebellar neurons in a wide variety of language, reasoning, affective, and behavioral tasks.

There are many speculative ideas regarding what the cerebellum contributes to nonmotor function, but this remains an open and very important—as well as controversial—area of investigation. The answer must conform to the following principles:

- The cerebellum is an associative learning specialist, using data to rapidly adapt brain function to changing conditions.

- The cerebellum receives an enormous amount of sensory information about the outside world and the body's internal state.

- The cerebellum receives an enormous amount of information from cortex about ongoing activities—movements, thoughts, mood.

- When functioning properly, the cerebellum modulates function in advance, in a feed-forward manner, guaranteeing proper function and preventing mistakes before they occur.

One speculative idea is that our "automatic" reactions—be they motor, affective, cognitive, or linguistic—are elicited by familiar situations, situations that have occurred countless times before. The cerebellum may associate a particular output—movement, feeling, thought, or language—to a particular set of internal and external stimuli. Just as one learns to smoothly serve a tennis ball or play a piano solo, one can presumably learn a cognitive strategy for solving a problem, constructing sentences, making instant judgments about people, evaluating the power structure in a group, or assessing one's safety.

In the past decade or two, evidence has accumulated that the cerebellum plays a causative role in at least some forms of *autism*. One of the strongest pieces of evidence for this idea is that neonatal damage to the cerebellum dramatically increases the chance of autism to a similar degree as smoking increases the risk of lung cancer. Neuroscientist Samuel Wang and colleagues synthesized the developmental *diaschisis* (from Greek *dia*, "to set against each other" and *chisis*, "to split"; meaning an action that occurs at one time but exerts its effects at a different time) hypothesis from a large number of experimental and clinical findings. Essentially, they propose that neonatal cerebellar damage has downstream organizing effects on neocortical circuits responsible for executive and limbic functions critical to social behavior. According to this hypothesis, early dysfunction of the cerebellum due to traumatic damage or environmental (e.g., gestational exposure to valproic acid, known as Depakote in the United States) and/or genetic (e.g., 15q11–13 maternal duplication) factors, changes neocortical development, particularly in areas important to social behavior, communication, emotional reciprocity, and *repetitive behavior* or *stereotypies*. One can imagine that the neonatal cerebellum's role in setting up distant brain circuits may bear relevance to a variety of developmental disorders. This is an exciting area for future investigation.

ADDITIONAL READING

Apps R, Garwicz M. Anatomical and physiological foundations of cerebellar information processing. *Nat Rev Neurosci.* 6: 297–311, 2005.

Apps R, Hawkes R. Cerebellar cortical organization: A one-map hypothesis. *Nat Rev Neurosc.* 10: 670–681, 2009.

Bastian AJ. Learning to predict the future: The cerebellum adapts feedforward movement control. *Curr Opin Neurobiol.* 16: 645–649, 2006.

Bhanpuri NH, Okamura AM, Bastian AJ. Predicting and correcting ataxia using a model of cerebellar function. *Brain.* 137: 1931–1944, 2014.

Bell CC. Evolution of cerebellum-like structures. *Brain Behav Evol.* 59: 312–326, 2002.

Bodranghien F, Bastian A, Casali C, et al. Consensus Paper: Revisiting the symptoms and signs of cerebellar syndrome. *Cerebellum.* 15: 369–391, 2016.

Dum RP, Li C, Strick PL. Motor and nonmotor domains in the monkey dentate. *Ann N Y Acad Sci.* 978: 289–301, 2002.

Gebhart AL, Petersen SE, Thach WT. Role of the posterolateral cerebellum in language. *Ann N Y Acad Sci.* 978: 318–333, 2002.

Gladwell M. *Blink.* New York: Back Bay Books, 2005.[1]

Sotelo C. Viewing the brain through the master hand of Ramón y Cajal. *Nat Rev Neurosci.* 4: 71–77, 2003.

Thach WT. What is the role of the cerebellum in learning and cognition? *Trends Cogn Sci.* 2: 331–317, 1998.

Therrien AS, Bastian AJ. Cerebellar damage impairs internal predictions for sensory and motor function. *Curr Opin Neurobiol.* 33: 127–133, 2015.

Tseng Y, Diedrichsen J, Krakauer JW, Shadmehr R, Bastian AJ. Sensory prediction errors drive cerebellum-dependent adaptation of reaching. *J Neurophysiol.* 98: 54–62, 2007.

Wang SS, Kloth AD, Badura A. The cerebellum, sensitive periods, and autism. *Neuron.* 83: 518–532, 2014.

---

1. Note that the word cerebellum is not mentioned in *Blink*. Yet, one may speculate that the unconscious and quick judgments discussed in this thought-provoking book could arguably employ cerebellar function.

25.

BASAL GANGLIA

ACTION SELECTION

he *striatum* and *pallidum* are the core participants in circuits that adapt behavioral output to conditions with continually changing priorities and dangers. As introduced in Chapter 7, functional and connectional considerations have led to grouping forebrain and midbrain nuclei—the *substantia nigra pars compacta, substantia nigra pars reticulata*, and the *subthalamic nucleus*—together with the striatum and *globus pallidus* as the basal ganglia. These regions operate via parallel but interacting loops with the cortex and brainstem to influence motor, oculomotor, motivational, emotional, and perceptual components of behavior. This chapter focuses on circuits through the dorsal striatum that contribute to skeletomotor *action selection*.

Although they are intimately involved in motor function, the basal ganglia exert their effects indirectly through projections to motor control centers of the brainstem and even more indirectly through projections, via thalamus, to cortex, primarily motor and prefrontal cortices. Targets of basal ganglia output in turn control the motivation, affect, strategy, and initiation of self-generated actions.

THE CORE FUNCTION OF THE BASAL GANGLIA IS TO CHOOSE BETWEEN MUTUALLY EXCLUSIVE ACTIONS

The striatum and pallidum are phylogenetically ancient structures, with the former present in the earliest vertebrates—think jawless fish, hagfish and lamprey—suggesting that the original, and potentially still core, function of the striatopallidal system solves a problem that all animals face. The ubiquitous and fundamental problem resolved by the basal ganglia is that *actions that use the same muscles differently simply cannot occur simultaneously.* A fish cannot swim to the left for food, to the right toward a mate, *and* forward to get farther away from a predator

circling behind. The fish has to choose one of these actions. Similarly, we cannot turn left to go to a fruit stand, right toward a friend's apartment, and accelerate forward in case the speeding car behind does not slow down. Just as fish do, we must choose one of several, mutually exclusive actions. *In fish, reptiles, birds, and mammals, including humans, striatopallidal circuits select and promote one action while suppressing competing actions.*

The process of choosing one action from many possible ones is termed *action selection*. Ideally, animals employ a strategy for action selection that favors their emotional and physical state. Actions that bring about favorable results are repeated and those that disappoint are avoided. Several neuropsychiatric disorders can be understood as problems of different sorts with action selection. For example, action selection breaks down when a person stays with an action beyond the point of that action's usefulness, a process termed *perseveration*. *Obsessive-compulsive* behavior represents perseverative action. A person who compulsively washes her hands until they are raw and bleeding perseverates, failing to select another action even though the hand-washing no longer provides any benefit. Alternatively, a person may not stick with an action long enough to derive full benefit. *Attention-deficit hyperactivity disorder* exemplifies this type of problem in which a child flits from one action to another or one focus to another. Motor disorders such as *Tourette syndrome* involve excess movements and may result from incomplete suppression, so that inappropriate, random movements break through the basal ganglia's suppressive blanket and interrupt appropriately selected actions. Basal ganglia dysfunction has been implicated in all of the above-mentioned disorders.

Although organized similarly in animals throughout the vertebrate tree, neurons and circuits of the basal ganglia achieve far greater complexity and vastly more connections in the cerebral cortex of mammals and especially in humans.

The increase in basal ganglia complexity from hagfish to human reflects:

- A much more complex body plan. Humans control limb, digit, laryngeal, and facial muscles that fish, sharks, and snakes do not possess.

- More complex interactions with gravity and the physical environment on land than in the sea.

- A larger behavioral repertoire. Fish swim this way and that, whereas humans swim, crawl, walk, hop, run, jump, and skip as well as play guitar, imitate bird calls, and so on.

- Our bipedal gait frees our hands. Humans are unique in having forelimbs and hands that can manipulate objects while hindlimbs take care of locomotion. This arrangement allows for behavioral multitasking during exploration that is not possible in other animals.

- An enormously complex social structure, in which individuals tailor their actions to specific persons or people. A child shares her favorite toy with a best friend but not with a stranger.

- The ability to learn from experience and match behavior to particular circumstances. An infant goes to pet the friendly cocker spaniel and unfamiliar pit bull alike, whereas, after acquiring some experience with dogs, she pets the friendly cocker spaniel and even the familiar pit bull, but walks away, hands in pockets, from the unfamiliar pit bull.

Humans not only face more options when considering what to do at any one time than do fish, but they also consider far more variables in making the decision than do fish. Nonetheless, the fundamental challenge of choosing between available options is the same whether one faces two or a thousand options, and therefore the same basic neuroarchitectural solution to the action selection problem works in hagfish, lamprey lizards, sparrows, elephants, and humans.

OUR DEFAULT CONDITION IS TO DO NOTHING

At rest, the basal ganglia suppress all movement, so that not moving is our default condition. One can think of the basal ganglia as one large wet blanket, greatly hindering movement—or thought or emotion—until and unless the importance of an action reaches a critical level. This is a

useful strategy because it prevents the arbitrary and potentially chaotic release of actions in inappropriate combinations or at inopportune times.

When a candidate action becomes imperative, the basal ganglia release only the imperative action from suppression while maintaining the wet blanket over all other possible and therefore competing actions. Determining which action to allow out from under the basal ganglia's suppressive clamp depends on the circumstances. The action judged most salient based on present conditions and past experiences wins the competition, and the basal ganglia release this action from inhibition. Other potential actions, losing competitors to the winning action, remain suppressed by the basal ganglia. If circumstances change and a different action becomes sufficiently imperative, the basal ganglia interrupt the current action and release the newly imperative action from inhibition. As we move through the world, the basal ganglia paces and sequences particular actions to fit with external conditions, our own judgments of urgency, and lessons learned from past actions.

THE BASAL GANGLIA RELEASE SELECTED ACTIONS FROM SUPPRESSION

Basal ganglia circuits choose an action from among the candidate actions possible for any given muscle. They then control how long an action continues, whether a different action is of sufficient urgency to interrupt the current ongoing action, and when to end an action. The basal ganglia exert limits on our movements that go far beyond the absolute constraints imposed by our body's mechanics. Everyone can pat their head and everyone can rub their stomach. However, patting the head with one hand and rubbing the stomach with the other does not come easily. It takes practice. Yet the component actions are easy and require no practice. There is no physical reason why patting the head and rubbing the stomach cannot occur at the same time. *The only obstacle to multiple simultaneous actions arises from the "chooser" within the brain, the basal ganglia.*

Consider a clerk at the grocery store. As the clerk scans through one customer's items, a shopper asks, "Where could I find chicken broth?" Clerks, particularly novices, typically stop scanning items as they look up, think for a moment, and then tell the shopper the aisle number where soups and broths are shelved. Yet *continuing to scan grocery items while answering a question presents no true physical challenge.* In other words, moving items past a scanner and speaking are both easy movements, and since they employ non-overlapping musculature, nothing prevents the two movements from occurring simultaneously. Only because of the basal ganglia's influence do the two nonconflicting movements not occur together. Put in anthropomorphic terms, it appears that, in their enthusiasm to prevent conflicting movements from occurring together, the basal ganglia have gone overboard in preventing even compatible movements from occurring together.

CHUNKING TOGETHER OFTEN REPEATED MOVEMENTS ENABLES SIMULTANEOUS ACTIONS

You may be frowning and shaking your head while also chewing gum at the idea that the basal ganglia prevent movements from occurring together. And, of course, you are right. Two or more movements occur together all the time, but only after they have been practiced and *chunked* by the striatum. To understand chunking, consider the eye movements that you make to view a face. You move your eyes to focus on the eyes, mouth, hair, and so on and thereby identify the individual. However, you do this so quickly that the time between saccades is insufficient to allow for sensory feedback from one saccade to trigger the next saccade. In other words, as one saccade completes, the next one is already programmed and ready to go. The sequencing of successive movements into a single chunk is a key function of the basal ganglia.

The term *chunking* was originally coined with reference to memory in recognition of our limited capacity to recall an increasing number of items. More than about seven items overloads the typical person's working memory. Packaging items together into chunks provides a solution. Thus, instead of remembering your social security number as nine separate numbers, you store and retrieve it—or fail to recall it—as a single piece of information. The number does not come back one number at a time but in an all-or-none burst. In the motor version of chunking, reducing an intrinsically complicated sequence of movements into one action provides great advantages over deliberately performing each component movement.

Chunking offers an enormous speed advantage. To illustrate this, we consider the task of typing or texting the word "the." For a person who is not an expert typist or texter, the key representing "t" will be searched for and then pressed. After checking that a "t" has appeared on the screen, the key representing "h" will be searched for, pressed, and the letter's appearance confirmed with a quick glance. Finally the "e" will be found and pressed (Fig. 25-1A). In stark contrast,

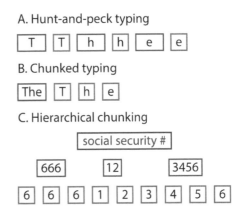

A. Hunt-and-peck typing

| T | T | h | h | e | e |

B. Chunked typing

| The | T | h | e |

C. Hierarchical chunking

social security #

| 666 | 12 | 3456 |

| 6 | 6 | 6 | 1 | 2 | 3 | 4 | 5 | 6 |

Figure 25-1 A: Without chunking, the keystroke (*red boxes*) for every letter in a word (*blue boxes*) is performed separately and deliberately after the completion of the previous keystroke. B: When typing a chunked word such as "The," keystrokes for each letter of the word are processed in parallel and occur without an intervening pause and in an automated fashion. C: Simple chunks are combined to make longer and more complex chunks. In this example, the hyphen-separated groupings of a social security number are chunked separately (for recall or articulation) and then combined into a higher-level chunk. Note that social security numbers cannot start with 6-6-6, and therefore this is not a usable number.

a habitual typist makes the three keystrokes needed to type "the" in one fluid, fast, and concatenated motion (Fig. 25-1B). The expert typist uses parallel processing of the component keystrokes so that as soon as the left index finger presses the t key, the right index finger is already in place and can press the h key. In this way, typing proceeds at a fast clip with minimal time between keystrokes. This is basal ganglia chunking in action. Prior to the ubiquity of autocorrect, anyone who needed to correct misspelled words employed the benefits of chunking. Even though it requires more movements to retype a simple word such as "that" than it does to fix one letter in a misspelled version such as "thet," the former is what we choose to do. Retyping "that" can be performed quickly as a chunk whereas replacing an "e" with an "a" requires slow and deliberate, focused action.

Beyond improved speed, chunking offers an additional advantage in that it reduces cognitive load. As a person hunts and pecks for letters on a keyboard, she is unable to think of much else. In contrast, an expert typist can talk and think while typing in an automated fashion. Grouping together all the movements needed to perform an action frees up the brain's capacity to perform additional cognitive tasks. For example, in one experiment, expert typists were given a set of five digits to recall before typing either a word or a nonword, a scramble of the letters in a word (e.g., brain to irnba). They were then asked to recall a string of five digits. Even experts cannot type nonwords automatically, in a chunk. Thus, this experiment compares working memory during chunked and unchunked actions. The average number of incorrectly recalled digits more than tripled while typing (unchunked) nonwords compared to (chunked) words. Moreover, the average number of typing errors quadrupled. Thus, chunked actions allow for concentrated focus on higher level thoughts, goals, and actions that would otherwise overwhelm an individual's cognitive capacity. They are also associated with reduced performance variability and thereby fewer errors.

Chunking results from plastic changes in the synapses that afferents make onto striatal neurons. Striatal learning occurs outside of cortical control and therefore automatically and not by conscious choice. One can no more consciously choose to chunk actions than choose not to. Sequential movements associated with positive outcomes are repeatedly selected. This repeated selection favors the future repetition of the same movement sequence through changes in synaptic strength. When a series of movements is selected over and over again, occurring in the same order time after time, synaptic changes reinforce the circuits that give rise to that sequence of related movements. Thus, component movements are chunked into an all-or-none action, enabling a series of movements to be relatively hard-wired together. In this way, *chunking permits a sequence of movements to occur without the need for deliberately intending each component movement.*

Once learned, chunks are combined with other chunks in a hierarchical structure in order to accomplish meaningful actions. For example, in opening a door, a person grips the doorknob, rotates the doorknob, pushes on the doorknob, holds the doorknob while walking over the threshold, and finally releases the doorknob. Each of these movements is itself a chunked action. These elemental chunks are themselves chunked into a single automatic action. When recalling a social security number, in the form of XXX-YY-ZZZZ, the first, second, and third number groupings are recalled as low-level chunks and then chunked together into a higher level chunk (Fig. 25-1C). Just as hierarchical chunking extends our ability to recall more digits, it also extends our capacity to make multiple simultaneous movements. This is highly relevant to safe driving. An experienced driver—one who has essentially chunked all of driving into one automatic action—may be able to change the radio station while driving on the expressway. In contrast, a student driver who still performs each component chunk of driving individually finds it challenging to add the simple movements involved in changing the radio station to the multitude of component driving chunks not yet grouped together within a "super-chunk" or *habit*. Although "habit" and "chunk" are synonymous terms, I will use *habit* to refer to high-level actions such as walking or driving and *chunks* to refer to low-level component actions. Hierarchical chunking allows for a modular approach to actions, repurposing low- or mid-level chunks for use in multiple habitual actions.

As the preceding examples show, concatenation of basic chunks into increasingly complicated chunks enables the assembly of complex behaviors. Such layered chunking allows action selection to work on loftier choices than would be possible in the absence of chunking. Thus, one chooses between taking a shower and fixing breakfast rather than between supination and pronation of the wrist. Now consider a store employee who has worked as a clerk for many years. After endless repetition, the clerk likely has grouped the movements involved in scanning items into one chunk. Therefore, when asked a question, the "over-trained" clerk can easily continue to scan items while answering a customer's question because scanning items is one action rather than a multitude of motions, as it is for a clerk new to the job. Multitasking becomes possible as long as only one of the tasks requires conscious control. For example, while walking—a chunked action—people can also chat with a friend, make a calculation, or catch a ball. In sum, *the basal ganglia allow multitasking when all but one task is performed as a chunk, thereby freeing cortex to initiate nonroutine actions.*

Along with the advantages of chunking comes a disadvantage—once started, a chunk is difficult to modify or interrupt. Chunks are inflexible. Once a signature is begun, very deliberate effort is required to alter the name signed. For example, to start signing Edwin and switch to Edward midway is challenging, particularly for someone who has signed *Edwin* a few thousand times previously. The habit is hard to change and difficult to break altogether. The difficulty in interrupting a chunk stems in large part from *the independence of that chunk from its outcome.* In other words, we complete chunks regardless of whether they produce positive, neutral, or negative results. A complete sentence is typed regardless of how many mistakes are made. *Freeing chunks from contingencies enables us to quickly perform complicated movements without focused thought and attention and allows people to achieve many of their goals on "automatic pilot."*

Dissociating habitual actions from resulting outcomes can promote completion of acts that may not always serve us well and may even lead to debilitating problems. People with obsessive-compulsive disorder feel compelled to perform a habit, such as washing hands, from its beginning and in its entirety. Since habits are freed from contingencies, they continue even when no longer useful or even harmful. Obsessive-compulsive patients replay the same habit over and over again even though it serves no purpose and, in many cases, causes injury or distress. It is in this context of reinforced habits that are *outcome-independent* that the basal ganglia greatly interest scientists interested in *substance abuse*. Drugs of abuse may initially produce pleasurable outcomes, but, upon becoming habits, they eventually wreak havoc on a user's life. Despite the adverse consequences, drug-using continues to be favored by the basal ganglia because it has been transformed into an outcome-independent habit. In other words, the habit of using a substance such as nicotine, alcohol, heroin, or cocaine persists even as that use causes personal wreckage.

PATHWAYS THROUGH THE BASAL GANGLIA EMPLOY THE SAME INPUT AND OUTPUT PORTS

Circuits resulting in action selection and chunking follow common pathways through the basal ganglia, which we explore in some detail here. In general, the basal ganglia process input from two area and return their verdict—the product of all their processing—to the same, and related, nearby areas. These *loops* through the basal ganglia moderate between competing candidate actions—or thoughts, perceptions, emotions—and then release the winning candidate from inhibition while ensuring that the losing candidates remain suppressed.

The architecture of basal ganglia loops is stereotyped across the different loops. At its root, the architecture is quite simple, involving two regions that receive input and two regions that project out of the basal ganglia to target structures. Afferents from outside of the basal ganglia project into and excite neurons in:

- Striatum

- Subthalamic nucleus

The output from the basal ganglia is carried by neurons in:

- Substantia nigra pars reticulata

- Internal globus pallidus

The projection neurons in both substantia nigra pars reticulata and the internal globus pallidus are inhibitory, utilizing γ-aminobutyric acid (GABA) as a fast neurotransmitter.

Features characteristic of loops through the striatum are ideally suited to selection regardless of whether the thing being selected is an action, thought, strategy, or emotion.

First, as with the cerebellum, *the striatum receives far more inputs than there are outputs.* This allows all "candidates" access to the selector—the striatum—while also maintaining the striatum's selection-making authority. One can think of the striatum as akin to the casting director of a drama who entertains as many hopeful actors as care to audition but chooses only one to play each part. Furthermore, the default state is that none of the candidates is selected, just as none of the actors has the part prior to auditions. The striatum maintains this default state through tonic GABAergic inhibitory output, provided by neurons in the internal globus pallidus and the substantia nigra pars reticulata, to all target structures.

More than 90% of the neurons in the striatum are GABAergic neurons of medium size with spine-covered dendrites; these cells are called *medium spiny neurons*. Input to the striatum converges onto medium spiny neurons. In the case of skeleto- and oculomotor loops, regions within motor control centers that influence movement of a specific body part converge on medium spiny neurons within a localized region of the striatum. For example, both frontal eye fields and the superior colliculus (cortical and subcortical sites that control eye movements) project into the caudate. In the same vein, medial parts of motor cortex project to the leg region of the putamen, which also receives input from the subcortical *mesencephalic locomotor region*.

Although allowing an open and full competition between synaptic inputs, the striatum, like the director of a play choosing the actor for a part, selects only one winner from the candidates bidding for control of each resource; the resource can be particular muscles, thought, attention, motivation, perception, or emotion. Selection takes the form of a focal relief of the inhibition exerted on the winning input. For example, a saccade toward a diving hawk may be released from inhibition while saccades to a building, cloud, or tree continue to be suppressed.

Cortical and subcortical sites connect with the striatum through different routes (Fig. 25-2). Cortical regions project directly into the basal ganglia but receive output from the basal ganglia only indirectly via the thalamus. In contrast, subcortical regions, such as the superior colliculus and the mesencephalic locomotor region, project indirectly, via the thalamus, to the basal ganglia but receive output directly. A thalamic area used as a way-station from subcortical sites to the striatum is the intralaminar nuclei, a group of about a dozen small thalamic nuclei with diverse functions. The intralaminar nuclei remain incompletely understood, but one view is that the intralaminar nuclei link attention and arousal to cognitive, motor, limbic, and sensory processes.

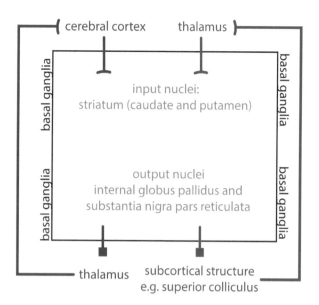

input nuclei:
striatum (caudate and putamen)

output nuclei
internal globus pallidus and
substantia nigra pars reticulata

cerebral cortex   thalamus

basal ganglia (left side)

basal ganglia (right side, top)

basal ganglia (right side, bottom)

basal ganglia (left side, bottom)

thalamus   subcortical structure
e.g. superior colliculus

Figure 25-2 Cortical loops (*brown on left*) involve direct projections to the basal ganglia coupled with indirect projections, via thalamus, from basal ganglia back to cortex. In contrast, subcortical structures reach the basal ganglia only through a synapse in thalamus but receive output from the basal ganglia directly (*blue on right*).

In a head-to-head competition, *subcortical inputs enjoy an advantage over cortical ones because the former synapse on striatal neurons more proximally and more densely than do the latter.* This advantage promotes subcortical goals such as orienting toward a streaker unexpectedly running across the front of the lecture hall—a movement mediated by the superior colliculus—over continuing to orient toward the lecturer—an action mediated by frontal eye fields. Indeed, most people would find *not* glancing at the streaker a most difficult task.

The power of subcortical inputs in guiding the striatum is revealed by experiments in which the cerebral cortex has been removed. Experimental animals left with only subcortical structures still seek and consume food, groom themselves, and even take care of their offspring. Thus, subcortical inputs to the basal ganglia are sufficient for many of the actions that mammals perform every day. In fact, most of our daily activities are packages of motor behavior that have been chunked by the basal ganglia and are performed by rote without cognitive oversight.

THE SKELETOMOTOR LOOP EMPLOYS EFFERENCE COPY AND SENSORY AND COGNITIVE INFORMATION TO ACHIEVE ACTION SELECTION

The basal ganglia influence actions using skeletal muscles through the *skeletomotor loop*. The notable exception to this

rule is that eye movements are modulated by the oculomotor loop of the basal ganglia. In this chapter, we focus on the skeletomotor loop through the basal ganglia before briefly discussing loops through the basal ganglia that influence cognitive and emotional function.

In order to select an action, the basal ganglia utilize information of three major types:

- *Efference copy* that provides a running record of current and imminent actions, as well as those in the immediate past (see Chapter 24 for a refresher on efference copy if needed)

- *Sensory, cognitive, and affective information* that conveys the current internal and external circumstances, as well as memories associated with those circumstances

- *Urgency or saliency of different actions*, including the action being currently performed

Efference copy from currently selected actions heavily biases basal ganglia selection. Thus, *without a compelling reason to stop, we typically continue doing what we are currently doing.* A person reading the newspaper at one moment is astronomically more likely to be reading the newspaper than to be doing sit-ups or any other action besides newspaper-reading a minute later. In this way, efference copy allows for *behavioral continuity* in our actions, lending great advantage to the current action over any other potential action. Of course, behavioral continuity also supports biological inertia, favoring the continuation of ongoing activity—or inactivity, as the case may be—for hours. In this regard, think of the great effort needed to start an activity, such as writing a term paper, in contrast to our ready ability to while away an entire afternoon continuing to "do nothing." When a selected action is completed— the newspaper has been read—efference copy stops, and basal ganglia selection is once again an open competition. *By biasing action selection heavily toward the currently selected action, efference copy input to the basal ganglia promotes sticking with an action for as long as it takes to complete the action while also preventing us from perseverating with an action already completed.*

Internal desires and external stimuli lend support to one action or another, tipping the basal ganglia's ultimate "decision" toward a particular action. Consider how grocery clerks would behave if, instead of working 8-hour shifts, they worked 1,000-scan shifts; viz., the clerk could leave work after scanning 1,000 items regardless of whether this took 2 or 12 hours. One can imagine that, working under this regime, many more clerks would quickly train themselves to group scanning items into a chunk. Sensations, thoughts, and emotions also influence action selection. Most people are far more likely to go bike-riding on a sunny day than on a rainy one, when their legs feel strong rather than when experiencing muscle cramps. People are more likely to exercise on January 2, propelled by New Year's resolve, than just a few days earlier in late December. We pick fights when angry or frustrated much more often than when we are happy or even sad. In sum, the solution to every instance of action selection—should I do a cartwheel, lift weights, or play with my cat?—depends on internal and external sensations, cognition, and affect.

OPERATIONAL LEARNING PROVIDES CRITERIA WITH WHICH TO CHOOSE BETWEEN ACTIONS

Every candidate action offers different advantages and disadvantages. To choose between candidate actions, action selection uses criteria, preferably criteria that serve an organism's survival needs. The selection criteria employed by the basal ganglia are based on operational learning, an unconscious associative process continuously executed by the basal ganglia. Operational learning is the process by which we learn to associate actions with the immediate consequences of those actions. Operational learning is also called *instrumental, procedural, operant,* or *reinforcement learning.* It is *an implicit type of learning in which we learn the effects of self-generated actions.* This information is used to bias behavior toward actions that produce positive effects over those that cause negative effects. In this type of learning, an individual acts and then learns the consequences of that action. A cat meows in the morning and is fed, a child who cries is picked up and comforted, a person walks outside with bare feet and sustains a foot injury, a basketball player does not play defense and is benched. As a consequence, the cat meows every morning, the child cries to get attention, the person wears shoes when venturing outdoors, and the player tries to block opposing teams' shots. Thus, actions that produce favorable outcomes recur, and those that produce immediately adverse effects are rarely repeated.

Operational learning works over a very short time frame so that *the immediate consequences of an action are the only consequences taken into account.* Consequences that occur some time later are not associated with actions through operational learning. Thus, a rat that presses a lever and receives an intravenous bolus of cocaine a second later learns to associate pressing the lever with the immediately positive feeling produced by the cocaine. Why not press the lever again and again? Indeed, rats do just that and may press a lever for a drug such as cocaine to the exclusion of eating and other critical survival behaviors. Operational learning does not take the "long view" but rather continues to favor continued lever-pressing over the wiser choice of eating, drinking, and sleeping. The start of drug abuse may be the product of operational learning. Once drug-taking becomes a habit, it is no longer constrained by contingencies, as described earlier. Moreover, the extinction or unlearning of operational learning is slow. How many days would you have to ignore a cat's meow or a baby's cry before the cat or the baby would stop trying to get your attention by meowing or crying? An individual who wants to unlearn the ultimately counterproductive behavior of drug abuse faces a difficult biological obstacle.

Rules learned through operational learning become the criteria and provide the evaluative structure that allows for selection between potential actions. When a visitor pushes a doorbell, a sound emanates from within the dwelling. When this first happens to a child, the *ding-dong* is unexpected. However, after learning this operational rule, the only unexpected outcome would be *not* hearing a sound after pressing a doorbell. One idea posits that a phasic burst of dopamine release accompanies unexpected sensory events and facilitates the association between the preceding motor command and the resulting sensory outcome.

All predictions emerging from operational learning exist unconsciously, although some rise to conscious levels as well. Some lessons derived from operational learning are both realistic and critical to survival—pet cats learn through operational learning that if they meow loud enough, they will be fed. Other lessons derived from operational learning are more hopeful than realistic—every time I touch my hand to my ear and then rub my chin, I make a foul shot. Operational learning is neither logical nor based on thought processes. Because of the highly subjective nature of operational learning, the basal ganglia do not always make wise choices that optimize benefit and minimize danger. One person having fond memories of beach vacations may excitedly jump into the ocean to swim and play whereas another person, remembering a past pummeling by surf, runs from every incoming wave, frightened to even wet her feet. Weighty actions—talking about a momentous event, running from perceived danger, eating when hungry—win the basal ganglia's attention far more often than do banal, tedious ones. *In sum, memories and associations formed by operational learning, more so than sensory details, tip the scales for or against candidate actions.*

Motor control regions that influence movement of a specific body part all project to a localized region of the striatum, within the putamen in the case of the skeletomotor loop. For example, in the oral region of the putamen, neurons might receive inputs from various cortical regions involved in generating a smile of enjoyment, a smile used for greeting, whistling, and kissing, all actions that require mouth muscles. As should be clear by now, only one of the mouth movements listed can occur at a time, and the basal ganglia select the winner.

Three major pathways loop through the basal ganglia, arbitrating between all potential movements to choose one action (Fig. 25-3). I list the three pathways here with their general function in action selection; subsequent sections describe each pathway in more detail:

- The *hyperdirect pathway* through the subthalamus provides a global stop signal that stops all movements. This is the *global inhibition* pathway.

- The *direct pathway* through the putamen and internal globus pallidus releases a selected action from suppression. This is the *action initiation* pathway.

- *Indirect pathways* through the putamen, subthalamus, and globus pallidus has the net effect of selectively suppressing specific movements but not all movements. This is the *selective inhibition* pathway.

In addition to these three pathways, local circuits are instrumental in shaping the final output of the basal ganglia. Local circuits within the striatum, internal globus pallidus, and substantia nigra pars reticulata use lateral inhibition to facilitate the bids of leading candidates while inhibiting loser candidate actions—the neural equivalent of jumping off the sinking ship to get on the bandwagon. *Lateral inhibition opposes indecision in action selection, preventing us and other animals from spending unproductive time deciding between candidate actions of nearly equal weights.*

Recall that neurons in the substantia nigra pars compacta are dopaminergic neurons that project to the caudate and putamen as the *nigrostriatal dopamine pathway*. Centered on the midline of the midbrain, between the left and right substantia nigra, is the *ventral tegmental area* that contains another group of dopaminergic cells. Dopaminergic cells in the ventral tegmental area supply dopamine to the *nucleus accumbens* (often called simply *accumbens*), also known as the limbic striatum. The accumbens occupies the ventral

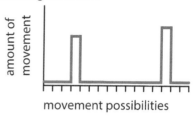

A. Starting condition

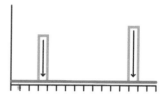

B. Hyperdirect pathway: global inhibition

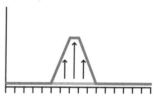

C. Direct pathway: initiate action

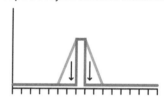

D. Indirect pathways: selective inhibition

Figure 25-3 A functional overview of basal ganglia pathways in cartoon. In each graph, the amount of movement (*y axis*) for a number of discrete action possibilities (*x axis*) is plotted. A: In the starting condition, two actions are in progress. Actions that occur simultaneously are typically both well practiced and use different muscles, for example, walking and chewing gum. B: When a high-priority action possibility arises, the first pathway engaged is the hyperdirect pathway. The effect of the hyperdirect pathway is to quickly stop all actions in process. C: Immediately following the hyperdirect pathway, the direct pathway is engaged, leading to focal disinhibition of a salient action. This disinhibition may not be perfectly focused on the chosen action. D: Indirect pathways provide an annulus, or donut, of inhibition around the chosen action. Thus, the indirect pathways sharpen the disinhibition produced by the direct pathway. Dopamine facilitates the direct pathways (*upward blue arrow*) through D_1 receptors and exerts a net inhibitory modulatory effect (*downward blue arrow*) on indirect pathways mediated by D_2 receptors.

region present at the rostral pole of the striatum. Dopamine arising from the ventral tegmental area is released in the nucleus accumbens. This release is thought to be critically important to naturally rewarding stimuli such as food, drink, and sex. Dopamine release also accompanies drug-taking, fast-paced video games, and so on.

The nigrostriatal dopamine pathway from substantia nigra pars compacta to the striatum is critically important to movement. Dopaminergic nigral cells densely innervate the striatum, firing tonically all the time. The *tonic release of dopamine within the striatum is necessary for movement just as oil is required for an engine to run.* Understanding dopamine's roles in movement has been aided greatly by research on transgenic mice. Mice engineered with an inactivated tyrosine hydroxylase gene do not make dopamine; these mice do not move around, do not feed, and die within a day or so of birth. Yet these mice breathe, evidence that dopamine affects certain movements but not others.

Dopamine strongly promotes movement in a graded fashion: more dopamine promotes more movement. People who lose more than 80–90% of their dopaminergic nigral cells move far less frequently than is normal, the cardinal sign of Parkinson's disease. Moving less than normal is termed *hypokinesia*, whereas a person who stops moving altogether, becoming "frozen," exhibits *akinesia* (see Chapter 7). Treatment with the dopamine precursor, L-Dopa, increases dopamine levels (see Chapter 12) and facilitates basal ganglia–mediated movement in both dopamine-deficient mice and parkinsonian patients. Just as a lack of dopamine causes akinesia, surplus dopamine causes excess movements. As a consequence, drugs that artificially increase the tonic level of dopamine, such as amphetamines or cocaine, greatly increase motor activity. Users appear jumpy and, because of this excess motor activity, are readily perceived as being "on something." In the same vein, conditions that augment dopaminergic transmission also cause excess movements. After receiving long-term treatment with dopamine receptor antagonists commonly used to treat psychiatric diseases, patients develop receptor supersensitivity to dopamine that operationally facilitates dopaminergic transmission. As a result, these patients develop an iatrogenic (i.e., caused by medical treatment) disorder called *tardive dyskinesia*, in which the patient makes excess movements particularly of facial and tongue musculature.

In addition to tonic firing, dopaminergic cells fire with a phasic burst of activity when something unexpected—a sound, a light, a touch, and so on—occurs. This phasic burst of activity plays an important and still incompletely understood role in basal ganglia learning, including assignment of reward value. At least in some patients with Parkinson's disease, dopamine-boosting drugs cause dramatic increases in repetitive and stereotypic behaviors such as picking at hairs or organizing household objects over and over again. This type of compulsive behavior, termed *punding*, takes a wide variety of expressions from taking apart and putting back together flashlights to weeding without breaks even to relieve oneself. Changes in therapeutic management are used to reverse these unfortunate side effects.

For our purposes here, it is important to recognize that (1) dopamine is absolutely required for goal-directed movements, and (2) dopamine facilitates the learning of motor sequences as chunks, as well as the modification of those chunks according to changing circumstances.

THE HYPERDIRECT PATHWAY OPPOSES MOVEMENTS

Input from motor cortex travels at high speed through myelinated axons to the subthalamic nucleus. In contrast, inputs from motor cortex to the striatum are conducted through unmyelinated axons. Therefore, motor cortex excites the subthalamic nucleus *before* it reaches striatum. This difference in timing gives rise to the term *hyperdirect* in comparison to the *direct* pathway that depends on motor cortex projections to striatum.

Subthalamic neurons are glutamatergic, the only glutamatergic neurons within the basal ganglia collective. They therefore excite target cells. Once excited by cortical input, subthalamic neurons excite internal globus pallidus neurons that, in turn, inhibit neurons in the ventral anterior and ventral lateral nuclei of the thalamus (VA/VL) regions involved in motor control that project back to motor cortex (Fig. 25-4). This hyperdirect pathway comprises the quickest route through the basal ganglia. It increases the inhibition of target nuclei beyond that provided by the pallidal neurons' tonic discharge and thereby greatly decreases discharge in target thalamic cells. The ultimate effect is a global depression of somatomotor activity.

Activity in the hyperdirect pathway opposes action, providing a global interrupt signal. Such an interrupt signal would be useful for interrupting an action for any number of reasons. Perhaps something else really important, such as a mosquito bite screaming to be scratched, has suddenly come up. Or a jogger sees a careening bicyclist approaching and does a full stop to avoid a collision. A clerk stops scanning items when a customer asks a question or a supervisor calls out his or her name. A global stop signal may also be helpful in switching from one movement to another. Starting a movement from a state of not-moving is far easier than switching from one movement to another. For example, to switch from running to skipping is far more difficult than initiating skipping directly from standing.

Finally, the subthalamic nucleus appears to play a major role in impulsivity. To understand this, consider that actions, the only outward expressions of an individual's choices, are the stuff of which decisions are made. As a region that has the ability to make a "full-stop," the subthalamic nucleus

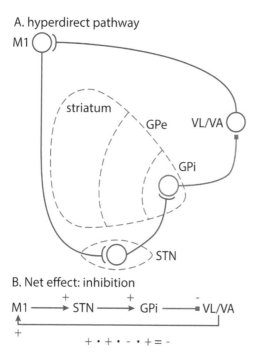

A. hyperdirect pathway

B. Net effect: inhibition

$$M1 \xrightarrow{+} STN \xrightarrow{+} GPi \xrightarrow{-} VL/VA$$

$$+ \cdot + \cdot - \cdot + = -$$

Figure 25-4 The hyperdirect pathway within the skeletomotor circuit is illustrated and its net effect diagrammed. A: Neurons in somatomotor cortex (*M1*) are normally inactive but discharge before initiating a movement. The myelinated axons of motor cortex neurons excite neurons in the subthalamic nucleus (*STN*) at short latency. Excitation of subthalamic neurons in turn causes an increase in the discharge of already active neurons in the internal globus pallidus (*GPi*). GABAergic cells in the internal globus pallidus inhibit the tonically active neurons in ventral lateral and ventral anterior thalamus (*VL/VA*). Since thalamic cells project to somatomotor cortex, the inhibitory effect of the hyperdirect pathway on thalamic firing is passed on to motor cortex. In sum, the hyperdirect pathway has an immediate but short-lasting effect of global suppression of somatomotor cortex. GABAergic neurons are shown in red, and their inhibitory terminals are shown as red squares. Excitatory neurons are shown in blue. B: The sign of each connection in the hyperdirect pathway is diagrammed at top. Below, the product of all connections produces a net inhibitory effect. GPe: external globus pallidus.

biases decisions away from fast, impulsive actions. When the subthalamic nucleus is active, more support for a candidate action is needed in the direct pathway. Interestingly, electrical stimulation of the subthalamic nucleus, termed *deep brain stimulation* (*DBS*), decreases subthalamic output, effectively acting as a lesion. Therefore, DBS of the subthalamic nucleus, used to treat the tremor in Parkinson's disease, can elicit dramatic and impulsive behavior in patients for whom these behaviors are wholly uncharacteristic. Compulsive gambling, shopping, eating, punding, and sexual activity have all been reported in patients who showed no previous predilections for such behaviors. The emotional and financial cost of these behaviors to affected patients and their loved ones is enormous. Patients may not realize that impulsive behaviors are a known side effect of DBS, and their own embarrassment may delay pursuit of

medical help. Clearly, presurgical education of the potential risks can alleviate this unfortunate situation. Once alerted, physicians can adjust stimulation parameters and therapeutic drug dosages to minimize impulsive behavior while retaining as much therapeutic effect (on movement) as possible.

HEMIBALLISMUS IS A HYPERKINETIC DISORDER INVOLVING INVOLUNTARY FLAILING MOVEMENTS EMPLOYING ARM, LEG, AND FACIAL MUSCLES

Hemiballismus or *hemiballism* is a movement disorder that can be viewed as a failure of the hyperdirect pathway. It is characterized by uncontrolled flinging, flailing, or other ballistic movements of the proximal arm, leg, and often the face. It is termed *hemi-* because the cause is invariably a unilateral telencephalic lesion with contralateral effects.

Over time, the movements in hemiballismus slow down to become *choreiform*, more writhing and dance-like than flailing. Some patients present initially with *hemichorea*, meaning involuntary writhing movements on one side of the body. Hemiballism and hemichorea are considered to represent two extremes of the same disorder. In most cases, the movements remit completely within several months, either spontaneously or following short-term pharmacological treatment. Treatment is aimed at the underlying cause of the lesion, which in most cases is a focal stroke. In addition, dopamine receptor antagonists help decrease the occurrence of excess movements and therefore aid patients, particularly in the initial weeks.

Hyperglycemia secondary to diabetes mellitus is the second most common cause of hemiballism. In hyperglycemic hemiballism, movements are transiently present for as long as blood sugar is abnormal. The pathophysiology of this recently recognized disorder, most prevalent in individuals of East Asian origin, is unknown and worthy of study. The third most common cause of hemiballism or hemichorea is a toxoplasmosis lesion in individuals with HIV disease.

For a relatively rare disorder, hemiballismus is very well known among medical professionals. For years, hemiballism was thought to result exclusively from a lesion of the subthalamic nucleus contralateral to the affected limbs. Certainly, there is both clinical and experimental evidence to support the idea that a lesion of the subthalamus in a healthy individual will produce a hyperkinetic disorder. The interpretation is that, due to loss of the global inhibition provided by the hyperdirect pathway, the somatomotor cortex becomes overly excitable. The predicted behavioral

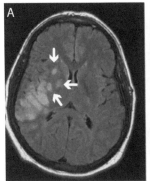
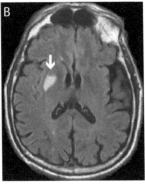

Figure 25-5 Magnetic resonance images (MRIs) from two individuals with hemiballism, neither of whom has a lesion in the subthalamus. A: A 34-year-old man with a stroke in the right middle cerebral artery presented with left-sided hemiballism. Affected areas include cerebral cortex and several small areas within the striatum and pallidum (*arrows*). B: A 69-year-old man with Parkinson's disease presented with left-sided hemiballism. A lesion in the right striatum (*arrow*) was found. The left-sided hemiballism coincided with an amelioration of this patient's symptoms of Parkinson's disease on the left side. Note that radiological convention is that the left side of the brain is illustrated on the right and right side of the brain on the left. Modified from Postuma RB, Lang AE. Hemiballism: Revisiting a classic disorder. *Lancet Neurol* 2: 661–668, 2003, with permission of the publisher, Elsevier.

consequence is an increase in movement. Essentially, hemiballism has been used for decades to teach students the role of the subthalamic nucleus in suppressing movement.

Unfortunately, this attractive teaching device can no longer be employed in good faith. It is now clear that more than 60% of patients with hemiballism have a lesion outside of the subthalamic nucleus (Fig. 25-5). Lesions that produce hemiballism are found in the putamen, thalamus, or deep white matter and occasionally, in about 20–25% of cases, in the subthalamic nucleus. Does this neuropathological finding mean that our interpretation of the role of subthalamic nucleus function is all wrong? Absolutely not. The idea that the subthalamus facilitates basal ganglia output and thereby depresses movements is still widely accepted. However, it is now clear that hyperkinetic disorders often result from lesions of subcortical structures in addition to the subthalamic nucleus. An understanding of the pathophysiology involved in these nonconventional but more representative cases of hemiballism represents an intriguing puzzle for future investigators.

THE DIRECT PATHWAY RELEASES
SELECTED MOVEMENTS
FROM ONGOING SUPPRESSION

The direct pathway provides a fast route through the basal ganglia, second in speed only to the hyperdirect pathway.

In the direct pathway, information from wide areas of sensorimotor cortex—somatosensory and primary motor cortices, supplementary motor and premotor areas—reaches the putamen through unmyelinated corticostriatal axons. Excitation of cells in the putamen causes an inhibition of internal globus pallidus neurons, which in turn disinhibits target cells in ventral anterior and ventral lateral thalamus (Fig. 25-6). *Through removal of the tonic inhibition of thalamic neurons, engagement of the direct pathway results in an increase in the discharge of thalamic neurons.* An increase in thalamic activity is passed on to motor control centers, facilitating the initiation of the selected action. The net effect of the direct pathway is the activation of a focused ensemble of cells in somatomotor cortex. The behavioral result is that one action is released from tonic inhibition and therefore occurs.

Recall that striatal and pallidal neurons both use GABA to inhibit target cells. Therefore, when placed in series, striatal inhibition of pallidal inhibition causes *disinhibition*,

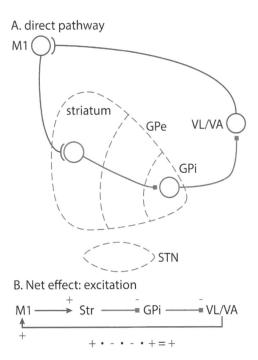

Figure 25-6 The direct pathway within the skeletomotor circuit. Neurons in somatomotor cortex (*M1*) are normally inactive but discharge before initiating a movement. A burst of activity in these motor cortex neurons excites GABAergic medium spiny neurons in the putamen (*striatum*). Neurons of the putamen in turn inhibit the discharge of tonically active neurons in the internal globus pallidus (*GPi*) that inhibit tonically active neurons in ventral lateral and ventral anterior thalamus (*VL/VA*). The resulting disinhibition of thalamic cells facilitates somatomotor cortex and ultimately movement. GABAergic neurons are shown in red, and their inhibitory terminals are shown as red squares. Excitatory neurons are shown in blue. B: Multiplying the sign of each connection in the direct pathway (*top*) yields a net facilitatory effect (*bottom*). GPe: external globus pallidus.

which, as you recall from Chapter 24, has the net effect of increasing discharge rate. The direct pathway only works because pallidal cells discharge tonically, rendering them sensitive to inhibitory influences from striatum. Indeed, pallidal cells as well as cells in substantia nigra pars reticulata discharge tonically at rates of 50–100 Hz.

In the direct pathway, the striatum, internal globus pallidus, and substantia nigra pars reticulata are the only nuclei that are considered part of the basal ganglia. Therefore, when cortical input engages the direct pathway, the output of the basal ganglia *decreases*. Because the basal ganglia output to thalamus is inhibitory, a decrease in basal ganglia output leads to more activity in thalamic and consequently cortical neurons, and things happen. In Parkinson's disease, the direct pathway is disfacilitated and movement rarely occurs.

PARKINSON'S DISEASE CAN BE VIEWED AS A DISORDER OF THE DIRECT PATHWAY

The cardinal sign of Parkinson's disease is a poverty of movement, often initially in one body part, such as one hand. Since dopaminergic neurons involved in boosting habitual actions mediated by the striatum are most vulnerable to neurodegeneration, the poverty of movement in patients with Parkinson's disease is specifically a deficit in initiating chunked or habitual actions. Without habits, every action becomes effortful. Imagine having to use a modified alphabet in which a is b, b is c, and so on until z is a. Typing or writing a single word (uif in place of the) would be feasible only through deliberate action. A full sentence would take enormous concentration, effort, and time. Then imagine having to employ the same level of conscious effort in order to walk across a room, speak, bring food to the mouth, and so on. That is the hourly and daily struggle of severe Parkinson's disease.

Most of the symptoms described for Parkinson's disease fall comfortably under the rubric of a reduction in either the number (hypokinesia) or speed (bradykinesia) of movements. There are few movements of the facial muscles, resulting in an expressionless face that is termed *masked facies*. The gait of affected individuals becomes shuffling, involving small steps with little or no clearance above the ground during the swing phase. This type of gait is termed *festinating*. The arms fail to swing normally during locomotion. Speech becomes strained, reduced in volume, and breathy. Postural stability is greatly impaired as adjustments either do not occur or occur too slowly to be effective.

There are two major symptoms beyond a poverty of movement in Parkinson's disease. First, there is *cogwheel rigidity*, which is a deficit in passive movement. When a physician tries to extend the arm of a patient with Parkinson's disease, there is resistance that yields in a ratcheting or cogwheel-like pattern. The other major symptom is a *resting tremor* of a few cycles per second. The *parkinsonian tremor* involves the thumb and forefinger moving as though rolling pills and thus has been called a *pill-rolling tremor*. Although perhaps the most widely known symptom of Parkinson's disease, a resting tremor is not experienced by roughly 30% of patients with Parkinson's disease.

As you are aware by now, Parkinson's disease results after dopaminergic neurons in the substantia nigra pars compacta die. There are two routes by which a loss of dopaminergic neurons could result in a poverty of movement. First, as mentioned earlier, tonic dopamine is necessary for movement. The exact mechanism of this absolute requirement is unclear. The second route through which a loss of dopaminergic tone could impact the initiation of movements is through dopaminergic modulation of the direct and indirect pathways. As a consequence of dopaminergic neuronal loss, the direct pathway is no longer facilitated through actions mediated by D_1 receptors. This renders movement initiation more difficult. Additionally, D_2 receptor-mediated depression of the indirect pathway declines with the loss of the dopaminergic nigrostriatal pathways. This results in excessive movement suppression. In sum, the behavioral results are (1) difficulty in initiating movements due to *disfacilitation*, meaning a decrease in excitation, of the direct pathway and (2) exuberant suppression of movements through disinhibition of indirect pathways.

Pharmacological treatment with L-Dopa, a dopamine precursor (see Chapter 12) has served as the standard therapy for Parkinson's disease for decades. This treatment aids most patients at least initially. Unfortunately, people treated with dopamine replacement over an extended period of time often stop responding well to the treatment. They may freeze up as the last dose of L-Dopa wears off, or they may develop excess tic-like movements due to drug-induced dyskinesia (tardive dyskinesia, as discussed earlier). In some patients, the freezing and hyperkinetic states alternate in a state of rapidly alternating *on* and *off states* with altogether too short periods of comfort between. The unfortunate consequences of long-term L-Dopa treatment increase in likelihood with treatment duration, leading some to delay L-Dopa treatment of patients in the early stages of disease. The logic of this tactic is clear: delaying the start of L-Dopa therapy will delay the arrival of debilitating side effects consequent to long-term use. Nonetheless, the efficacy of this tactic remains unknown.

Deep brain stimulation of either the subthalamic nucleus or internal globus pallidus is approved as a treatment for Parkinson's disease in the United States and is efficacious in reducing resting tremor, rigidity, and bradykinesia. When effective, DBS reduces the time that patients spend immobile in the off state and thereby reduces the required dose of dopaminergic drugs. This in turn moderates the risk of developing dyskinesia and decreases the dosage of dopaminergic drugs that a patient requires. A neuroprotective effect of DBS has been postulated but is unproven as of now.

As beneficial as DBS can be in ameliorating parkinsonian symptoms, it sometimes does not result in a subjective improvement in the patient's quality of life, in either the personal sphere or on the job. One possible explanation for this finding stems from the fact that the motor symptoms ameliorated by DBS are only a subset of the many symptoms of Parkinson's disease. Even if DBS "cures" a patient's tremor and bradykinesia, postural instability, deficits in verbal fluency, and so on may be untouched or even worsened by the surgical intervention. Insensitive to this difference, it is easy to imagine that family members could view a patient without a tremor as cured and be impatient for that individual to return to the person he or she was before the first symptoms of the disease appeared, an expectation that is beyond the proven reach of DBS. These issues highlight the difference between disease and illness, with illness representing the impact of a disease on a person's life, a topic we return to in the final chapter. In sum, treatments such as DBS that are aimed at treating disease symptoms may not be helping an individual manage his or her illness completely. There is no foolproof way to foretell the wisdom of choosing to undergo DBS surgery. However, clear benefits in performing daily living activities, bodily comfort, and emotional well-being have been demonstrated in young (~50 years old) patients with mild Parkinson's disease treated with DBS. Moreover, current guidelines have greatly advanced methods of patient selection for DBS. More questions remain. For example, whether DBS can lead to personality changes is intensely discussed amongst bioethicists who will play an important role in maximizing the chances for patient satisfaction.

Parkinson's disease is a common neurological disorder, affecting as many as 5–10% of people over the age of 50. There is little chance of making it through life, and certainly through life as a physician, without encountering an individual with Parkinson's disease. Parkinson disease ranges from mild to severe. Unfortunately, Parkinson's disease involves a process of progressive degeneration, and symptoms worsen over time. The development of dopamine replacement therapy in the 1960s was revolutionary because it greatly improved the lives of patients and continues to do so to this day. Nonetheless, as discussed earlier, dopamine replacement therapy is not a cure. An actual cure for Parkinson disease remains a hope for the future but is only likely to come after an understanding of why dopamine cells die is achieved.

INDIRECT PATHWAYS KEEP RIVAL MOVEMENTS SUPPRESSED

The indirect pathways comprise a varied group of polysynaptic routes through the basal ganglia. We focus on the main indirect pathway in which somatomotor cortex cells project to striatal cells that project into the external globus pallidus (Fig. 25-7). External globus pallidus cells in turn inhibit

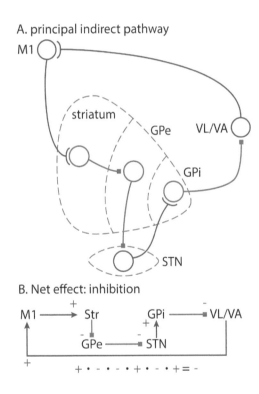

Figure 25-7 Using the same conventions as in Figures 25-4 and 25-6, the main indirect pathway of the skeletomotor circuit is illustrated and its net effect diagrammed. A: Neurons in somatomotor cortex (*M1*) project to neurons in the putamen (striatum) that project to and inhibit neurons in the external globus pallidus (*GPe*). The inhibitory projection from external globus pallidus to the subthalamic nucleus (*STN*) produces a disinhibition. Subthalamic cells excite cells in the internal globus pallidus (*GPi*). An increase in the discharge of neurons in the internal globus pallidus leads to an inhibition of thalamic cells (*yellow highlight*). As a result, the conventional indirect pathway serves to suppress somatomotor cortex and, ultimately, movement. The net effect of the family of indirect pathways also appears to be net inhibition of thalamic cells and, consequently, a suppression of movement.

subthalamic neurons, causing a net disinhibition due to the back-to-back inhibitory signals. Disinhibited subthalamic neurons discharge at an increased rate and thereby provide a greater than normal excitation of output neurons in the internal globus pallidus. In turn, the excited neurons of the internal globus pallidus deliver an exaggerated inhibition of thalamic target neurons. The result is less movement emanating from somatomotor cortex.

Huntingon's disease is a disorder of the indirect pathways, at least in its initial stages. The first neurons to die in Huntington's disease are striatal neurons that project to the external globus pallidus. Thus, neurons in the indirect pathways are affected first. This accounts for the initial hyperkinesia characterized by an excess of *choreiform* (from the Greek *khoreia* for a chorus dancing together) or "dance-like" movements observed in Huntington's disease patients. More and more striatal cells and eventually pallidal and nigral cells die over time. At death, the lateral ventricles of Huntington's patients have enlarged to occupy most of the territory of the striatum and globus pallidus. As neuronal death progresses beyond the initially vulnerable population of striatal neurons that project to the external globus pallidus, hyperkinetic symptoms are increasingly replaced by akinesia, a cessation in self-initiated movements.

Huntington's disease is an autosomally inherited genetic disorder with 100% penetrance. The first symptoms typically appear in the fourth or fifth decade of life. Because the mutation is dominant, patients have typically watched a parent suffer through the 10- to 20-year decline that characterizes Huntington's disease. Initially, involuntary choreiform movements are present intermittently and, with time, nearly constantly. A progressive dementia develops, with memory loss and eventually a nearly total loss of cognition. There is a wasting component to Huntington's disease; it is still not clear whether this symptom stems from increased energy expenditure due to excess movements or from a primary metabolic effect. On average, death occurs 15 years after diagnosis of Huntington's disease, by which time akinesia has replaced hyperkinesia.

The genetic defect responsible for Huntington's disease was identified in 1983. Individuals with more than 40 copies of the trinucleotide repeat CAG in the huntingtin gene develop Huntington's disease (see Chapter 2). The onset of the disease is earliest and disease progression most rapid in patients with the greatest number of CAG repeats. The mechanism by which the mutant protein huntingtin kills neurons remains unknown but is under active investigation.

There is a genetic test for Huntington's disease but no cure. Therapy is aimed at relieving the symptoms of patients and is frankly insufficient in the face of such a relentless and debilitating disease. Consequently, a diagnosis of Huntington's disease is devastating in its promise of an inexorable decline and erosion of the life that an individual has enjoyed up until that point. The lack of either a cure or an effective treatment is often cited as the reason that the vast majority of individuals at risk for Huntington's disease have chosen not to take the available genetic test.

ALL BASAL GANGLIA PATHWAYS WORK TOGETHER TO ACHIEVE MEANINGFUL ACTIONS

The hyperdirect, direct, and indirect pathways operate in concert to produce one action at a time and to allow for "clean" switching between actions. Switching may be particularly aided by global action inhibition provided by the hyperdirect pathway. Then, when action selection yields to action initiation, the direct and indirect pathways are simultaneously engaged so that one action is selected and similar actions or potential distractions are selectively inhibited.

This chapter has described the motor loop through the basal ganglia in some detail. The basal ganglia also receive and process information about feelings, perceptions, thoughts, and emotions through loops that resemble the skeletomotor loop in their *basic* architecture. All loops use some part of the striatum and a region of subthalamic nucleus as entry ports into the basal ganglia and either the internal globus pallidus or substantia nigra pars reticulata as the exit port. Yet the different loops differ in terms of many specifics, such as the part of striatum, cortex, brainstem, or thalamus involved. Of course, the loops also serve different functions. In addition to the skeletomotor loop described in this chapter, other circuits that loop through the basal ganglia and thalamus include:

- *Oculomotor circuit*: Connects frontal and parietal eye fields as well as superior colliculus with intralaminar thalamic nuclei, caudate, and substantia nigra pars reticulata to control gaze and orienting movements

- *Dorsolateral prefrontal circuit*: Connects the head of the caudate, the substantia nigra pars reticulata, and ventral anterior and medial dorsal nuclei of the thalamus with dorsolateral prefrontal cortex to influence executive function and cognition, such as the strategic planning of movements needed to solve a problem

- *Orbitofrontal circuit*: Connects the caudate, substantia nigra pars reticulata, and medial dorsal nucleus with the orbitofrontal cortex to influence motivation and the ability "to play well with others"

- *Limbic or anterior cingulate circuit*: Connects the ventral striatum, including the nucleus accumbens, ventral pallidum, and medial dorsal nucleus of the thalamus with the anterior cingulate gyrus and temporal lobe cortex to influence emotionality and motivated behavior

Additional loops, less well characterized, also exist. For example, a loop involving the mesencephalic locomotor region and the substantia nigra places locomotion and postural control within the purview of basal ganglia function. Dysfunction within this loop is likely largely responsible for the festinating gait and loss of postural stability in Parkinson's disease.

Although subcortical inputs to the dorsolateral prefrontal and orbitofrontal circuits are poorly characterized and widely omitted from consideration, subcortical inputs to nonmotor circuits exist, arising from the midbrain periaqueductal gray, amygdala, and brainstem reticular nuclei. Recall that inputs originating in subcortical sites terminate more densely and more proximally on striatal medium spiny neurons than do inputs from cortex. Now, imagine that subcortical and cortical inputs excite different neuronal ensembles within the caudate territory of the orbitofrontal circuit. Chances are that the subcortically excited ensemble will win over the cortically excited ensemble resulting in social behavior determined by noncognitive inputs. In this way, we may experience a "gut" dislike of someone for which we cannot articulate a logical reason, we may panic at the sight of a garter snake that we cognitively understand is harmless, and so on.

Two mechanisms support a consistent bias of action selection toward reactions to unexpected events over pre-planned or anticipated inputs. First, brainstem neurons, such as those in the superior colliculus, carry inputs related to unexpected events, and, as mentioned earlier, subcortical excitation dominates cortical excitation of striatal cells. Second, unexpected events excite a phasic burst of activity in dopaminergic nigrostriatal cells, which in turn strengthens striatal responses to such inputs. A point worth explicit consideration is the speculation that the bias toward reactions to unexpected, sudden events contributes to the short attention span prevalent in our modern world. In the natural world, rapidly paced and unexpected events are relatively rare and are noteworthy, typically signaling a potential meal or mate or an impending danger, all of which are actionable items. However, in our communication-rich world, cell phones, text messages, radio and TV news flashes all capitalize on the biological penchant to orient and pay attention to new, quick, and unexpected stimuli. These stimuli continuously invade our environment, repeatedly challenging us to switch our direct pathway focus from our current action to one that responds to the novel stimulus.

Loops supporting cognitive, motivational, and emotional function provide the integrated platform needed for the initiation, planning, and execution of self-generated movements. A common scenario may be that *the goal of a possible action is selected within the limbic or orbitofrontal circuit, passed on to the dorsolateral prefrontal circuit for selection of the implementation strategy, and finally passed to the skeletomotor loop for selection of a motor plan to execute the action.* Although the basal ganglia loops operate in parallel, information can flow between loops through, for example, promiscuous connections from thalamus to multiple areas of cortex. One illustration of this possibility is the projection from neurons in the ventral anterior nucleus of thalamus to cortical regions that participate in both executive function and movement execution loops.

Since information may, but does not always, flow between basal ganglia loops, movement can proceed with or without an associated thought or feeling. One can readily discern the difference between a phone conversation with a friend who is reading e-mail while talking to you and one with a friend focused entirely on conversing with you. To accomplish this variety of behaviors, the basal ganglia can, but does not always, couple action selection to emotions or thoughts. We can imagine that when all the loops engage in concert toward a common goal, we act with "heart," reflecting "single-minded" engagement. Perhaps when only the dorsolateral prefrontal and skeletomotor loops act in concert, we act methodically and deliberately, and when the skeletomotor loop operates solo, we "go through the motions." Thus, the basal ganglia can link movement with feeling or allow movement to proceed without accompanying affect.

Some habitual actions may not need motivational or emotional support under most circumstances—a chef dices carrots at rapid speed while happily thinking about an enjoyable date the night before or an upcoming trip, a commuter drives home while thinking about the past day. However, there may be circumstances incompatible with successful completion of the same, normally automatic chunks—the same talented chef goes to work worried about a gravely ill mother and ends up cutting a finger instead of carrots, the commuter drives homeward after hearing bad news and crashes. Other actions clearly require motivational and emotional commitment for successful completion—an actor performing in a play, a parent trying to calm a child, an athlete competing in a championship game. In sum, between-loop crosstalk allows coupling of movement with emotion, intent, and focus.

Neuropsychiatric disorders may result from deficits in one or more of the nonmotor basal ganglia loops. Basal ganglia dysfunction is implicated in neuropsychiatric diseases such as obsessive compulsive disorder and schizophrenia. Since the basal ganglia are involved in the selection of thoughts, strategies, perceptions, motivations, emotions, and goals, their heavy involvement in psychological function should come as no surprise. People with obsessive-compulsive disorder perseverate, continuing to select a single action (compulsion) or thought (obsession) over and over, long after the action or thought has outlived its utility. Patients with schizophrenia may incompletely switch between rival thoughts. If true, the simultaneous selection of multiple thoughts would result in a confusing mélange of concurrent thoughts and perceptions. We should also note that many, but certainly not all, patients with basal ganglia–centered movement disorders have neuropsychiatric complications. For example, nonmotor symptoms afflict a proportion of patients with Parkinson's disease.

THE BASAL GANGLIA AND CEREBELLUM WORK IN CONCERT

Every time that we act, the cerebellum and basal ganglia, the two great loops in the brain, receive information about the action generated from cortex. Both structures communicate indirectly with the motor hierarchy, only affecting motor neurons and motor interneurons through an indirect route. Both structures receive at least an order of magnitude more information than they send out to target structures, making them processing bottlenecks that reduce an overwhelming confusion of conflicting input to a concise and decisive winner-takes-all output. Furthermore, the basal ganglia are critical to, and the cerebellum may influence, many nonmotor functions, processing thoughts, emotions, and memories, all of which, of course, ultimately influence movements. Even the functions of the two, in sequencing movements and learning associations, overlap.

In marked contrast to the case with the cerebellum, the basal ganglia do not receive peripheral or spinal input. Instead, input to the basal ganglia comes from virtually all areas of the cerebral cortex, as well as from subcortical regions that can themselves direct movement, such as the superior colliculus. Thus, the cerebellum receives information about muscle contractions, whereas the basal ganglia only receive input about movements and actions. Sensory input to the cerebellum comes from the spinal cord and represents the sensory consequences of movement. In contrast, neurons in cortical and brainstem regions interpret and then present sensory information about the world to the basal ganglia. Consider the sequential versions of an action, from motivation and selection of a goal in prefrontal cortex to action in motor cortex, to movement in the ventral horn interneurons, and muscle control in the α-motoneurons. *The basal ganglia receive motor information biased toward goal selection and action, whereas the cerebellum receives information biased toward movement and muscle contraction.*

The cerebellum smoothes out movements, important and trivial ones alike, whereas the skeletomotor loop of the basal ganglia ensures that salient actions take priority over automatic, mundane ones. The nonmotor functions of the cerebellum and basal ganglia may similarly diverge, with the cerebellum focusing on automatic associations and the basal ganglia on matching motivation, thought, emotion, strategy, and movement to urgency and circumstance.

Both the cerebellum and basal ganglia support operational learning. The cerebellum associates sensory input with motor output, so that a set of inputs related to the body and the outside world—an entire sensory gestalt—becomes associated with a particular *movement*. In contrast, the basal ganglia associate self-generated *actions* with their consequences, biasing present and future selection of actions toward previously rewarding ones. Ultimately, our actions are those dictated by the cerebellum *and* the basal ganglia, incorporating influences from the sensory world as well as from our cognitive, motivational, and emotional states.

ADDITIONAL READING

Albin RL, Young AB, Penney JB. The functional anatomy of basal ganglia disorders. *Trends Neurosci.* 12: 366–375, 1989.

Demetriades P, Rickards H, Cavanna AE. Impulse control disorders following deep brain stimulation of the subthalamic nucleus in Parkinson's disease: Clinical aspects. *Parkinsons Dis.* 2011: 658415, 2011.

Doya K. Complementary roles of basal ganglia and cerebellum in learning and motor control. *Curr Opin Neurobiol.* 10: 732–739, 2000.

Fernandez HH, Friedman JH. Punding on L-dopa. *Mov Disord.* 14: 836–838, 1999.

Graybiel AM. The basal ganglia and chunking of action repertoires. *Neurobiol Learn Mem.* 70: 119–136, 1998.

Grillner S, Robertson B. The basal ganglia downstream control of brainstem motor centres--an evolutionarily conserved strategy. *Curr Opin Neurobiol.* 33: 47–52, 2015.

Haber SN. The primate basal ganglia: Parallel and integrative networks. *J Chem Neuroanat.* 26: 317–330, 2003.

Havemann J. *A Life Shaken: My Encounter with Parkinson's Disease.* Baltimore: Johns Hopkins University Press, 2002.

Hernández LF, Redgrave P, Obeso JA. Habitual behavior and dopamine cell vulnerability in Parkinson disease. *Front Neuroanat.* 9: 99, 2015.

Israel Z, Bergman H. Pathophysiology of the basal ganglia and movement disorders: From animal models to human clinical applications. *Neurosci Biobehav Rev.* 32(3): 367–377, 2008.

Jin X, Costa RM. Shaping action sequences in basal ganglia circuits. *Curr Opin Neurobiol.* 33: 188–196, 2015.

Liu Y, Postupna N, Falkenberg J, Anderson ME. High frequency deep brain stimulation: What are the therapeutic mechanisms? *Neurosci Biobehav Rev.* 32 (3): 343–351, 2008.

Marin O, Smeets WJ, Gonzalez A. Evolution of the basal ganglia in tetrapods: A new perspective based on recent studies in amphibians. *Trends Neurosci.* 21: 487–494, 1998.

McHaffie JG, Stanford TR, Stein BE, Coizet V, Redgrave P. Subcortical loops through the basal ganglia. *Trends Neurosci.* 28: 401–407, 2005.

Posturna RB, Lang AE. Hemiballism: Revisiting a classic disorder. *Lancet Neurology.* 2: 661–668, 2003.

Redgrave P, Prescott TJ, Gurney K. The basal ganglia: A vertebrate solution to the selection problem? *Neuroscience.* 89: 1009–1023, 1999.

Reiner A, Medina L, Veenman CL. Structural and functional evolution of the basal ganglia in vertebrates. *Brain Res Brain Res Rev.* 28: 235–285, 1998.

Schuepbach WM, Rau J, Knudsen K, et al. Neurostimulation for Parkinson's disease with early motor complications. *N Engl J Med.* 368: 610–622, 2013.

Schüpbach M, Gargiulo M, Welter ML, et al. Neurosurgery in Parkinson disease: A distressed mind in a repaired body? *Neurology.* 66: 1811–1816, 2006.

Tewari A, Jog R, Jog MS. The striatum and subthalamic nucleus as independent and collaborative structures in motor control. *Front Syst Neurosci.* 10: 17, 2016.

Yamaguchi M, Logan GD. Pushing typists back on the learning curve: Revealing chunking in skilled typewriting. *J Exp Psychol Hum Percept Perform.* 40: 592–612, 2014.

SECTION 6

HOMEOSTASIS

Every organ system in the body must pay its dues to sustaining cardiorespiratory life, and the nervous system is no exception. What is exceptional about the nervous system is all that the brain does beyond simply sustaining life: perception, action, thought, emotion. We view the liver, skin, pancreas, heart, and so on through a single lens: how well do they support the life of the owner? The nervous system, which also makes enormous contributions to sustaining life, is rarely viewed through this lens. Yet we cannot live without a functioning nervous system.

Without a pathway from hindbrain to spinal cord to diaphragm muscle, life ceases. Without a hypothalamus to drive food- and water-seeking and consumption, life ends. Without distributed thermoregulatory defenses, the body overheats during a summer walk around the block and life is over. In this section, we examine several ways in which the nervous system sustains life. Breathing does not simply happen in one stereotyped sequence but occurs in a manner that fits one's mood and conscious objectives. Eating does not simply meet caloric needs. As the modern epidemic of overweight makes clear, rational, emotional, and perceptual factors strongly influence food acquisition and consumption. Effectors of thermoregulation such as sweating and cutaneous vasodilation do double duty as both defenders of core temperature and as emotional reactions.

In the end, you may come to admire, or at least appreciate, the brain's unique style of life-support, stamped as it is with ultimately lofty and cerebral end goals even as it performs mundane, uncelebrated tasks.

26.

INTRODUCTION TO HOMEOSTASIS

omeostasis is a concept attributed to Walter Cannon, an influential American physiologist of the early 20th century who coined the term as well as the phrases *fight-or-flight* and *rest-and-digest*. Cannon wrote a book titled *The Wisdom of the Body*, which popularized the idea that the body contains an organized system of defenses that maintain physiological variables such as body temperature and blood glucose within optimal ranges. Homeostasis is defined as the collection of physiological processes and behavioral actions that keep the internal milieu of the body steady or sufficiently so to support good health. The physiological actions of both neural and non-neural tissues contribute to the body's defenses, but the neural contribution is special because it can anticipate changes prior to deviations occurring and because it operates in a context-specific way.

The nervous system anticipates threats to homeostasis on several time scales. On an immediate time scale, the sight of food, the intention to stand up, and the like elicit nervous system–mediated reactions that anticipate and prevent the body from deviating from homeostasis. On a daily time scale, the nervous system sets a circadian rhythm that organizes the timing of many physiological processes, such as ingestion, digestion, and hormone secretion. On a seasonal time scale, homeostatic limits are adjusted to the seasonal environment so that, for example, we feel chilly during the summer at an ambient temperature that is perceived as balmy in wintertime. Finally, our bodies continue to operate even as we move through our life cycle, growing, maturing, and aging from birth to death.

HOMEOSTASIS IS ANTICIPATORY

A popular notion of homeostasis is that it operates as a servomechanism—in other words, a feedback error correction system analogous to a thermostat-controlled heating system. However, a servomechanism only effects corrective actions *after* the controlled variable has deviated from a tolerance zone (Fig. 26-1A). In stark contrast, the nervous system has the unique ability to mount anticipatory or preemptive defenses against changes that could potentially push the body's physiology out of homeostatic range.

To take an example from thermoregulation, consider the core body temperature of a person (or pet) that leaves a heated house to walk into subfreezing temperatures. If mammalian thermoregulation functioned as a home-heating system does, this person's core body temperature would have to dip below the tolerable range before cold defense mechanisms were engaged. This is not what happens. Instead, the dip in core body temperature never occurs. Deviations are

A. Thermostat-controlled heating system

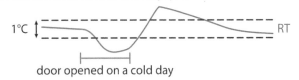

B. Human nervous system

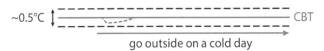

Figure 26-1 A: A servomechanism such as a thermostat-controlled home heating system only corrects room temperature (*RT, red line*) after it has deviated from the desired set point. Therefore, when a house door is opened on a cold wintry day, the heating system kicks in *after* room temperature has already dipped below the set temperature range. B: In contrast, a human (or pet mammal) who leaves the temperature-controlled environment of a building benefits from the brain's thermoregulatory system to keep core body temperature (*CBT, red line*) steady. Anticipatory mechanisms typically prevent any deviation of core body temperature. Small changes in core body temperature (*dotted red line*) that are quickly opposed may occur in very cold conditions.

prevented before they ever could happen through anticipatory thermoregulatory adjustments. Thus, our core temperature and other physiological variables do not oscillate in and out of the healthy range but rather are maintained within restricted limits primarily by *anticipatory* adjustments (Fig. 26-1B).

Neural adjustments initiated by sensory input, circadian zeitgeist, or cognitive experience effectively prevent large deviations from homeostasis. Homeostatic changes tend to be slow. For example, even as one moves from one temperature extreme to another, core body temperature does not change instantaneously; we are insulated beings after all. The lag in time allows for cutaneous thermoreceptors to send a message that elicits thermoregulatory adjustments before core temperature has a chance to budge. Thus, core temperature never changes. A circadian example of an anticipatory adjustment is the insulin release that *precedes* eating at roughly the same time as the day before. This is aptly termed the *cephalic phase*, as it requires the brain. As a result of homeostatic mechanisms, physiology is remarkably steady across a wide variety of conditions.

DISPELLING MYTHS ABOUT HOMEOSTASIS

A common misconception about homeostatic regulation is that homeostasis stems entirely from the hypothalamus. Continuing the example of thermoregulation, it is true that neurons within the hypothalamus are directly sensitive to temperature. Yet hypothalamic temperature does not vary by even 0.5°C across variations in ambient temperature of 10°C –50°C. Thermoreceptive neurons that innervate the skin sense ambient temperature changes and initiate physiological and behavioral reactions before the hypothalamus temperature ever changes. A second line of defense is a set of deep thermoreceptors surrounding internal organs including the spinal cord. Thus, peripheral sensory afferents serve as thermoregulatory sentries that, fortunately, prevent even small changes in brain temperature that can produce adverse effects such as extreme lethargy, confusion, and disorientation.

The hypothalamus is certainly important to homeostasis and is a key site where hormones act to engage physiological adjustments. The hypothalamus also serves as an integrator for the coordination of different homeostatic systems so that, for example, a lower core body temperature is tolerated during sleep. Yet, the hypothalamus only achieves homeostasis by working in concert with neurons in the telencephalon, brainstem, spinal cord, and periphery.

Another misconception, namely that homeostatic functions depend entirely on the autonomic nervous system, is so entrenched that many use autonomic and homeostatic as synonyms. Such an equivalency is simply not true. The most obvious example that exposes the fallacious equivalency between autonomic and homeostatic is breathing. Breathing, absolutely critical to life, depends primarily on the diaphragm, which is skeletal musculature and under voluntary control.

Most homeostatic function requires cooperation between skeletomotor and autonomic neurons. For example, micturition depends on the contraction of the detrusor muscle, a *smooth muscle controlled by parasympathetic neurons*, and the voluntary relaxation of the external urethral sphincter, a *skeletal muscle* controlled by sacral motoneurons. And this does not even speak to the need for an appropriate voiding posture that is entirely dependent on skeletomotor muscle control.

In sum, the following are principles of homeostatic regulation:

- Homeostatic regulation can be, and often is, anticipatory. In any case, a deviation outside of the acceptable range is not required for homeostatic adjustments to occur.

- Neurons throughout the brain, including but not restricted to the hypothalamus, are critical to homeostasis.

- Anticipatory and feedback influences of the brain on the body's physiology can be triggered by either external stimuli, such as temperature, internal stimuli, such as hormones, or circadian cues.

- To effect homeostasis, the brain employs changes in behavior (skeletal muscle), autonomic output (smooth muscle, cardiac muscle, glandular release), and hormonal release.

THE ALLOSTATIC PERSPECTIVE

I have defined homeostasis as a system that keeps the internal milieu of the body steady. The idea that homeostasis keeps the body in a constant, invariant state is rooted in its etymology because the Greek root *homolos* means "same" or "like." Yet it is patently obvious that our body's physiology changes all the time. The pounding heart and dilated pupils that precede a bungee jumping adventure would not accommodate an afternoon nap on a rainy afternoon. Nor would the warm relaxed body that yields to an afternoon nap support bungee jumping. Neither the pounding heart nor the warm lethargy is right or wrong. Each is simply appropriate for some sets of activities and entirely inappropriate for others.

Allostasis is a term that acknowledges the changing nature of body physiology, with *allo* coming from the Greek root for "variable." The importance of approaching the brain's contribution to staying alive through an allostatic rather than a homeostatic lens can be illustrated with a clinical example. The homeostatic approach to high blood pressure is to prescribe pharmacological drugs such as diuretics, β-blockers, and the like. These drugs act on the actual mechanisms that elevate blood pressure. In contrast, the allostatic perspective holds that an elevation in blood pressure is the proper response to a brain state of heightened arousal, perceived danger, or the like. Exactly this response has evolved over thousands of years and has served humans and other mammals extraordinarily well through evolutionary time.

Now consider that a person lives with a perception of danger, stemming from a military war, crime, poverty, social isolation, or the like. Further suppose that that sense of threat persists day in and day out. To put it in colloquial terms, the brain is not stupid. After a steady need for vigilance during the past stretch of time, the brain has learned to predict that vigilance will again be needed today, tomorrow, next week, and next month. In other words, given the brain's penchant for anticipatory adjustments, a *persistent* elevation of blood pressure is the natural, evolutionarily approved outcome. According to this view, therapy should be directed toward a modification of the brain state that has essentially put an individual into a chronic state of heightened fight-or-flight readiness. It should not be directed at downstream players, such as peripheral sympathetic neurons or cardiac muscle, which are simply and correctly following orders.

Taking the allostatic approach to disease necessarily widens the purview of medicine. It suggests that the conditions that put people into steady states of fear and danger are the true causes of at least some modern scourges. The allostatic lens further suggests that the cure for diseases such as hypertension and diabetes may be found in public parks, access to fresh food, and economic opportunities before it is found in molecular moieties.

ADDITIONAL READING

Sterling P. Allostasis: A model of predictive regulation. *Physiol Behav.* 106: 5–15, 2011.
Zajicek G. Wisdom of the body. *Med Hypotheses.* 52: 447–449, 1999.

27.

HOMEOSTATIC SYSTEMS

STAYING ALIVE

n this chapter, we start with a look at several hypothalamic functions before examining thermoregulation, cardiovascular function, breathing, micturition, and digestion. Finally, we consider sleep and the circadian rhythm.

THE HYPOTHALAMUS REGULATES FLUID BALANCE THROUGH VASOPRESSIN RELEASE

The hypothalamus can be considered the head ganglion for neural control of the body's physiology. As introduced in Chapter 7, a group of neurons that controls hormone release is present in animals from worms to mammals. In vertebrates, hormone release is the core function of the hypothalamus around which many embellishments arose. We start with the hypothalamic control of *antidiuretic hormone* (*ADH*) or *vasopressin* release.

Normally, when blood osmolarity increases—evidence of dehydration—ADH acts on the kidneys to increase the salt concentration of urine. This minimizes the fluid that is excreted. Without ADH, the hypothalamus cannot regulate kidney function. In the absence of even baseline levels of ADH, the kidneys work harder and more urine is voided, termed *polyuria*. Moreover, voided urine is far more dilute than usual. Excessive voiding of dilute urine leads to insufficient hydration, marked by elevated plasma osmolarity and a feeling of thirst. The affected person drinks more than usual, termed *polydipsia*. (Note that whereas ADH contributes to the motivation to drink in response to thirst and dehydration, it is not the only factor. As a result, people continue to drink even without ADH.) The water ingested further dilutes the urine voided and so on. Increased voiding of dilute urine causes a further increase in plasma osmolarity, which again cannot be rectified because of the lack of ADH. This vicious cycle leads

to high plasma osmolarity and low urine osmolarity, the cardinal signs of *diabetes insipidus*. The end result is greatly increased intake and output of fluid as though the affected person were a *siphon*, the Greek word for which is the root of the word "diabetes." The term "insipidus" reflects the insipid or tasteless water that is siphoned through in affected individuals.

Diabetes insipidus is distinct from diabetes mellitus, a condition in which glucose is not appropriately processed by insulin. A major difference between the two conditions is that the urine in patients with diabetes mellitus contains elevated levels of glucose (*mellitus* is derived from Greek words meaning "honey sweet"), whereas the urine in patients with diabetes insipidus does not. A further difference is that diabetes mellitus is a pancreatic disorder whereas diabetes insipidus is due to hypothalamic or pituitary dysfunction. Diabetes insipidus is therefore termed central or neurogenic. It can result from a tumor in the pituitary or hypothalamus. Iatrogenic cases of central diabetes insipidus can also be the unintentional result of surgical removal of a space-occupying pituitary tumor. Diabetes insipidus can be a reversible condition, in which case it does not require lifelong treatment as is the case for type 1 diabetes mellitus.

THE HYPOTHALAMUS PRODUCES A HORMONAL ENVIRONMENT THAT SUPPORTS POSTPARTUM MATERNAL CARE

The period in a female's life after the birth of a child is biologically stressful. The mother must adapt to a baby's crying and needs, to her own sleep deprivation, and to radical changes in her body's physiology while also tolerating repeated nursing. Although in modern life some mothers have access to nannies and the like, natural selection has left us with a system evolved under conditions in which babies were wholly dependent on mother, day in and day out. Cultural challenges piggy-back upon biological ones. Whether having her first or fifth child, a modern woman faces the additional stress of changing family dynamics during an already challenging postpartum period.

To promote maternal well-being and, in turn, a child's development, nature has armed mothers with ammunition against the difficulties of the postpartum period. The ammunition comes in two forms. First, contact with her baby improves a mother's mood. Second, a flood of neurochemical and hormonal changes lead to improved mood, reduced anxiety, and reduced reactivity to stress, virtually a neural version of a "chill pill." For example, *oxytocin* and another neuropeptide *prolactin* are both released from hypothalamic neurons, and both reduce anxiety and reactivity to stress. The apparently redundant effects of the two neuropeptides likely reflect the extremely critical need for a mother to maintain a stable, upbeat mood. Imagine how helpful an upbeat attitude would be to a woman who is nursing and caring for a completely helpless baby all the time, 24/7 in the modern vernacular. Furthermore, buoying a mother's mood and ability to cope with challenges will inevitably facilitate the child's normal and healthy development.

In a number of well-publicized tragic cases, women suffering from either *postpartum depression* or *postpartum psychosis* have harmed, abandoned, or even killed their babies. Thankfully, such extreme types of *postpartum mood disorders* are rare. The most common form of postpartum mood disorder is in fact *postpartum anxiety*. Unfortunately, since plasma levels of neurotransmitters do not reflect brain levels, we know little about the neurochemistry of the postpartum period directly from women. However, we have learned a great deal about the roles of prolactin, oxytocin, and the like from findings in laboratory animals. Oxytocin, which can be administered intranasally to women, may prove to be a useful and effective treatment for some postpartum disorders, although this remains controversial. On the other hand, contact with her baby demonstrably improves a woman's mood and reduces her anxiety, providing a simple method for cutting a mother's risk of developing a mood or anxiety disorder.

In contrast to our burgeoning knowledge regarding the role of the hypothalamus in postpartum maternal behavior and maternal care, we know very little about the brain and paternal care. Our lack of information is not evidence that fathers are or are not biologically inclined to provide parental or spousal care—it is simply a hole in our knowledge that we need to fill.

OVERPRODUCTION OF CORTISOL CAUSES SEVERE WEIGHT GAIN AND OTHER PROBLEMS, WHEREAS CORTISOL INSUFFICIENCY CAN BE FATAL

Cushing's disease occurs when a pituitary adenoma (see Chapter 8) causes overproduction of *adrenocorticotropic hormone* (*ACTH*), which in turn leads to excess *cortisol* production (see Chapter 2). When the same end result—excessive cortisol—results from an adrenal tumor, intake of a steroidal medication, or other cause, it is termed *Cushing's syndrome*. High levels of cortisol cause severe weight gain, particularly in the face and trunk. Treatments for Cushing's syndrome and disease are aimed at removing the source of cortisol production and surgical removal of the pituitary adenoma, respectively.

Although modern vernacular views *stress* as a negative and the absence of stress as desirable, an insufficient amount of the stress hormone cortisol, a condition known as *Addison's disease*, is potentially fatal. Without cortisol, individuals are fatigued, have little appetite, and are hypotensive. Most importantly, people with Addison's disease cannot react appropriately to homeostatic challenges. As a result, stressors can trigger a potentially fatal *Addisonian crisis*, which is marked by sudden back and leg pain, low blood pressure, vomiting, and unconsciousness. Most cases of Addison's disease stem from the autoimmune destruction of adrenal tissue and are treated by supplying drugs that substitute for the missing adrenal hormones.

Contrasting Addison's disease with Cushing's syndrome tells us something important. The concentration of hormones, such as cortisol, needs to be just right, neither too high nor too low. Furthermore, the appropriate amount of cortisol is different across varying conditions. We need more cortisol during periods of stress, and, without it, our body cannot rise to the challenges presented.

SECRETING PITUITARY TUMORS LEAD TO HORMONE OVERPRODUCTION

As you learned in Chapter 2, pituitary tumors are relatively common neoplastic growths, typically benign, in the anterior pituitary. Most people with such pituitary adenomas never experience any adverse symptoms. Beyond causing symptoms through occupying too much space, some pituitary adenomas cause excess secretion of one or more

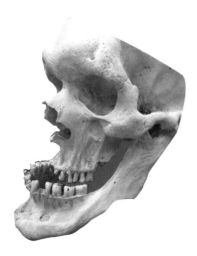

Figure 27-1 In acromegaly, bones grow even though the affected individuals are adults long past the normal time of growth and development. The brow and jaw are particularly accentuated.

adenohypophyseal hormones. The most typical hormones involved are prolactin, growth hormone, and adrenocorticotropic hormone (ACTH). Excess levels of each of these hormones can produce symptoms that lead an affected individual to seek medical advice. For example, excess secretion of growth hormone in an adult causes excessive and painful growth, termed *acromegaly*. Visible signs of acromegaly include protrusive growth in the hands, brow, and jaw (Fig. 27-1). If excess amounts of growth hormone are secreted in a prepubertal child, gigantism will result if the condition is not treated.

Although some secreting pituitary tumors can be shrunk using medications targeting the oversecreting cells, many patients undergo trans-sphenoidal (i.e., via an approach through the nose) surgery, which is usually successful.

THE BIGGEST THREAT TO THERMOREGULATION IS OVERHEATING

Thermoregulation is perhaps the easiest homeostatic system to visualize and understand. The goal of thermoregulation is to maintain the body at roughly 37°C during waking. Core temperature is defended against both cold stress, termed *cold defense*, and heat stress, termed *heat defense*. Effectors of cold defense include *heat production* and *heat conservation*, whereas *heat defense is accomplished only through heat loss*. There is no mechanism for active cooling. In other words, we can dissipate body heat by sweating, panting, and vasodilation, but we lack a physiological refrigeration process. Consequently, overheating can be a dangerous threat to the body.

Heat production is accomplished by *shivering* using skeletal muscle and by increasing metabolic activity and therefore *metabolic heat production*. The effectors of heat conservation are *cutaneous vasoconstriction* and postural adjustments that decrease the body's surface area. An example of the latter is a huddling posture. Heat loss is accomplished by sweating, panting, cutaneous vasodilation, and postural adjustments that increase the body's surface area. In addition to the physiological thermoregulatory effectors inherited through evolution, modern humans have added cultural behavioral effectors for thermoregulation. Examples include donning more or less clothing, seeking shelter or covering blankets, turning on air conditioning or a heater, running through a sprinkler, or building a fire.

The behavioral effectors of thermoregulation—postural adjustments, clothing, and so on—depend on skeletal muscle activity. In addition, skeletal muscles are responsible for shivering and panting to produce and lose heat, respectively. The remaining thermoregulatory effectors—vasomotor changes, metabolic rate, and sweating—are under sympathetic control.

VASOMOTION DEFINES THE THERMONEUTRAL ZONE

The range of the thermoneutral zone is some measurable fraction of a degree centigrade, roughly 0.4°C (<1°F), in the healthy human. The thermoneutral zone is centered at a defended temperature termed the *set point*. As the body temperature varies within the thermoneutral zone, the only thermoregulatory effectors active are vasomotor. Within this range, sweating, panting, shivering, and metabolic adjustments contribute little if at all to determining core body temperature. The range where vasomotion is the only active thermoregulatory effector is the *thermoneutral zone* (Fig. 27-2A).

Vasomotor effectors can be triggered by changes in core temperature and by local changes in skin temperature. Changes in core temperature are sensed by sensory neurons, processed by the central nervous system (CNS), and lead to changes in sympathetic output. Local changes in skin temperature also directly feedback on to the peripheral circulation, leading to either vasoconstriction or vasodilation, without participation of the CNS. Mechanisms to alter vasomotion include:

- Noradrenergic sympathetic fibers innervate cutaneous arterioles and, when stimulated, cause vasoconstriction.

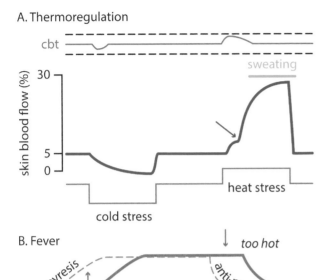

A. Thermoregulation

B. Fever

Figure 27-2 A: At thermoneutral temperatures, thermoregulation is accomplished by vasomotion. In response to a drop in temperature, skin blood flow (*dark blue line*) drops from a resting value of about 5% of cardiac output to near zero. Conversely, in response to heat stress, skin blood flow increases. At first, the increase is due to a relaxation of active vasoconstriction. If that response is insufficient, an active vasodilation occurs (starting at the inflection point indicated by the *arrow*). In addition, in response to moderate heat stress, sweating occurs (*light blue line*). These vasomotor adjustments keep core body temperature (*cbt, red line*) within the thermoneutral zone (*dashed black lines*). B: During a fever, the set point (*dashed gray line*) increases in response to a pyrogen. The increase in set point activates heat production effectors, shivering, and increased metabolism, and therefore core body temperature (*red line*) increases after a delay. While core body temperature is increasing but is still below the set point, the subjective feeling is one of being too cold. When core body temperature reaches set point, the chills subside. When the fever breaks, either naturally or in response to an antipyretic, the set point decreases and heat loss responses, such as sweating and throwing off blankets, are engaged. While core body temperature is decreasing but still above set point, the subjective feeling is one of being too warm.

- Cholinergic sympathetic fibers innervate cutaneous arterioles in the *glabrous*, or nonhairy, skin. Stimulation of these fibers causes vasodilation.

- Local increases in temperature elicit vasodilation that is mediated by sensory neurons and the local release of nitric oxide.

- In response to local cooling, cold-sensitive sensory fibers facilitate norepinephrine release from sympathetic vasoconstrictor fibers, leading to increased vasoconstriction.

Ultimately, vasomotion changes the blood flow through the skin, either increasing or decreasing blood flow through vasodilation and vasoconstriction, respectively (Fig. 27-2A).

The more blood flow at the surface of the body, the more heat is lost to the environment.

The normal operation of thermoregulation works something along the lines of the following. As body temperature approaches the lower end of the thermoneutral zone or when skin temperature cools, cutaneous vasoconstriction reduces skin blood flow. The basal level of skin blood flow is about 5% of cardiac output and can go to 0% in response to cold. As body temperature approaches the upper end of the thermoneutral zone or when skin temperature warms, the initial response is a reduction in vasoconstriction. If the warming persists, active cutaneous vasodilation occurs, and this greatly increases skin blood flow to comprise a large proportion of cardiac output. Along with active vasodilation, sweating is triggered, and the combination of vasodilation and sweating is typically effective in preventing overheating. The width and absolute range of the thermoneutral zone differs across age, seasonal temperatures, hormonal status, and a myriad of other factors. For example, the thermoneutral zone of perimenopausal women who suffer from hot flashes is so narrow that it is not measurable.

There is a key vulnerability to the vasomotor system of thermoregulation. Any change in temperature due to vasomotion depends on the transfer of heat between the skin and the environment. At very cold temperatures, below freezing, letting the skin equilibrate to the environment causes *frostbite*. Frostbite can produce permanent changes in skin, circulation, innervation, and bone structure. The first line of defense against frostbite is a *paradoxical vasodilation* to extreme cold. This vasodilation warms the exposed tissue and prevents frostbite, at least for some time. Vasodilation is not effective in individuals with compromised circulation, such as diabetics, who therefore are at a higher risk for frostbite.

At very warm temperatures, there is a strong risk of gaining heat through vasodilation. Yet, warm temperatures, even very warm temperatures, do not elicit vasoconstriction. In other words, there is no paradoxical vasoconstriction at very warm temperatures analogous to the paradoxical vasodilation that occurs at freezing temperatures. For this reason, *ambient temperatures above skin temperature and certainly those above body temperature are medical dangers and can lead to death in those without access to cooling devices.* The only effective responses are sweating and relocating to a cooler environment. Consequently, it is a matter of life and death that governments and municipalities set up cooling centers where individuals without access to air conditioning can go during the increasing number of heat waves affecting our planet.

THE SET POINT VARIES ACROSS CIRCUMSTANCES

The center of the thermoneutral zone is the *set point*, an empirically defined temperature that the body defends against change. This set point is very important because the *perception* of one's temperature is always *in relation* to the set point. For example, a body temperature of 39°C is perceived as mildly hot when, as is true under normal circumstances, the set point is at 37°C. In contrast, when the set point is at 39°C, a body temperature of 39°C does not feel hot. As another example, the set point falls during sleep relative to during waking. This gives rise to the common experience of feeling quite warm upon unexpectedly waking up in the middle of a sleep, despite the core temperature's being lower during sleep than during waking.

Fever is characterized by an increase in the set point (Fig. 27-2B). A *pyrogen* is a substance that elicits *pyresis*, the medical term for a fever. During the development of pyresis, set point increases before core temperature does. Consequently, febrile individuals feel cold; this corresponds to the familiar chills that foreshadow a fever. During a fever, shivering and an increase in metabolic rate drive core temperature up, toward the elevated set point. *Antipyresis*, referring to a fever breaking, is characterized by a lowering of the set point. Consequently, people feel too warm when a fever breaks.

The concept of a defended set point makes it very important to know the underlying cause of an elevated body temperature. *Hyperthermia* refers to a body temperature that is greater than set point. Hyperthermia often results from excessive environmental heat or overexertion. With the exception of *malignant hyperthermia*, a thankfully rare and now treatable condition (see Box 27-1), hyperthermia is effectively treated with lots of fluids and active cooling of the body. However, the same treatment for an individual with a fever would simply increase the body's drive to increase core temperature. Therefore, a person with a high fever must be treated with *antipyretic drugs* to bring the set point down. Conversely, antipyretics are ineffective in treating a person with hyperthermia.

Nonsteroidal anti-inflammatory drugs double as antipyretics. Circulating pyrogens reach the brain through the *organum vasculosum of the lamina terminalis* (see Chapter 8), with the result that prostaglandin E2 is released into the *medial preoptic area* in the rostral hypothalamus. The effect of *prostaglandin E2* is to elevate the set point. Therefore, drugs that block prostaglandin synthesis, such as aspirin, also prevent or reverse the elevation in set point that defines fever.

Malignant hyperthermia is a rare reaction to commonly used inhalational general anesthetics such as isoflurane. Mutations in the *ryanodine receptor* are the known cause of malignant hyperthermia. The ryanodine receptor plays an important part of coupling excitation to contraction in skeletal muscles by pairing the influx of calcium ions with a massive release of calcium ions from intracellular stores. The mutations that lead to malignant hyperthermia render the ryanodine receptor more sensitive to calcium ions in the presence of triggering general anesthetics. Thus, calcium ions flood into skeletal muscles, triggering muscle contraction and adenosine triphosphate (ATP) consumption, which in turn lead to excessive heat production.

Malignant hyperthermia was fatal in a majority of cases 50 years ago. Fortunately, today, *dantrolene*, a drug that blocks ryanodine receptor–mediated release of intracellular calcium ion stores, prevents most fatalities from malignant hyperthermia. Nonetheless, malignant hyperthermia is appropriately treated as a serious medical emergency. General anesthetic administration must be discontinued and dantrolene administered immediately.

We usually do not know whether a person is susceptible to malignant hyperthermia before the first "experiment" of general anesthesia is tried. On the other hand, an individual who has been exposed to triggering general anesthetics without showing malignant hyperthermia is considered to be free of a susceptibility mutation. Since malignant hyperthermia runs in families, a careful history may be helpful in identifying potentially susceptible individuals.

Hypothermia refers to a body temperature that is below set point. There are no clinical conditions in which set point is clearly lowered. In other words, there is no analogy to fever for a regulated decrease in body temperature. Therefore, hypothermia is always treated by rewarming using progressively more aggressive methods depending on the severity of the drop in core temperature.

The thermoneutral zone narrows tremendously in peri- and postmenopausal women. Up to 80% of perimenopausal and postmenopausal women experience hot flushes, hot flashes, or night sweats. Collectively, these three symptoms are referred to as *vasomotor disorders* because they all include an initial vasodilation event followed by the sensation of being far too hot and behaviors aimed at reducing core temperature. The best characterized of the vasomotor disorders, a hot flash is a short-lived, rapid-onset, subjective feeling of being excessively and uncomfortably hot. Physiologically, the first and core event in a hot flash is a spontaneous increase in cutaneous blood flow that is usually accompanied by an increase in heart rate. Within a minute or two of the increase in skin blood flow, women report the subjective sensation of having a hot flash and try to cool off by removing clothes, opening a window, turning on a fan, or the like. After a further lag, sweating, a powerful and rapidly effective heat loss process, starts. Sweating produces a large decrease, typically more than a degree centigrade, in core temperature.

The core temperature of unaffected men and women can vary within a 0.4°C range without eliciting a thermoregulatory reaction. In contrast, in an individual with a vasomotor disorder, thermoregulatory reactions are elicited in the absence of any measurable change in core temperature. This constriction of the thermoneutral zone results in symptomatic menopausal women feeling alternately too cold and too hot. Thus, hot flashes and night sweats are just the most uncomfortable manifestations of a more general dysfunction of thermoregulation in menopausal women.

It should be noted that since testosterone stimulates prostate cell growth, men with prostate cancer receive treatment to reduce testosterone production or to block the effect of testosterone. Most men receiving androgen suppression therapy suffer from hot flashes, suggesting that loss of testosterone, as with loss of estrogen, leads to hot flashes. Similarly, vasomotor disorders in both men and women are effectively treated by estrogen replacement therapy. Unfortunately, estrogen increases the risk of breast cancer and has uncomfortable side effects in men. Fortunately, the frequency of hot flashes and night sweats diminishes within a year or two of menopause in women or within months of treatment's end for men.

THE BAROREFLEX STABILIZES BLOOD PRESSURE ACROSS A SHORT TIME SCALE

The brain regulates blood pressure across a short time scale of seconds to minutes through the *baroreflex*. The baroreflex is a feedback reflex that serves to stabilize blood pressure in response to increases or decreases. It is essentially the blood pressure version of a stretch reflex. *Baroreceptors* are primary afferents that sense the pressure (*baro* is Greek for "weight") within the carotid sinus and aortic arch. Baroreceptors fire at rest so that the discharge rate of baroreceptors increases when blood pressure increases and decreases when blood pressure decreases. Baroreceptors carry information about

blood pressure into the medulla through the glossopharyngeal and vagus nerves and terminate in the caudal portion of the nucleus tractus solitarius (Fig. 27-3). Nucleus tractus solitarius neurons that receive baroreceptive input send this information to neurons in the caudal ventrolateral medulla, which in turn inhibit neurons in the rostral ventrolateral medulla (rVLM). Through this circuit, increases in blood pressure cause inhibition of neurons in the rVLM, whereas decreases in blood pressure disinhibit rVLM neurons.

The rVLM is a *sympathoexcitatory* region. This means that stimulation in the rVLM increases sympathetic outflow. Neurons in the rVLM influence sympathetic activity through direct projections that excite preganglionic sympathetic motor neurons in the intermediolateral cell column of the thoracic cord. The sympathetic effects through which activation of the rVLM a leads to an elevated blood pressure include increases in heart rate, myocardial contractility, and the peripheral resistance of arterioles.

A steady blood pressure may serve us well under many circumstances. Yet there are conditions when the increase in

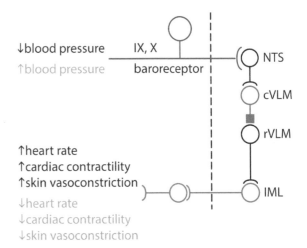

Figure 27-3 The baroreflex serves to dampen changes in blood pressure. Baroreceptors that innervate the carotid sinus and aortic arch enter the nervous system through the glossopharyngeal and vagus nerves (*IX, X*) and excite cells in the nucleus of the tractus solitarius (*NTS*). Cells in the nucleus of the tractus solitarius excite cells in the caudal ventrolateral medulla (*cVLM*), which in turn inhibit cells in the rostral ventrolateral medulla (*rVLM*). Cells in the rostral ventrolateral medulla are sympathoexcitatory because they excite preganglionic sympathetic neurons in the intermediolateral cell column of the thoracic cord (*IML*). Increasing sympathetic outflow increases heart rate, cardiac contractility, and skin vasoconstriction. These three effects lead to an elevation in blood pressure because blood pressure is a function of cardiac output (in turn dependent on heart rate) and peripheral resistance. There is one *sign switch* in this circuit due to the inhibitory neuron in the caudal ventrolateral medulla. Therefore, a decrease in blood pressure leads to a reflexive increase in blood pressure (*black*), whereas an increase in blood pressure leads to a reflexive decrease in blood pressure (*gray*). Note that the arrangement of neurons in this diagram does not accurately reflect the anatomic relationships between the areas involved.

oxygen and nutrients afforded by an elevation of blood pressure is adaptive. For example, during a fight-or-flight reaction, skeletal muscles are active and are best served by more blood flow. Several mechanisms exist to suppress the baroreceptor reflex so that a greater increase in blood pressure is required to trigger a reflexive adjustment. Noxious input and signals from the hypothalamus related to exercise, feeding, and strong emotions all can lead to baroreceptor reflex modulation.

ORTHOSTATIC HYPOTENSION OCCURS COMMONLY IN THE ELDERLY

Orthostatic hypotension refers to an episode of low blood pressure associated with standing up. Most people have experienced at least a mild form of orthostatic hypotension when rising rapidly from a recumbent position or a squat. However, orthostatic hypotension is a chronic problem that afflicts a large number of elderly individuals. As you recall from Chapter 8, low blood pressure may prevent adequate cerebral blood flow, and, consequently, there may be a feeling of lightheadedness associated with orthostatic hypotension. People often report seeing spots, and, if cerebral blood flow decreases sufficiently, syncope occurs (see Chapter 8).

Under normal circumstances, the motor command to stand up is accompanied by an anticipatory signal to leg skeletal muscles that leads to their contraction. This contraction prevents blood from pooling in the lower limbs and ensures sufficient cerebral perfusion pressure. However, in a person with low blood volume, often secondary to dehydration, sustaining cerebral blood flow is simply not possible. Another possible cause of orthostatic hypotension is neurogenic, stemming from a loss of either central or peripheral norepinephrine in association with, for example, Parkinson's disease or *multiple systems atrophy*. Without adequate support from sympathetic outflow, a person cannot maintain adequate cerebral blood flow while in an upright posture. Treatment for orthostatic hypotension is tailored to the underlying cause.

INSPIRATION IS THE KEY COMPONENT OF NORMAL BREATHING

Breathing is a patterned skeletomotor movement that is critical to keeping us alive. The skeletal muscles used for respiration are under volitional control. Despite our ability to voluntarily take command of respiration, most of the 500 million or so breaths in an 80-year lifespan, even those that occur during wakefulness, are performed without conscious thought.

Breathing has three phases: *inspiration, postinspiration,* and *expiration.* Inspiration is accomplished by two pump muscles, the diaphragm and the external intercostal muscles, with the diaphragm playing the critical role. The diaphragm is innervated by spinal motoneurons in C3–C5, which send their axons through the *phrenic nerve.* Contraction of the diaphragm expands the thoracic cavity, creating a low-pressure sink into which air floods (Fig. 27-4A). However, resistance in the upper airway tempers the flow of air, decreasing inspiratory volume. Upper airway resistance is

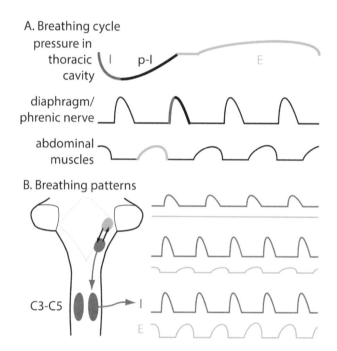

Figure 27-4 A: A single cycle of breathing consisting of inspiratory (*I*), postinspiratory (*p-I*), and expiratory (*E*) phases is shown at the top. The bottom two traces show that inspiration (*red*) is accomplished by activation of phrenic motoneurons that innervate the diaphragm. Contraction of the diaphragm expands the thoracic cavity and decreases the pressure therein. For quiet breathing, the ribcage recoils to its starting position to support passive expiration. During increased energy expenditure and increased CO_2 formation, active expiration using abdominal muscles occurs (*blue*), thereby increasing the thoracic pressure and forcing air out of the lungs. B: Eupnea (*top pair of traces*) consists of inspiration (*red*) and passive expiration. The pre-Bötzinger complex (*upper red area in cartoon at left*) produces the rhythm required for eupnea. The output of the pre-Bötzinger complex reaches phrenic motoneurons (*red area marked C3–C5*) in the upper cervical cord. Phrenic motoneurons control the diaphragm and produce the basic breathing rhythm. A disconnection between the pre-Bötzinger complex and the phrenic motoneurons in the upper cervical cord renders an individual dependent on a respirator. As energy demands increase (*middle pair of traces*), respiratory frequency increases, tidal volume increases, and active expiration (*blue*) occurs. With further energy expenditure, active expiration (*E*) increases in effort (*bottom pair of traces*). The breathing rhythm is produced by interactions between the pre-Bötzinger complex and the parafacial respiratory group (*blue area*). The output of the parafacial respiratory group controls active expiration through projections to the abdominal muscles (not shown).

governed by oral and pharyngeal muscles innervated by cranial nerves VII, IX, X, and XII (see Chapters 5, 16).

Expiration can occur passively as the lungs and thoracic cavity relax back to their starting position. Indeed, during normal breathing, termed *eupnea*, inspiration is followed by the passive recoil of the lungs, and there is *no* active expiratory phase (Fig. 27-4B). In other words, as we sit quietly, our breathing consists almost exclusively of periodic contractions of the diaphragm. However, when carbon dioxide (CO_2) production increases, for example during exercise, passive expiration is replaced by active expiration. Essentially, active expiration rids the body of excess CO_2 generated by activity.

A COLLAPSE OF THE UPPER AIRWAY DURING SLEEP PRODUCES REPEATED EPISODES OF APNEA

Upper airway muscles relax during sleep. In some individuals, the upper airway actually collapses during inspiration when the pressure in the airway is lowest. This collapse results in *apnea*, a cessation of breathing. Individuals with *obstructive sleep apnea* can experience hundreds of apneic episodes, each lasting 10 seconds to 2 minutes, every night. The accumulated effects of repeated, intermittent apnea are severe. Individuals develop daytime sleepiness, hypertension, and are at high risk for cardiac arrest and stroke.

The first line of treatment for obstructive sleep apnea is to increase the pressure in the airway, either during inspiration alone or during both inspiration and expiration, using a device such as a *continuous positive airway pressure* (*CPAP*) device. The CPAP machine has a mask that fits over the patient's mouth, nose, or both. Positive air pressure is maintained within the mask, thus preventing airway collapse.

Obesity, smoking, and diabetes are risk factors for obstructive sleep apnea. As the incidence of obesity and diabetes continue to climb in industrialized societies, so too has the incidence of obstructive sleep apnea. In the United States, 5–10% of the population suffers from obstructive sleep apnea, much of it as of yet undiagnosed.

SIGHS OCCUR PERIODICALLY AND PREVENT ALVEOLAR COLLAPSE

Gas exchange in the lungs occurs through hundreds of millions of structures called *alveoli* (singular is alveolus). The alveoli are hollow spherical formations, about 1 millimeter in diameter. The inside of the alveoli is coated by a monolayer of surfactant that reduces the surface tension on the alveoli. A reduction of alveolar surface tension decreases the work needed to expand the alveoli and achieve gas exchange. However, over time, there is a tendency for the alveoli to collapse. When the alveoli collapse, the surface surfactant on the inner surface of the alveoli sticks together and is difficult to separate. Imagine trying to inflate a collapsed water balloon. As this analogy makes apparent, reinflating collapsed alveoli is difficult.

Mammals use the tactic of *preventing* alveolar collapse before it occurs. To do this, we *sigh* about 10–12 times per hour. A sigh is an augmented inspiration, a hyperinflation, which inflates the alveoli by creating a very-low-pressure sink within the thoracic cavity. This periodic superinflation of the alveoli counters the natural tendency for alveolar collapse and prevents *atelectasis*, or lung collapse. Because of the importance of periodic sighing to lung health, artificial respirators are programmed to produce periodic hyperinflations in individuals unable to breathe on their own. This greatly reduces the incidence of atelectasis in patients dependent on a respirator.

Sighs not only serve the physiological function of preventing alveolar collapse but also are used and understood as emotional expressions. Sighs are understood by others as expressions of sadness, boredom, weariness, resignation, or as a sign that the sigher finds something stupid or hopeless. Interestingly, people do not always understand sighs as they are intended. Sighs are primarily produced to express resignation or boredom. Both of these emotions reflect a disconnect between expectation and actuality and the acceptance that the disconnect is out of one's control. For example, resignation happens when hopes and desires become unattainable, and people are forced to let them go. Boredom results when one's expectation to be entertained and amused is dashed. Individuals trying to solve very difficult puzzles sigh as they try various solutions that do not work.

To paraphrase the Nobel Prize winning ethologist Niko Tinbergen, we will never know whether a rooster crows because it is happy, or because it wants to wake the hens, or because it hates its neighbor. Similarly, sighs serve a variety of physiological and emotional functions, and, at present, it is not possible to distinguish a sigh that is "intended" to prevent alveolar collapse from one that serves to express an emotion such as resignation or relief.

BREATHING IS PRODUCED BY A CENTRAL PATTERN GENERATOR IN THE MEDULLA

Fundamentally, *eupnea* consists of a repeated pattern of bursting activity in the phrenic nerve that leads to periodic contraction of the diaphragm and external intercostal muscles and associated changes in upper airway muscles that modulate the patency of the airway. This fundamental pattern is produced by a central pattern generator network known as the *pre-Bötzinger complex* located in the ventrolateral medulla (Fig. 27-4B). The pre-Bötzinger complex sends out a pattern of activity to motoneurons in cranial nerve nuclei and the spinal ventral horn. Essentially, the pre-Bötzinger complex is the source of the breathing rhythm—and probably of sighs—during eupnea.

Damage to the pre-Bötzinger complex itself may result in disordered breathing specifically during sleep. Experiments in rodents show that the first consequence of damage to the pre-Bötzinger complex is apnea during rapid eye movement (REM) sleep. After more time, apneic episodes start to occur during non-REM sleep. In both Parkinson's disease and amyotrophic lateral sclerosis, there is neuropathological evidence for a loss of neurons in the region of the pre-Bötzinger complex. In both of these diseases, breathing is disordered during sleep but not during waking. The loss of neurons in the pre-Bötzinger complex may in fact cause a disruption of breathing specifically during sleep. Accumulated damage from a lifetime of random insults and cell deaths may reduce the number of neurons in the pre-Bötzinger complex and contribute to the increasing incidence of sleep apnea with age.

Injury to the spinal cord above the level of phrenic motoneurons (i.e., in either C1 or C2) may, depending on the location and extent of the lesion, disconnect the pre-Bötzinger complex from the phrenic motoneurons in the upper cervical cord. The consequence of such disconnection is paralysis of either half or all of the diaphragm. As introduced in Chapter 4, people with high cervical spinal cord injuries typically need nighttime ventilator assistance at the very least, and some employ a respirator during waking hours as well. Spinal cord injuries as low as the high thoracic cord damage the brainstem connections to external intercostal muscles, which may produce adverse consequences on breathing.

BREATHING IS MODULATED BY THE LEVELS OF OXYGEN AND CARBON DIOXIDE IN THE BLOOD

Eupnea serves us and other mammals well as long as we are resting quietly and remain unstressed by environmental factors such as heat. However, during activity or in challenging environments, energy demands increase, and, as a result, the body needs more oxygen. During exertion, as we use our muscles or increase metabolic rate, the production of CO_2 also increases. Breathing changes to accommodate the needs to inspire more oxygen and to eliminate the buildup of CO_2. Deeper and more rapid inspirations bring in more oxygen (Fig. 27-4B). Moreover, active expiration replaces passive expiration and is able to eliminate the excess CO_2.

Active expiration depends on a second central pattern generator distinct from that in the pre-Bötzinger complex. The central pattern generator critical to active expiration is found just medial to the facial nucleus, in a region that we will call the *parafacial respiratory group* (Fig. 27-4B). Neurons in the parafacial respiratory group are sensitive to the concentration of CO_2. Elevated levels of CO_2 directly activate neurons in the parafacial respiratory group, with the result that active expiration begins. There is parsimony in this arrangement. Exertion is accompanied by active expiration, mediated by the parafacial respiratory group. The automatic engagement of active expiration when inadequate ventilation results in a buildup of CO_2 is particularly important during sleep. Individuals with a congenital insensitivity to CO_2 are severely affected, and many require artificial ventilation during sleep.

Congenital central hypoventilation syndrome, also called *Ondine's curse*, is a genetic disease that is caused by either expanded trinucleotide repeats, as in Huntington's disease (see Chapter 2), or missense mutations in the gene for a homeobox factor, *PHOX2B*. Homeobox genes are critical to patterning the developing embryo, and the loss of *PHOX2B* specifically causes a failure of CO_2-sensitive neurons in the parafacial respiratory group to develop. Additional neuronal populations, such as neurons of the enteric nervous system, also fail to develop. Nonetheless, the breathing abnormalities associated with congenital central hypoventilation syndrome are the most striking and most debilitating aspect of congenital central hypoventilation syndrome.

Individuals with congenital central hypoventilation syndrome are insensitive to elevated levels of CO_2. They therefore are insensitive to asphyxiation. They have a very difficult time exercising because they do not make appropriate breathing adjustments in the face of inadequate ventilation. The inability of parafacial respiratory neurons to detect elevated levels of CO_2 requires that artificial ventilatory assistance be employed during sleep. The restrictions on normal life experienced by individuals with congenital central hypoventilation syndrome dramatically illustrate the debilitating effects of an inability to sense CO_2 and highlight the everyday importance of this neural function.

Recall that the onset of Huntington's disease is earliest and disease progression is most rapid in patients with the greatest number of trinucleotide repeats in *huntingtin*. Similarly, it appears that the number of trinucleotide repeats in *PHOX2B* determines age of onset and severity of congenital central hypoventilation syndrome. Thus, an adult with a borderline number of trinucleotide repeats may be largely symptom-free, but his or her offspring may have a more classic presentation of respiratory inadequacy at birth. This scenario suggests that it is worthwhile to clinically evaluate the parents of a baby with congenital central hypoventilation syndrome.

The inspiratory rhythm generated by the pre-Bötzinger complex and the active expiration generated by the parafacial respiratory group are coordinated. Projections between the two central pattern generator networks accomplish this coordination (Fig. 27-4B).

MUSCLES USED FOR BREATHING ARE SHARED WITH MANY OTHER MOTOR PATTERNS

Although breathing may have first dibs on the diaphragm, external intercostal muscles, and muscles of the upper airway, many other motor patterns use at least some of the same muscles. During nonbreathing movements, muscles shared with breathing are controlled by a combination of reconfigured breathing central pattern generators and other central pattern generators specific to nonbreathing movements. For example, there are many different breathing patterns such as gasping, sighing, breathing at different rates, and so on. A reconfiguration of the respiratory central pattern generators in the pre-Bötzinger complex and the parafacial respiratory group are adequate to produce these different breathing patterns. This is analogous to the manner in which reconfigurations of the mesencephalic locomotor region produce walking, trotting, running, and sprinting (see Chapter 22). Coughing is a motor pattern that largely relies on a reconfiguration of the breathing central pattern generators with a small contribution from other areas. Motor patterns more distinct from than similar to breathing include swallowing, speech, vomiting, gagging, and sneezing. In these cases, additional central pattern generators work with the breathing pattern generators to suspend breathing during incompatible movements such as vomiting.

URINE STORAGE DOMINATES OUR LIVES BUT BLADDER-EMPTYING MUST OCCUR REGULARLY

We store urine in our bladder for virtually all of our lives. Bladder-emptying requires little time, rarely longer than 10 seconds and occupies well under 1% of our lifetime. Nonetheless, the bladder must be emptied regularly. Urinary retention is a medical emergency and can be fatal. Although critical to survival, micturition is incapacitating in the sense that it prevents an individual from making other movements. It is probably for this reason that forebrain control over the timing of micturition has evolved in most territorial mammals. Modern humans utilize the control circuits inherited from evolution and marry them to social norms, so that the switch from urine storage to micturition occurs at a socially appropriate time and place. The failure to void in accordance with social norms—incontinence—has devastating effects on both an affected individual and on his or her loved ones.

In adults, control over the timing of micturition is accomplished by the medial prefrontal cortex. The prefrontal cortex tonically suppresses micturition in accordance with social and environmental conditions. Strokes in the medial orbitofrontal cortex often produce urinary incontinence that is accompanied by a bizarre lack of concern on the part of the patient over the inappropriate voiding.

BLADDER CONTROL DEPENDS ON THE COORDINATED ACTIVITY OF VOLUNTARY AND SMOOTH MUSCLES

Afferent input from the bladder that signals bladder filling reaches both sacral circuits that are in immediate control of the bladder and higher centers responsible for initiating voiding at appropriate times. Using information about bladder distension, prefrontal cortex does not engage the pontine micturition center when the bladder is empty. When the bladder fills and micturition is released from inhibition by the forebrain, neurons in the pontine micturition center are activated. The pontine micturition center, located just caudal to the periaqueductal gray, is essentially a central pattern generator for micturition. Neurons in the pontine micturition center project to the sacral cord where they contact (1) preganglionic parasympathetic neurons that innervate the *detrusor* muscle and (2) inhibitory interneurons that contact the motoneurons that innervate the external urethral sphincter. The effect of pontine micturition center activity is (1) detrusor contraction and (2) external urethral sphincter relaxation. This allows urine to flow out of the bladder (Fig. 27-5A, B). It should be noted that although the preganglionic parasympathetic neurons may be influenced by descending inputs, the detrusor muscle cannot be controlled voluntarily. Thus, the voluntary control over voiding occurs at the level of the external urethral sphincter muscle.

Since micturition requires a start signal from the pons reaches sacral cord, the vast majority of spinal cord injuries impair micturition. Whenever the connection from the pontine micturition center to the sacral cord is cut, a disordered activation of both the detrusor *and* the external urethral sphincter results (Fig. 27-5C). Essentially, the entire reflex changes, so that, upon filling, increases in bladder afferent input result in excitation of both the detrusor and the external urethral sphincter. Although leakage may occur under these circumstances, normal micturition does not. This is termed *bladder–sphincter dyssynergia* and represents a significant problem for spinal cord injured patients.

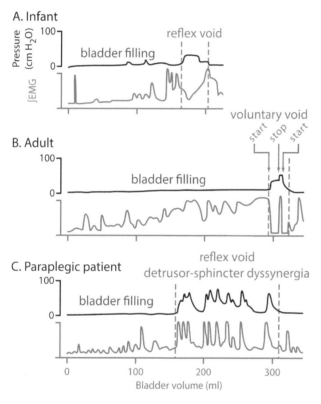

Figure 27-5 Three different patterns of human micturition are shown. The top trace in each panel shows the pressure within the bladder that is exerted on the detrusor muscle (which forms the wall of the bladder). The bottom trace is an electromyograph (EMG) trace from the external urethral sphincter. A: Infants do not have forebrain control over voiding. They void purely by reflex. Thus, when the detrusor pressure reaches a threshold level, the infant voids. Note that the infant does not fully relax the sphincter during voiding. B: Healthy adults void under voluntary control. Moreover, adults can start and stop a void by voluntarily relaxing and contracting the external urethral sphincter. Thus, as the bladder fills, activity in the urethral sphincter increases until the subject willfully relaxes it (*start*), thereby initiating a void. C: In a patient with spinal cord injury, the detrusor and the external urethral sphincter are contracted simultaneously. The result is that the bladder pressure is increased but the outflow is blocked. This phenomenon is termed *detrusor sphincter dyssynergia* and requires medical intervention.   Adapted from Fowler CJ, Griffiths D, de Groat WC. The neural control of micturition. *Nature Rev Neurosci* 9: 453–466, 2008, with permission of the publisher, Macmillan Publishers Ltd.

THE ENTERIC NERVOUS SYSTEM IS A LITTLE NERVOUS SYSTEM UNTO ITSELF

The *enteric nervous system* comprises roughly 200–600 million neurons located in the lining of the gut. It is influenced and in turn influences CNS function. This remarkable nervous system within the gut is able to generate the gut motility and secretions needed for digestion. The enteric nervous system is able to function nearly independently because it consists of sensory neurons, motor neurons, and interneurons. This is in stark contrast to the sympathetic and parasympathetic divisions of the autonomic nervous system, which only consist of preganglionic and postganglionic motor neurons.

The neurons and glia of the enteric nervous system are grouped into thousands of small ganglia distributed along the length of the gastrointestinal tract, an arrangement reminiscent of invertebrate neural nets. Most neurons are odd looking by CNS standards and have appearances more like invertebrate neurons than central vertebrate neurons. For instance, although some enteric cells have a prominent axon, others have processes that resemble invertebrate processes in that they are neither axons nor dendrites.

A prominent feature of the enteric nervous system is the multitude and diversity of neurotransmitters including acetylcholine, γ-aminobutyric acid (GABA), and serotonin. In addition, there are a multitude of peptides, many of which were first identified in the gut before eventually being found in the brain. Enteric neuropeptides include cholecystokinin, vasoactive intestinal peptide, neurotensin, bombesin, galanin, and substance P, all of which are also present in the brain.

One population of enteric cells, the enterochromaffin cells, contains more than 95% of the serotonin found in the body! When excited by intraluminal pressure, enterochromaffin cells secrete serotonin, which then initiates peristalsis. Because of the involvement of serotonin in the control of peristalsis, it is not surprising that *selective serotonin reuptake inhibitors* (*SSRIs*) have effects on gastric motility (see Chapter 12). At low doses or early in therapy, SSRIs augment serotonergic transmission, resulting in increased peristalsis and diarrhea. At higher doses or later in the therapy with SSRIs, there is a desensitization of serotonin receptors. As a result, constipation may occur.

The enteric nervous system allows the gut to function largely independently of the CNS. There are two major locations of enteric neurons:

- *Auerbach's* or *myenteric plexus*: These cells sit between the outer layer of longitudinal muscles and the middle layer of circular muscles and are present throughout the gastrointestinal tract from the esophagus to the internal anal sphincter.

- *Meissner's* or *submucosal plexus*: These cells sit between the middle layer of circular muscles and the inner mucosa and are present only in the small and large intestines.

As may be obvious from their different locations, these two plexi have different functions. The myenteric plexus controls gut motility, and the submucosal plexus controls secretions into the lumen of the gut.

Connections between the CNS and the enteric nervous system are bidirectional. Anatomically, axons bringing information from the gut to the CNS outnumber axons taking information from the CNS to the gut by 10:1. Information *from* the gut is used to sense distension, satiety, nausea, and so on. Although relatively few in number, connections from the CNS to the gut can exert powerful control over the enteric nervous system, altering gut function in accordance with changing emotional states. The vagus nerve innervates and has the greatest influence on movements of the esophagus and stomach and little influence over intestinal and colonic motility. Sympathetic nerves innervate the lower gastrointestinal tract and influence both motility and secretion.

There is a range of patterns of gut motility. The most common is peristalsis, the propulsive movement of lumen contents toward the anus that is associated with normal digestion. Other motility patterns include mixing, the peristaltic rush that rapidly propels noxious contents toward the anus, and the backward peristalsis that accompanies vomiting. The interstitial cell of Cajal is a *pacemaker cell*, meaning that it fires rhythmically on its own. It is the rhythmic discharge of the interstitial cell of Cajal that largely drives gut peristalsis. In the absence of enteric cells, the gut is hypomotile.

The most common disorder of the enteric nervous system is *Hirschsprung disease*, also termed *megacolon* or *congenital aganglionic megacolon*. Hirschsprung disease results when neural crest cells fail to migrate into the distal colon. The severity of the disease varies, but it can be serious and demanding of immediate surgical intervention. The severity of the disease is dependent on how much of the colon is *aganglionic*, meaning lacking collections of enteric neurons. Newborns with this problem present with constipation and are typically treated surgically. The normal part of the colon is pulled down and sewed over the aganglionic portion. In many cases, this procedure resolves the problem. In others, careful dietary management is needed for life.

Secretory reflexes of the enteric nervous system are responsible for returning about 9 liters—more than 2 gallons—of water to the lumen of the gastrointestinal tract each day. The sympathetic nervous system can influence the amount of water secreted. This is one pathway through which emotion, via an effect on sympathetic outflow, plays out in the motility of our guts, a common experience.

SLEEP IS CLEARLY A BIOLOGICAL NECESSITY, EVEN IF WE DO NOT UNDERSTAND ITS FUNCTION

Sleep can be characterized as a reversible state of decreased mobility and decreased sensitivity to external stimulation. It is an innate behavior that neither requires nor benefits from learning. Sleepiness is rampant and is a factor in roughly one fifth of all vehicular crashes that occur in the United States, an impact that is on a par with the effect of alcohol intoxication. Drowsiness also negatively impacts work performance and productivity, increasing for example, the number of medical errors.

Recently, Jerome Siegel and his colleagues studied three preindustrial groups of people and reported two particularly interesting findings. First, the people studied slept for an average of just under 6 and 7 hours per night. This suggests that the fashionably prescribed 8 hours of sleep may not be a magical number or goal. Second, the timing of the sleep was tightly tied to ambient temperature. Sleep began when ambient temperature fell, roughly 3 hours after sunset. Waking occurred during an active vasoconstriction that coincided with the lowest temperature of the morning. These results suggest that sleep is timed to temperature changes that modern life has largely evened out. Hopefully, these data can be used to improve sleep among people living in industrialized conditions.

Depriving an animal or person from sleeping by keeping them awake increases the pressure to sleep, often termed *sleep drive*. Extended *sleep deprivation* has serious adverse consequences, including death if prolonged long enough. The finding that animals throughout phylogeny from flies to fish to mammals exhibit a sleep-like state, show evidence of sleep drive, and are adversely affected by sleep deprivation leads to the conclusion that *sleep is a necessary process*. This firm conclusion is unaffected by continued controversy over the purpose of sleep that is so universal across animals.

THE SLEEP–WAKE CYCLE IS SYNCHRONIZED TO THE CIRCADIAN RHYTHM

Given that we need to sleep and that sleep is a vulnerable state, the most adaptive organization of sleep and wake would be to consolidate sleep during periods when food availability is lowest and to be most refreshed, awake, and active when food and mates are obtainable. Indeed, the normative pattern for adult humans is to sleep in a single bout during the night. Recall from Chapter 15 that neurons in the *suprachiasmatic nucleus* receive information about light levels from intrinsically photosensitive retinal ganglion cells and behave like an internal clock. In the absence of any light cues, we keep a diurnal rhythm of greater than 24 hours. Damage to the suprachiasmatic nucleus abolishes this internal clock.

Connections from the suprachiasmatic nucleus to sleep-regulating regions of the hypothalamus entrain sleep–wake cycles to light–dark cycles. At night, the lack of light leads, via the suprachiasmatic nucleus, to the release of *melatonin* from the *pineal gland*. Because the circadian facilitation of wakefulness is entrained by light stimulation, repeated exposure to light during the evening will delay the melatonin increase and prolong the influence of the circadian facilitation of wakefulness. Thus, sleepiness is postponed. This has recently become an issue as people increasingly read from back-lit electronic devices while in bed and trying to fall asleep.

Because the circadian rhythm is entrained almost entirely by light in people, totally blind people with no light sensitivity cannot entrain to the day–night cycle of the Earth. Instead, blind people "free run," with a period of more than 24 hours so that their subjective nighttime shifts forward in time. Accordingly, the blind often have difficulty sleeping. Fortunately, nightly treatment with *melatonin*, a hormone critical to circadian entrainment, has been efficacious in improving sleep among the blind.

The interaction between sleep drive and circadian rhythm controls the sleep–wake cycle. The idea is that sleep drive builds during the day and dissipates during a night spent sleeping. Opposing the sleep drive is a circadian facilitation of wakefulness during the daytime hours. A simple, probably familiar, example can illustrate the way in which the opposing processes interact. After spending all night writing a paper or studying for an exam, morning arrives. Because the night before was not spent sleeping, the sleep drive is strong. Yet the sleep drive is mitigated by the circadian drive to be awake in morning time. Of course, the outcome of these dueling physiological processes varies across individuals, age, and context.

ADULT HUMAN SLEEP CONSISTS OF TWO FUNDAMENTALLY DIFFERENT STATES

Humans and most other mammals exhibit two very different types of sleep: REM sleep, also called *paradoxical sleep* or *active sleep*, and non-REM sleep, also called *slow-wave sleep*. Because sleep states are difficult to judge by behavioral observations alone, the differences between non-REM and REM sleep are determined and described in electrophysiological terms by the amount of activity in neurons of the cerebral cortex, postural muscles, and extraocular muscles.

The *electroencephalogram* (*EEG*) measures *synchronized* activity in the cerebral cortex. As cells fire more and more synchronously, the EEG grows in amplitude. During non-REM sleep, cortical neurons are synchronously active so that the EEG shows slow rhythmic oscillations at a rate of about 1–4 Hz; these oscillations are termed δ waves. When the cerebral cortex shows δ waves, it is unresponsive to outside stimulation. Because many neurons are all firing at the same time during non-REM sleep, EEG recordings have a characteristic *high-amplitude, low-frequency* appearance.

During wakefulness, neurons respond to outside stimuli and fire asynchronously. This results in a distributed pattern of activity and a low-amplitude EEG. During REM sleep, most regions of cortex look "awake." However, the hippocampus is different from other areas of cortex because it shows synchronized activity that appears as 4–8 Hz θ waves. Some postulate that hippocampal θ waves play a role in memory consolidation during sleep, but this intriguing idea remains controversial.

During sleep, there is a paucity of voluntary movements. Humans usually sleep in a recumbent position, and the lack of activity in physiological extensors is particularly accentuated during sleep. During non-REM sleep, there is some, but certainly a minimal amount, of muscle activity. The amount of muscle activity, revealed by electromyograph (EMG) recordings, decreases across time as sleep deepens. During REM sleep, the EMG becomes virtually flat, reflecting atonia, a total lack of muscle activity. Associated with this atonia is a profound hyperpolarization of motoneurons that greatly increases the threshold needed to activate these neurons. Interspersed within the period of atonia are brief muscle twitches that differ dramatically from organized voluntary movements. REM sleep is, as its name suggests, characterized by rapid eye movements that can be measured with an electrooculogram (EOG) that measures extraocular muscle activity. Rapid eye movements are associated with the occurrence of *dreaming*, although dreaming also can occur during non-REM sleep. The concurrence of most dreaming with atonia during REM sleep prevents us from acting out our dreams (see Box 27-2).

The sleep drive exerts independent pressures for non-REM and for REM sleep. This means that a lack of non-REM sleep from a lost night's sleep will trigger a demand for a compensatory increase in non-REM sleep. Similarly, a lack of REM sleep, even if the full complement of non-REM sleep was obtained, leads to additional REM sleep during the next sleep period.

Box 27-2 **IN RAPID EYE MOVEMENT (REM) SLEEP BEHAVIOR DISORDER, ATONIA DOES NOT OCCUR**

Rapid eye movement sleep behavior disorder is a bizarre condition characterized by the absence of muscle atonia during REM and the consequent acting out of dreams. Patients are typically middle-aged or older men. During REM sleep, they make loud and angry vocalizations that are usually quite distinct from their waking demeanor. Since patients kick, punch, and flail about, a common problem is injury to a sleeping partner. The dreams that patients act out are almost universally antagonistic, with the patient typically on the receiving end of an attack. Note that REM sleep behavior disorder is entirely distinct from *sleepwalking*. Sleepwalking is a relatively benign condition that occurs during non-REM sleep.

The atonia during REM is produced by brainstem networks. Neurons in the hindbrain reticular formation inhibit motoneurons to produce atonia. In REM sleep behavior disorder, these neurons are not activated and consequently do not inhibit motoneurons to produce atonia. REM sleep behavior disorder shares significant comorbidity with Parkinson's disease and several other neurodegenerative diseases, suggesting that it may be an early sign of neurodegeneration.

Many brain regions participate in various aspects of sleep–wake regulation. The hypothalamus is a key area, and damage to the hypothalamus can produce either a fatal *insomnia* or a state of continuous sleep, termed *somnolence*. Neurons in the posterior hypothalamus, basal forebrain, and histaminergic *tuberomammillary nucleus* all promote wakefulness. Conversely, activity in neurons within the ventral lateral preoptic nucleus of the anterior hypothalamus leads to sleep, in part by inhibition of the regions that promote wakefulness. The brain region or regions that mediate sleep drive remain unclear. Yet widespread cortical excitation, as occurs in response to stimulants such as caffeine or amphetamine, dampens the sleep drive. Conversely, widespread cortical inhibition, as occurs in response to hypnotics such as benzodiazepines, facilitates the sleep drive.

SLEEP STATES OCCUR IN A PREDICTABLE SEQUENCE

Sleep follows a stereotypical pattern, which is termed *sleep architecture*. Sleep begins with light stages of non-REM sleep that progress into stages of increasing EEG synchrony. *REM sleep is only entered into from non-REM sleep* in the healthy individual (see Box 27-3). A normal night of sleep involves four to six cycles of non-REM sleep to REM sleep. In each succeeding cycle, non-REM sleep becomes progressively more synchronous and then switches into REM sleep for 5–10 minutes. Within a single night's sleep, there is more EEG synchrony during the initial few hours and far less by morning. This gradual reduction in EEG synchrony and amplitude from the evening to the morning is associated with a decrease in sleep drive.

Insomnia is among the most common and also heterogeneous health-related complaints. Individuals with insomnia may have difficulty initiating sleep, staying asleep, or may have unsatisfying sleep. Unsatisfying sleep is usually associated with less EEG synchronization than normal and a multitude of arousals each night.

Associated with different sleep stages are consistent changes in homeostasis. For example, gastric motility increases during sleep. There is a decrease in the temperature set point during non-REM sleep, and thermoregulation is turned off during REM sleep. Luckily, we do not spend much time in REM sleep, and so body temperature is in free-fall for a minimum of time. There are also consistent changes in cardiovascular function and breathing. During sleep, certain behaviors, such as voiding, are not supposed to happen. Many patients experience the failure of a homeostatic process during nighttime sleep before any daytime

Narcolepsy is a sleep disorder characterized by daytime *sleep attacks* that involve a transition from wakefulness to REM sleep, a transition that is not observed in healthy individuals. The cardinal features of narcolepsy are extreme daytime sleepiness and sleep attacks during the day. Sleep attacks are accompanied by a loss of muscle tone, termed *cataplexy*, which can cause injury to the patient. Fragmented sleep at night and hallucinations upon falling asleep or waking from sleep are frequent symptoms. In addition, atonia, which normally only accompanies REM sleep, can occur upon falling into non-REM sleep or when waking from sleep. This produces a frightening sensation of being aware, in a drowsy kind of way, but unable to move.

Insight into the circuits governing wakefulness, REM sleep, and atonia derive from the identification of mutations that cause narcolepsy in dogs. The mutations identified are in a receptor for a neuropeptide, *orexin*, which is at higher levels during wakefulness than during sleep. Although mutations in the gene responsible for narcolepsy in dogs are not found in humans with narcolepsy, the pathophysiology appears related since humans with narcolepsy have low levels of orexin and a loss of hypothalamic neurons containing orexin. Thus, a deficiency in orexin signaling appears to be a common cause of narcolepsy in dogs and humans. Human narcolepsy may be an autoimmune disorder because it is far more prevalent in people with a particular histocompatability profile. Treatment is aimed at reducing daytime sleepiness and preventing cataplexy.

symptoms appear. For example, people with urinary incontinence due to a stroke often have nighttime enuresis long before losing control over voiding during the daytime.

By entraining sleep–wake cycles to the entirely predictable circadian rhythm, changes in homeostatic physiology can be made in *anticipation* of waking. Reliably, before we wake up, core temperature, sympathetic nerve activity, and cortisol release increase while gut motility decreases. These changes in physiology enable us to perform voluntary actions, perceive the world, and be cognitively alert. What more could one ask for?

THE INSIGHTFUL AND INSPIRED OBSERVATIONS OF A PHYSICIAN LED TO OUR MODERN UNDERSTANDING OF SLEEP AND WAKE REGULATION

Long before the modern interest in sleep, before EEG recordings or the discovery of REM sleep, Constantin von

Economo had the revolutionary idea to search for the neuroanatomical locus of sleep. Von Economo was a Romanian of Greek descent who practiced psychiatry and neurology in the early 20th century. In 1916, he saw 13 patients whose symptoms did not fit into any known disease at the time. Nor were the complaints of these patients uniform. One group of patients slept too much and exhibited ptosis, another group could not sleep, and the third group did not move.

From carefully examining a modest number of patients, von Economo described three forms of *encephalitis lethargica*: (1) an ophthalmoplegic form associated with hypersomnolence, (2) a hyperkinetic form associated with insomnia, and (3) an akinetic form that we now term *postencephalitic parkinsonism*. Von Economo did not stop at simply describing three clinical syndromes. He carefully studied the brains of patients. By combining his pathological observations with his meticulous clinical analysis, von Economo was able to postulate: (1) a sleep region in the anterior hypothalamus and (2) a waking region at the midbrain-diencephalic border. Damage to the latter area would produce somnolence and oculomotor deficits due to involvement of rostral portions of the oculomotor complex. Lesion of the former area would produce insomnia. As an aside, von Economo even linked the akinetic form of encephalitis lethargic to damage in the substantia nigra.

Remarkably, von Economo's insights have largely been borne out by modern research. It should be noted that encephalitis lethargica has disappeared since von Economo's time. Thus, long after the disease that occupied so much of his career has vanished, von Economo lives on because of his remarkable contributions to our understanding of the biological basis of sleep and wake.

The story of von Economo and encephalitis lethargica is intended to demonstrate the importance of the inquisitive physician to the advancement of our understanding of the brain. Each patient represents a unique combination of history, physiology, genetics, and anatomy asking for help and offering up individual traits to the physician to use as tools. The alert and curious physician holds the potential to help patients while also advancing medicine, and indeed biology, forward just as von Economo did.

ADDITIONAL READING

Bianchi AL, Gestreau C. New perspectives on the brainstem respiratory network: An overview of a half century of research. *Resp Physiol Neurobiol.* 168: 4–12, 2009.

Boeve BF. REM sleep behavior disorder. Updated review of the core features, the REM sleep behavior disorder-neurodegenerative disease association, evolving concepts, controversies, and future directions. *Ann NY Acad Sci.* 1184: 15–54, 2009.

Carroll MS, Patwari PP, Weese-Mayer DE. Carbon dioxide chemoreception and hypoventilation syndromes with autonomic dysregulation. *J Appl Physiol.* 109: 978–988, 2010.

Institute of Medicine (US) Committee on Sleep Medicine and Research (Colten HR, Altevogt BM, eds.). *Sleep Disorders and Sleep Deprivation: An Unmet Public Health Problem.* Washington, DC: National Academies Press (US), 2006.

Dauvilliers Y, Arnulf I, Mignot E. Narcolepsy with cataplexy. *Lancet.* 10: 499–511, 2007.

Feldman JL, Del Negro CA. Looking for inspiration: New perspectives on respiratory rhythm. *Nat Rev Neurosci.* 7: 232–242, 2006.

Fowler CJ, Griffiths D, de Groat WC. The neural control of micturition. *Nat Rev Neurosci.* 9: 453–466, 2008.

Freedman RR, Norton D, Woodward S, Cornelissen G. Core body temperature and circadian rhythm of hot flashes in menopausal women. *J Clin Endocrinol Metab.* 80: 2354–2358, 1995.

Fuller PM, Gooley JJ, Saper CB. Neurobiology of the sleep-wake cycle: Sleep architecture, circadian rhythms and regulatory feedback. *J Biol Rhythms.* 21: 482–493, 2006.

Furness JB. *The Enteric Nervous System.* Malden, MA: Blackwell Publishing, 2006.

Guyenet PG. The sympathetic control of blood pressure. *Nat Rev Neurosci.* 7: 335–346, 2006.

Holstege G. The emotional motor system and micturition control. *Neurourol Urodynamics.* 29: 42–48, 2010.

Kellogg DL Jr. In vivo mechanisms of cutaneous vasodilation and vasoconstriction during thermoregulatory challenges. *J Appl Physiol.* 100: 1709–1718, 2006.

Max DT. *The Family that Couldn't Sleep: A Medical Mystery.* New York: Random House, 2006.

Romanovsky AA, Ivanov AI, Shimansky YP. Selected contribution: Ambient temperature for experiments in rats: A new method for determining the zone of thermal neutrality. *J Appl Physiol.* 92: 2667–2679, 2002.

Simon E. Temperature regulation: The spinal cord as a site of extra-hypothalamic thermoregulatory functions. *Rev Physiol Biochem Pharmacol.* 71: 1–76, 1974.

Skene DJ, Arendt J. Circadian rhythm sleep disorders in the blind and their treatment with melatonin. *Sleep Med.* 8: 651–655, 2007.

Tataryn IV, Lomax P, Bajorek JG, Chesarek W, Meldrum DR, Judd HL. Postmenopausal hot flushes: A disorder of thermoregulation. *Maturitas.* 2: 101–107, 1980.

Teigen KH. Is a sigh "just a sigh"? Sighs as emotional signals and responses to a difficult task. *Scand J Psychol.* 49: 49–57, 2008.

Triarhou LC. The signalling contributions of Constantin von Economo to basic, clinical and evolutionary neuroscience. *Brain Res Bull.* 69: 223–243, 2006.

Triarhou LC. The percipient observations of Constantin von Economo on encephalitis lethargic and sleep disruption and their lasting impact on contemporary sleep research. *Brain Res Bull.* 69: 244–258, 2006.

Weese-Mayer DE, Berry-Kravis EM, Zhou L. Adult identified with congenital central hypoventilation syndrome—mutation in *PHOX2b* gene and late-onset CHS. *Resp Crit Care Med.* 171: 88, 2005.

Yetish G, Kaplan H, Gurven M, et al. Natural sleep and its seasonal variations in three pre-industrial societies. *Curr Biol.* 25: 2862–288, 2015.

Zajicek G. Wisdom of the body. *Med Hypotheses.* 52: 447–449, 1999.

SECTION 7

YOU AND THE BRAIN

If you are actually reading this chapter, you have worked hard and engaged with the nervous system. You have read, thought, and talked about the nervous system. Conversations about "myasthenia gravis," "sodium channel inactivation," "outer hair cells," and a myriad of other topics are now understandable to you. For those of you who began reading this book knowing nothing about the nervous system, I recognize how much you have learned, and I hope you do, too. And for those of you who knew quite a bit before reading a page, my hope is that you have deepened both your knowledge and interest. You all deserve congratulations for your respective accomplishments. In the first part of this final chapter, we revisit what you have learned. Later, we imagine how you may be able to expand our collective understanding of the nervous system in your future careers as physicians.

In this chapter, we also consider the difference between disease and illness. As Sherwin Nuland said, "There's a big difference between what we call 'disease' and what we call 'illness'. A disease is a pathological entity; an illness is the effect of the disease on the patient's entire way of life." You deserve to celebrate your mastery of the basis for neurological disease gained from this book. Yet individuals seek medical care within the context of a disease's meaning to their own lives. Using detailed knowledge of disease to treat illness is the challenge and promise of medicine.

28.

THE BRAIN IN A PHYSICIAN'S LIFE

YOU HAVE LEARNED A GREAT DEAL

We started this course by considering the simultaneously tragic and uplifting story of Jean-Dominique Bauby. With your acquired knowledge of neuroanatomy, you can now reconstruct Bauby's lesion. What Bauby tells us in his book is that he had a pontine lesion. Indeed, a pontine stroke is the typical cause of the locked-in syndrome.

How does a pontine stroke explain Bauby's symptoms? Bauby's most striking symptom was the inability to willfully move or speak. This stems from a lesion of the corticospinal and corticobulbar tracts traveling through the basis pontis. Bauby also became deaf in his left ear as a result of his stroke. The only central lesion with that effect is one that knocks out the cochlear nuclei on one side. Bauby also suffered from paresthesia of his body and face, a positive sign indicating a lesion of the ascending sensory tracts bilaterally. The stroke must have damaged portions of the midbrain, too, to explain Bauby's nearly total ophthalmoplegia and right-sided blown pupil.

Bauby also suffered from hyperacusis, likely the result of facial nucleus damage. It is striking that Bauby "writes" more about hyperacusis than he complains that he cannot walk. Hyperacusis *demands* Bauby's attention. Bauby's inability to walk is a constant that fades into the background and about which he writes little that is specific. Bauby's describes hyperacusis as, "My left ear amplifies and distorts all sounds farther than ten feet away. When a plane tows an ad for the local theme park over the beach, I could swear that a coffee mill has been grafted onto my eardrum . . . [even] more disturbing is the continuous racket that assails me from the corridor whenever they forget to shut my door . . . [sending] out an auditory foretaste of hell."

It is also important to consider what is working well in Bauby. Bauby does not write of deficits in olfaction, vision, sleep, circadian rhythm, memory, language, thought, or executive function. He certainly demonstrates a remarkable consideration for others, exhibiting immense concern for the minor inconveniences of others. He appears to have retained his personality, replete with a wry sense of humor.

At one point, he requests a particular sweater, remarking, "If I must drool, I may as well drool on cashmere."

The abstract functions of thought, executive function, language (albeit through the unusual outlet of a blinking eyelid), and memory all appear unaffected in Bauby. What about the final telencephalic output of emotion or affect? How did Bauby experience emotions after his stroke? Bauby certainly had the forebrain circuits needed for affect and motivation—cingulate, insular, and prefrontal cortices, amygdala, and hypothalamus. But when Bauby felt sad and produced tears, he could not sob or lean his head upon another. He could not gasp when shocked, laugh when amused, or smile contentedly when seeing a loved one. He was thus unable to match his skeletomotor and autonomic output to his forebrain-generated feeling. How did this alter his emotional experience?

Bauby's blunted body experience comes across in the emotional content of his book. In reminisces about the past, he wrote, "My old life still burns within me but more and more of it is reduced to the ashes of memory." He narrates the day and immediate aftermath of his stroke with a palpable lack of immediacy in his emotional reactions. He reports that, on his first trip back to Paris from the rehabilitation hospital in the south of France where he stayed, his "emotions got the better of me" but 4 months later, on another such trip, he "was unmoved by it." At times, a reader feels more because of the facts of his case than because he writes of dismay and despair. In other words, we feel more as we—inevitably—place ourselves in Bauby's position than we do from the emotional immediacy of his words.

The idea that the sensory feelings of the body contribute to our full expression and experience of emotion is a concept that was promulgated by the great American psychologist, William James, who wrote, "we feel sorry because we cry, angry because we strike, afraid because we tremble. . . . Without the bodily states following on the perception, the latter would be purely cognitive in form, pale, colorless, destitute of emotional warmth." In the popular abbreviation of this idea, we see a bear, we run and therefore feel fear, rather than we see a bear, feel fear, and then run. Since Bauby was unable to move and had very little forebrain access to his autonomic system, his bodily sensations were reduced. A Jamesian prediction would be that, as a result, Bauby's emotional experiences would be blunted.

However, that may not be the case. Myriam White-Le Goff, an expert of medieval literature and native French speaker, analyzed the emotional content of Bauby's book. She concludes that rather than not feeling full emotions, Bauby felt more emotion than his imprisoned body was able to tolerate. His diving bell-existence placed him perpetually in the realm of feeling too much. His ability to express himself could not match the depth of his feelings. Moreover, Bauby felt a profound need to express his emotions as he wrote, "As much as I need breathing, I need to be moved, to love and to admire. The letter from a friend, a Balthus painting on a postcard, a page of Saint-Simon gives meaning to the passing hours. But to stay on the alert and not to sink into a warm resignation, *I keep a dose of fury, hatred, neither too much nor too little, just as the pressure cooker has a safety valve that keeps it from exploding* [emphasis added]." The inability to emote and show affect was so overwhelming that Bauby was forced to distance himself from his emotions. Thus, Bauby's emotions were deeply felt but simultaneously battled against.

When Bauby was successful at keeping his emotions in check, he viewed himself from a detached perspective with a sense of "gallows humor." For example, he wrote, "Not only was I exiled, paralyzed, mute, half deaf, deprived of all pleasures and reduced to the existence of a jellyfish, but I was also horrible to see. I was taken by nervous laughter . . . [and] decided to treat it as a joke." At times, Bauby simply was not capable of distancing himself, and he chose a version of silence by abruptly ending a story or a chapter, leaving the reader to imagine the indescribable.

In the end, Bauby shows us that embodying emotion not only facilitates our feelings but also dissipates them. Without the safety valve of bodily expression, affect can overwhelm. In a healthy individual, the body works as the brain's able partner to both facilitate and dissipate emotion, enabling a rich life.

BRAIN DAMAGE AND DISEASE PRODUCE HIGHLY PERSONAL EFFECTS

Clive Wearing, an accomplished music conductor who suffered from encephalitis presents a complementary clinical picture to that of Bauby. After a long recovery from the acute illness, Wearing is able to walk, conduct choral groups, read and play music, to breathe, listen to music, void, and stand up without feeling light-headed. Yet, he has one enduring and devastating deficit—memory. He has no ability to form new explicit memories. Every moment, he feels that he is awakening for the first time. The following transcript of one of many nearly identical conversations between Mr. Wearing and his wife Deborah dramatically reveals the enormity of Mr Wearing's deficit:

Clive Wearing (CW) asks Deborah Wearing (DW), "How long have I been ill?"

DW: Nine weeks.

CW: Nine weeks? I haven't heard anything, seen anything, touched anything, smelled anything. It's like being dead. What's it like being dead? Answer: Nobody knows. How long's it been?

DW: Nine weeks.

CW: Nine weeks? [He shakes his head] I haven't heard anything, seen anything, touched anything, smelled anything. It's like one long night lasting . . . how long?

DW: Nine weeks.

CW: Nine weeks? . . . One long night lasting . . . how long?

DW: Nine weeks.

CW: Nine weeks? I haven't heard anything, seen anything, touched anything, smelled anything. It's just like being dead. What's it like being dead? Answer: Nobody knows. How long's it been? I haven't heard anything, seen anything, felt anything, smelled anything, touched anything. It's been one long night lasting . . . how long?

The pathos of Wearing's condition is evident to us, and it is clearly evident to Wearing. When pressed to consider the inconsistencies in his belief of repeatedly waking anew—the fact that the diary is filled with entries, in his own handwriting, documenting previous awakenings—he *rages*. You can see this in numerous videos available on the Internet. Wearing's life is devastated, and he knows it fully, albeit *implicitly*.

Clive Wearing's and Jean-Dominique Bauby's conditions are dramatically different and together encompass only the tiniest proportion of possible neural dysfunctions. The lesson to derive from their disparate stories is not a general principle about brain function or specific information about two rare clinical conditions, but rather the idea that *the impact of brain dysfunction is particularly poignant when it attacks our essence, who we are to ourselves*. People with cancer, heart disease, or diabetes may suffer both physically and psychologically with reduced quality of life and the knowledge of a fast-approaching end, but their sense of self does not fundamentally change. After Bauby's brain stopped functioning correctly, he felt that he "faded away." When pressed to acknowledge that he has a problem with memory, Wearing asserts that he is missing consciousness, "I wasn't conscious, I have no knowledge of it at all! Consciousness has to involve ME!!" Wearing was devastated, unable to function, unable to think, unable to stitch together two moments in his life.

THE MEANING OF DISEASE DIFFERS ACROSS INDIVIDUALS

Patients' interpretations of disease are not homogenous. One disease does not elicit a uniform reaction in all individuals and no one person's singular experience is predictable. Instead, patients' reactions to disease are filtered through their personality, temperament, past experiences, current life circumstances, and social resources; sometimes with surprising results. For example, JR was a man in his seventies who had just been diagnosed with Parkinson's disease. When asked to rate his disease on a scale of one, a curse, to ten, a growth experience; JR rated his Parkinson's disease as an eight or nine. He explained, "My first reaction to the diagnosis was one of relief. I knew what I was dealing with. . . . My PD has brought [my spouse] and me closer together . . . [and] has also rendered me more sympathetic to the trials and tribulations of others. . . . Upon reflection, I think that my PD has made me a better person with respect to my own self and to others about me."

JR is not unique in realizing growth from disease or injury. Lauren Scruggs, a young woman who lost her left hand and eye to a plane propeller exemplifies the difficulty of imagining another individual's reaction to disease or injury. She told *People* magazine, "My accident was bad, but I think it's deepened me as a person and increased my compassion for people and intensified my joy. It's kind of weird to say but I wouldn't trade it. I have seen it as a miracle. I've been through a lot but I'm living." Similarly, upon looking back on a stroke that occurred in her fifties, AH calls it her "stroke of luck." After the stroke, AH reunited with her husband and began to write poetry, finding deep satisfaction and joy from her renewed relationship and fulfilling mode of artistic expression.

Not all patients interpret their diseases with the equanimity of JR, Ms. Scruggs, or AH. A roughly 40-year-old neuroscience professor with Parkinson's disease has a different perspective, writing, "I am living in the P closet.

I'm not really sure why . . . I am unclear what the shame or need to hide is all about." Of a past experience with crippling obsessive-compulsive disease at the age of 13, one individual wrote, "It stole my life. It ruled what I could do, where I could go—no, it ruled what I couldn't do, where I couldn't go. It paralyzes and while I was alive inside I was locked up, locked away. . . . I am shriveling as I type this, the memory of mental anguish that tortured 24/7."

For the physician, two take-home messages from these stories stand out. First, a diagnosis, even when not accompanied by a cure, effective treatment, or positive prognosis, has a powerfully positive effect on patients. A diagnosis represents valuable information upon which to base future choices. It tells a patient that she or he is not imagining symptoms; that the patient is not "crazy." Prognosis provides a roadmap to future possibilities, greatly lessening the surprises in store for the patient.

The second take-home message is that two individuals can react to the same condition in vastly different ways.

THE IMPACT OF ILLNESS ON OTHERS

As John Dunne said, "no man is an island." William James considered that "*a man's Self is the sum total of all that he CAN call his,* not only his body and his psychic powers, but his clothes and his house, his wife and children, his ancestors and friends, his reputation and works, his lands and horses, and yacht and bank-account" [emphasis in original]. This formulation of "self" draws from the common experience of individuals reacting to the fortunes of their loved ones as they would if the same fortune or misfortune befell one's self. A mother's joy at her child's happiness and a woman's dismay at her friend's illness are examples of the extended self in action.

The extension of the self toward pets holds particular power, as shown by the ameliorative effect of pets on wellbeing and the unwillingness to leave beloved pets behind during times of imminent danger. The relationship between humans and their pets appears to be of comparable strength to the relationship between individual humans. When the disastrous Hurricane Katrina struck New Orleans, most people who failed to evacuate made that choice in part to stay with animals for whom shelters made no accommodation at the time. As a consequence of these experiences, a new law was passed that authorized the US Federal Emergency Management Agency (FEMA) to spend public monies to rescue and accommodate pets during federal emergencies. Both pet ownership and visits from humans with stranger dogs increase social interaction, elevate mood, and buffer the response to stressors. Although no causal relationship has been established, people with pets make fewer visits to physicians and enjoy generally better health, as evidenced by lower cholesterol levels and the like than do people without pets.

The social context within which we live affects illness and health care in a number of ways. Those of you, likely the majority, who will go into internal medicine or oncology will see in great and tragic detail how mood and affect can impact outcome. Of two patients who come to you with similar physical findings, we know that the one who is happy and engaged in life will fare better than the one who is depressed and unhappy. Strong social ties and support bring better health outcomes than does social isolation. Remarkably, the simple communication that treating a patient's pain is important to a health care provider predicts patient satisfaction with pain management to a comparable extent as does sustained pain relief using pharmacological treatment. In other words, communicating that you care about a patient can be an efficacious treatment.

On a practical level, patients who feel connected with their health care providers are more compliant—they take their physician's advice—and have better health outcomes than patients without such a connection. The challenge to the physician is to express genuine empathic concern toward patients while avoiding personal distress that, if unchecked, leads ultimately to burnout. Effective clinical empathy involves a true understanding of the patient's emotional state. This requires that a physician distinguish how a medical condition has affected *another* (the patient) with enough detachment to recognize that the patient's reaction may be quite distinct from what the physician imagines his or her own emotional state would be given the same disease or medical circumstances. Moreover, empathic concern requires that the empathizer feel at least some degree of the distress of the other. This places physicians who want to employ empathic concern in their practice at great risk for burnout. To prevent burnout and create a sustainable habit of medical empathy requires down-regulation of personal distress on the physician's part.

Finally, one person's illness affects all the people connected to the sick individual. In essence, all the people for whom an ill individual is part of their extended selves are affected by that individual's illness. People with terminal conditions cannot survive disability and dying alone. Families take on the personal and financial costs of caring for patients. In the United States, the average personal cost to care for an Alzheimer's patient during the 5 years preceding death was $287,000. The emotional effects

of a loved one's illness and disability ripple through the circle of extended selves, through friends and family, continuing to have ramifications even past a patient's death (Fig. 28-1).

The involvement of family and friends is particularly poignant in the case of unconsciousness patients. When a patient is not competent to make decisions, family members are asked to make choices about health care. A typical scenario is of a person, young or old, who has suffered trauma, anoxia, or a stroke and suddenly becomes unconscious. Family members must process this highly upsetting and completely unexpected turn of events while simultaneously becoming conversant with complex medical issues. Imagine trying to learn the difference between brain dead, vegetative state, and minimally conscious state with absolutely no medical or even science background. And imagine doing this in the middle of the night after being called to the hospital where you find your parent, spouse, or child—who was fine yesterday—unresponsive and full of "tubes." Then imagine that you must make the decision whether or not to place your loved one on a ventilator. Making such a momentous decision is never easy but in the circumstances that surround brain injury, the decision can be overwhelming.

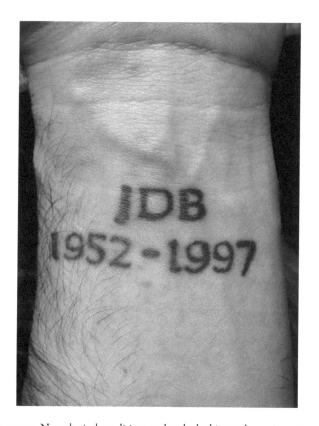

Figure 28-1 Neurological conditions such as locked-in syndrome impact patients, loved ones, and caregivers alike. A tattoo on the arm of Jean-Dominique Bauby's son speaks with quiet eloquence. Photograph is courtesy of Theophile Bauby.

Fewer than 10% of medical students will go into fields directly related to neurobiology—neurology, neurosurgery, and psychiatry. For the rest of you, beyond passing the boards, what are my hopes for what you will take away from this book?

First, I hope you see that neurobiology is all around you. When you go to the gym and watch your own and other's efforts to dissipate body heat—that is neurobiology. When you get up too fast in the middle of the night and feel light-headed, "go vagal"—that is neurobiology. When you deliberately look for a dim light in your peripheral visual field because you know that there are no rods in your fovea—that is neurobiology. When you watch a person over 45 read a restaurant menu at arm's length. Should you ever imbibe a substantial amount of liquor, move your head, and feel the room spin. When you watch a toddler on the move, practicing and practicing locomotion, all of that is neurobiology. When you are at the check-out counter at the grocery store and watch a clerk stop making change to answer a question—that is neurobiology.

This book has not covered every neural function that is important, interesting, or often negatively impacted by disease or trauma. Rather, my goal has been to give you a framework with which to understand nervous function. For instance, you learned how early visual experience is critical to the development of normal visual perception. This will be invaluable to those of you who become pediatricians and ophthalmologists as you see young patients with misaligned eyes.

It is also my hope that you have learned from this book a way to think of neural function and dysfunction and that this will translate into an ability to explain to patients in understandable terms the symptoms they are experiencing and the disease processes from which they suffer. There is not a single one of you who will not encounter at least one patient who presents with pain. Explaining to a patient how pain arises and your strategy for treating the pain will mitigate even a gloomy prognosis. People want to understand what is happening to them. Explaining to a postmenopausal woman how a hot flash works and a few simple strategies to avoid triggering them will make her feel better, even if hormone replacement therapy is contraindicated and she understands that no other method exists for the prevention of hot flashes.

Beyond being doctors to your patients, you are individuals with friends and family, and, in many cases, you may be the only doctor in your social group. I am the lone scientist among my family and friends, and I am called upon to explain all things neurobiological and most things medical. So, I imagine that for many of you, your family and friends will expect you to explain all things medical regardless of your future specialty. This is likely already happening, as the detail that you are still students is as ignored as is the detail that I am a Ph.D. rather than a M.D. Although very few of you will ever see a locked-in person or a case of global amnesia, I would venture to say that all of you will know, or already do know, someone who develops Parkinson's disease, multiple sclerosis, or has a stroke. You will also meet people with diseases that are not primarily neurological but which impact on nervous function: HIV disease, diabetes, and cancer patients on chemotherapy are obvious examples. Whether you encounter people with such diseases personally or in the clinic, you can help them by explaining their illness to them. Even a person with a devastating disease such as amyotrophic lateral sclerosis will feel relief at knowing and understanding that the symptoms he or she is experiencing are the expected ones—in essence, that he or she is not "crazy." Such patients will want to know their prognosis, however dismal, because knowledge translates to a feeling of control.

Finally, I hope that you will use your knowledge of the power and potential of the nervous system to improve your chosen discipline, to further our understanding of a myriad of problems that have traditionally resided in non-neuronal specialties. Let me take a moment here to tell you a story. A patient comes in to a dermatologist with alopecia, meaning loss of hair. She also has reduced cortisol secretion. Two years later, she develops memory problems. A magnetic resonance image (MRI) reveals a gross enlargement of the temporal horn of the lateral ventricle, at the expense of the hippocampus. Another patient with the same three problems comes in. I am not sure when the physicians realized that the alopecia, hypocortisolemia, and amnesia stemmed from one disease process, but they did and published a report describing the two cases and postulating a pathophysiology of an autoimmune attack on a molecule common to hair follicles, corticotrophs, and hippocampus. Put yourself in their position. What would you do? Could you make the connections between dermatology, endocrinology, and neurology? Could you help the patient and deepen our understanding of biology at the same time?

There are also far more common problems to be solved. Individuals who suffer from schizophrenia smoke cigarettes. Does nicotine addiction hold a clue to the pathophysiology of this tragic and baffling disease? Can we stem the tide of myopia, already at epidemic proportions in many communities and bound to get worse as children increasingly stay inside to use hand-held devices? We know that women are flooded with oxytocin after giving birth, allowing them to nurse, and, from animal experiments, we infer that this same hormone facilitates a new mother's bond with her child and family. Does this release fail in women who develop postpartum depression? Can we prevent the damaging effects of chronic activation of airway afferents while still enabling the acute protective functions? There are a myriad of such questions that are waiting for new, innovative thinkers.

I hope that those of you who go into sports medicine will think of motor units and cerebellar circuits and imagine new, brain-friendly ways to improve upon the more traditional treatments of immobilization and rest to treat your patients. Today, in the early years of the 21st century, the most common effective "treatment" for incontinence is clothing, namely diapers. The potential of treating various types of incontinence with therapies directed at the central nervous system has hardly been tapped. The most common treatment for sleep apnea is a mask with positive pressure. Again, this is a peripheral, mechanical treatment that fails to utilize the power of the central nervous system.

So, I leave you with the message, "Go forth and be innovative." The brain is spectacularly powerful. Use yours for good and compassionate care of your patients.

ADDITIONAL READING

Bauby J-D. *The Diving Bell and the Butterfly*. New York: Alfred A. Knopf, 1997.

Beetz A, Uvnäs-Moberg K, Julius H, Kotrschal K. Psychosocial and psychophysiological effects of human-animal interactions: The possible role of oxytocin. *Front Psychol.* 3: 234, 2012.

Dawson R, Spross JA, Jablonski ES, Hoyer DR, Sellers DE, Solomon MZ. Probing the paradox of patients' satisfaction with inadequate pain management. *J Pain Symptom Manage.* 23: 211–220, 2002.

Fins JJ. *Rights Come to Mind*. New York: Cambridge University Press, 2015.

Fox M. Lia Lee dies; Life went on around her, redefining care. *NY Times.* Sept 14, 2012.

Gleichgerrcht E, Decety J. Empathy in clinical practice: How individual dispositions, gender, and experience moderate empathic concern, burnout, and emotional distress in physicians. *PLoS One.* 8: e61526, 2013.

Halpern J. Clinical empathy in medical care. In: Decety J, ed. *Empathy: From Bench to Bedside*. Cambridge, MA: MIT Press, 2012: 229–244.

Ichiki K, Nakamura T, Fujita N, et al. An endocrinopathy characterized by dysfunction of the pituitary-adrenal axis and alopecia universalis: Supporting the entity of a triple H syndrome. *Eur J Endocrinol.* 147: 357–361, 2002.

Kelley AS, McGarry K, Gorges R, Skinner JS. The burden of health care costs for patients with dementia in the last 5 years of life. *Ann Intern Med.* 63: 729–736, 2015.

Mason P. Embodying affect for emotional release. Retrieved from https://thebrainissocool.com/2014/11/02/embodying-affect-for-emotional-release/

Wearing D. *Forever Today: A Memoir of Love and Amnesia*. New York: Doubleday, 2005.

INDEX

Voluntary actions, 363–68, 365*f,* 398–404, 401*f,* 403*f,* 406–07
  vs. emotional actions, 366–68, 392–93, 399, 402*f,* 403–04, 403*f,* 406–07
  and gaze shifts, 141, 352–53, 357–58
  and homeostasis, 5, 55, 446, 457–58, 458*f*
  impairment of, 366–68, 367*f,* 403–06, 404*t,* 405*f* (*see also* Paralysis)
  and locked-in syndrome, 3, 5, 398
  pathways, 7–8, 8*f,* 41*f,* 42, 47, 118, 140–42, 141*f,* 365, 393, 398–403 (*see also* Corticobulbar pathway; Corticospinal pathway)
  recruitment during, 376–78, 377*f,* 382
  and somatosensation, 55, 379
von Economo, Constantin, 462
von Recklinghausen neurofibromatosis, 87

Waardenburg syndrome, 11
Wakefulness, 5, 126–28. *See also* Sleep; Sleep–wake cycle
  brain regions important to, 91, 126–28, 128*f,* 210, 461–62
  circadian rhythm, 460, 462
  disorders of, 461–62, 462*b*
  and disorders of consciousness, 3, 43, 90–91, 468
  eye-opening, 81
  and homeostasis, 452, 456, 459, 462
  neurotransmitters, 126–28, 127*f,* 208, 210–12, 240–41
  reflex modulation, 383
Walking, 388–91, 388*f,* 390*f,* 409–10. *See also* Gait
  and basal ganglia, 428, 436
  central pattern generator for, 365–66, 365*f,* 379, 387–89, 388*f,* 457
  cerebellar involvement, 409, 417, 420, 422
  command to initiate, 398
  feedback reflexes during, 379, 383, 389–90, 390*f,* 398
  head acceleration during, 332, 340–41, 343
  homeostasis during, 363
  impairment of, 89, 379, 388, 391, 393, 397, 399, 404, 436, 439, 467
  learning, 390–91, 409–10
  across life cycle, 390–91
  muscle fibers and motor units involved, 370–71, 370*f,* 375, 375*f*
  vs. robotic locomotion, 395*b*
  and somatosensory input, 363, 379
Wallenberg syndrome. *See* Lateral medullary stroke
Waterman, Ian, 363, 379
Watershed zone, 153*f,* 154
Wearing, Clive, 468–69
Weber's law, 252, 252*f,* 268, 296
  motor version, 375
Weber test, 296, 296*t,* 297*f*

Wetness, 311
White matter, 15, 33*f*
Whooping cough, 236*b*
Withdrawal reflex
  evoked by painful stimulation, 314*f,* 366, 385–86, 386*f*
  cough as a, 319
  circuits for, 385–86, 386*f*
Working memory, 141, 143, 145, 427

Xerophthalmia, 269

Yaw (plane), 330*f,* 335–37, 336*f,* 338
  and canal orientations, 337, 337*t*
  and VOR, 347–49, 347*f,* 348*f,* 348*t*